MOSBY'S
PEDIATRIC
NURSING
REFERENCE

MOSBY'S
PEDIATRIC
NURSING
REFERENCE

FIFTH EDITION

Cecily Lynn Betz, PhD, RN, FAAN

Director, Nursing Training
Research Coordinator
USC University Affiliated Program
Childrens Hospital Los Angeles
Los Angeles, California

Linda A. Sowden, MN, RN

Location Director
Pediatric Services of America
Kids Medical Club
West Palm Beach, Florida

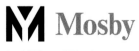 Mosby

An Affiliate of Elsevier

M Mosby

An Affiliate of Elsevier

11830 Westline Industrial Drive
St. Louis, Missouri 63146

NOTICE

Pharmacology is an ever-changing field. Standard safety precautions must be followed, but as new research and clinical experience broaden our knowledge, changes in treatment and drug therapy may become necessary or appropriate. Readers are advised to check the most current product information provided by the manufacturer of each drug to be administered to verify the recommended dose, the method and duration of administration, and contraindications. It is the responsibility of the licensed prescriber, relying on experience and knowledge of the patient, to determine dosages and the best treatment for each individual patient. Neither the publisher nor the author assumes any liability for any injury and/or damage to persons or property arising from this publication.

Previous editions copyrighted 1989, 1992, 1996, 2000

Library of Congress Cataloging-in-Publication Data

Mosby's pediatric nursing reference / [edited by] Cecily Lynn Betz, Linda A. Sowden.—5th ed.
    p. ; cm.
    Includes bibliographical references and index.
    ISBN 0-323-01979-X
    Pediatric nursing—Handbooks, manuals, etc. I. Title: Pediatric nursing reference. II. Betz, Cecily Lynn. III. Sowden, Linda A.
    [DNLM: 1. Pediatric Nursing—Handbooks. 2. Pediatrics—Handbooks. WY 49 M8944 2004]
    RJ245.M675 2004
    610.73'62—dc21

Executive Editor: Loren S. Wilson
Senior Developmental Editor: Michele D. Hayden
Publishing Services Manager: Deborah L. Vogel
Project Manager: Deon Lee
Design Manager: Teresa McBryan Breckwoldt

Printed in the United States of America

Last digit is the print number: 9   8   7   6   5   4   3   2   1

Contributors

Susan Givens Bell, MS, RNC
Staff Nurse
All Children's Hospital
St. Petersburg, Florida

Joan Calandra, RN, PhD
Clinical Nurse Specialist, Psychiatry
Licensed Clinical Psychologist
Los Angeles, California

Sharon DiSano, MS, ARNP
Director, Transplant Administration
All Children's Hospital
St. Petersburg, Florida

Bonnie F. Gahn, MSN, MA, RNC
Director, Pediatric Nursing Services
Ross Products Division, Abbott Labs
Auxiliary Faculty
College of Nursing
The Ohio State University
Columbus, Ohio

Rita A. Giordano, MSN, ARNP
Clinical Nurse Specialist
Sarasota Memorial Hospital
Sarasota, Florida

Cindy Grainey, RN, MSN, CPNP
District Nurse
South Kitsap School District
Port Orchard, Washington

Valerie Hammel, RN, MSN, CNS
Clinical Educator
Kaiser Permanente Southern California
  Medical Group
Fontana, California

Maureen T. Jakocko, RN, MN
Laguna Niguel, California

Mary Kaminski, RNC, MS, NNP
Advanced Practice Nurse
Clinical Instructor
Children's Hospital, Columbus
The Ohio State University
Columbus, Ohio

Sally Valentine Kimpel, RN, MN, CNS
Clinical Nurse Specialist—Pediatrics
Kaiser Foundation Hospital
San Diego, California

Kay Frances Lawrence, RN, ARNP
Nursing Education Specialist
All Children's Hospital
St. Petersburg, Florida

Norma L. Liburd, RN,C, MN
Clinical Nurse Specialist
All Children's Hospital
St. Petersburg, Florida

Gay A. Redcay, RN, MN, FNP-C
Family Nurse Practitioner
Transition Service Coordinator
South Pasadena, California

Joanne Rothblum, RN, MN
Assistant Professor
Nursing Program
William Rainey Harper College
Palatine, Illinois

Linda A. Sciuto, ARNP, RNCS, MSN
Pediatric Nurse Practitioner
Pediatric Critical Care Medicine
Jackson Memorial Hospital
Miami, Florida

Noreene Clark Sheehan, RN, MSN
Nurse Researcher
Children's Hospital, Los Angeles
Los Angeles, California

Wendy A. Stuart, MSN, RN, CDE
Director, Pediatrics and Pediatric Intensive Care
Plantation General Hospital
Plantation, Florida

Ellen Tappero, RNC, MN, NNP
Neonatal Nurse Practitioner
Exempla Lutheran Medical Center
Wheat Ridge, Colorado

Beverly Noble Vandercook, MSN, RN, CPNP, CLC
Nurse Practitioner, Administrator
University of Phoenix
Southern California Campus
Fountain Valley, California

Teresa Vaughn-Davies, RN, MSN
School Nurse
Los Angeles County Office of Education
Covina, California

Michele Wolff, RN, MSN, CCRN
Professor of Nursing
Saddleback College
Mission Viejo, California

Ronda M. Wood, RNC, MN, EdD
Professor of Nursing
Long Beach City College
School of Health and Science
Long Beach, California

Reviewers

Ann Bennett, RN, MSN
Director of Nursing
Scioto County Joint Vocational School
Lucasville, Ohio

Catherine F. Noonan, RN, MS, CPNP
Nurse Practitioner
Children's Hospital Boston
Boston, Massachusetts

Elizabeth L. Pruitt, RN, MEd
Instructor
Arkansas Valley Technical Institute
Ozark, Arkansas

Trena R. Shouse, RN, MSN
Assistant Professor
Kentucky State University
Frankfort, Kentucky

Lisa South, RN, DSN
Clinical Assistant Professor
University of Alabama, Huntsville
College of Nursing
Huntsville, Alabama

Marguerite E. Wright, RN, MSN, RDMS
Assistant Professor
Maternal-Child Health Nursing
Gordon College
Barnesville, Georgia

◆

Preface

Mosby's Pediatric Nursing Reference, fifth edition, is designed to serve nurses and nursing students who care for children and their families. Its small size and concise format were purposefully created for the nurse who wants an easily accessible reference. This book is divided into two parts. Part I contains information about frequently encountered medical and surgical conditions in the pediatric population and includes the most current clinical updates. Several chapters have undergone significant revisions, such as the chapters on cleft lip and palate, mental retardation, child abuse and neglect, chronic lung disease of infancy, and suicide. Part II presents diagnostic tests and procedures. For the user's convenience, the chapters in each part are listed in alphabetical order. In the appendixes, the nurse will find valuable information about growth and development, immunizations, laboratory values, and guidelines for taking blood pressure measurements and conducting complete nursing assessments for each body system. Appendixes on community services and breast-feeding have been updated, as have the appendixes on growth charts and taking a blood pressure.

The organization of the care-planning guidelines reflects our philosophical orientation of a family-centered approach. The needs of the child and family are addressed from a biopsychosocial perspective. The care-planning guidelines reflect a holistic approach to the child's and family's short-term and long-term needs.

It is our hope that this compact yet authoritative tool will prove a useful resource in the delivery of high-quality nursing care for children and the associated care required by their families.

Cecily L. Betz
Linda A. Sowden

A Note on Pediatric Drug Dosages

Because children vary widely in weight, age, body surface area, and their ability to absorb, metabolize, and excrete medications, extreme caution should be used when determining the proper dosage for a particular patient. Although the physician is responsible for writing the order correctly, the nurse is responsible for administering medications, always being careful to determine whether the dosage is correct. The nurse is urged to use the body surface method for calculating dosages (see Appendix G, West Nomogram).

The authors of this reference have endeavored to provide pediatric dosages consistent with safe practice. The nurse is advised, however, to rely on her or his own calculations, experience, judgment, and authoritative pharmacologic sources when administering drugs to specific patients.

Contents

Part I
Pediatric Medical and Surgical Conditions, 1

1	Anorexia Nervosa,	3
2	Aplastic Anemia,	10
3	Apnea,	16
4	Apparent Life-Threatening Event,	20
5	Appendicitis and Appendectomy,	25
6	Asthma,	31
7	Attention-Deficit/Hyperactivity Disorder,	36
8	Bronchiolitis,	43
9	Bulimia Nervosa,	47
10	Burns,	52
11	Cellulitis,	60
12	Cerebral Palsy,	64
13	Child Abuse and Neglect,	68
14	Chronic Lung Disease of Infancy,	77
15	Cleft Lip and Cleft Palate,	85
16	Coarctation of the Aorta,	93
17	Congestive Heart Failure,	100
18	Croup,	105
19	Cystic Fibrosis,	110
20	Cytomegaloviral Infection,	117
21	Developmental Dysplasia of the Hip,	123
22	Diabetes Mellitus: Insulin-Dependent,	129
23	Disseminated Intravascular Coagulation,	138

24 Drowning and Near-Drowning, 144

25 Epiglottitis, 150

26 Foreign Body Aspiration, 155

27 Fractures, 160

28 Gastroenteritis, 167

29 Gastroesophageal Reflux, 177

30 Glomerulonephritis, 181

31 Hemolytic-Uremic Syndrome, 186

32 Hemophilia, 192

33 Hepatitis, 200

34 Hernia (Inguinal) and Hernia Repair, 208

35 Hirschsprung's Disease, 212

36 Hodgkin's Disease, 219

37 HIV Infection and AIDS, 226

38 Hydrocephalus, 238

39 Hyperbilirubinemia, 244

40 Hypertension, 248

41 Hypertrophic Pyloric Stenosis, 253

42 Idiopathic Thrombocytopenic Purpura, 258

43 Imperforate Anus, 263

44 Inborn Errors of Metabolism, 270

45 Inflammatory Bowel Disease, 288

46 Iron Deficiency Anemia, 300

47 Juvenile Rheumatoid Arthritis, 306

48 Kawasaki Disease, 317

49 Lead Poisoning, 325

50 Learning Disabilities, 334

51 Leukemia, Childhood, 340

52 Meconium Aspiration Syndrome, 357

53   Meningitis, 362

54   Mental Retardation, 369

55   Muscular Dystrophy, 385

56   Necrotizing Enterocolitis, 391

57   Nephrotic Syndrome, 400

58   Neuroblastoma, 410

59   Nonaccidental Trauma, 416

60   Non-Hodgkin's Lymphoma, 422

61   Osteogenic Sarcoma and Amputation, 429

62   Osteomyelitis, 437

63   Otitis Media, 443

64   Patent Ductus Arteriosus, 452

65   Pneumonia, 460

66   Poisoning, 466

67   Renal Failure: Acute, 469

68   Renal Failure: Chronic, 480

69   Respiratory Distress Syndrome, 490

70   Respiratory Syncytial Viral Infection, 497

71   Reye's Syndrome, 500

72   Rheumatic Fever: Acute, 507

73   Scoliosis, 513

74   Seizure Disorders, 520

75   Serious Bacterial Infection, 528

76   Short Bowel Syndrome, 532

77   Sickle Cell Anemia, 543

78   Spina Bifida, 552

79   Substance-Related Disorders, 562

80   Sudden Infant Death Syndrome, 570

81   Suicide, 576

82 Tetralogy of Fallot, 582

83 Transplantation: Bone Marrow (Hematopoietic Stem Cell Transplantation), 593

84 Transplantation: Organ, 603

85 Traumatic Brain Injury, 608

86 Urinary Tract Infections, 616

87 Ventricular Septal Defect and Repair, 621

88 Wilms' Tumor, 628

Part II
Pediatric Diagnostic Tests and Procedures, 635

General Nursing Action, 637

89 Cardiac Catheterization, 639

90 Computed Tomography, 642

91 Electrocardiography, 644

92 Endoscopy, 646

93 Intracranial Pressure Monitoring, 648

94 Intravenous Pyelogram, 650

95 Magnetic Resonance Imaging, 654

96 Peritoneal Dialysis, 656

97 pH Probe Monitoring, 661

98 Pneumogram Sleep Studies, 663

Appendixes, 665

A Nursing Assessments, 667

B Growth and Development, 673

C Immunizations, 699

D Standardized Method for Taking Blood Pressure in Children, 706

E Laboratory Values, 714

F Abbreviations, 722

G West Nomogram, 728

H Pain in Children, 730

I Height and Weight Growth Curves, 743

J Psychosocial Interventions, 750

K Home Care, 754

L Community Services, 757

M Breast-Feeding, 769

I

◆

Pediatric Medical
and
Surgical Conditions

◆

1

◆

Anorexia Nervosa

◆

PATHOPHYSIOLOGY

Anorexia nervosa is an eating disorder characterized by the refusal to maintain a body weight within the minimal range of normal for height, weight, and body frame. The seriousness of weight loss is denied, and the individual has a distorted body image. Despite being dangerously thin, the individual feels fat. In addition, there may be a focus on the shape and size of particular body parts (Box 1-1).

Two general subtypes of anorexia nervosa exist. The restricting type involves severe restriction of food intake and compulsive exercising. The binge eating and purging type involves restricted dietary intake coupled with intermittent episodes of binge eating, followed by purging. Self-induced vomiting and use of ipecac, laxatives, diuretics, or enemas are common means of purging. The excessive use of appetite suppressants or diet pills is seen in both types.

Purging and semistarvation may induce electrolyte imbalance and cardiac problems, which may ultimately lead to death. Starvation creates a range of medical symptoms. Changes in growth hormone levels, diminished secretion of sex hormones, defective development of bone marrow tissue, structural abnormalities of the brain, cardiac dysfunction, and gastrointestinal difficulties are common. A notable problem associated with anorexia in adolescents is the potential for growth retardation, delay of menarche, and peak bone mass reduction. When normal eating is reestablished and laxative use is stopped, the child may develop peripheral edema.

A variety of psychologic factors are associated with anorexia nervosa. Low self-esteem often plays a significant role.

3

BOX 1-1
Diagnostic Criteria for Anorexia Nervosa

- Refusal to maintain body weight at or above a minimally normal weight for age and height (e.g., weight loss leading to maintenance of body weight less than 85% of that expected; or failure to make expected weight gain during period of growth, leading to body weight less than 85% of that expected).
- Intense fear of gaining weight or becoming fat, even though underweight.
- Disturbance in the way in which one's body weight or shape is experienced, undue influence of body weight or shape on self-evaluation, or denial of the seriousness of the current low body weight.
- Amenorrhea in postmenarchal females, i.e., the absence of at least three consecutive menstrual cycles. (A woman is considered to have amenorrhea if her periods occur only following hormone, e.g., estrogen, administration.)

Restricting Type
During the current episode of anorexia nervosa, the person has not regularly engaged in binge eating or purging behavior (i.e., self-induced vomiting or the misuse of laxatives, diuretics, or enemas).

Binge Eating and Purging Type
During the current episode of anorexia nervosa, the person has regularly engaged in binge eating or purging behavior (i.e., self-induced vomiting or the misuse of laxatives, diuretics, or enemas).

From American Psychiatric Association: *Diagnostic and statistical manual of mental disorders*, ed 4, text revision (DSM-IV-TR), Washington, DC, 2000, The Association, p 589.

Weight loss is viewed as an achievement, and self-esteem becomes dependent on body size and weight. A relationship also is seen between eating disorders and mood disorders. In some cases, major depression may result from nutritional deprivation. Individuals with anorexia nervosa may lack spontaneity in social situations and may be emotionally restrained.

Family dynamics may play a role in development of symptoms. Parents may be controlling and overly protective.

Eating behaviors may emerge in an unconscious attempt to gain control. In some cases, diminished weight and loss of secondary sexual characteristics may be related to difficulty accepting maturation into adulthood. Disordered eating that is not severe enough to meet criteria for anorexia nervosa is common among United States adolescent girls and reflects a sociocultural ideal of thinness.

INCIDENCE
1. Cardiac complications occur in 87% of affected youth.
2. Renal complications occur in approximately 70% of affected youth.
3. More than 90% of individuals with anorexia are females.
4. Rate of incidence among those aged 15 through 24 years is 14.6% for females and 1.8% for males.
5. Mortality rates range between 6% and 15%. Half the deaths result from suicide.
6. Prevalence continues to be higher in Western industrialized nations of white ethnicity and among middle- and upper-class females. Increasing diversity in the ethnic and socioeconomic groups of those affected is being reported. For immigrants, degree of acculturation may play a role.

CLINICAL MANIFESTATIONS
1. Sudden, unexplained weight loss
2. Emaciated appearance, loss of subcutaneous fat
3. Changes in eating habits, unusual eating times
4. Excessive exercise and physical activity
5. Amenorrhea
6. Dry, scaly skin
7. Lanugo on extremities, back, and face
8. Yellowish discoloration of skin
9. Sleep disturbances
10. Chronic constipation or diarrhea, abdominal pain, bloating
11. Esophageal erosion (from frequent vomiting)
12. Depressed mood
13. Excessive focus on high achievement (becomes distressed when performance is not above average)

14. Excessive focus on food, eating, and body appearance
15. Erosion of tooth enamel and dentin on lingual surfaces (late effects from frequent vomiting)

COMPLICATIONS

1. Cardiac: bradycardia, tachycardia, arrhythmias, hypotension, cardiac failure
2. Gastrointestinal: esophagitis, peptic ulcer disease, hepatomegaly
3. Renal: serum urea and electrolyte abnormalities (hypokalemia, hyponatremia, hypochloremia, hypochloremic metabolic alkalosis), pitting edema
4. Hematologic: mild anemia and leukopenia (common) and thrombocytopenia (rare)
5. Skeletal: osteoporosis, pathologic fractures
6. Endocrine: reduced fertility, elevated cortisol and growth hormone levels, elevated gluconeogenesis
7. Metabolic: decreased basal metabolic rate, impaired temperature regulation, sleep disturbances
8. Death caused by complications, including cardiac arrest and electrolyte imbalance, and suicide

LABORATORY AND DIAGNOSTIC TESTS

1. Electrocardiogram—bradycardia is common
2. Erect and supine blood pressure—to assess for hypotension
3. Serum urea, electrolyte, creatinine levels (in severe cases, monitor every 3 months)—may show low blood urea nitrogen level due to dehydration and inadequate protein intake; metabolic alkalosis and hypokalemia due to vomiting
4. Urinalysis, urine creatinine clearance (in severe cases, monitor annually)—pH may be elevated; ketones may be present
5. Complete blood count, platelet count (in severe cases, monitor every 3 months)—usually normal; normochromic, normocytic anemia may be present
6. Serum glucose level (in severe cases, monitor every 3 months)

7. Liver function tests (in severe cases, perform every 3 months)
8. Thyroid-stimulating hormone, cortisol levels (in severe cases, monitor semiannually)
9. Bone density (in severe cases, monitor annually)— demonstrates osteopenia
10. Body composition (in severe cases, monitor annually using calipers or water immersion)
11. Presence of hypercarotenemia (causes yellowing of skin, also known as pseudojaundice)—due to vegetarian diet or decreased metabolism

MEDICAL MANAGEMENT

Treatment is provided on an outpatient basis unless severe medical problems develop. An interdisciplinary approach is needed to ensure optimal outcome. Outpatient treatment includes medical monitoring, dietary planning to restore nutritional state, and psychotherapy. Therapeutic approaches include individual, family, and group therapy. Family involvement is crucial. Use of psychotropic medication should be considered only after weight gain has been established. Medication may be used to treat depression, anxiety, and obsessive-compulsive behaviors. Hospitalization is indicated if the adolescent weighs less than 20% of ideal body weight or is unable to adhere to the treatment program on an outpatient basis, or if neurologic deficits, hypokalemia, and cardiac arrhythmias are present. Hospitalization is limited to brief stays focusing on acute weight restoration and refeeding.

The following medications may be given:

1. Antidepressants—the selective serotonin reuptake inhibitors (e.g., fluoxetine, sertraline, paroxetine) may be used if compulsive exercising is a component of the illness.
2. Estrogen replacement—may be used for amenorrhea.

NURSING ASSESSMENT

1. Assess psychologic status with psychologic inventories. The Eating Disorder Examination is designed for structured interviews. Clinical self-reports include the Eating Disorder

Inventory (for ages 14 years and older). The Eating Attitudes Test and the Kids Eating Disorder Survey may be used for school-aged children. The Children's Depression Inventory may be used to assess level of depression in 7- to 17-year-olds.

2. Assess height and weight using growth charts and body mass index (weight measurements are taken after the individual has undressed and voided).
3. Assess pattern of elimination.
4. Assess exercise pattern for type, amount, and frequency.
5. Assess for signs of depression.

NURSING DIAGNOSES

- Nutrition: less than body requirements, Imbalanced
- Self-esteem, Chronic low
- Body image, Disturbed
- Fluid volume, Risk for deficient
- Activity intolerance
- Coping, Ineffective

NURSING INTERVENTIONS

1. Include family in developing dietary supplementation plan.
2. Provide information about adequate nutritional intake and effect of inadequate intake on energy level and psychologic well-being.
3. Initiate specific plan of exercise to reinforce positive behavioral outcomes.
4. Establish trusting relationship that promotes disclosure of feelings and emotions.
5. Organize eating of meals with others, record amount of food eaten, and monitor activity for 2 hours after eating.
6. Promote individual's sense of responsibility and involvement in recovery and treatment.
7. Participate in interdisciplinary team that uses multiple modalities such as individual and group psychotherapy, assertiveness training, music and/or art therapy, and nutritional education.
8. Support involvement of family members who are vital to recovery.

🛆 Discharge Planning and Home Care

1. Recommend psychotherapy for treatment of distorted body image and self-concept.
2. Refer adolescent and family to community resources, e.g., support groups and mental health professionals.

CLIENT OUTCOMES

1. Individual's physical health status will improve with steady, reasonable weight gain (about 1 pound every 4 days).
2. Individual will establish healthy pattern of nutritional intake.
3. Individual will establish increased self-esteem and improvement in psychologic functioning.

REFERENCES

American Psychiatric Association Work Group on Eating Disorders: Practice guideline for the treatment of patients with eating disorders (revision), *Am J Psychiatry* 157(1 suppl):1, 2000.

American Psychological Association: *Diagnostic and statistical manual of mental disorders*, ed 4, text revision (DSM-IV-TR), Washington, DC, 2000, The Association.

Atkins D, Silber T: Clinical spectrum of anorexia nervosa in children, *J Dev Behav Pediatr* 14(4):211, 1993.

Carpenito L: *Handbook of nursing diagnosis*, ed 9, Philadelphia, 2001, JB Lippincott.

Gillberg C, Rastam M, Gillberg I: Anorexia nervosa: physical health and neurodevelopment at 16 and 21 years, *Dev Med Child Neurol* 36(7):567, 1994.

Irwin E: A focused overview of anorexia nervosa and bulimia. II. Challenges to the practice of psychiatric nursing, *Arch Psychiatr Nurs* 7(6):347, 1993.

Nussbaum M: Nutritional conditions: anorexia nervosa. In McArnarney E et al, editors: *Textbook of adolescent medicine*, Philadelphia, 1994, WB Saunders.

Sharp C, Freeman C: The medical complications of anorexia nervosa, *Br J Psychiatry* 162:452, 1993.

Steiner H, Lock J: Anorexia nervosa and bulimia nervosa in children and adolescents: a review of the past ten years, *J Am Acad Child Adolesc Psychiatry* 37:352, 1998.

Steinhausen H: *Eating disorders in adolescence: anorexia and bulimia nervosa*, New York, 1995, DeGruyter.

2

◆

Aplastic Anemia

◆

PATHOPHYSIOLOGY

Aplastic anemia is a disorder of bone marrow failure resulting in the depletion of all marrow elements. The production of blood cells is decreased or lacking. Pancytopenia and hypocellularity of the marrow occur. The manifestation of symptoms is dependent on the extent of the thrombocytopenia (hemorrhagic symptoms), neutropenia (bacterial infections, fever), and anemia (pallor, fatigue, congestive heart failure, tachycardia). Severe aplastic anemia is characterized by a granulocyte count of less than 500/mm^3, a platelet count of less than 20,000/mm^3, and a reticulocyte count of less than 1%. Aplastic anemia can be acquired or inherited. Acquired forms can be caused by drugs (chloramphenicol), chemicals (benzene), radiation, or viral infection (hepatitis virus, Epstein-Barr virus), and, in rare instances, are associated with paroxysmal nocturnal hemoglobinuria. Fanconi's anemia is the most common inherited type. Prognosis is grave. Fifty percent of affected individuals die within 6 months of diagnosis. With more than 70% nonhematopoietic cells, the prognosis is poor.

INCIDENCE

1. Aplastic anemia may occur at any age.
2. Fifty percent of cases are idiopathic.
3. Long-term survival rate with bone marrow transplant from histocompatible donors is as high as 70% to 90% in children.
4. Incidence of acquired aplastic anemia is 1 in 1 million. The disorder occurs equally in males and females.

5. Males and females are affected equally with Fanconi's anemia. Most cases are diagnosed at about 7 years of age, although the disorder may be diagnosed in infancy or as late as 30 to 40 years of age.

CLINICAL MANIFESTATIONS

1. Petechiae, ecchymoses, epistaxis (occur first)
2. Oral ulcerations, bacterial infections, fever (occur later in course)
3. Anemia, pallor, fatigue, tachycardia (late signs)
4. Café-au-lait spots, melanin-like hyperpigmentation, absent thumbs (Fanconi's anemia)

COMPLICATIONS

1. Sepsis
2. Sensitization to cross-reacting donor antigens resulting in uncontrollable bleeding
3. Graft versus host disease (occurs after bone marrow transplantation)
4. Failure of marrow graft (occurs after bone marrow transplantation)
5. Acute myelogenous leukemia (associated with Fanconi's anemia)

LABORATORY AND DIAGNOSTIC TESTS

1. Bone marrow aspiration and biopsy—hypocellular
2. Complete blood count with differential—macrocytic anemia; decreased granulocytes, monocytes, and lymphocytes
3. Platelet count—decreased
4. Reticulocyte count—decreased
5. Hemoglobin electrophoresis—elevated fetal hemoglobin level
6. Serum folate and B_{12} levels—normal or elevated
7. Chromosome breakage test—positive result for Fanconi's anemia

MEDICAL MANAGEMENT

The first-choice treatment for aplastic anemia is bone marrow transplant from a sibling donor who is human lymphocyte antigen (HLA) matched. In more than 70% of cases there will be no sibling match. However, there is an increased chance of a match between one parent and the child with aplastic anemia. If bone marrow transplantation is to be done, HLA typing of the family is performed immediately, and blood products are used as little as possible to avoid sensitization. Also to avoid sensitization, blood should not be donated by the child's family. Blood products should always be irradiated and filtered to remove white blood cells before being given to a child who is a candidate for bone marrow transplantation.

Immunotherapy with either antithymocyte globulin or antilymphocyte globulin is the primary treatment for children who are not candidates for bone marrow transplantation. The child will respond within 3 months or not at all to this therapy. Cyclosporin A is also an effective immunosuppressant that can be used in the treatment of aplastic anemia. Androgens are rarely used unless no other treatment is available.

Clinical trials exploring the use of granulocyte-macrophage colony-stimulating factor (GM-CSF) in pediatric clients have shown some hematologic improvement. Further research is required to determine the role of GM-CSF in treating aplastic anemia and Fanconi's anemia.

Supportive therapy includes use of antibiotics and administration of blood products. Antibiotics are used to treat fever and neutropenia; prophylactic antibiotics are not indicated for the asymptomatic child. Blood product administration may include the following:

1. Platelets—to maintain platelet count higher than 20,000/mm^3. Use single-donor platelet pheresis to decrease the number of HLA antigens to which the child is exposed.
2. Packed red blood cells—to maintain hemoglobin level (chronic anemia is often well tolerated). For long-term therapy, use deferoxamine as a chelating agent to prevent complications of iron overload.
3. Granulocytes—to transfuse to the child who has sepsis caused by gram-negative organisms.

NURSING ASSESSMENT

1. See the Hematologic Assessment section in Appendix A.
2. Assess for sites of bleeding and hemorrhagic symptoms.

3. Assess for signs of infection.
4. Assess activity level.
5. Assess developmental level.

NURSING DIAGNOSES

- Injury, Risk for
- Infection, Risk for
- Activity intolerance
- Fatigue
- Growth and development, Delayed

NURSING INTERVENTIONS

1. Identify and report signs and symptoms of hemorrhage.
   a. Vital signs (increased apical pulse, thready pulse, decreased blood pressure)
   b. Bleeding sites
   c. Skin color (pallor) and signs of diaphoresis
   d. Weakness
   e. Decreased level of consciousness
   f. Decreased platelet count
2. Protect from trauma.
   a. Do not administer aspirin or nonsteroidal antiinflammatory drugs.
   b. Avoid use of intramuscular injection and suppositories.
   c. Administer contraceptive to decrease excessive menstruation.
   d. Provide good oral hygiene with soft toothbrush.
3. Protect from infection.
   a. Limit contact with potential sources of infection.
   b. Use strict isolation precautions (refer to institution's policies and procedures).
4. Administer blood products and monitor child's response to their infusion (after bone marrow transplantation to avoid sensitization to donor transplantation antigen).
   a. Observe for side effects or untoward response (transfusion reaction).
   b. Observe for signs of fluid overload.
   c. Monitor vital signs before transfusion, 15 minutes after infusion has started, as needed during infusion (or

based on institution's policies), and upon completion of transfusion.

5. Provide frequent rest periods. Organize nursing care to increase activity tolerance and prevent fatigue.
6. Monitor child's therapeutic and untoward response to medications; monitor action and side effects of administered medications.
7. Prepare child and family for bone marrow transplantation.
8. Monitor for signs of bone marrow transplant complications (see the Complications section in this chapter).
9. Provide age-appropriate diversional and recreational activities (see relevant section in Appendix B).
10. Provide age-appropriate explanation before procedures.

Discharge Planning and Home Care

1. Instruct parents about measures to protect child from infection.
   a. Limit contact with infectious agents.
   b. Identify signs and symptoms of infection.
2. Instruct parents to monitor for signs of complications (see the Complications section in this chapter).
3. Instruct parents about administration of medication.
   a. Monitor child's therapeutic response.
   b. Monitor for untoward response.
4. Provide child and family with information about community support systems for long-term adaptation.
   a. School reintegration
   b. Parent groups
   c. Child and sibling groups
   d. Sources of financial advice

CLIENT OUTCOMES

1. Child will have gradual increase in red blood cells, white blood cells, and eventually platelets.
2. Child will have fewer infections.
3. Child will have minimal bleeding episodes.

4. Child and family will understand home care and follow-up needs.

REFERENCES

Alter BP, Young NS: The bone marrow failure syndromes. In Nathan DG, Orkin SH, editors: *Nathan and Oski's hematology of infancy and childhood,* ed 5, Philadelphia, 1998, WB Saunders.

Kojima S et al: Immunosuppressive therapy using antithymocyte globulin, cyclosporine, and danazol with or without human granulocyte colony-stimulating factor in children with acquired aplastic anemia, *Blood* 96(6):2049, 2000.

Marsh JCW: Results of immunosuppression in aplastic anemia, *Acta Haematol* 103:26, 2000.

Williams DM: Pancytopenia, aplastic anemia and pure red cell aplasia. In Lee GR et al, editors: *Wintrobe's clinical hematology,* ed 10, Baltimore, 1999, Williams & Wilkins.

3

❖

Apnea

❖

PATHOPHYSIOLOGY

Apnea is the cessation of respiration for more than 20 seconds with or without cyanosis, hypotonia, or bradycardia. Apnea may be a symptom of another disorder that resolves when the latter is treated. Such disorders may include infection, gastroesophageal reflux, hypoglycemia, metabolic disorders, drug toxicity, hydrocephalus, or thermal instability in newborns. *Central apnea* is a respiratory pause, the cause of which is related to the failure of the excitatory mechanisms to function properly in the respiratory center in the brain. Immaturity of the central nervous system frequently accounts for apnea of the newborn, which occurs most frequently during active sleep. *Obstructive apnea* occurs when an obstruction of the airway exists, usually at the level of the pharynx, and occurs most frequently during sleep. Here, there is continuation of respiratory effort without air flow in the airway because of the obstruction. This condition may be due to enlarged tonsils and adenoids, congenital disorders such as Pierre Robin syndrome, or muscular hypotonia. Apnea can also occur in premature infants during certain normal activities, such as feeding.

INCIDENCE

1. Idiopathic apnea rarely occurs in term infants.
2. About one third of infants younger than 32 weeks' gestation have apnea episodes.
3. More than 50% of infants weighing less than 1.5 kg require treatment for recurrent prolonged apneic episodes.
4. Obstructive apnea is most often caused by hypertrophy of the adenoids and tonsils.

CLINICAL MANIFESTATIONS

1. Cessation of respiration for more than 20 seconds with or without cyanosis, bradycardia, or hypotonicity
2. Snoring

COMPLICATIONS

Complications associated with apnea are dependent on the underlying cause as described in the Pathophysiology section. If apnea is due to developmental factors, this condition will resolve as the child grows. However, if the infant's apnea is caused by another etiology (mentioned in the Pathophysiology section), treatment, diagnosis, and long-term prognosis will be dependent on the cause. An important consideration is the psychosocial implications for the family as identified in the Nursing Interventions and Discharge Planning and Home Care sections.

LABORATORY AND DIAGNOSTIC TESTS

1. Polysomnography
2. Apnea monitoring
3. Pulse oximetry

MEDICAL MANAGEMENT

Infants with suspected or documented apnea are monitored using either a cardiorespiratory or an apnea monitor. The immediate management of an apneic episode is to provide gentle stimulation by rubbing the child's back or feet. Shaking vigorously or creating loud noises should be avoided. If the infant or child does not respond, the airway should be opened, and cardiopulmonary resuscitation (CPR) should be initiated.

The management of central apnea, most frequently seen in premature infants, includes minimizing potential causes such as temperature variances and feeding intolerance. The use of xanthine medications such as caffeine and theophylline provide central nervous system stimulation. Pulmonary function support may include the use of supplemental oxygen and continuous positive airway pressure (CPAP) at low pressures. Indications for home apnea monitoring in newborns with apnea include a history of severe apneic episodes, documentation of apnea during polysomnography, severe feeding difficulties with apnea and bradycardia, and sibling relationship with a victim of SIDS.

The management of obstructive apnea may include the use of specific positioning techniques, the use of CPAP or inspiratory and expiratory positive airway pressure (BiPAP), tracheostomy to bypass the area of obstruction, or adenotonsillectomy. Aggressive surgical management to widen the caliber of the trachea has eliminated the need for tracheostomy in some cases.

NURSING ASSESSMENT

1. See the Respiratory Assessment section in Appendix A.
2. Provide early identification of apneic event.

NURSING DIAGNOSES

- Ventilation, Impaired spontaneous
- Tissue perfusion, Ineffective
- Sleep pattern, Disturbed
- Family processes, Interrupted
- Caregiver role strain, Risk for

NURSING INTERVENTIONS

1. Perform routine monitoring of heart rate and respiratory rate in preterm infants.
2. Gently rub infant's back or feet, which will stop some apneic episodes if they are caught early.
3. Allow parents to verbalize feelings.
4. Provide instruction on all equipment to be used by parents, i.e., apnea monitor or BiPAP unit.

Discharge Planning and Home Care

1. Educate parents in use of monitor and proper application of electrodes or belt, as well as in infant safety and infant CPR.
2. Educate parents in how to position child to prevent airway obstruction.

CLIENT OUTCOMES

1. Child will maintain adequate oxygenation.
2. Child's apneic events will be identified early to minimize complications.

REFERENCES

Bhatia J: Current options in the management of apnea of prematurity. *Clin Pediatr* 39(6), 2000.

Chernick V, Boat TF, editors: *Kendig's disorders of the respiratory tract in children,* ed 6, Philadelphia, 1998, WB Saunders.

Cohen SR et al: Alternatives to tracheostomy in infants and children with obstructive sleep apnea, *J Pediatr Surg* 34(1):182, 1999.

Hockenberry M: *Wong's nursing care of infants and children,* ed 7, St Louis, 2003, Mosby.

Kenner C et al: *Comprehensive neonatal nursing,* ed 3, Philadelphia, 2002, Mosby.

4

◆

Apparent Life-Threatening Event

◆

PATHOPHYSIOLOGY

An apparent life-threatening event (ALTE) is an episode that may occur in infants and that is characterized by some combination of the following: apnea (usually central, but occasionally obstructive), color change (cyanosis, pallor, erythema, or sometimes plethora), marked change in muscle tone (usually marked hypotonia or limpness), and choking or gagging. In some cases the infant appears to have died. Previously used terminology such as *near-miss sudden infant death syndrome* should be avoided. Many causes for ALTE have been identified, including pathologic apnea, sepsis, seizures, gastroesophageal reflux, upper airway obstruction, hypoglycemia, and inborn error of metabolism or other metabolic problem. Only in approximately 50% of cases of ALTE can a specific cause be determined.

INCIDENCE

1. ALTE occurs in 0.5% to 6.0% of all infants in the general public.
2. Peak age of incidence is 8 to 14 weeks.
3. Incidence is higher in boys.
4. Incidence is higher in premature infants (less than 34 weeks' gestation).
5. Infants who have had a previous ALTE are at increased risk for sudden infant death syndrome (SIDS); they constitute between 7% and 15% of all SIDS victims.

The existence of numerous studies with different designs, particularly with regard to inclusion and exclusion criteria, makes it very difficult to determine the exact incidence.

CLINICAL MANIFESTATIONS

1. Apnea—respiratory pause longer than 20 seconds
2. Marked color change—particularly cyanosis or pallor
3. Hypotonia or limpness
4. Hyperactive gag reflex
5. Often, need for cardiopulmonary resuscitation (CPR) and/or "vigorous" stimulation to elicit response

COMPLICATIONS

Complications of ALTE are dependent on appropriate identification and evaluation of the specific cause. If ALTE etiology is not attributable to an underlying condition, there are no long-term effects. However, if ALTE is caused by another etiology (mentioned in the Pathophysiology section), treatment, diagnosis, and long-term prognosis will be dependent on the cause. An important consideration is the psychosocial implications for the family as identified in the Nursing Interventions and Discharge Planning and Home Care sections.

LABORATORY AND DIAGNOSTIC TESTS

1. Complete blood count with differential and platelet count—to rule out anemia and infection
2. Arterial blood gas values—to assess respiratory status and detect metabolic acidosis
3. Blood chemistry tests (levels of electrolytes, serum glucose, phosphorus, magnesium, blood urea nitrogen, and creatinine)—to assess for metabolic abnormalities
4. Chest radiographic study—to detect respiratory infection
5. Continuous cardiorespiratory monitoring

Further laboratory and diagnostic tests, such as an upper gastrointestinal tract study, 12-lead electrocardiography, or lumbar puncture, can be performed if the initial tests suggest a specific diagnosis.

MEDICAL MANAGEMENT

Medical management focuses on care of the immediate problem and appropriate identification and evaluation of the specific cause. Initial management includes checking airway, breathing, and circulation, with restoration of cardiorespiratory function. Once stabilized, the infant should be admitted to the hospital for careful observation and further evaluation. A meticulous history taking and physical examination are performed, laboratory and diagnostic test results are obtained, and the infant is observed for 24 to 48 hours. These steps are essential in determining the specific cause of the ALTE. Further evaluation of the infant is performed as indicated by the initial assessment and test results. Therapeutic interventions consist of the treatment of any underlying disorder and the education of the primary caregivers (e.g., the parents).

NURSING ASSESSMENT

1. See the Cardiovascular Assessment and Respiratory Assessment sections in Appendix A.
2. Assess complete history—in particular, infant's state before, during, and after the event; duration of the episode; and associated changes in color, muscle tone, movements, and respiratory efforts during the episode.

NURSING DIAGNOSES

- Ventilation, Impaired spontaneous
- Breathing pattern, Ineffective
- Gas exchange, Impaired
- Infection, Risk for
- Injury, Risk for
- Anxiety
- Knowledge, Deficient
- Therapeutic regimen management, Ineffective
- Family processes, Interrupted
- Caregiver role strain, Risk for

NURSING INTERVENTIONS

1. Assist in resuscitative efforts.
   a. Provide CPR, bag or mask breathing, or medication administration as directed by team leader.

    b. Provide neutral thermal environment.

    c. Ensure proper documentation of all resuscitative events.

2. Assess infant's cardiovascular and respiratory status.

    a. Ensure continuous cardiorespiratory monitoring.

    b. Monitor and record vital signs, including blood pressure in the four extremities.

    c. Check peripheral pulses, mucous membrane color, and capillary refill.

    d. Administer oxygen therapy or other respiratory treatments as ordered.

3. Ensure that proper diagnostic tests are ordered and results obtained (see the Laboratory and Diagnostic Tests section in this chapter).

4. If specific diagnosis is confirmed, administer therapeutic interventions as ordered.

5. Assess ability of family members to participate in home apnea monitoring program (if applicable).

6. Teach family about home apnea monitoring.

    a. Assess need for monitoring.

    b. Instruct family in use of the monitor.

    c. Instruct parents on duration of monitoring.

    d. Provide 24-hour support, both medical and technical, for home monitoring.

7. Teach parents and other caregivers infant CPR.

8. Reinforce family's knowledge of medical condition.

9. Encourage parents to seek out respite care as needed.

🏠 Discharge Planning and Home Care

1. Teach parents to administer any medications.

2. Teach parents to perform any therapeutic interventions that may be prescribed (e.g., seizure interventions if neurologic disorder is diagnosed).

3. Teach parents and other caregivers what signs of ALTE are and how to perform infant CPR.

4. Provide training in home apnea monitoring if needed.

5. Refer family to community resources (e.g., home care specialists, early intervention programs, and parent support groups).

6. Stress importance of follow-up care.

CLIENT OUTCOMES

1. Infant will be episode free.
2. Parents will understand reason for monitoring, use of monitor, and required duration of monitoring.
3. Parents will be able to perform infant CPR if necessary.

REFERENCES

Arad-Cohen N et al: The relationship between gastroesophageal reflux and apnea in infants, *J Pediatr* 137(3):321, 2000.

Chernick V, Boat TF, editors: *Kendig's disorders of the respiratory tract in children,* ed 6, Philadelphia, 1998, WB Saunders.

McGrath NE et al: Pediatric update. Infants with apparent life-threatening event (ALTE): recognizing the symptoms, the seriousness, *J Emerg Nurs* 28(3):255, 2002.

Perkins R et al: Apparent life-threatening events: recognition, differentiation, and management, *Pediatr Emerg Med Rep* 3:99, 1998.

Steinschneider A et al: Clinical characteristics of an apparent life-threatening event (ALTE) and the subsequent occurrence of prolonged apnea or prolonged bradycardia, *Clin Pediatr* 37:223, 1998.

5

❖

Appendicitis and Appendectomy

❖

PATHOPHYSIOLOGY

Appendicitis is the most common condition that requires surgical intervention during childhood. Appendicitis is caused by the obstruction of the appendiceal lumen and results in edema, inflammation, venous engorgement, increased intraluminal pressure, and ischemia. It may lead to bacterial invasion, necrosis, perforation, and peritonitis.

Causes for obstruction of the lumen include hyperplasia of the submucosal lymphoid tissue, appendiceal fecaliths, foreign bodies, and parasites. In most cases, no definitive cause can be identified at the time of surgery. The prognosis is excellent, especially when surgery is performed before perforation occurs.

INCIDENCE

1. Incidence is slightly higher in males.
2. Incidence is highest in later childhood, age 10 to 12 years.
3. Occurrence is unusual in children younger than 4 years of age and is rare in children younger than 1 year old.
4. Likelihood of perforation is related to age—it occurs more frequently in younger children, most probably because of difficulty in diagnosis.

CLINICAL MANIFESTATIONS

1. Pain—cramping located in periumbilical area migrating to right lower quadrant, with most intense pain at McBurney's point (located midway between right anterior superior iliac crest and umbilicus).

2. Anorexia
3. Nausea
4. Vomiting (common early sign; less common in older children)
5. Fever—low-grade early in disease; can rise sharply with peritonitis
6. Rebound tenderness
7. Decreased or absent bowel sounds
8. Constipation
9. Diarrhea (small, watery evacuations)
10. Difficulty walking or moving
11. Irritability

COMPLICATIONS (IF NOT DIAGNOSED)

1. Perforation
2. Peritonitis

LABORATORY AND DIAGNOSTIC TESTS

1. Complete blood count—leukocytosis, neutrophilia, absence of eosinophils
2. Urinalysis—to exclude urinary tract infection
3. Abdominal radiographic study—concave curvature of spine to right, calcified fecaliths
4. Ultrasonography—noncalcified fecaliths, nonperforated appendix, appendiceal abscess

SURGICAL MANAGEMENT

Children with suspected appendicitis are admitted to hospital, given intravenous (IV) fluids and antibiotics, and observed; the rapid progression of symptoms will make the diagnosis obvious. A nasogastric tube is inserted if the child is vomiting. The appendix is removed through an incision in the right lower quadrant or may be removed laparoscopically. If the appendix has perforated, the abdominal cavity is irrigated. A drain may be inserted and the wound left open to prevent wound infection and abscess formation. In some cases a small catheter may be left in place to instill antibiotics. Postoperatively the child is put in semi-Fowler position for the first 24 hours. Gastric drainage and administration of IV fluids and antibiotics are continued.

Narcotic/analgesic medications are used for pain. Oral feedings are started within 1 or 2 days and increased as tolerated when bowel function has returned.

NURSING ASSESSMENT

1. See the Gastrointestinal Assessment section in Appendix A.
2. Assess for rapid progression in severity of symptoms.
3. Assess for preoperative and postoperative pain.
4. Assess for symptoms of perforation, including sudden relief from pain.
5. Assess for bowel sounds and abdominal distention postoperatively.
6. Assess wound for drainage and signs of infection.

NURSING DIAGNOSES

- Pain
- Fluid volume, Risk for deficient
- Infection, Risk for
- Anxiety
- Knowledge, Deficient

NURSING INTERVENTIONS

Preoperative Care

1. Provide pain relief and comfort measures.
   a. Positioning for comfort
   b. Avoidance of unnecessary movements and unnecessary palpation of abdomen
   c. Administration of pain medications if ordered
2. Maintain fluid and electrolyte balance.
   a. Maintain nothing by mouth (NPO) status.
   b. Monitor infusion of intravenous solution at maintenance rate.
   c. Monitor and record output of vomitus, urine, stool, and nasogastric drainage.
3. Monitor child's status for progression of symptoms and complications.
   a. Signs of shock—decreased blood pressure, decreased respiratory rate, pallor, diaphoresis, rapid thready pulse

   b. Perforation or peritonitis—absent bowel sounds, increased apical pulse, increased temperature, increased respiratory rate, abdominal splinting, diffuse abdominal pain followed by sudden relief from pain
   c. Intestinal obstruction—decreased or absent bowel sounds, abdominal distention, pain, vomiting, no stools
4. Prepare child for surgery.
   a. Maintain NPO status.
   b. Collect specimens for analysis preoperatively.
   c. Prepare child for and support child during laboratory and diagnostic testing.
   d. Explain anticipated preoperative and postoperative events (e.g., dressing, nasogastric tube).

Postoperative Care

1. Assess pain and institute pain relief measures as needed.
   a. Administer analgesics as needed.
   b. Use distraction to alleviate pain with toys and games.
   c. Use comfort measures such as cold and positioning (e.g., right side lying or low to semi-Fowler position).
2. Prevent and monitor for abdominal distention.
   a. Maintain NPO status.
   b. Maintain patency of nasogastric tube.
   c. Assess abdominal tenseness (firm, soft).
3. Monitor hydration status.
   a. Monitor intake and output.
   b. Maintain NPO status, then advance as tolerated.
   c. Maintain IV infusions and IV site as ordered.
4. Monitor for signs of infection and prevent spread of infection.
   a. Monitor vital signs as ordered.
   b. Observe wound for signs of infection—warmth, drainage, pain, swelling, and redness.
   c. Administer antibiotics; monitor child's response.
   d. Perform wound care as indicated and appropriate disposal of dressings.
   e. Have child ambulate when able.
5. Promote wound healing.
   a. Perform wound care—maintain site, keeping it clean and dry.

   b. Position child in semi-Fowler position to promote drainage if drain is present.
6. Support child and parents to help them deal with emotional stresses of hospitalization and surgery.
   a. Provide age-appropriate information before and after procedures.
   b. Encourage quiet diversional activities.
   c. Promote family contacts and visits with peers.
   d. Incorporate child's home routine into daily activities.

Discharge Planning and Home Care

1. Instruct parents to observe for and report signs of complications.
   a. Infection
   b. Obstruction
2. Instruct parents regarding wound care.
3. Instruct parents to have child avoid strenuous activities for a few weeks.
4. Instruct parents about follow-up appointment.
   a. Name and phone number of physician
   b. Date and time of follow-up appointment

CLIENT OUTCOMES

1. Child will have return to normal gastrointestinal function, including presurgery dietary intake and normal bowel function.
2. Child will have minimal pain.
3. Child will be free from infection.
4. Child and family will understand home care and follow-up needs.

REFERENCES

Burd RS, Whalen TV: Evaluation of the child with suspected appendicitis, *Pediatr Ann* 30(12):720, 2001.

Mequerditchian AN et al: Laparoscopic appendectomy in children: a favorable alternative in simple and complicated appendicitis, *J Pediatr Surg* 37(5):695, 2002.

Pelosi L: The role of the advanced practice nurse in pediatric general surgery, *Nurs Clin North Am* 35(1):159, 2000.

Peterson-Smith AM: Gastrointestinal disorders. In Burns CE et al, editors: *Pediatric primary care: a handbook for nurse practitioners,* ed 2, Philadelphia, 2000, WB Saunders.

6

◈

Asthma

◈

PATHOPHYSIOLOGY

Asthma is a lung disease in which there is airway obstruction, airway inflammation, and airway hyperresponsiveness or spasm of the bronchial smooth muscle. An exacerbation of asthma may be precipitated by specific allergens (e.g., pollen, mold, animal dander, dust, or foods) or by other factors such as weather changes, respiratory infections, exercise, gastroesophageal reflux, or emotional factors. Asthma results from complex interactions among the inflammatory cells and mediators in the airways and autonomic neural regulation of the airway, in which the following occur:

1. Bronchial smooth muscle contraction
2. Bronchospasm
3. Mucosal edema from inflammatory cells in the airways with injury to the epithelium
4. Increased mucus production
5. Mucus plugging
6. Trapping of air behind occluded or narrowed airways
7. Insufficient oxygenation and ventilation
8. Air hunger responses, which result in anxious behavior

INCIDENCE

1. Asthma affects 10% to 15% of all children.
2. Asthma accounts for 25% of school absences caused by chronic illness (leading cause of absenteeism).
3. Asthma mortality rates are increasing by 6% per year.

CLINICAL MANIFESTATIONS

1. Clinical evidence of airway obstruction—obstruction may be gradual or acute; severity of acute exacerbations is

      classified as mild intermittent, mild persistent, moderate persistent, or severe persistent

2. Dyspnea with prolonged expiration
3. Expiratory wheezing, progressing to inspiratory and expiratory wheezing, progressing to inaudibility of breath sounds
4. Grunting respirations in infancy
5. Nasal flaring
6. Cough
7. Accessory muscle use
8. Anxiety, irritability, decreasing level of consciousness
9. Cyanosis
10. Drop in arterial partial pressure of carbon dioxide (Pa_{CO_2}) initially from hyperventilation; then rise in Pa_{CO_2} as obstructive process worsens

COMPLICATIONS

1. Status asthmaticus
2. Chronic persistent bronchitis, bronchiolitis, pneumonia
3. Chronic emphysema
4. Cor pulmonale with right-sided heart failure
5. Atelectasis
6. Pneumothorax
7. Death

LABORATORY AND DIAGNOSTIC TESTS

1. White blood cell count—increased with infection
2. Arterial blood gas values (for severe cases)—initially increased pH, decreased Pa_{O_2}, and decreased Pa_{CO_2} (mild respiratory alkalosis from hyperventilation); subsequently decreased pH, decreased arterial partial pressure of oxygen (Pa_{O_2}), and increased Pa_{CO_2} (respiratory acidosis)
3. Eosinophil count—increased in blood, sputum
4. Chest radiographic study—to rule out infection or other cause of worsening respiratory status
5. Pulmonary function tests—decreased tidal volume, decreased vital capacity, decreased maximal breathing capacity
6. Peak flow meter monitoring—decreased peak expiratory flow volumes

MEDICAL MANAGEMENT

Medical management is targeted at preventing asthma exacerbations by avoiding asthma triggers and by decreasing airway obstruction, inflammation, and reactivity with medications. Medication choices and combinations depend on the severity classifications indicated in the Clinical Manifestations section in this chapter. Because prevention of exacerbations is the mainstay of treatment of this chronic illness, two medication classifications have emerged: long-term control and quick relief.

Long-Term Control

1. Corticosteroids—antiinflammatory; oral, inhaled, and intranasal forms
2. Cromolyn sodium and nedocromil—antiinflammatory; inhaled form; used to reduce exercise-induced asthma
3. Long-acting β_2-agonists—bronchodilator; inhaled form; used to reduce exercise-induced asthma and nocturnal symptoms
4. Methylxanthines—bronchodilator; all dosage forms
5. Leukotriene modifiers—improve lung function and reduce need for short-acting β_2-agonists; oral form

Quick Relief

1. Short-acting β_2-agonists—bronchodilator; inhaled form
2. Anticholinergics—improve smooth muscle tone; inhaled form
3. Corticosteroids—antiinflammatory; intravenous form

NURSING ASSESSMENT

1. See the Respiratory Assessment section in Appendix A.
2. Assess breathing pattern.
3. Assess for anxiety/agitation.
4. Assess fluid volume status.
5. Assess child and family coping strategies.

NURSING DIAGNOSES

- Airway clearance, Ineffective
- Gas exchange, Impaired
- Fluid volume, Risk for deficient

- Anxiety
- Family processes, Interrupted

NURSING INTERVENTIONS

1. Promote pulmonary function.
   a. Administer and assess response to oxygen for respiratory distress.
   b. Administer and assess response to aerosolized bronchodilators and antiinflammatory agents.
   c. Elevate head of bed.
   d. Avoid use of sedatives in child with asthma experiencing respiratory distress.
2. Assess and monitor child's hydration status.
   a. Monitor intake and output.
   b. Assess for signs of dehydration.
   c. Monitor infusion of intravenous solution.
   d. Monitor urine specific gravity.
3. Alleviate or minimize child's and parents' anxiety, in manner appropriate for developmental level.
4. Assess child's and parents' feelings about child's having asthma and taking medications.
5. Assess willingness to participate in education programs and refer family to support groups as needed.

🔺 Discharge Planning and Home Care

1. Begin client education at time of diagnosis and integrate it with continuing care.
2. Reinforce understanding of asthma.
3. Provide specific instructions about medications, equipment, and adverse effects.
4. Instruct on monitoring signs and symptoms and peak expiratory flow rate, and recognizing indications for treatment modifications.
5. List steps in managing an acute episode of asthma and instruct on when to seek emergency medical care.
6. Instruct in how to identify asthma triggers and how to avoid, eliminate, or control them.
7. Discuss fears and misconceptions concerning treatments.

CLIENT OUTCOMES

1. Child will have optimal pulmonary function.
2. Child will be able to perform daily activities.
3. Child will be able to participate in endurance activities (e.g., swimming, tennis).

REFERENCES

Behrman R, Kliegman R, Jenson HB: *Nelson textbook of pediatrics*, ed 16, Philadelphia, 2000, WB Saunders.

Guidelines for the diagnosis and management of asthma: national asthma education program—expert panel report 2, Bethesda, Md, February 1997, National Institutes of Health.

Hockenberry M: *Wong's nursing care of infants and children*, ed 7, St Louis, 2003, Mosby.

Kavura M, Wiedemann H: *Diagnosis and management of asthma*, ed 2, Cleveland, 1998, PCI.

Kwong J, Jones C: Chronic asthma therapy, *Pediatr Rev* 20(10):327, 1999.

Ladebauche P: Managing asthma: a growth and development approach, *Pediatr Nurs* 23(1):37, 1997.

7

❖

Attention-Deficit/ Hyperactivity Disorder

❖

PATHOPHYSIOLOGY

Attention-deficit/hyperactivity disorder (ADHD) is a chronic neurobiologic disorder characterized by problems in regulating activity (hyperactivity), inhibiting behavior (impulsivity), and attending to tasks (inattention). The *Diagnostic and Statistical Manual of Mental Disorders,* fourth edition, text revision (DSM-IV-TR), outlines specific observable behavioral symptoms in these three areas (Box 7-1). To meet the criteria for ADHD, symptoms must be present across settings. In other words, if the child is hyperactive at home but not at school, ADHD is not diagnosed.

Although ADHD symptoms are present before age 7 years, a diagnosis is not usually made until the child begins school, when behavior interferes with academic and social functioning. Children with ADHD are prone to physical injury. Sensorimotor coordination may be impaired, and clumsiness and problems with spatial orientation are common. Disruptiveness, temper outbursts, and aimless motor activity often irritate peers and family members. Secondary problems such as oppositional behavior, mood and anxiety disorders, and communication problems are common. Learning may be delayed as a result of chronic inability to attend to educational tasks.

As children enter adolescence, observable symptoms are less obvious. Restlessness and jitteriness replace the excessive activity seen during childhood. Adolescents with ADHD have difficulty complying with behavioral expectations or rules normally

BOX 7-1
Diagnostic Criteria for Attention-Deficit/ Hyperactivity Disorder

A. Either (1) or (2):

(1) Six (or more) of the following symptoms of **inattention** have persisted for at least 6 months to a degree that is maladaptive and inconsistent with developmental level:

Inattention

(a) Often fails to give close attention to details or makes careless mistakes in schoolwork, work, or other activities

(b) Often has difficulty sustaining attention in tasks or play activities

(c) Often does not seem to listen when spoken to directly

(d) Often does not follow through on instructions and fails to finish schoolwork, chores, or duties in the workplace (not due to oppositional behavior or failure to understand instructions)

(e) Often has difficulty organizing tasks and activities

(f) Often avoids, dislikes, or is reluctant to engage in tasks that require sustained mental effort (such as schoolwork or homework)

(g) Often loses things necessary for tasks or activities (e.g., toys, school assignments, pencils, books, or tools)

(h) Is often easily distracted by extraneous stimuli

(i) Is often forgetful in daily activities

(2) Six (or more) of the following symptoms of **hyperactivity- impulsivity** have persisted for at least 6 months to a degree that is maladaptive and inconsistent with developmental level:

Hyperactivity

(a) Often fidgets with hands or feet or squirms in seat

(b) Often leaves seat in classroom or in other situations in which remaining seated is expected

(c) Often runs about or climbs excessively in situations in which it is inappropriate (in adolescents or adults, may be limited to subjective feelings of restlessness)

(d) Often has difficulty playing or engaging in leisure activities quietly

(e) Is often "on the go" or often acts as if "driven by a motor"

(f) Often talks excessively

Continued

BOX 7-1
Diagnostic Criteria for Attention-Deficit/ Hyperactivity Disorder—cont'd

Impulsivity
(g) Often blurts out answers before questions have been completed
(h) Often has difficulty awaiting turn
(i) Often interrupts or intrudes on others (e.g., butts into conversations or games)
B. Some hyperactive-impulsive or inattentive symptoms that caused impairment were present before age 7 years.
C. Some impairment from the symptoms is present in two or more settings (e.g., at school [or work] and at home).
D. There must be clear evidence of clinically significant impairment in social, academic, or occupational functioning.
E. The symptoms do not occur exclusively during the course of a pervasive developmental disorder, schizophrenia, or other psychotic disorder and are not better accounted for by another mental disorder (e.g., mood disorder, anxiety disorder, dissociative disorder, or a personality disorder).

Code based on type:
314.01: Attention-deficit/hyperactivity disorder, combined type: if both criteria A1 and A2 are met for the past 6 months
314.00: Attention-deficit/hyperactivity disorder, predominantly inattentive type: if criterion A1 is met but criterion A2 is not met for the past 6 months
314.01: Attention-deficit/hyperactivity disorder, predominantly hyperactive-impulsive type: if criterion A2 is met but criterion A1 is not met for the past 6 months
Coding note: For individuals (especially adolescents and adults) who currently have symptoms that no longer meet full criteria, "in partial remission" should be specified.

From American Psychiatric Association: *Diagnostic and statistical manual of mental disorders,* ed 4, text revision (DSM-IV-TR), Washington, DC, 2000, The Association.

observed in educational and work settings. Conflicts with authority figures are also noted. Symptoms may persist into adulthood. These individuals may be described as "on the go," always busy, and unable to sit still.

No signal cause of ADHD exists. Genetic influences are likely, but to date, no specific genetic link has been found.

Neurodevelopmental and genetic risk factors do exist. Most notable are fetal risk factors, which include exposure to alcohol, nicotine, lead, and nutrient deficiencies (i.e., deficiency of iron, calcium).

INCIDENCE

1. Studies suggest a higher incidence of ADHD in children with first-degree biologic relatives with diagnosed ADHD.
2. The incidence rate among school-aged children is 3% to 5%.
3. Incidence is higher in males than in females (roughly three times higher in boys than in girls).

CLINICAL MANIFESTATIONS

Clinical manifestations are listed in Box 7-1.

COMPLICATIONS

1. Secondary diagnoses—conduct disorder, depression, and anxiety disorder
2. Academic underachievement, school failure, reading and/or arithmetic difficulties (frequently resulting from attentional problems)
3. Poor peer relationships (frequently due to impulsive behaviors such as aggressive behavior and verbal outbursts)

LABORATORY AND DIAGNOSTIC TESTS

1. Take behavioral history—obtain historical data from parents and teachers. This is the most important method of gathering information.
2. For accurate diagnosis of ADHD, symptoms must meet specific criteria outlined in *DSM-IV* (see Box 7-1).
3. Use ADHD checklist (i.e., Copeland Symptom Checklist for Attention-Deficit Disorders, Attention-Deficit Disorders Evaluation Scale).
4. Intelligence and achievement testing provides information about overall intellectual functioning and academic achievement (ADHD is likely to affect achievement and cognitive performance). Assessment report should include child's strengths and weaknesses.

5. The following neuropsychologic tests may be used to assess and monitor treatment. (No neuropsychologic instrument can be relied upon exclusively to diagnose.)
   - Continuous Performance Test
   - Matching Familiar Figures Test
   - Paired Associates Learning Task
6. The Child Behavior Checklist (Achenbach, 1991) is an assessment tool completed by parents for children aged 4 to 18 years. It measures withdrawal, somatic complaints, anxiety and depression, social problems, thought problems, attention problems, sex problems, delinquent behavior, and aggressive behavior.

MEDICAL MANAGEMENT

The treatment plan for ADHD should be carefully tailored to each child. Treatment options generally include medications (most commonly stimulants) and specific behavioral treatments. The various behavioral treatments include psychotherapy, cognitive-behavioral therapy, social skills training, support groups, and parent skills training. Behavioral rating scales and neuropsychologic tests may be used for baseline measurement and monitoring of treatment effectiveness.

Medication

Psychostimulant medications, including methylphenidate (Ritalin) and amphetamines (Dexedrine, Dextrostat, and Adderall), are the first line of treatment. Antidepressant medications are used for children who cannot tolerate or show poor response to stimulants, or for treatment of comorbid symptoms. Parents may express concern about using medication. Risks and benefits of medication must be explained to parents, including prevention of potential ongoing scholastic and social problems through the use of medications. When taken as prescribed for ADHD, stimulants are not addictive, nor do they lead to substance abuse. For most children medication alone may not be the best strategy.

NURSING ASSESSMENT

1. Assess family history via interview and/or genogram.
2. Assess child's behavioral history.

NURSING DIAGNOSES

- Social interaction, Impaired
- Self-concept, Disturbed
- Therapeutic regimen management, Ineffective
- Parenting, Risk for impaired
- Violence, Risk for other-directed
- Injury, Risk for

NURSING INTERVENTIONS

Nursing interventions are generally implemented in outpatient and community settings.

1. Assist parents in implementing a behavior program, including positive reinforcement.
2. Provide daily structure.
3. Administer stimulant medication as ordered.
   a. Stimulants may be temporarily discontinued on weekends and holidays.
   b. Stimulants are not given after 3 or 4 PM.

Discharge Planning and Home Care

1. Educate and support parents and family members.
2. Collaborate with teachers and involve parents. Encourage parents to ensure that teacher and school nurse are aware of medication name, dosage, and times of administration.
3. Ensure that child receives necessary academic evaluation and tutoring. Placement in special education class is often required.
4. Monitor child's progress and response to medication.
5. Refer to behavioral and parenting specialists to develop and implement a behavior plan.

CLIENT OUTCOMES

1. School performance will improve, as evidenced by classroom grades and work completed.
2. Improvement of child's behavior according to teacher and parent rating will be noted.
3. Child will display positive peer relationships.

REFERENCES

Achenbach T: *Manual for the child behavior checklist/4-18 and 1991 profile,* Burlington, Vt, 1991, University of Vermont Department of Psychiatry.

American Psychological Association: *Diagnostic and statistical manual of mental disorders,* text revision (DSM-IV-TR), Washington, DC, 2000, The Association.

Arnold LD et al: National Institute of Mental Health collaborative multimodal treatment study of children with ADHD (the MTA): design challenges and choices, *Arch Gen Psychiatry* 54:865, 1997.

Goldman LS et al: Diagnosis and treatment of attention-deficit/hyperactivity disorder in children and adolescents. Council on Scientific Affairs, American Medical Association, *JAMA* 279:1100, 1998.

Niebuhr V, Smith L: The school nurse's role in attention deficit hyperactivity disorder, *J Sch Health* 63(2):112, 1993.

Swanson JM et al: Effect of stimulant medication on children with attention deficit disorder: a review of reviews, *Except Child* 60:154, 1995.

8

❖

Bronchiolitis

❖

PATHOPHYSIOLOGY

Bronchiolitis is a lower respiratory tract illness characterized by inflammation of the small bronchi and smaller bronchioles. Edema of the mucous membranes lining the walls of the bronchioles plus cellular infiltrates and increased mucus production result in obstruction of the bronchioles. The obstruction causes hyperinflation of the affected areas as expired air is trapped distally, resulting in hypoxemia. The obstructions do not occur uniformly throughout the lung. In addition, resistance to airflow increases. This leads to dyspnea, tachypnea, and lower tidal volumes, which may result in hypercarbia in severely affected individuals. Symptoms are more severe in infants because the diameter of their bronchiole lumina is smaller. The infection is most commonly caused by the respiratory syncytial virus (RSV). RSV is transmitted by way of droplets. Other causative agents include adenovirus and parainfluenza virus. Prognosis is generally good.

INCIDENCE

1. Bronchiolitis is one of the most frequent reasons for hospitalization of infants younger than 1 year old.
2. Mortality rate is determined by the presence of underlying disease; the rate is higher if RSV is present.
3. Bronchiolitis occurs most frequently in winter and early spring.

CLINICAL MANIFESTATIONS

1. Upper respiratory tract infection for 1 to 4 days; then acute phase for 2 to 6 days; resolution in 7 to 14 days

2. Labored and rapid respirations
3. Nasal flaring and retractions
4. Expiratory wheezing of acute onset
5. Difficulty feeding or refusal to eat
6. Hacking, harsh paroxysmal cough
7. Cyanosis (may or may not be present)
8. Audible and palpable rhonchi
9. Malaise
10. Increased mucus production
11. Irritability

COMPLICATIONS

1. Atelectasis (acute)
2. Apnea (acute)
3. Respiratory fatigue or failure (acute)
4. Recurrent pulmonary infection (long term)

LABORATORY AND DIAGNOSTIC TESTS

1. Chest radiographic study—hyperinflation with air trapping, atelectasis, slight perihilar infiltrate; widely varied diagnostic criteria
2. Rapid viral diagnostic techniques for RSV—to detect RSV
3. Arterial blood gas values—to assess gas exchange
4. White blood cell count—normal or mild elevation

MEDICAL MANAGEMENT

Mild cases of bronchiolitis can usually be managed at home with fluid administration, humidification, and rest. Progressive respiratory distress and apnea are common indicators for inpatient admission and possible admission to the intensive care unit, and might require the use of mechanical ventilation. Supportive therapy includes administration of humidified oxygen, intravenous hydration, and rest. The only specific pharmacologic therapy is the use of ribavirin for RSV infection. This medication is not always used due to cost, benefit, safety, and efficacy. Antibiotics are not indicated unless a bacterial infection is detected.

NURSING ASSESSMENT

1. See the Respiratory Assessment section in Appendix A.
2. Assess respiratory status.
3. Assess for signs and symptoms of dehydration.
4. Assess for signs and symptoms of fluid overload.

NURSING DIAGNOSES

- Airway clearance, Ineffective
- Breathing pattern, Ineffective
- Gas exchange, Impaired
- Fluid volume, Risk for deficient
- Nutrition: less than body requirements, Imbalanced
- Anxiety
- Knowledge, Deficient

NURSING INTERVENTIONS

1. Monitor respiratory status (including vital signs).
   a. Assess vital signs every 2 hours until stable, then every 2 to 4 hours, and as necessary.
   b. Assess for and report signs of increased respiratory distress and changes in respiratory status.
   c. Perform cardiorespiratory monitoring.
   d. Monitor oxygen status with pulse oximetry.
2. Monitor child's response to humidified oxygen therapy through hood, tent, or nasal cannulae (improving respiratory status).
3. Promote respiratory function.
   a. Administer antiviral medications as ordered.
   b. Place in semiprone or side-lying position, avoiding neck hyperextension.
   c. Promote opportunities for rest.
4. Monitor hydration status.
   a. Monitor intake and output and urine specific gravity.
   b. Monitor weight.
   c. Monitor laboratory values.
   d. Assess for signs of dehydration or fluid overload.
5. Assess child for untoward therapeutic response to medications if indicated.

6. Encourage intake of diet high in calories and protein.
   a. Serve favorite foods if possible.
   b. Arrange food attractively on tray (for older child).
   c. Encourage use of routine feeding practices (e.g., usual mealtimes, presence of parents, or favorite cup).
7. Encourage age-appropriate quiet play (see the relevant section in Appendix B).
8. Alleviate or minimize child's and parents' anxiety during hospitalization (see Appendix J).
9. Provide consistent nursing care to promote trust and to alleviate anxiety.

🔺 Discharge Planning and Home Care

Instruct parents about the following for home care of child:
1. Use of humidifiers (may use moisture from hot shower)—cold versus warm mists
2. Rationale for treatments (medication administration)
3. Signs of secondary infection
4. Infection control and prevention measures
5. Provision of adequate fluid intake

CLIENT OUTCOMES

1. Infant or child will maintain patent airway with easy respiratory effort.
2. Infant or child will exhibit appropriate weight gain and hydration status.
3. Infant or child will exhibit no signs of anxiety or apprehension.

REFERENCES

Coto JA: Protocols in practice. Pediatric lower airway disease: do not be blown away by cost, *Nurs Case Manag* 3(2):75, 1998.

James S, Ashwill JW, Droske SC: *Nursing care of children—principles and practice*, ed 2, Philadelphia, 2002, WB Saunders.

Wohl MEB: Bronchiolitis. In Chernick V, Boat TF, editors: *Kendig's disorders of the respiratory tract in children*, ed 6, Philadelphia, 1998, WB Saunders.

Wong DL et al: *Wong's essentials of pediatric nursing*, ed 6, St Louis, 2001, Mosby.

9

❖

Bulimia Nervosa

❖

PATHOPHYSIOLOGY

Bulimia nervosa is a nutritional and psychologic disorder characterized by rapid consumption of large quantities of food (bingeing), followed by any number of behaviors used to prevent weight gain. Eating occurs during discrete periods of time. Self-induced vomiting is the most commonly used method to avoid weight gain. Other purging methods include use of laxatives, enemas, and diuretics. Fasting and excessive exercise may also be used as an attempt to compensate for intake and prevent weight gain. Most individuals develop a chronic pattern of binge/purge behavior. Bingeing may be triggered by dysphoria, stress, or negative feelings related to body image. Due to associated feelings of shame, bingeing is often done in secrecy. Individuals typically feel out of control during bingeing episodes. For some, vomiting becomes the goal in and of itself. Impulse control problems such as alcohol abuse and shoplifting often coexist with bulimia. As in individuals with anorexia nervosa, there is an excessive focus on one's body. Self-worth is connected to physical appearance. Unlike the individual with anorexia, the bulimic individual is likely to be within the normal weight range for age and height. The diagnostic criteria of the *Diagnostic and Statistical Manual of Mental Disorders,* fourth edition, text revision (DSM-IV-TR), are presented in Box 9-1.

INCIDENCE

1. Bulimia nervosa affects about 3% of adolescent girls and fewer than 1% of adolescent boys.
2. Most individuals with bulimia manifest symptoms in the latter half of adolescence.
3. Female/male ratio is 10:1.

BOX 9-1

Diagnostic Criteria for Bulimia Nervosa

1. Recurrent episodes of binge eating occur. An episode of binge eating is characterized by both of the following:
   a. Eating, in a discrete period of time (e.g., within any 2-hour period), an amount of food that is definitely larger than most people would eat during a similar period of time and under similar circumstances
   b. A sense of lack of control over eating during the episode (e.g., a feeling that one cannot stop eating or control what or how much one is eating)
2. Recurrent inappropriate compensatory behavior occurs to prevent weight gain, such as self-induced vomiting; misuse of laxatives, diuretics, enemas, or other medications; fasting; or excessive exercise.
3. The binge eating and inappropriate compensatory behaviors both occur, on average, at least twice a week for 3 months.
4. Self-evaluation is unduly influenced by body shape and weight.
5. The disturbance does not occur exclusively during episodes of anorexia nervosa.

Purging Type

During the current episode of bulimia nervosa, the person has regularly engaged in self-induced vomiting or the misuse of laxatives, diuretics, or enemas.

Nonpurging Type

During the current episode of bulimia nervosa, the person has used other inappropriate compensatory behaviors, such as fasting or excessive exercise, but has not regularly engaged in self-induced vomiting or the misuse of laxatives, diuretics, or enemas.

From American Psychiatric Association: *Diagnostic and statistical manual of mental disorders*, ed 4, text revision (DSM-IV-TR), Washington, DC, 2000, The Association, pp 544-545.

4. Incidence is greater in higher socioeconomic groups.
5. Fifty percent of bulimic individuals have an alcoholic relative.

CLINICAL MANIFESTATIONS

1. Binge eating done in secret as means of dealing with anxiety and stress

2. Hiding or stealing of food
3. Excusing of self to use bathroom during or after meals
4. Compulsive dieting and exercise
5. Preoccupation with weight and physical appearance
6. Impaired body image and self-concept
7. Depression and dysthymia
8. Food cravings

COMPLICATIONS

1. Parotid and submaxillary gland swelling (sialadenosis)
2. Facial fullness
3. Russell's sign—scarring of and callus formation on knuckles
4. Erosion of tooth enamel
5. Abdominal tenderness or pain
6. Esophagitis, gastritis
7. Impairment of school and social functioning due to preoccupation with food

LABORATORY AND DIAGNOSTIC TESTS

1. Thorough physical examination
2. Serum electrolyte levels—hypokalemia, hyponatremia, hypochloremic metabolic alkalosis
3. Serum amylase level—possible elevation
4. Evaluation of psychologic factors

MEDICAL MANAGEMENT

Treatment is provided on an outpatient basis unless severe medical problems emerge. An interdisciplinary approach is needed to ensure optimal outcomes. Outpatient treatment includes medical monitoring, initiation of a dietary plan to restore nutritional state, and individual and family psychotherapy. Treatment involves helping the individual learn to self-monitor and to identify distorted thinking patterns about weight, food, body image, and relationships. The goal of treatment is to restore normal eating. Psychopharmacologic treatment (i.e., antidepressants) may also be used. Prognosis is better if the condition is treated early, before purging is reinforced by weight loss.

NURSING ASSESSMENT

1. Perform thorough nursing history taking and assessment, including history of bulimic episodes, information related to family dynamics, and psychosocial functioning.
2. Assess psychologic status with psychologic inventories. The Beck Depression Inventory (adolescent version) can be used to assess level of depression. For structured interviews, the Eating Disorder Examination is available. Self-report measures include the Eating Disorder Inventory for ages 14 years and older. The Eating Attitudes Test and the Kids Eating Disorder Survey are applicable for school-aged and middle school–aged children, respectively.

NURSING DIAGNOSES

- Nutrition: less than body requirements, Imbalanced
- Self-esteem, Chronic low
- Fluid volume, Risk for deficient
- Coping, Ineffective
- Family processes, Interrupted
- Social interaction, Impaired

NURSING INTERVENTIONS

1. Provide information about adequate nutritional intake and effect of inadequate intake on energy level and psychologic well-being.
2. Establish trusting relationship that promotes disclosure of feelings and emotions.
3. Promote individual's sense of responsibility and involvement in recovery and treatment.
4. Promote cognitive restructuring and self-esteem through counseling.
5. Incorporate family-centered approach in providing services.

🔺 Discharge Planning and Home Care

Recommend psychotherapy for treatment of distorted body image and self-concept.

CLIENT OUTCOMES

1. Adolescent will maintain weight within normal range for age.
2. Adolescent will use more effective mechanisms to cope with negative emotions.
3. Adolescent will practice normal patterns of eating.

REFERENCES

American Psychiatric Association Work Group on Eating Disorders: Practice guideline for the treatment of patients with eating disorders (revision), *Am J Psychiatry* 157(1 suppl):1, 2000.

American Psychological Association: *Diagnostic and statistical manual of mental disorders,* ed 4, text revision (DSM-IV-TR), Washington, DC, 2000, The Association.

Boumann CE, Yates WR: Risk factors for bulimia nervosa: a controlled study of parental psychiatric illness and divorce, *Addict Behav* 19(6):667, 1994.

Heebink DM et al: Anorexia nervosa and bulimia nervosa in adolescence: effects of age and menstrual status on psychological variables, *J Am Acad Child Adolesc Psychiatry* 34(3):378, 1995.

Irwin EG: A focused overview of anorexia nervosa and bulimia. I. Etiological issues, *Arch Psychiatr Nurs* 7(6):342, 1993.

Position of the American Dietetic Association: nutrition intervention in the treatment of anorexia nervosa, bulimia nervosa, and binge eating, *J Am Diet Assoc* 94(8):902, 1994.

Steiner H, Lock J: Anorexia nervosa and bulimia nervosa in children and adolescents: a review of the past ten years, *J Am Acad Child Adolesc Psychiatry* 37:352, 1998.

Steinhausen H: *Eating disorders in adolescence: anorexia and bulimia nervosa,* New York, 1995, DeGruyter.

10

◆

Burns

◆

PATHOPHYSIOLOGY

Burns are the tissue damage that results from contact with thermal, chemical, or electrical agents. Burn severity is determined by (1) the depth of burn injury, (2) percentage of body surface area affected, and (3) involvement of specific body parts. There are four main types of burns: thermal, chemical, electrical, and radioactive. See Box 10-1 and Figure 10-1 for descriptions of burn severity and depth.

The severity of the burn determines the degree of change seen in the body's organs and systems. A thermal injury creates an open wound as a result of destruction of the skin. Following the burn, skin perfusion is decreased as blood vessels are occluded and vasoconstriction occurs. Intravascular volume decreases as fluids are leaked from the intravascular to interstitial space as a result of increased capillary permeability. Pulmonary injury may occur as a result of inhalation of smoke, steam, or irritants. With a major burn, cardiac output decreases and blood flow to the liver, kidney, and gastrointestinal tract is compromised. The child with a major burn is in a hypermetabolic state, consuming oxygen and calories at a rapid rate.

Prognosis is dependent on the severity of the burn that is sustained.

INCIDENCE

1. Burns are the second leading cause of accidental injury and death in children younger than 14 years of age.
2. Burns caused by thermal agents are the most common and usually occur in the kitchen or bathroom.

BOX 10-1
Burn Classification According to Depth

First Degree (Superficial)
- Superficial; involves only superficial epidermis (e.g., sunburn)
- Symptoms: pain, redness, no tissue or nerve damage

Second Degree (Partial Thickness)
- Superficial to deep dermal; involves entire epidermis and varying amounts of dermis (e.g., scald)
- Symptoms: pain; red, edematous skin; vesicles

Third Degree (Full Thickness)
- Epidermis and dermis destroyed; involves subcutaneous adipose tissue, fascia, muscle, and bone (e.g., fire)
- Symptoms: no pain; white, red, or black skin; edematous skin

3. Electrical and chemical burns are common in the toddler age group.
4. Three fourths of all burns are thought to be preventable.

CLINICAL MANIFESTATIONS

The following are initial manifestations of moderate to severe burn:

1. Tachycardia
2. Decreased blood pressure
3. Cold extremities and poor perfusion
4. Change in level of consciousness
5. Dehydration (decreased skin turgor, decreased urinary output, dry tongue and skin)
6. Increased rate of respirations
7. Pallor (not present with second- and third-degree burn)

COMPLICATIONS

1. Renal failure
2. Metabolic acidosis
3. Hyperkalemia
4. Hyponatremia
5. Hypocalcemia

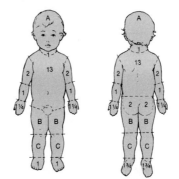

RELATIVE PERCENTAGES OF AREAS AFFECTED BY GROWTH

AREA	BIRTH	AGE 1 YR	AGE 5 YR
A = ½ of head	9½	8½	6½
B = ½ of one thigh	2¾	3¼	4
C = ½ of one leg	2½	2½	2¾

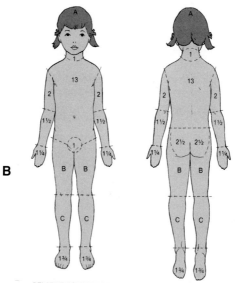

RELATIVE PERCENTAGES OF AREAS AFFECTED BY GROWTH

AREA	AGE 10 YR	AGE 15 YR	ADULT
A = ½ of head	5½	4½	3½
B = ½ of one thigh	4½	4½	4¾
C = ½ of one leg	3	3¼	3½

Figure 10-1 Estimated distribution of burns in children. **A,** Children from birth to age 5 years. **B,** Older children. (From Hockenberry M: *Wong's nursing care of infants and children,* ed 7, St Louis, 2003, Mosby.)

6. Pulmonary problems
   a. Pulmonary edema
   b. Pulmonary insufficiency
   c. Pulmonary embolus
   d. Bacterial pneumonia
7. Infection
8. Curling's ulcer

LABORATORY AND DIAGNOSTIC TESTS

1. Complete blood count—decreased
2. Arterial blood gas values—metabolic acidosis (decreased pH, increased partial pressure of carbon dioxide [Pco_2], and decreased partial pressure of oxygen [Po_2])
3. Serum electrolyte levels—decreased because of loss to traumatized areas and interstitial spaces
4. Serum glucose level—increased because of stress-invoked glycogen breakdown or glyconeogenesis
5. Blood urea nitrogen level—increased because of tissue breakdown and oliguria
6. Creatinine clearance—increased because of tissue breakdown and oliguria
7. Serum protein levels—decreased because of protein breakdown for massive energy needs
8. Chest radiographic study

MEDICAL MANAGEMENT

Burn treatment is based on the size and severity of the burn along with consideration as to its cause. Fluid resuscitation is critical in remedying intravascular fluid losses. Oxygen is delivered by mask or artificial ventilation. The burn itself may be covered with either moist or dry sterile dressings. Addition of topical medications may also be indicated. Severe burns require débridement of the wound and grafting. The child will receive analgesics or narcotics for pain. With severe burns, nutritional requirements are met with either a high-calorie diet or intravenous nutritional support.

NURSING ASSESSMENT

1. See Appendix A.
2. Assess fluid volume status.

3. Assess for adequate oxygenation and tissue perfusion.
4. Assess for pain.
5. Assess cause, extent, and depth of burns.

NURSING DIAGNOSES

- Gas exchange, Impaired
- Fluid volume, Deficient
- Pain, Acute
- Infection, Risk for
- Skin integrity, Impaired
- Nutrition: less than body requirements, Imbalanced
- Disuse syndrome, Risk for
- Anxiety
- Growth and development, Delayed
- Family processes, Interrupted

NURSING INTERVENTIONS
First Aid and Emergency Care

Prevent further injury.

1. Scald burn—stop burning process; remove individual's clothing and jewelry; apply moist or dry sterile dressing.
2. Flame burn—have individual drop and roll to extinguish; remove nonadherent clothing; apply moist or dry sterile dressing.
3. Chemical burn—flush eyes and skin for 20 minutes with water.
4. Electrical burn—turn off power sources; initiate cardiopulmonary resuscitation.

Hospital Care

1. Maintain patent airway.
   a. Monitor and report signs of respiratory distress (dyspnea, increased respiratory rate, air hunger, nasal flaring).
   b. Provide thorough pulmonary care.
   c. Elevate head of bed—administer oxygen as necessary; keep intubation kit at bedside.
   d. Administer corticosteroids as prescribed.

2. Monitor child for signs and symptoms of hypovolemic shock.
   a. Monitor vital signs and capillary refill time every hour or more frequently until stable.
   b. Monitor input and output hourly (output—20 to 30 ml/hr, >2 years; 10 to 20 ml/hr, <2 years).
3. Monitor child for signs and symptoms of electrolyte imbalances (Box 10-2).
4. Monitor child for signs and symptoms of hemorrhage.
   a. Changes in vital signs (monitor every hour or more frequently when first admitted [during critical period], then every 2 hours until stable, then every 4 hours)
      i. Rapid, thready pulse
      ii. Decreased blood pressure
   b. Bleeding
5. Provide pain relief measures to alleviate or control child's pain (see Appendix H).
   a. Use comfort measures (pillow, bed, cradle).
   b. Position for comfort.
   c. Medicate before wound care or dressing changes.
   d. Use distraction, guided imagery, hypnosis.
   e. Monitor child's therapeutic response to medications.
6. Protect child from potential infections.
   a. Administer tetanus booster as ordered.
   b. Monitor child's therapeutic and untoward response to antibiotics.
   c. Maintain and monitor use of protective isolation.
   d. Use sterile technique during wound care.
   e. Monitor for wound infections (offensive odor, redness at site, increased temperature, warmth, purulent drainage).
7. Promote adequate nutritional intake to counteract nitrogen loss and potential gastrointestinal complications.
   a. Provide diet high in calories and protein (total caloric requirement equals 60 calories times weight in kilograms plus 60 calories times percentage of burn).
   b. Monitor for signs of Curling's ulcer (decreased hemoglobin level, decreased red blood cell count [anemia], coffee-ground emesis, abdominal distention).
   c. Administer antacids as needed.
   d. Monitor bowel sounds for ileus.

8. Promote optimal healing of wounds (see Medical Management section in this chapter).
   a. Use sterile technique when dressing wound.
   b. Observe for cellulitis or area that is trapping pus.
9. Promote maximal function of joints.
   a. Use splints appropriately to prevent contractures.
   b. Check splints every 4 hours for pressure sores.
   c. Direct performance of range-of-motion exercises and passive range-of-motion exercises for extremities.
   d. Encourage ambulation when child is able.
   e. Encourage participation in self-care activities.
10. Encourage verbalization of feelings regarding altered body image.
    a. Depression (associated with injury and pain)
    b. Anxiety (associated with treatments)
    c. Shame (associated with appearance)
11. Provide for child's developmental needs during hospitalization.
    a. Encourage use of age-appropriate toys (see the relevant section in Appendix B); modify according to child's condition (e.g., use passive coloring—child directs nurse in coloring pictures).
    b. Encourage contact with peers (as appropriate).
    c. Provide age-appropriate roommate as dictated by condition.
    d. Encourage academic pursuits.
12. Provide emotional and other support to family.
    a. Encourage airing of concerns.
    b. Refer to social services as necessary.
    c. Refer to other parents in comparable situation as appropriate.
    d. Provide for physical comforts (e.g., place to sleep and bathe).
    e. Refer to support group (e.g., parent, religious) as needed.

🔺 Discharge Planning and Home Care

1. Instruct child and/or parents in wound care.
2. Provide burn prevention education.

BOX 10-2
Electrolyte Imbalances

Hyperkalemia
- Oliguria or anuria
- Diarrhea
- Muscle weakness
- Arrhythmias
- Intestinal colic

Hyponatremia
- Abdominal cramps
- Diarrhea
- Apprehension

Hypocalcemia
- Tingling in fingers
- Muscle cramps
- Tetany
- Convulsions

3. Make referrals for outpatient physical and occupational therapies as indicated.

CLIENT OUTCOMES
1. Child will be free from infection.
2. Child will have adequate intravascular fluid volume.
3. Child will demonstrate adequate respiratory function.
4. Child will experience little to no pain.

REFERENCES

Behrman R, Kleigman R, Jenson HB: *Nelson textbook of pediatrics*, ed 16, Philadelphia, 2000, WB Saunders.

Emergency Nurses Association: Burns. In *Emergency Nurses Pediatric Course*, pp 207-222, Des Plaines, Il, 1998, The Association.

Hansbrough J, Hansbrough W: Pediatric burns, *Pediatr Rev* 20(4):117, 1999.

Hazinski MF: *Manual of pediatric critical care*, St Louis, 1999, Mosby.

Hockenberry M: *Wong's nursing care of infants and children*, ed 7, St Louis, 2003, Mosby.

11

◆

Cellulitis

◆

PATHOPHYSIOLOGY

Cellulitis is an infection that affects the skin and subcutaneous tissue. The site of involvement is most commonly an extremity, but cellulitis may also occur on the scalp, head, and neck. Organisms causing cellulitis include *Staphylococcus aureus*, group A streptococci, and *Streptococcus pneumoniae*. Invasive infection caused by *Haemophilus influenzae* type B, once common, is now rare due to childhood immunization. A history of trauma or, in young children, an upper respiratory tract infection or sinusitis is often reported. The site of infection is characterized by a swelling with indistinct margins that is tender and warm. Infection may extend to deeper tissues or spread systemically. See Box 11-1 for orbital and periorbital cellulitis symptoms. Outcome is excellent with treatment.

INCIDENCE

1. Most children with periorbital or facial cellulitis are under the age of 2 years.
2. Cellulitis of the extremities occurs at a median age of 5 years.

CLINICAL MANIFESTATIONS
Local Reaction

1. Lesion with indistinct margins
2. Usually red, warm, and painful site of involvement
3. Indurated tissue

For orbital and periorbital reactions, see Box 11-1.

BOX 11-1
Orbital and Periorbital Cellulitis Symptoms

Orbital Cellulitis

- Infection easily spreads from sinuses because orbit shares common wall with ethmoid, maxillary, and frontal sinuses (caused by group A streptococci, *Staphylococcus aureus*, and *Streptococcus pneumoniae*)
- Symptoms: exophthalmos, ophthalmoplegia, and loss of visual acuity

Periorbital Cellulitis

- Caused by trauma, infected wound, or insect bite
- Symptoms: rapid onset of fever and swelling; area is warm, indurated, and tender

Systemic Reaction

1. Fever
2. Malaise
3. Chills
4. Red streak along lymphatic drainage path
5. Enlarged and painful lymph glands

COMPLICATIONS

1. Systemic involvement, septicemia
2. Osteomyelitis
3. Septic arthritis
4. Meningitis
5. Loss of visual acuity (orbital cellulitis)
6. Potential for brain abscess (orbital, periorbital cellulitis)

LABORATORY AND DIAGNOSTIC TESTS

1. Complete blood count—elevated white blood cell count
2. Blood cultures—positive result
3. Tissue aspirate culture—positive result
4. Radiographic study of paranasal sinuses (periorbital cellulitis)—opacification of sinuses
5. Computed tomographic scan of orbit and paranasal sinuses—to rule out orbital involvement

MEDICAL MANAGEMENT

Children with cellulitis may be treated with oral antibiotics as outpatients if they have localized symptoms without fever. When systemic symptoms are present, the child is admitted to the hospital for a course of intravenous (IV) antibiotics. Warm compresses are applied to the site. The site is elevated and immobilized whenever possible. Acetaminophen is given as needed to manage fever and pain. For the first 24 to 36 hours after effective antibiotic therapy is begun, it is not unusual for the cellulitis to appear to progress. Antibiotic administration may be changed from IV to oral administration when symptoms of redness, warmth, and swelling have significantly improved. A total 10- to 14-day course of antibiotics is given. Incision and drainage may be performed if the area becomes suppurative.

NURSING ASSESSMENT

1. Assess for local and systemic reactions.
2. Assess for pain.

NURSING DIAGNOSES

- Tissue integrity, Impaired
- Pain
- Anxiety

NURSING INTERVENTIONS

1. Monitor child's status for progression of symptoms and complications.
   a. Assess skin locally for changes; minimize palpation because of pain.
   b. Assess for signs of systemic infection.
   c. Monitor therapeutic and untoward responses to antibiotics.
2. Provide pain relief and comfort measures.
   a. Bed rest; immobilization and elevation of affected extremity
   b. Warm compresses to site for 10 to 20 minutes daily or more frequently
   c. Pain medications as needed

3. Provide emotional support to child and family.
   a. Provide age-appropriate explanations before procedures.
   b. Incorporate home routine into care.
   c. Encourage parental verbalization of concerns.
   d. Refer to social services as needed.

🏠 Discharge Planning and Home Care

1. Instruct parents about importance of continuing full course of antibiotics even though symptoms have resolved.
2. Instruct parents about follow-up appointment.
3. Instruct parents to observe for and report signs of infection spread.

CLIENT OUTCOMES

1. Child will have decreased redness, swelling, and warmth at cellulitis site.
2. Child will be free of pain.
3. Child and family will understand home care and follow-up needs.

REFERENCES

Bradley JS: Cellulitis. In Jenson HB, Baltimore RS, editors: *Pediatric infectious diseases: principles and practice,* Norwalk, Conn, 1995, Appleton & Lange.

Givner LB et al: Pneumococcal facial cellulitis in children, *Pediatrics* 106(5):E61, 2000.

Jain A, Rubin PAD: Orbital cellulitis in children, *Int Ophthalmol Clin* 41(4):71, 2001

Starkey CR, Steele RW: Medical management of orbital cellulitis, *Pediatr Infect Dis J* 20(10):1002, 2001.

12

❖

Cerebral Palsy

❖

PATHOPHYSIOLOGY

Cerebral palsy (CP) is a nonspecific term used to characterize abnormal muscle tone, posture, and coordination caused by a nonprogressive lesion or injury that affects the immature brain. CP may result from prenatal brain abnormalities, birth asphyxia, or premature birth. The actual brain abnormality may arise from a variety of causes: anatomical malformations of the brain, atrophy, vascular occlusion, loss of neurons, or low brain weight. Predisposing risk factors include multiple-gestation births, maternal infections, and maternal and fetal thrombophilic conditions. CP is frequently classified according to functional categories noted to describe the neuromuscular abnormalities. The two most common forms are the following:

1. *Spastic* CP is the most common form (80% of cases). It is characterized by hypertonicity and poor postural control, balance, and coordination. Gross and fine motor skills are impaired. Spastic CP is further classified according to the part of the body affected.
   a. Diplegia—involves the legs and occurs most often in those who were premature infants and who had an intraventricular hemorrhage or ischemic leukomalacia. Mild upper extremity uncoordination of the arms may also be seen.
   b. Monoplegia—involves just one extremity
   c. Hemiparesis—usually affects the arm more than the leg
   d. Quadriparesis—involves all extremities, with the legs having more impairment

2. *Dyskinetic* CP is characterized by a movement disorder and results from Rh incompatibility and hypoxic ischemic encephalopathy.
   a. Athetosis—slow writhing movements involving the face and extremities
   b. Dystonia—rhythmic twisting distortions involving the trunk and proximal extremities
   c. Chorea—rapid irregular movements of the face and extremities
   d. Ballismus—flailing movements of the extremities

INCIDENCE

1. CP is the most common permanent physical disability of childhood.
2. Incidence is 2 to 3 cases in every 1000 live births.
3. The prevalence of CP has risen with the increased survival of very low birth weight infants.
4. Spastic CP is the most common type.

CLINICAL MANIFESTATIONS

1. Delay in reaching motor developmental milestones
2. Abnormal motor performance and loss of selective motor control
3. Alterations of muscle tone
4. Abnormal posture
5. Reflex abnormalities

COMPLICATIONS

1. Impaired intellectual function
2. Seizures
3. Communication disorders
4. Drooling, feeding and swallowing difficulties
5. Joint contractures
6. Perceptual dysfunction
7. Learning disabilities

LABORATORY AND DIAGNOSTIC TESTS

1. Clinical examination to identify tone abnormalities, frequently hypotonicity followed by hypertonicity, postural abnormalities, and delayed motor development

2. Cranial ultrasonography to detect hemorrhagic and hypoxic ischemic insults
3. Computed tomographic scan to detect central nervous system lesions
4. Magnetic resonance imaging to detect small lesions
5. Positron emission tomography and single photon emission computed tomography to visualize brain metabolism and perfusion

MEDICAL MANAGEMENT

The overall goal of medical management is to develop a rehabilitation plan to promote optimal functioning. This includes assisting the child to gain new skills and anticipating potential complications. A multidisciplinary team approach is required. Most children identified with a delay or risk for delay are enrolled in an early intervention program (EIP) and receive physical, occupational, and speech therapy as indicated. As children grow from the infancy/toddler stage, treatments support the functional goals set. These treatments include therapeutic exercises, splinting, serial casting, bracing, and use of mobility aids and adaptive devices to provide functional independence. Surgical procedures such as osteotomies or tendon lengthening or tendon transfer may be performed. Antispasmodic drugs may be given orally or injected into the nerves to decrease spasticity. Selective posterior rhizotomy and botulinum toxin A can be used in the treatment of spasticity.

NURSING ASSESSMENT

1. See the Musculoskeletal Assessment section in Appendix A.
2. Assess for delay in motor skills.

NURSING DIAGNOSES

- Growth and development, Delayed
- Mobility, Impaired physical
- Self-esteem, Chronic low
- Social interaction, Impaired

NURSING INTERVENTIONS

1. Promote maximal functioning of joints.
2. Provide adaptive equipment for activities of daily living.

3. Ensure compliance with use of ambulatory aids (i.e., walker, crutches, orthoses).
4. Position to prevent contractures.
5. Direct performance of active and passive range-of-motion exercises.
6. Encourage verbalization of feelings about altered body image.
7. Encourage social interaction with peers.
8. Collaborate with educational specialist in EIP and/or 504 planning to promote achievement of educational goals.

🔺 Discharge Planning and Home Care

1. Refer to EIP or outpatient physical, occupational, and/or speech therapy.
2. Obtain adaptive equipment.
3. Teach individual and family how to maintain individual's optimum functional independence.
4. Identify appropriate support groups for individual and family.

CLIENT OUTCOMES

1. Child will achieve functional independence and mobility within physical limitations.
2. Child will avoid further disability.

REFERENCES

Gormley ME Jr: Treatment of neuromuscular and musculoskeletal problems in cerebral palsy, *Pediatr Rehabil* 4(1):5, 2001.

Hanna DL et al: Cerebral palsy—an update. Part I: Classification and etiology; Part II: Clinical presentation and early intervention, *Nebr Med J* 80(7):174, 1995.

Kerr GH: Botulinum toxin A in cerebral palsy: functional outcomes, *J Pediatr* 137(3):300, 2000.

Molnar GE: Cerebral palsy. In Molnar E, editor: *Pediatric rehabilitation,* ed 2, Baltimore, 1992, Williams & Wilkins.

Petersen MC, Palmer FB: Advances in prevention and treatment of cerebral palsy, *Ment Retard Dev Disabil Res Rev* 7(1):30, 2001.

Turnbull JD: Early intervention for children with or at risk of cerebral palsy, *Am J Dis Child* 147(1):54, 1993.

13

❖

Child Abuse and Neglect

❖

PATHOPHYSIOLOGY

The Child Abuse Prevention and Treatment Act amendments of 1996 define child abuse and neglect as, at a minimum, "any recent act or failure to act on the part of a parent or caretaker, which results in death, serious physical or emotional harm, sexual abuse or exploitation, or an act or failure to act which presents an imminent risk of serious harm." There are four major types of abuse: physical abuse, sexual abuse, emotional abuse (psychologic/verbal/mental injury), and child neglect. It is of interest to note that emotional abuse is almost always present when other forms are identified. The most recent research suggests several other types or subcategories of maltreatment, including congenital child abuse, sibling abuse, and child abandonment.

Child maltreatment crosses all areas of society and all cultural, racial/ethnic, religious, socioeconomic, and professional groups. It is most common, however, among adolescent parents and in low-income families. Risk factors and statistics associated with child maltreatment are categorized as they relate to parents, children, families, and the environment.

Perpetrator Characteristics

Perpetrators of child maltreatment are the persons responsible for a child's well-being, such as parents or caretakers, who have abused or neglected the child. Parents account for 78.8% of perpetrators.

1. Maltreating parents consistently report having been physically, sexually, or emotionally abused or neglected as children. However, not all maltreated children grow up to be abusive parents.

2. Common characteristics identified in abusive parents include low self-esteem, low intelligence, social isolation, depression, low frustration tolerance, immaturity, lack of parenting/coping skills, lack of knowledge of child development, marital problems, single or adolescent parenthood, closely spaced pregnancies, substance abuse, physical illness, and criminal behavior.

Child Characteristics

1. Children who are born prematurely and/or with congenital anomalies or who have difficult-to-soothe temperaments, frequent illness, or special needs are at greater risk for abuse.
2. Girls were sexually abused three times more often than boys.
3. Boys had a higher risk of emotional neglect and serious injury than girls.
4. Children are consistently vulnerable to sexual abuse from age 3 years and up.
5. There have been no significant racial differences in the incidence of maltreatment reported in the NIS-2 or NIS-3.

Family Characteristics

1. Children of single-parent families had a 77% higher risk of physical abuse, an 87% higher risk of physical neglect, and an 80% higher risk of serious injury or harm from abuse or neglect than children living with both parents.
2. Children in the largest families were physically neglected nearly three times more often than those from single-child families.
3. Children from families with annual incomes below $15,000 were more than 22 times more likely to suffer some form of maltreatment as defined by the Harm Standard and more than 25 times more likely to experience some form of maltreatment as defined by the Endangerment Standard than were children from families with annual incomes above $30,000.
4. Children from the lowest income families were 18 times more likely to be sexually abused, almost 56 times more likely to be educationally neglected, and over 22 times more likely to suffer serious injury as defined by the Harm Standard than were children from higher income families.

Environmental Characteristics

Environmental factors related to child abuse include ethnic/ racial prejudices, poor living conditions, lack of community and family resources, poor access to health care and follow-up services, economic pressure, varied cultural beliefs concerning the role of the child in the family, and varied cultural attitudes toward use of physical punishment. Ineffective child protection laws are another culprit in the environment. Studies have shown that nearly half of the children killed by caretakers are killed after they come to the attention of the child welfare service. Keeping the family intact may no longer be the goal if maltreatment is significant.

INCIDENCE

1. In 2000, child protective services investigated more than 3 million reports alleging maltreatment of more than 5 million children.
2. The national rate of victimization was 11.8 victims per 1000 children in the population.
3. An estimated 1200 child maltreatment fatalities occurred in the 50 states and District of Columbia in 2000. Children younger than 1 year old accounted for 44% of all deaths, and 85% of child fatalities were in children younger than 6 years of age.
4. More than half of all victims (63%) suffered neglect (including medical neglect), 19% suffered physical abuse, and about 10% of victims were sexually abused. Victims of emotional maltreatment accounted for 8% of all victims. Other types of maltreatment, including abandonment, congenital drug addiction, and threats to harm the child, accounted for 16% of victims. (Percent totals are higher than 100% because some children suffered multiple types of abuse.)
5. Sexual abuse is most common among girls, stepfamilies, and children living with one parent or a primary caregiver who is an unrelated male.
6. More than half of all abuse victims were white (51%), a quarter (25%) were African American, and 15% were Hispanic. American Indians and Native Alaskans accounted for 2% of victims, and Asians and Pacific Islanders accounted for 1% of victims.

CLINICAL MANIFESTATIONS

See Box 13-1 for a list of the clinical manifestations.

COMPLICATIONS

1. Attention-deficit/hyperactivity disorder (ADHD)
2. Learning difficulties

BOX 13-1

Clinical Manifestations of Child Abuse and Neglect

Skin Injuries

Skin injuries are the most common and easily recognized signs of maltreatment in children. Human bite marks appear as ovoid areas with tooth imprints, suck marks, or tongue thrust marks. Multiple bruises or bruises in inaccessible places are indications that the child has been abused. Bruises in different stages of healing may indicate repeated trauma. Bruises that take the shape of a recognizable object are generally not accidental.

Traumatic Hair Loss

Traumatic hair loss occurs when the child's hair is pulled or used to drag or jerk the child. The result of the pulling on the scalp can cause the blood vessels under the skin to break. An accumulation of blood can help differentiate between abusive and nonabusive loss of hair.

Falls

If a child is reported to have had a routine fall but has what appear to be severe injuries, the inconsistency of the history with the trauma sustained indicates suspected child abuse.

External Head, Facial, and Oral Injuries

Cuts, bleeding, redness, or swelling of the external ear canal; facial fractures; tears or scarring of the lip; oral, perioral and/or pharyngeal lesions; loosened, discolored, or fractured teeth; dental caries; tongue lacerations; unexplained erythema or petechiae of the palate; and bilateral black eyes without trauma to the nose all may indicate abuse.

Deliberate or Unexplained Thermal Injuries

Immersion burns, with clear line of demarcation; multiple small circular burns, in varying stages of healing; iron burns (show iron pattern); diaper area burns; and rope burns suggest intentional harm.

Continued

BOX 13-1

Clinical Manifestations of Child Abuse and Neglect—cont'd

Shaken Baby Syndrome

A shaken baby may suffer only mild ocular or cerebral trauma. The infant may have a history of poor feeding, vomiting, lethargy, and/or irritability that occurs periodically for days or weeks prior to the initial health care consult. In 75% to 90% of cases, unilateral or bilateral retinal hemorrhages are present but may be missed unless the child is examined by a pediatric ophthalmologist. Shaking produces an acceleration-deceleration (shearing) injury to the brain, causing stretching and breaking of blood vessels that results in subdural hemorrhage. Subdural hemorrhage may be most prominent in the interhemispheric fissure. However, cerebral edema may be the only finding. Serious insult to the central nervous system may result, without external evidence of injury.

Unexplained Fractures and Dislocations

Posterior rib fractures in different stages of healing, spiral fractures, or dislocation from twisting of an extremity may provide evidence of nonaccidental injury in children.

Sexual Abuse

Abrasions or bruising of the inner thighs and genitalia; scarring, tearing, or distortion of the labia and/or hymen; anal lacerations or dilatation; lacerations or irritation of external genitalia; repeated urinary tract infections; sexually transmitted disease; nonspecific vaginitis; pregnancy in the young adolescent; penile discharge; and sexual promiscuity may provide evidence of sexual abuse.

Neglect

The symptoms of neglect reflect a lack of both physical and medical care. Manifestations include failure to thrive without a medical explanation, multiple cat or dog bites and scratches, feces and dirt in the skin folds, severe diaper rash with the presence of ammonia burns, feeding disorders, and developmental delays.

3. Mental health problems (e.g., depression, post-traumatic stress disorder, eating disorders)
4. Aggressive behaviors (fighting)
5. Developmental delays
6. Difficulties with social relationships
7. Inappropriate sexual behaviors
8. Substance abuse
9. Increased risk for sexually transmitted diseases (e.g., AIDS)

LABORATORY AND DIAGNOSTIC TESTS

1. Skeletal (bone) survey radiographic studies, in two planes, for all children with suspected abuse injuries. Repeat in 2 weeks for children for whom there is a strong suspicion of abuse. Rationale: Metaphyseal ("corner-chip") fractures have high specificity for abuse but may be difficult to see initially. Healing fractures form a callus (bump of bone) that is apparent within 2 weeks of an acute injury. Skeletal surveys also provide information about the age of the injuries.* Multiple fractures at various stages of healing are common in child abuse.
2. Computed tomography/magnetic resonance imaging of affected areas
3. Ophthalmologic examination—to detect retinal hemorrhages (result from severe shaking or slamming of head)
4. Color photographs of injuries
5. Head circumference, abdominal circumference
6. Examination of cerebrospinal fluid
7. Pregnancy test
8. Screens for sexually transmitted diseases, human immunodeficiency virus
9. Evidentiary examination (specimen collection and examination should comply with the recommendations of child protective services or local coroner or medical examiner)

---

*The "bodygram" or partial skeletal surveys are no longer acceptable because of the newer total skeletal bone survey technology.

MEDICAL MANAGEMENT

The first priority in the care of the abused child is resuscitation and stabilization as deemed necessary depending on the injuries sustained. Confirmation of the abuse is achieved through thorough history taking, complete physical examination with detailed inspection of the child's entire body, and collection of laboratory specimens. All injuries should be documented with color photographs and recorded carefully in the written medical record.

Every state has a child abuse law that specifies legal responsibilities for reporting suspected abuse. Suspected abuse must be reported to the local child protective service agency. Mandated reporters include nurses, physicians, dentists, podiatrists, psychologists, speech pathologists, coroners, medical examiners, child day care center employees, children's services workers, social workers, and schoolteachers. Failure to report suspected child abuse can result in a fine or other punishment, depending on individual statutes.

NURSING ASSESSMENT

1. Conduct comprehensive history taking and parent (or caregiver) interview. Verification and documentation of circumstances associated with the injury event are critical. Therefore nurse should make a written checklist of who, what, when, where, why, and how questions and answers.
2. Perform comprehensive physical examination as well as social, emotional, and cognitive assessment.
3. Observe parent-child interactions, including frequency of contact and length of time parent visits child.
4. Assess emotional status of parents.

NURSING DIAGNOSES

- Injury, Risk for
- Pain
- Fear
- Growth and development, Delayed
- Coping, Compromised family

NURSING INTERVENTIONS

1. Resuscitate and stabilize as necessary.
2. Protect from further injury.
3. Assist with diagnosis of abuse.
4. Report suspected abuse.
5. Provide supportive care.
6. Document assessment of physical findings, parent interactions, and child's verbal disclosures.
7. Provide explanations of normal child growth and development, and compliment parent for behaviors that indicate appropriate responses to child's needs.
8. Discuss, encourage, and role-model behaviors that foster maternal-child attachment and positive parenting skills.
9. Discuss alternative methods of discipline and encourage positive reinforcement for good behavior in child.
10. Discuss family stress and review coping strategies (positive versus negative).
11. Discuss need for community resources and make appropriate referrals (child life specialist; child protective services; social worker; home visiting nurse; parenting classes; women, infants, and children [WIC] services; fuel assistance; Section 8 housing assistance; Parents Anonymous).

🏠 Discharge Planning and Home Care

1. Refer parents to multidisciplinary community resources that will assist with improving impulse control, increase knowledge of child's growth and development, aid in setting realistic expectations, and provide alternatives to physical abuse (Box 13-2).
2. Refer family to support groups, family therapy, or parenting effectiveness classes.

CLIENT OUTCOMES

1. Child will be protected from further injury or harm.
2. Child will demonstrate minimal long-term sequelae as a result of abuse.
3. Parents will develop effective parenting skills.

BOX 13-2
Resources

American Academy of Pediatrics website: http://www.AAP.org

Child Abuse and Neglect Database Instrument System (CANDIS) on the website of the National Crime Victims Research and Treatment Center: http://www.musc.edu/cvc/ candis.htm

National Child Abuse Reporting Hotline: 800-522-3511

National Clearinghouse on Child Abuse and Neglect Information
330 C St., SW
Washington, DC 20447
Phone: 800-FYI-3366 or 703-385-7565
Fax: 703-385-3206
e-mail: nccanch@calib.com
website: http://www.calib.com/nccanch

National Data Archive on Child Abuse and Neglect website: http://www.ndacan.cornell.edu/

REFERENCES

DePanfilis D, Salus MK: *A coordinated response to child abuse and neglect: a basic manual*, US Department of Health and Human Services Pub No (ACF) 92-30362, Washington, DC, 1992, US Government Printing Office.

National Clearinghouse on Child Abuse & Neglect Information: *Focus: understanding the effects of maltreatment on early brain development 2001*, available online at http://www.calib.com/nccanch/pubs/focus/earlybrain.cfm#effects, accessed June 6, 2003.

Nester CB: Prevention of child abuse and neglect in the primary care setting, *Nurse Pract* 23(9):61, 1998.

Patterson M: Advanced practice. Protocol for detecting child abuse, *Nurs Spectrum* (Washington, DC/Baltimore metro edition) 8(8):4, 1998.

US Department of Health and Human Services, Children's Bureau, Administration on Children, Youth and Families: *National child abuse and neglect data system (NCANDS) summary of key findings from calendar year 2000*, Washington, DC, April 2002, US Government Printing Office.

14

❖

Chronic Lung Disease of Infancy

❖

PATHOPHYSIOLOGY

Chronic lung disease (CLD) of infancy, formerly known as bronchopulmonary dysplasia (BPD), is a disorder seen in infants born with severe respiratory distress syndrome. The disease occurs in both full-term and preterm infants who have been treated with prolonged mechanical ventilation and/or oxygen therapy. It is the most common complication in the care of infants who weigh less than 1 kg at birth. Clinical presentation is characterized by ongoing respiratory distress, persistent oxygen requirement (with or without ventilatory support) at 36 weeks' postconceptual age, and a classically abnormal chest radiographic study. More recently, CLD has been categorized into three levels of severity in those younger than 32 weeks' gestation:

1. Mild: supplemental oxygen required at 28 days of age but not at 36 weeks of age
2. Moderate: supplemental oxygen required at 28 days of age but less than 30% oxygen required at 36 weeks of age
3. Severe: supplemental oxygen required at 28 days of age and more than 30% oxygen or ventilator therapy required at 36 weeks of age

The four major risk factors that contribute to the development of CLD are prematurity, presence of respiratory distress or failure, severe initial respiratory illness, and lack of antenatal treatment with steroids. Other important risk factors include exposure to mechanical ventilation, exposure to high air leaks, fluid overload, sepsis, and a patent ductus arteriosus.

Pulmonary changes typical of infants with CLD include alterations in lung structure, increased airway resistance, increased airway reactivity, decreased lung compliance, increased mucus production, and increased work of breathing. Although pulmonary function often improves significantly in early childhood, recent research demonstrates that some pulmonary problems may persist into adult life. Survival rate is dependent on the infant's birth weight, gestational age, and severity of CLD (Table 14-1).

INCIDENCE

1. Incidence varies among neonatal intensive care units because of differences in diagnostic criteria, client populations, and client management.
2. The suggestion has been made that the incidence has increased due to improved infant survival rates.

CLINICAL MANIFESTATIONS

1. Hypoxia
2. Hypercapnia

TABLE 14-1
Percentage of Surviving Infants with CLD in Different Birth Weight Groups

Birth Weight (g)	Oxygen Dependence at 28 Days' PNA	Oxygen Dependence at 36 Weeks' PCA for Infants Born at <32 Weeks' Gestation
<750	90-100%	54%
750-999	50-70%	33%
1000-1249	30-60%	20%
1250-1499	6-40%	10%

From Nievas F, Chernick V: Bronchopulmonary dysplasia (chronic lung disease of infancy): an update for the pediatrician, *Clin Pediatr (Phila)* 41(2):77, 2002.
CLD, Chronic lung disease; *PCA*, postconceptual age; *PNA*, postnatal age.

3. Tachypnea
4. Retractions
5. "Seesaw" breathing (due to decreased lung compliance)
6. Wheezing
7. Rhonchi
8. Cough
9. Increased work of breathing

COMPLICATIONS

1. Persistent changes in pulmonary function
2. Respiratory infections
3. Pulmonary hypertension
4. Right ventricular failure
5. Intraventricular hemorrhage
6. Cor pulmonale
7. Systemic hypertension
8. Altered growth and nutrient needs
9. Delayed development
10. Activity intolerance
11. Long-term need for supplemental oxygen
12. Cerebral palsy
13. Cognitive delay
14. Hearing loss requiring amplification
15. Bilateral blindness

LABORATORY AND DIAGNOSTIC TESTS

1. Chest radiographic studies—may include spectrum of findings, including bilateral diffuse interstitial thickening (mild to very severe) and normal to increased lung expansion
2. Arterial and venous blood gas values—hypercapnia and compensated respiratory acidosis are common findings
3. Pulmonary function testing
4. Serum electrolyte levels—useful when monitoring effects of long-term diuretic therapy
5. Serial electrocardiograms—useful to monitor for cor pulmonale

MEDICAL MANAGEMENT

The goals of medical management for infants with CLD are (1) treatment of the complications and symptoms with oxygen therapy and medication, and (2) enhancement of lung healing through adequate nutrition and promotion of respiratory stability (stable oxygenation and prevention of infection).

Therapies commonly used include the following:

1. Oxygen
2. Bronchodilators—decrease pulmonary resistance and increase lung compliance
3. Diuretics—prevent fluid overload and pulmonary edema
4. Corticosteroids—decrease inflammatory responses and promote lung healing
5. Nutrition—adequate nutrition promotes lung and total body healing, growth, and development
6. Palivizumab (Synagis), used prophylactically, protects against respiratory syncytial virus (RSV)

NURSING ASSESSMENT

1. See the Respiratory Assessment section in Appendix A.
2. Assess infant's cardiorespiratory status.
3. Assess for signs and symptoms of fluid overload.
4. Assess infant's oral intake and growth.
5. Assess developmental level.
6. Assess infant-parent interactions.
7. Assess parents' discharge readiness and ability to manage home care and access community resources.

NURSING DIAGNOSES

- Gas exchange, Impaired
- Fluid volume, Excess
- Nutrition: less than body requirements, Imbalanced
- Growth and development, Delayed
- Activity intolerance
- Family processes, Interrupted
- Parent-infant attachment, Risk for impaired
- Knowledge, Deficient
- Therapeutic regimen management, Ineffective

NURSING INTERVENTIONS

1. Maintain cardiorespiratory stability.
   a. Establish infant's baseline respiratory assessment and monitor for changes.
   b. Monitor responsiveness to medical interventions.
   c. Monitor trends in oxygenation through oximetry.
   d. Monitor action and side effects of medications.
      i. Bronchodilators
      ii. Corticosteroids
      iii. Diuretics
2. Evaluate for signs and symptoms of fluid overload.
   a. Monitor intake (ml/kg/day) and output (ml/kg/hr).
   b. Administer diuretic and/or fluid-restrictive therapy as ordered.
3. Monitor for adequate caloric intake and growth over time.
   a. Weight gain should be approximately 20 to 30 g/day.
   b. Monitor infant's ability to maintain adequate oral intake. (Infants who are tachypneic and have increased work of breathing may not be able to take in food orally because of risk of aspiration.)
   c. Monitor for increased oxygen requirements during and immediately after oral feedings; provide increased oxygen as needed.
   d. Provide supplementation to oral feedings through gavage or gastrostomy tube feedings.
4. Prevent infection.
   a. Provide RSV prophylaxis as recommended.
   b. Ensure that immunizations are given on schedule.
5. Promote growth and development through integration of play and positive stimulation into care routine (see relevant section of Appendix B).
   a. Provide opportunities for developmentally appropriate visual, auditory, tactile, and kinesthetic stimulation—when infant is alert and stable.
   b. Integrate pattern and routine into care, including undisturbed night sleep and predictable daytime activities.

6. Monitor infant's response to caregiving and developmental activities.
   a. Assess for increased oxygen requirements during and immediately following activity.
   b. Assess for patterns of response to activities and caregivers.
   c. Develop list of likes, dislikes, and comfort measures from assessed patterns of response.
   d. Decrease environmental and caregiver stimulation during periods of agitation and/or stress.
7. Facilitate integration of infant into his or her family.
   a. Assist parents in recognizing infant's responses to activity.
   b. Teach parents how they can best interact with and provide care for their child.
   c. Develop parents' confidence in caring for their child.
   d. Promote visitation and caregiving by other key family members, including siblings, as soon as appropriate.

🔺 Discharge Planning and Home Care

1. Evaluate readiness for discharge. Factors to assess include presence of the following:
   a. Stable respiratory status
   b. Adequate nutritional intake and growth
   c. Stable medication needs
   d. Medical treatment plan that is realistic for the home
      i. Parents or other caregivers can provide needed care.
      ii. Needed home equipment and monitoring are provided.
      iii. Parents have necessary social and/or financial supports.
      iv. Provision is made for respite or home nursing needs.
2. Provide discharge instruction for parents covering the following:
   a. Explanation of CLD (BPD)
   b. Monitoring for signs of respiratory distress and other medical problems
   c. Individualized feeding needs

  d. Well-baby needs
  e. Guidelines on when to call doctor
  f. Method of performing cardiopulmonary resuscitation
  g. Use of home equipment and monitoring
  h. Administration of medications and monitoring of their effects
  i. Infection prevention
  j. Importance of smoke-free environment
  k. Appropriate developmental activities
  l. Recognition of infant's stress and interaction cues
  m. Available community resources and supportive services (see Appendix L)
3. Provide follow-up to monitor ongoing respiratory, nutritional, and developmental needs; administer RSV prophylaxis; and address other specialized needs.
  a. Help parents make first follow-up appointments; provide written documentation of when appointments are scheduled.
  b. Make referral for in-home nursing visits or care based on needs of infant and family.
  c. Ensure that infant is referred to an early intervention program.

CLIENT OUTCOMES

1. Infant will have optimal lung functioning, with gas exchange and oxygenation sufficient for tissue perfusion, growth, and healing.
2. Infant will reach maximum potential for growth and development.
3. Parents will be competent in the care of their child.

REFERENCES

American Lung Association: *BPD: parent guide to bronchopulmonary dysplasia,* New York, 1987, The Association.

Barrington KJ, Finer NN: Treatment of bronchopulmonary dysplasia: a review, *Clin Perinatol* 25(1):177, 1998.

Committee on Infectious Disease and Committee on Fetus and Newborn: Prevention of respiratory syncytial virus infections: indications for the use of palivizumab and update on the use of RS-IGIV, *Pediatrics* 102:1211, 1998.

Davis GP et al: Evaluating "old" definitions for the "new" bronchopulmonary dysplasia, *J Pediatr* 140(5):555, 2002.

Ellsbury D et al: Variability in the use of supplemental oxygen for bronchopulmonary dysplasia, *J Pediatr* 140(2):247, 2002.

Farrell PA, Frasone JM: Bronchopulmonary dysplasia in the 1990's: a review for the pediatrician, *Curr Probl Pediatr* 27:133, 1997.

Howard G: Transition to home: discharge planning for the oxygen-dependent infant with bronchopulmonary dysplasia, *J Perinat Neonat Nurs* 6(2):85, 1992.

Mitchell S: Infants with bronchopulmonary dysplasia: a developmental perspective, *J Pediatr Nurs* 11(3):145, 1996.

Nievas F, Chernick V: Bronchopulmonary dysplasia (chronic lung disease of infancy): an update for the pediatrician, *Clin Pediatr (Phila)* 41(2):77, 2002.

Northway WH: Bronchopulmonary dysplasia: twenty-five years later, *Pediatrics* 89(5):969, 1992.

15

❖

Cleft Lip and Cleft Palate

❖

PATHOPHYSIOLOGY

Cleft lip and cleft palate are the outcomes of the failure of the soft tissue and/or bony structure to fuse during embryonic development. Cleft lip is a separation of the two sides of the lip. It may affect both sides of the lip as well as the bone and soft tissue of the alveolus. Cleft palate is a midline opening of the palate that results from the failure of the two sides to fuse during embryonic development. The exact cause is unknown, but in most cases it is thought to be multifactorial (a combination of environmental and genetic factors). Clefting is usually an isolated event but may occur as part of a syndrome. A good physical examination is very important to identify any other signs.

INCIDENCE

1. Cleft lip with or without cleft palate occurs in 1 in 700 live births.
2. Clefting is more common in Hispanic and Asian groups but may be seen in all ethnic groups.

CLINICAL MANIFESTATIONS

1. Visible unilateral or bilateral cleft lip (may be a complete cleft through the nares or an incomplete cleft of part of the lip)
2. Palpable and/or visible cleft palate
3. Cleft of the alveolus (gum line, may affect bone and soft tissue)
4. Nasal distortion
5. Feeding difficulties

COMPLICATIONS

1. Speech difficulties may include hypernasality, compensatory articulation.
2. Malocclusion may occur, with abnormal tooth eruption pattern and abnormal development of the way the mandible and maxilla meet.
3. Excessive dental decay is not unusual.
4. Chronic otitis media, secondary to eustachian tube dysfunction, may result in hearing loss.
5. Altered self-esteem and body image may occur.

LABORATORY AND DIAGNOSTIC TESTS

1. Multidisciplinary team evaluation to counsel parents on the condition and to prepare them for the surgical plan
2. Laboratory and diagnostic tests if other anomalies exist
3. Audiologic evaluation to determine if hearing loss is present and if the use of pressure-equalizing tubes is warranted

SURGICAL MANAGEMENT: CLEFT LIP AND CLEFT PALATE REPAIR

Cleft lip is repaired at 8 to 12 weeks of age if the baby has demonstrated good weight gain. The usual suggestion is that the baby weigh 10 pounds at the time of cleft lip repair. Cleft lip repair is usually done by a plastic surgeon specially trained in the repair of clefts. The plastic surgeon may choose among several methods for repair of the cleft lip, depending on his or her training and experience. Some surgeons choose the Millard repair, which results in a zigzag scar on the lip. Others choose to place the suture lines where the lines of the columella would have been if the clefting had not occurred. Still others choose among other types of repairs. The goal of all cleft lip surgery is the same, however—to achieve lip competence and to create the most natural-appearing lip.

Cleft palate repair is usually performed when the child is 9 to 12 months of age, weighing 18 to 20 pounds. Palatoplasty involves reconstruction of the palatal musculature with the goal of allowing normal speech development.

NURSING ASSESSMENT

1. Assess feeding to determine if the baby is receiving adequate caloric intake for growth and work with the family to develop the best feeding method for that baby. The following are broad guidelines for determining infant calorie* requirements:

   a. Newborns require about 100 kcal/kg/day to grow. (Multiply the weight in kilograms by 100 to obtain the daily calorie requirements. For example, 2.87 kg × 100 kcal/kg/day = 287 kcal/day. Standard infant formula and breast milk have 20 kcal/oz.

   b. Daily intake (number of ounces needed in a 24-hour period) is determined by first calculating total kilocalories needed per day (as indicated earlier), then dividing by 20. For example, 287 kcal/day divided by 20 kcal/oz = 14.35 oz/day.

   c. Most infants feed every 3 or 4 hours, which amounts to six to eight feedings per day. To determine the volume of each feeding, calculate the number of ounces per day and divide by the number of feedings. For example, 14.35 oz divided by 6 (feeding every 4 hours) is 2.4 oz or about 2½ oz every 4 hours. If the infant is fed more frequently—every 3 hours—divide the ounces per day by 8. In this example, feedings would be 8 oz or about 2 oz every 3 hours.

2. Assess parents' interactions with infant.
3. Assess respiratory status.
4. Assess for signs of infection.

NURSING DIAGNOSES

- Parenting, Risk for impaired
- Knowledge, Deficient (regarding clefting)
- Nutrition: less than body requirements, Imbalanced
- Pain (related to surgical procedure)

---

*Note: The term *calorie* is commonly used to mean the kilocalorie, the standard unit of measure for the energy value of food. Kilocalories (kcal) are used in formulas throughout this text.

NURSING INTERVENTIONS
Preoperative Care

1. Facilitate parents' positive adjustment to infant.
   a. Assist parents in dealing with their feelings about having a child with a visible difference. Encourage expression of feelings.
   b. Discuss treatment plan for child, answering parents' questions.
   c. Provide information that instills hope and positive feelings for infant (e.g., comment on infant's positive features, note positive aspects of parent-child interactions).
   d. Encourage parents to engage in caregiving activities.
   e. Model acceptance of and delight in the baby, congratulate family on birth of their baby.
   f. Arrange meeting with other parents who have undergone surgical and medical treatment experience.
2. Refer to cleft palate team. Local team listings may be found by contacting the American Cleft Palate–Craniofacial Association (ACPA/CPF), 104 South Estes Drive, Suite 204, Chapel Hill, NC 27514, (919) 933-9044, http://www.info@cleftline.org.
3. Provide information and resources to families regarding cause and treatment of clefting.
   a. Provide information on etiology of cleft lip and palate that explains when during embryonic development clefting occurred.
   b. Explain concept of team care and assist family with referral to local cleft palate team.
   c. Explain timing of surgical intervention.
   d. Educate parents on feeding techniques.
4. Maintain adequate nutritional intake to promote optimal growth.
   a. Babies with isolated cleft lips can usually feed at the breast. It is important to encourage and provide support to a new mother in breast-feeding her baby with a cleft lip.
   b. Babies with cleft palates have a difficult time breast-feeding. Most babies with cleft palates cannot generate enough suction at the breast to obtain the necessary

nutrition. Mothers of babies with cleft palates are encouraged to pump their breast milk and feed it to their babies via a special nipple and bottle.

c. A variety of bottle-nipple combinations may be used. No single method is best. What is best is what works for the family and allows the infant to finish feeding within 20 to 30 minutes, so that the feeding experience is satisfying for the family.

   i. Most babies with a cleft palate can be fed successfully using a soft nipple with an added crosscut (about ⅛ inch each way).

   ii. Another feeding system is the Pigeon nipple-bottle system. The Pigeon system has a squeeze bottle and a soft nipple with a valve, which prevents the baby from ingesting excess air during the feeding.

   iii. The Mead Johnson cleft lip/palate nurser can also be used. It is a compressible bottle.

d. Feeding instructions are as follows:

   i. Place the infant in an upright position (almost sitting).

   ii. Place the nipple in the baby's mouth, trying to position the nipple where there is more palatal tissue.

   iii. Use chin support with your pinky finger to improve the oral seal.

   iv. Assess the infant's response to feeding.

   v. If the baby arches and turns away, the flow of milk may be too rapid. The X cut may be too large. Use a nipple with a smaller X cut. If the baby does not get enough milk you may need to enlarge the X cut or compress the bottle.

   vi. If a squeeze bottle is used, parents are taught to compress the bottle in time with the infant's chewing motions and allow for rest periods when the infant rests. The parents should be taught the infant's cues.

   vii. Burp the baby about halfway through the feeding. The feeding should not last more than 20 to 30 minutes; otherwise the calories taken in will be expended by the feeding effort.

      viii. Monitor weight at least twice weekly until weight gain is at least an ounce per day.

5. Monitor respiratory status (respiratory effort, breath sounds, vital signs).

Preoperative Home Care

1. There is no special instruction for preoperative care. Bathe infant as usual.
2. Refer to institutional regimen for preoperative procedure, including when to stop feeding prior to surgery.

Postoperative Care
Cleft lip repair

1. Promote adequate nutritional fluid intake.
   a. Give breast milk/formula as tolerated (or per institution policy).
2. Promote healing and maintain integrity of child's incision site.
   a. Cleanse suture line gently if required by institutional protocol.
   b. Many surgeons use Dermabond skin adhesive to close outer layer of lip (skin). Antibiotic ointment and hydrogen peroxide should *not* be used in such cases, as they break down the Dermabond.

Cleft palate repair

1. Offer clear liquid (when recovered from anesthesia) with same feeding device used prior to surgery (or per surgeon's orders). Advance to blenderized or soft diet as tolerated.
2. Avoid placing objects in child's mouth (suction catheters, tongue depressors, straws, ice chips).
3. Remove toys that are hard or pointed.
4. Monitor for signs of infection or bleeding.

Both types of repair

1. Monitor infant's level of pain and need for nonpharmacologic interventions (e.g., holding, rocking) and/or pharmacologic interventions (see Appendix H). *Ensure that you have a current infant pain scale, either the FLACC (face, legs, activity, cry, consolability) or NPASS (Neonatal Pain, Agitation and Sedation Scale).*

🔺 Discharge Planning and Home Care

1. Instruct parents about care of surgical site.
2. Instruct parents about feeding techniques.
3. Instruct parents about signs of infection.
4. Instruct parents on how to position child.
5. Encourage parents to discuss feelings and concerns about caring for baby at home as well as about long-term care.
6. Reinforce to parents importance of long-term team care for early treatment of problems, which may include abnormalities in speech, language, hearing, dentition, and occlusion.
7. Inform parents of agencies and support groups for children with cleft lip and/or palate.

CLIENT OUTCOMES

1. Infant's or child's incision will heal properly without complications.
2. Infant or child will have appropriate weight gain.
3. Feeding will be pleasurable experience for infant and parent.
4. Parents will demonstrate correct feeding techniques.
5. Parents will demonstrate acceptance of infant or child.

REFERENCES

Andrews-Casal M et al: Cleft lip with or without cleft palate: effect of family history on reproductive planning, surgical timing, and parental stress, *Cleft Palate Craniofac J* 35(1):52, 1998.

Golden AS: Cleft lip and cleft palate. In Hoekelman RA et al, editors: *Primary pediatric care,* ed 3, St Louis, 1997, Mosby.

Grow JL, Lehman JA: A local perspective on the initial management of children with cleft lip and palate by primary care physicians, *Cleft Palate Craniofac J* 39(5):535, 2002.

Heidbuchel KL et al: Dental maturity in children with a complete bilateral cleft lip and palate, *Cleft Palate Craniofac J* 39(5):509, 2002.

Nelson WE et al: *Nelson textbook of pediatrics,* ed 15, Philadelphia, 1996, WB Saunders.

Resnick JI, Zarem HA: Diseases and injuries of the oral region. In Burg FD et al, editors: *Gellis and Kagan's current pediatric therapy,* ed 16, Philadelphia, 1999, WB Saunders.

Savage HE: An early intervention guide to infants born with clefts. Infant-toddler intervention, *Transdisciplinary J* 7(4):271, 1997.

Smahel Z et al: Changes in craniofacial development due to modifications of the treatment of unilateral cleft lip and palate, *Cleft Palate Craniofac J* 35(3):240, 1998.

Wong DL et al: *Wong's essentials of pediatric nursing,* ed 6, St Louis, 2001, Mosby.

16

❖

Coarctation of the Aorta

❖

PATHOPHYSIOLOGY

Coarctation of the aorta is a localized narrowing of the aortic lumen. Narrowing increases pressures in the ascending aorta, which results in higher pressures to the coronary arteries and vessels that arise from the aortic arch. There are three basic types of coarctation: (1) juxtaductal—narrowing at the level of the ductus arteriosus; (2) preductal—narrowing proximal to the ductus arteriosus; and (3) postductal—narrowing distal to the ductus arteriosus. Coarctation of the aorta is associated with several other defects, including anomalies of the left side of the heart, bicuspid aortic valve defect, and ventricular septal defect. Two thirds of children with this defect are asymptomatic. Severe cases can become apparent in infancy; many cases are discovered during a physical examination when hypertension of the upper extremity is noted. Prognosis is excellent with surgical intervention.

INCIDENCE

1. Coarctation of the aorta accounts for 10% of congenital cardiac defects.
2. Electrocardiogram (ECG) is normal in 50% of cases.

CLINICAL MANIFESTATIONS
Infants

Most infants are asymptomatic; initially, symptoms may be associated with severe sudden onset of congestive heart failure.

Children

1. Absent or diminished lower-extremity pulses
2. Hypertension of upper extremities, with bounding pulses
3. Systolic or systolic and diastolic murmurs
4. Leg muscle cramps during exercise (tissue anoxia)
5. Headache
6. Epistaxis
7. Cool lower extremities

COMPLICATIONS

1. Hypertension
2. Cerebrovascular accident
3. Ruptured aorta
4. Aortic aneurysm
5. Bacterial endocarditis

LABORATORY AND DIAGNOSTIC TESTS

1. ECG—normal or may reveal left ventricular hypertrophy and ST- and T-wave abnormalities
2. Chest radiographic study—to determine cardiac size or detect pulmonary venous congestion (in infants, consistent with clinical findings; in older individuals, normal)
3. Cardiac catheterization—to diagnose associated defects and abnormal pressure gradient
4. Echocardiogram—to examine size, shape, and motion of heart structures; may reveal reduced ejection fraction
5. Preoperative laboratory data
   a. Complete blood count, urinalysis, serum glucose level, blood urea nitrogen level
   b. Baseline electrolyte levels—sodium, potassium, chloride, carbon dioxide
   c. Blood coagulation studies—prothrombin time, partial thromboplastin time, platelet count

SURGICAL MANAGEMENT: COARCTECTOMY

Repair of a coarctation may be accomplished through several methods, depending on the age of the child and the degree of constriction. Elective repair in early childhood is generally preferred; infants with congestive heart failure who do not respond to medical treatment have surgical correction in infancy.

Repair is designed to reduce risks of restenosis. The left subclavian artery may be ligated distally and sutured over an opening in the aorta to provide for a patch enlargement of the aorta. A subclavian flap aortoplasty reduces the number of cases of restenosis because the natural tissue will grow with the child, which causes less tension than an end-to-end anastomosis. By 4 to 8 years of age the aorta is nearly adult size, and hypertension is still reversible. Many surgeons prefer this age for repair; other physicians believe that performing the procedure in 1- to 4-year-olds has results that are just as good and leads to fewer later complications. Postoperative complications increase if surgery is delayed until the child is older than 8 to 10 years.

The area of coarctation is patched with Teflon material, with some natural material left to grow with the child. Some surgeons excise the area of coarctation, but that procedure may lead to repeat coarctation. For both age groups entry to the thoracic cavity is performed through a left posterolateral thoracotomy incision. Bypass is not necessary, although adequate flow to the lower extremities must be maintained through collateral circulation, hypothermia, a temporary shunt, grafts connecting the ascending and descending aorta, or a partial cardiopulmonary bypass.

Complications

1. Chylothorax as a result of injury to thoracic duct or lymphatics
2. Congestive heart failure
3. Hemothorax caused by bleeding from the collateral network or aortic anastomosis
4. Repeat coarctation (5% to 10%) in children who underwent surgical repair as infants
5. Vomiting resulting from increased circulation to the gastrointestinal tract
6. Increased incidence of cardiovascular disease 11 to 25 years after surgery
7. Less than 5% mortality rate in children with isolated coarctation; increased risk with coexisting cardiac defects

Antihypertensive Medications

1. Sodium nitroprusside (Nipride)—used to treat postoperative hypertension; acts on the smooth muscle to produce peripheral vasodilation, causing decreased arterial pressures
2. Propranolol (Inderal)—used to treat postoperative hypertension; acts as a beta-blocker of cardiac and bronchial adrenoreceptors, resulting in decreasing heart rate and myocardial irritability and potentiating contraction and conduction pathway
3. Reserpine—used to treat postoperative hypertension; acts as a sympathetic inhibitor, resulting in decreased blood pressure and cardiac output
4. Captopril (Capoten)—used to treat postoperative hypertension; works on the renin-angiotensin system to reduce afterload

NURSING ASSESSMENT

1. See the Cardiovascular Assessment section in Appendix A.
2. Assess for paradoxical hypertension.
3. Perform frequent assessment for bowel sounds, abdominal tenderness, distention, and vomiting; notify physician immediately if any changes occur.

NURSING DIAGNOSES

- Activity intolerance
- Cardiac output, Decreased
- Injury, Risk for
- Fluid volume, Risk for imbalanced
- Gas exchange, Impaired
- Family processes, Interrupted
- Knowledge, Deficient

NURSING INTERVENTIONS
Preoperative Care

1. Monitor infant's or child's cardiac status.
   a. Color of mucous membranes and nail beds
   b. Quality and intensity of peripheral pulses

    c. Capillary refill time

    d. Temperatures of extremities

    e. Apical pulse

    f. Blood pressure

    g. Respiratory rate

2. Assist child in understanding by use of age-appropriate terminology (see Appendix J).

3. Provide information and assist parents in understanding child's condition.

Postoperative Care

1. Monitor infant's or child's cardiac status every hour for first 24 to 48 hours, then every 2 to 4 hours.

    a. Apical pulse, respiratory rate, temperature

    b. Arterial blood pressure—hypertension often present initially (no blood pressure present in left arm if subclavian artery used for surgery)

    c. Capillary refill time

    d. Cardiac arrhythmias

2. Monitor for signs and symptoms of hemorrhage.

    a. Measure chest tube output every hour—more than 3 to 5 ml indicates problems.

    b. Assess for clot formation in chest tube (increased output of blood followed by abrupt decrease).

    c. Assess bowel sounds and monitor for abdominal distention.

    d. Assess for bleeding from other sites (e.g., nose, mouth, gastrointestinal tract).

    e. Strictly record input and output (refer to institutional procedure manual).

3. Monitor infant's or child's hydration status.

    a. Dry mucous membranes

    b. Bulging or depressed fontanelles

    c. Decreased tearing, dry mouth

    d. Poor skin turgor

    e. Specific gravity (urine will be concentrated immediately after surgery)

    f. Daily weight

    g. Intake and output

    h. Fluids—intravenous at 50% to 75% of maintenance fluids first 24 hours postoperatively

4. Promote optimal respiratory status.
   a. Have child turn, cough, and deep breathe.
   b. Perform chest physiotherapy.
   c. Humidify air.
   d. Monitor for chylothorax (assess breath sounds; note chest tube drainage).
   e. Keep thoracotomy tray at bedside for emergency use.
   f. Monitor chest tube for patency to prevent pneumothorax; keep two chest tube clamps at bedside to prevent pneumothorax if tubing separates.

5. Monitor child's response to medications and blood products.
   a. See the Antihypertensive Medications section in this chapter.
   b. Assist with collection of laboratory data.

6. Use no cuff pressure or arterial punctures in left arm if left subclavian flap was performed, because only collateral vessels are providing arterial circulation.

7. Resume oral feedings slowly; monitor abdominal status.

8. Control hypertension through medications and anxiety relief measures.

9. Relieve postoperative pain: pain adds stress to suture lines (see Appendix H).

10. Provide age-appropriate diversional activities (see the relevant section in Appendix B).

11. Provide age-appropriate explanations before treatments and painful procedures (see the Preparation for Procedures and Surgery section in Appendix J).

🔺 Discharge Planning and Home Care

Stress importance of follow-up to screen for residual or premature cardiovascular problems, including development of calcific aortic stenosis. Antibiotic prophylaxis may be required during infectious periods.

CLIENT OUTCOMES

1. Child will be free of postoperative complications.
2. Child will demonstrate sense of mastery of the surgical experience as evidenced by expression of feelings and resumption of normal activity level.
3. Child will participate in physical activities appropriate for age.

REFERENCES

Gersony W: Coarctation of the aorta, *Hosp Med* 27(5):53, 1991.

Hockenberry M: *Wong's nursing care of infants and children,* ed 7, St Louis, 2003, Mosby.

McConnaha M: Surgery for congenital heart defects: a different world, *Semin Perioper Nurs* 6(3):170, 1997.

Park M: *Pediatric cardiology for practitioners,* ed 4, St Louis, 2002, Mosby.

Wood MK: Acyanotic cardiac lesions with normal pulmonary blood flow, *Neonatal Netw* 17(3):5, 1998.

17

❖

Congestive Heart Failure

❖

PATHOPHYSIOLOGY

Congestive heart failure (CHF) occurs when the heart cannot pump the blood returning to the right side of the heart or provide adequate circulation to meet the needs of organs and tissues in the body. The components of CHF include preload and circulating volume, afterload, and contractility. Causes include the following:

1. High-output state, usually related to congenital heart diseases in which there is increased pulmonary blood flow returning to the right side of the heart and, subsequently, lungs; common defects producing this volume overload are patent ductus arteriosus and ventricular septal defect.

2. Low-output state, related to (1) congenital heart diseases in which there are left-side heart obstructions causing the heart to pump harder to bypass the restrictive area, such as coarctation of the aorta or aortic valve stenosis, (2) a primary heart muscle disease, such as the cardiomyopathies, or (3) rhythm disturbances, either tachycardia or bradycardia dysrhythmias.

If the heart fails for any reason and cardiac output is not sufficient to meet the metabolic needs of the body, the sympathetic nervous system responds by trying to increase circulating blood volume by diverting blood from nonessential organs. This decreases renal blood flow, activates the renin-angiotensin-aldosterone mechanism, and increases sodium and water retention. Catecholamine release with decreased cardiac output causes increased heart rate, increased vascular tone, and sweating. These initial compensatory mechanisms for maintaining cardiac output (increased circulating blood volume, increased heart rate, and vascular tone) eventually lead to clinical manifestations of CHF.

INCIDENCE

1. Ninety percent of infants with congenital heart defects develop CHF within the first year of life.
2. The majority of affected infants manifest symptoms within the first few months of life.

CLINICAL MANIFESTATIONS

1. Tachycardia
2. Cardiomegaly
3. Increased respiratory effort
4. Tachypnea
5. Hepatomegaly
6. Edema
7. Diaphoresis
8. Feeding difficulty and poor weight gain
9. Irritability

COMPLICATIONS

Low cardiac output syndrome refractory to medications may develop.

LABORATORY AND DIAGNOSTIC TESTS

Diagnosis is made on the basis of physical examination revealing signs and symptoms previously noted. The following can assist in further evaluation:

1. Electrocardiogram (ECG)—for diagnosis of tachycardia or bradycardia dysrhythmias (a 12-lead ECG may show ventricular hypertrophy)
2. Chest radiographic study—heart will be enlarged and pulmonary infiltrates will be present
3. Echocardiogram
4. Cardiac catheterization

MEDICAL MANAGEMENT

The initial management of CHF is accomplished by the use of pharmacologic agents that act to improve the function of the heart muscle and/or reduce the workload on the heart. Digitalis is given to increase cardiac output by slowing conduction through the atrioventricular node to make each contraction stronger. Diuretics decrease preload volume because their actions result in decreased extracellular fluid volume. Venous, arterial, and mixed dilators may be given to decrease preload volume by reducing systemic or pulmonary vascular resistance. Fluids are usually restricted to two thirds of maintenance levels, and attention is given to nutrition and rest. Medical management continues with the plan for interventional cardiac catheterization or surgical intervention if indicated.

NURSING ASSESSMENT

1. See the Cardiovascular Assessment and Respiratory Assessment sections in Appendix A.
2. Assess activity level.
3. Assess extremities for edema.
4. Assess feeding pattern and weight gain history.
5. Assess family coping patterns.

NURSING DIAGNOSES

- Cardiac output, Decreased
- Breathing pattern, Ineffective
- Activity intolerance
- Fluid volume, Excess
- Nutrition: less than body requirements, Imbalanced
- Knowledge, Deficient
- Family processes, Interrupted

NURSING INTERVENTIONS

1. Promote cardiac output.
   a. Continue cardiovascular assessments, including evaluation of vital signs, pulses, color, capillary refill, and lung sounds.
   b. Administer medications and assess and record effects.
2. Promote oxygenation and ventilation.
   a. Maintain patent airway and assess effect of oxygen if provided.

    b. Elevate head of bed or place infant in infant seat to promote systemic venous return.

3. Provide rest and comfort measures.
   a. Maintain quiet environment with quick response to crying of infant or child.
   b. Swaddle infants.
   c. Provide neutral thermal environment, maintaining constant temperature for least oxygen consumption.
   d. Schedule activities to provide extended rest periods.
4. Promote and maintain child's fluid and electrolyte balance.
   a. Assess intake and output.
   b. Assess edema.
   c. Measure and record child's weight daily.
   d. Restrict fluids, usually to two thirds of maintenance fluid levels.
   e. Follow potassium levels closely if child is on diuretics.
5. Promote child's nutritional status.
   a. Assess and record infant's tolerance of and response to feedings.
   b. Provide small, frequent feedings for conservation of energy.
   c. Collaborate with nutrition services to provide optimal diet for maximal calories and minimal fluids.
6. Assist family in understanding, accepting, and working through emotions of having a child a with chronic condition.

🔺 Discharge Planning and Home Care

1. Educate on specific condition.
2. Provide specific instructions about medications and adverse effects.
3. Although caregivers of infants with chronic CHF are usually quite skilled in assessing for signs and symptoms of CHF, reinforce as necessary.
4. Instruct in feeding techniques and nutritional requirements.
5. Refer as indicated to infant stimulation programs or parent support groups.

CLIENT OUTCOMES

1. Child will have adequate cardiac output.
2. Child will have normal growth and development.
3. Caregivers will demonstrate ability to handle all facets of infant's home care.

REFERENCES

James SR et al: *Nursing care of children: principles and practice,* Philadelphia, 2002, WB Saunders.

Kay JD et al: Congestive heart failure in pediatric patients, *Am Heart J* 142(5):923, 2001.

Merle C: Nursing considerations of the neonate with congenital heart disease, *Clin Perinatol* 28(1):223, 2001.

Suddaby EC: Contemporary thinking for congenital heart disease, *Pediatr Nurs* 27(3):233, 2001.

18

◆

Croup

◆

PATHOPHYSIOLOGY

Croup, or acute laryngotracheobronchitis, is a viral infection that affects the larynx and the trachea. Subglottic edema with upper respiratory tract obstruction results, accompanied by thick secretions. Children are susceptible to airway obstruction because the diameter of the subglottic area is narrow. Croup can be caused by any virus associated with upper respiratory tract infection. The most common causative agents include parainfluenza virus types 1, 2, and 3; less frequent causes include respiratory syncytial virus and influenza virus types A and B. Onset occurs 1 to 2 days after the symptoms of upper respiratory tract infection begin. Fever may or may not be present.

Spasmodic croup is a sudden attack of croup, which usually occurs during the night and may be associated with an upper respiratory tract infection, fever, or allergies. This type of attack is recurrent in nature.

INCIDENCE

1. Incidence is seasonal—higher in late fall and early winter.
2. Age range of occurrence is 6 months to 6 years; peak age of onset is 2 years.
3. Although the condition is rare, significant airway obstruction may develop, and airway support may be needed.

CLINICAL MANIFESTATIONS
Initial Phase

1. Cold that lasts for 1 to 2 days
2. Rhinorrhea or nasal congestion

3. Persistent barking cough that worsens
4. Hoarse cry
5. Stridor (progression of stridor is an indicator of the severity of the disease)

Acute Phase

1. Increased respiratory rate
2. High-pitched inspiratory stridor
3. Cough
4. Retractions at rest, nasal flaring
5. Signs of respiratory failure (agitation, restlessness, listlessness, decrease in stridor and retractions without clinical improvement, and cyanosis)

COMPLICATIONS

Potential respiratory failure resulting from airway obstruction is the main complication of croup.

LABORATORY AND DIAGNOSTIC TESTS

1. Pulse oximetry for evaluation of hypoxia
2. Throat specimen culture
3. Posteroanterior and lateral neck radiographic study—steeple sign; also to rule out epiglottitis and foreign bodies
4. Chest radiographic study
5. Complete blood count—normal

MEDICAL MANAGEMENT

Mildly ill children who are well hydrated, have minimal stridor or retractions, and have parents who can recognize changes in condition and transport the child to a medical facility may be managed as outpatients.

When a child with suspected croup is presented at the hospital, supplemental humidified oxygen is given as indicated by the child's appearance and by pulse oximetry values and vital signs. The child can be treated with bronchodilators, usually racemic epinephrine if humidification alone is ineffective.

The use of corticosteroids is controversial. In controlled studies, children who received corticosteroids needed endotracheal intubation less frequently, and their stridor more quickly resolved. Antibiotics are administered if secondary bacterial infection is suspected.

The treatment of croup is mostly supportive, but if the child does not respond, use of an artificial airway may be indicated to support the child until the airway inflammation subsides. Intravenous fluid administration may also be indicated, depending on the child's hydration status.

NURSING ASSESSMENT

1. See the Respiratory Assessment section in Appendix A.
2. Assess oxygenation status—pulse oximetry, signs of increased respiratory distress.
3. Assess hydration status.
4. Assess child and parent anxiety level.

NURSING DIAGNOSES

- Breathing pattern, Ineffective
- Airway clearance, Ineffective
- Fluid volume, Deficient
- Anxiety

NURSING INTERVENTIONS

1. Provide humidification via mask; oxygen is administered if pulse oximetry reading is less than 92%.
2. Allow child to maintain position of comfort.
3. Monitor respiratory status (vital signs—use of accessory muscles, position, pulse oximetry values, and color).
4. Report signs of increased respiratory distress such as increased respiratory rate, labored breathing, wheezing, stridor, intercostal retractions, and circumoral cyanosis.
5. Monitor and observe effects of oxygen therapy with nebulized racemic epinephrine, mist tent with humidified oxygen.
6. Encourage oral feedings.
7. Monitor action and side effects of medications.
   a. Bronchodilators (i.e., racemic epinephrine)
   b. Corticosteroids—for antiinflammatory properties
   c. Antibiotics—for treatment of secondary bacterial infection if present

8. Provide age-appropriate quiet play and recreational activities (see the relevant section in Appendix B).
9. Provide for child's developmental needs during hospitalization.
   a. Encourage contact with siblings and parents.
   b. Incorporate home routines into hospital stay (e.g., feeding practices, night routine).
10. Provide emotional and other support to family.
    a. Encourage verbalization of concerns.
    b. Provide for physical comforts (e.g., place to sleep and bathe).
    c. Provide explanations before performing procedures.

Discharge Planning and Home Care

Instruct parents about home management.

1. Possible worsening of signs of croup at night or when child sleeps
2. Use of humidifiers (including use of shower)
3. Signs of secondary infection (increased temperature, signs of cold or respiratory infection)
4. Administration of medications (see Medical Management section in this chapter)
5. Infection control
   a. Avoid large groups of people.
   b. Avoid cold temperatures.
6. Need to call or return for additional care if condition is worsening

CLIENT OUTCOMES

1. Child will return to normal respiratory function.
2. Child will be hydrated adequately.
3. Child and/or family will demonstrate understanding of home care and follow-up.

REFERENCES

Brown JC: The management of croup, *Br Med Bull* 61:189, 2002.

Coakley-Maller C, Shea M: Respiratory infections in children: preparing for the fall and winter, *Adv Nurse Pract* 5(9):20, 1997.

Wong DL, Hess CS: *Wong and Whaley's clinical manual of pediatric nursing,* ed 5, St Louis, 2000, Mosby.

Wright RB et al: New approaches to respiratory infections in children: bronchiolitis and croup, *Emerg Med Clin North Am* 20(1):93, 2002.

19

◆

Cystic Fibrosis

◆

PATHOPHYSIOLOGY

Cystic fibrosis (CF) is inherited as an autosomal-recessive trait due to a mutation of the CF gene on chromosome 7. The disorder affects the exocrine glands, causing the production of viscous mucus leading to obstruction of the small passageways of the bronchi, the small intestine, and the pancreatic and bile ducts. The effects of this biochemical defect on the involved organs are as follows:

1. Lungs
   a. Bronchial and bronchiolar obstruction from excessive pooling of secretions causes generalized hyperinflation and atelectasis.
   b. Pooled mucous secretions increase the susceptibility to bacterial infections (*Pseudomonas aeruginosa* and *Staphylococcus aureus* are the predominant organisms found in sputum and lungs. *Burkholderia cepacia* is associated with later-life infection in the CF lung, causing devastating infection, It is highly transmissible from the infected person with CF to others with CF; those with known infection should not have contact with an uninfected individual with CF.)
   c. Altered oxygen and carbon dioxide exchange can cause varying degrees of hypoxia, hypercapnia, and acidosis.
   d. Fibrotic lung changes take place, and, in severe cases, pulmonary hypertension and cor pulmonale can occur.
2. Pancreas
   a. Degeneration and fibrosis of acini occur.

    b. Secretion of pancreatic enzymes is inhibited, which causes impaired absorption of fats, proteins, and, to a limited degree, carbohydrates.

3. Small intestine—absence of pancreatic enzymes (trypsin, amylase, lipase) causes impaired absorption of fats and proteins, which results in steatorrhea and azotorrhea.
4. Liver—biliary obstruction, fibrosis
5. Skeleton
   a. Growth and onset of puberty are retarded.
   b. Retardation of skeletal maturation results in delayed bone aging and shortness of stature (38% to 42% of children with CF).
6. Reproductive system
   a. Female—late menses; possible infertility because of thickness of cervical mucus
   b. Male—vas deferens often absent; sterility but not impotency

INCIDENCE

1. CF affects 1 in 3200 white infants each year.
2. It affects 1 in 15,000 African American infants each year.
3. It rarely affects infants of Asian descent (1 in 31,000).
4. Odds are one in four (25%) that each subsequent pregnancy after birth of child with CF will result in a child with CF.
5. CF affects males and females equally.
6. Newborn screening testing for CF could lead to early treatment and improved outcomes for the child with CF but has not been universally accepted at present.
7. Symptoms vary greatly, resulting in variable life span—95% survival rate to age 16 years, with a median survival of about 32 years.
8. Length and quality of life have greatly increased in recent years, but disease is ultimately terminal.

CLINICAL MANIFESTATIONS

1. Dry, nonproductive cough initially, changing to loose and productive

2. Viscous sputum, increasing in amount, with yellow-gray color normally and greenish color during infection
3. Wheezy respirations, moist crackles
4. Cyanosis (late sign)
5. Clubbed fingers and toes
6. Increased anteroposterior diameter of chest
7. Steatorrhea
8. Bulky, loose, foul-smelling stools
9. Distended abdomen
10. Thin extremities
11. Failure to thrive (below norms for height and weight despite large food intake)
12. Meconium ileus (infants)
13. Profuse sweating in warm temperature
14. Salty-tasting skin
15. Excessive loss of sodium and chloride

COMPLICATIONS

1. Pulmonary: emphysema, pneumothorax, pneumonia, bronchiectasis, hemoptysis, cor pulmonale, respiratory failure
2. Gastrointestinal: cirrhosis, portal hypertension, esophageal varices, fecal impactions, enlarged spleen, intussusception, cholelithiasis, pancreatitis, rectal prolapse
3. Endocrine: CF-related diabetes mellitus, poor bone mineralization leading to osteopenia and osteoporosis, poor growth, heat prostration

LABORATORY AND DIAGNOSTIC TESTS

1. Sweat test—to measure concentration of sodium and chloride in sweat; most definitive diagnostic test; not reliable for newborns younger than 1 month old (two positive results on sweat tests are diagnostic; value higher than 60 mEq/L represents positive result for CF)
2. Pulmonary function testing—used to assess respiratory status and severity of condition, and to determine therapy
3. Genetic blood testing for CF marker
4. Chest radiographic study—for evaluation of pulmonary complications

MEDICAL MANAGEMENT

The child with symptoms of CF is hospitalized for the diagnostic workup, initiation of treatment, clearing of any respiratory tract infection symptoms, and education of the child and family. The goal of this hospitalization is to stabilize the child's condition so that care can be managed for long periods at home.

Antibiotics are given based on the suspected organisms, sensitivity to antibiotics, severity of infection, and child's response to therapy. The course of therapy is usually at least 14 days. After the initial admission, when respiratory tract infections are not responsive to intensive home treatment measures or oral antibiotic therapy, the child may either be readmitted for intravenous (IV) antibiotic therapy or have home IV antibiotic therapy.

Pulmonary toilet includes adequate hydration to loosen secretions and chest percussion and postural drainage to clear mucus from the small airways. Breathing exercises and devices designed to loosen and mobilize pulmonary secretions are also used. Aerosol generators may be used to administer normal saline, bronchodilators (such as albuterol or other β-agonist drugs), antibiotics, and sometimes mucolytics. Dornase alfa has been used to reduce the viscosity of sputum and improve lung function in some children with CF. Some bronchodilators are administered through a metered-dose inhaler with or without a spacer. Intermittent positive pressure breathing does not improve drug delivery and may aggravate the pulmonary status.

Pancreatic enzyme supplements are given with meals and snacks; dosages are individualized for the child and generally increase as the child gets older. Supplements of fat-soluble vitamins (A, D, and E) are needed in greater than the normal dosage because they are not well absorbed. Vitamin K supplementation may be needed by the infant or if there is hemoptysis or surgery. Diet is modified to increase the number of calories provided (up to 150% more than normal needs based on age, weight, and activity). High levels of protein and normal amounts of fat (about 30%) should be included in the child's diet.

Lung or heart-lung transplantation may be an option for end-stage CF lung disease. The waiting period for donor organs is between 6 months and 2 years; it is increasing at all transplant centers. Referral criteria include progressive respiratory function impairment with severe hypoxemia and hypercarbia, increasing functional impairment, major life-threatening pulmonary complications, and antibiotic resistance of bacteria infecting the lungs. Individual transplant centers may have additional criteria or restrictions. The current 5-year survival rate for lung transplant in individuals with CF is 48%. The child with CF who undergoes transplantation is at risk for the same complications as other child transplant recipients (effects of immunosuppression, infection, acute rejection, and bronchiolitis obliterans). In addition, due to CF, such a child may have malabsorption of the immunosuppressive agents.

NURSING ASSESSMENT

1. See the Respiratory Assessment and Gastrointestinal Assessment sections in Appendix A.
2. Assess amount of sputum and its color and characteristics.
3. Assess activity level.
4. Assess height and weight for age of child.

NURSING DIAGNOSES

- Airway clearance, Ineffective
- Activity intolerance, Risk for
- Nutrition: less than body requirements, Imbalanced
- Infection, Risk for
- Coping, Compromised family
- Growth and development, Delayed

NURSING INTERVENTIONS

1. Monitor respiratory status and report any significant changes (in respiratory rate, presence of intercostal retractions, presence of cyanosis, and color and amount of sputum).
2. Monitor effects of aerosolized treatment (performed before postural drainage).
3. Administer and evaluate effects of postural drainage and percussion.
4. Administer and monitor side effects and actions of medications.
   a. Antibiotics
   b. Pancreatic enzymes

    c. Fat-soluble vitamins

    d. Bronchodilators

5. Teach and supervise breathing exercises (exhalation, inhalation, and coughing), although these are not a substitute for percussion and postural drainage.

6. Encourage physical activity as condition permits.

7. Obtain baseline information about dietary habits (food preferences and dislikes, eating attitudes, developmental abilities).

8. Monitor and record characteristics of stool (color, consistency, size, frequency).

9. Promote nutritional status.

    a. Administer high-protein, high-calorie, normal-fat diet.

    b. Administer supplemental fat-soluble vitamins.

    c. Administer pancreatic enzymes before meals and snacks.

    d. Assess need for supplemental protein formula.

10. Observe for and report signs of complications (see the Complications section in this chapter).

11. Provide emotional support to child and parents during hospitalization.

12. Provide guidance related to independence, self-care, sexuality, and educational planning as adolescent undergoes transition to adulthood.

Discharge Planning and Home Care

1. Instruct parents and child about techniques of home management.

    a. Dietary needs

    b. Postural drainage and percussion

    c. Aerosol treatments

    d. Breathing exercises

    e. Administration of medications

    f. Avoidance of exposure to respiratory tract infections

    g. Management of constipation or diarrhea

2. Monitor family's compliance with home management.

    a. Monitor child's clinical course.

    b. Monitor frequency of hospital admissions.

    c. Assess family's level of knowledge.

3. Assist family in contacting support systems for financial, psychologic, and medical assistance (e.g., Cystic Fibrosis Foundation).
4. Provide genetic counseling.
5. Immunize annually against influenza.

CLIENT OUTCOMES

1. Child's ability to clear airway will improve.
2. Child will gain weight.
3. Parents will administer home care regimen and provide for medical follow-up.

REFERENCES

Davis PB: Cystic fibrosis, *Pediatr Rev* 22(8):257, 2001.

Hamutcu R, Woo MS: Advanced cystic fibrosis lung disease in children, *Curr Opin Pulm Med* 7(6):448, 2001.

Moran A: Endocrine complications of cystic fibrosis, *Adolesc Med* 13(1):145, 2002.

Nasr SZ: Cystic fibrosis in adolescents and young adults, *Adolesc Med* 11(3):589, 2000.

Robinson RF, Nahata MC: Prevention and treatment of osteoporosis in the cystic fibrosis population, *J Pediatr Health Care* 15(6):308, 2001.

Rosenstein BJ, Cutting GR: The diagnosis of cystic fibrosis: a consensus statement, *J Pediatr* 132(4):589, 1998.

Yankaskas JR, Mallory GB, the Consensus Committee: Lung transplantation in cystic fibrosis: consensus conference statement, *Chest* 113(1):217, 1998.

Young SS et al: Cystic fibrosis screening in newborns: results from existing programs, *Curr Opin Pulm Med* 7(6):427, 2001.

20

❖

Cytomegaloviral Infection

❖

PATHOPHYSIOLOGY

Cytomegalovirus (CMV) is the leading cause of congenital viral infections in North America. A number of related strains of CMV exist. The virus is a member of the herpes family. CMV is probably transmitted through direct person-to-person contact with body fluids or tissues, including urine, blood, saliva, cervical secretions, semen, and breast milk. The period of incubation is unknown. The following are estimated incubation periods: after delivery—3 to 12 weeks; after transfusion—3 to 12 weeks; after transplantation—4 weeks to 4 months. The urine often contains CMV months to years after infection. The virus can remain dormant in individuals and be reactivated. Currently, no immunizations exist to prevent infection with the virus.

Three types of CMV infection exist:

1. Congenital—acquired transplacentally in utero. Approximately 40% of infants born to women experiencing a primary (first) CMV illness during pregnancy will be infected. The most severe form of this infection is cytomegalic inclusion disease.

2. Acute acquired—acquired anytime during or after birth through adulthood. Symptoms resemble those of mononucleosis (malaise, fever, pharyngitis, splenomegaly, petechial rash, respiratory symptoms). Infection is not without sequelae, especially in young children, and can result from transfusions.

3. Generalized systemic disease—occurs in individuals who are immunosuppressed, especially if they have undergone organ transplantation. Symptoms include

117

pneumonitis, hepatitis, and leukopenia, which can occasionally be fatal. Previous infection does not produce immunity and may result in reactivation of the virus.

INCIDENCE

1. Among live births, 0.5% to 3% of infants have congenital infection.
2. Premature infants are affected more often than full-term infants.
3. Ten percent of infected infants are symptomatic at birth; by 2 years of age another 10% develop serious sequelae (e.g., deafness or ocular abnormalities).
4. Twenty-five percent of severely infected infants die by 3 months of age; the remaining 60% to 75% will have some form of intellectual impairment or developmental delays. Approximately 10% will be normal in late childhood.
5. Prevalence of CMV infection is approximately 80% in children younger than 2 years of age who attend child care centers.
6. Sixty percent of adult women are seropositive.
7. Incidence is higher in lower socioeconomic groups.
8. Approximately 2% to 2.5% of susceptible women acquire infection during pregnancy.

CLINICAL MANIFESTATIONS

In the newborn period, an infant infected with CMV is usually asymptomatic. Onset of symptoms from congenitally acquired infection can occur from immediately after birth to as late as 12 weeks after birth.

There are no predictable indicators, but the following symptoms are common:

1. Petechiae and ecchymoses
2. Hepatosplenomegaly
3. Neonatal jaundice; direct hyperbilirubinemia
4. Microcephaly with periventricular calcifications
5. Intrauterine growth retardation
6. Prematurity
7. Small size for gestational age

Other symptoms can occur in the newborn or older child:
1. Purpura
2. Hearing loss
3. Chorioretinitis; blindness
4. Fever
5. Pneumonia
6. Tachypnea and dyspnea
7. Brain damage

COMPLICATIONS
1. Variable hearing loss
2. Lower intelligence quotient
3. Visual impairment
4. Microcephaly
5. Sensorineural handicaps

LABORATORY AND DIAGNOSTIC TESTS
1. Viral cultures of urine, pharyngeal secretions, and peripheral leukocytes
2. Polymerase chain reaction and DNA hybridization testing—to detect CMV in urine, amniotic fluid, fetal blood
3. Microscopic examination of urinary sediment, body fluids, and tissues—to detect virus in large quantities (examining urine for intranuclear inclusions is not helpful; verification of congenital infection must be accomplished within first 3 weeks of life)
4. Toxoplasmosis, other infections, rubella, CMV infection, and herpes (TORCH) screen—used to assess presence of other viruses
5. Serologic tests
   a. Immunoglobulin G (IgG) and immunoglobulin M (IgM) antibody titers (elevated IgM level indicates exposure to virus; elevated neonatal IgG level indicates prenatally acquired infection; negative maternal IgG result and positive neonatal IgG result indicate postnatal acquisition)
   b. Rheumatoid factor assay (result is positive in 35% to 45% of cases)

6. Radiologic studies—skull radiographic studies or computed tomographic scans of head used to reveal intracranial calcifications

MEDICAL MANAGEMENT

Only symptomatic relief is available at this time (e.g., fever management, transfusions for anemia, respiratory support). Some evidence exists that CMV immune globulin given intravenously in combination with the drug ganciclovir can reduce the severity of an infection in immunocompromised individuals. A live CMV vaccine has been available for over 30 years. It does not prevent infection but rather reduces the severity of the illness in immunocompromised individuals such as bone marrow and organ transplant recipients. Clinical trials have not been performed in women of childbearing age because of the risk of infection of the fetus and possible tumor formation later in life. Chemotherapy offers some promise, but the toxicity and immunosuppression associated with these drugs raise concerns about their use in newborns. No special precautions are necessary. However, caregivers should wear gloves, employ good hand-washing techniques, and use universal precautions.

NURSING ASSESSMENT

1. See the Respiratory Assessment and Neurologic Assessment sections in Appendix A.
2. Assess nutritional status.
3. Assess developmental level.
4. Assess for history of impaired vision and hearing.

NURSING DIAGNOSES

- Infection, Risk for
- Nutrition: less than body requirements, Imbalanced
- Growth and development, Delayed
- Sensory perception, Disturbed
- Home maintenance, Impaired

NURSING INTERVENTIONS

1. Monitor action and side effects of medications.
2. Monitor response to and side effects of blood transfusions.

3. Assess age and developmental level.
4. Weigh child upon admission and daily.
5. Monitor urine and serum electrolyte and glucose levels as needed.
6. Provide age-appropriate stimulation.
7. Review and reinforce with parents importance of maintaining adequate caloric intake.
8. Promote process of attachment between parents and infant.
9. Identify community resources that may be helpful in dealing with long-term sequelae.

🔖 Discharge Planning and Home Care

1. Instruct parents about methods to prevent spread of infection.
   a. Advise parents of possibility that virus is secreted for more than 1 year.
   b. Pregnant friends should not perform child care (e.g., changing child's diapers).
   c. Care should be taken to perform thorough hand washing after each diaper change and to dispose of diapers properly.
2. Instruct parents about long-term management of condition.
   a. Reinforce information about virus.
   b. If neurologic, cognitive, or developmental sequelae are evident, refer to community-based services.
   c. Emphasize importance of medical monitoring after an acute episode.

Presence of sequelae will necessitate further interventions beyond the scope of this section.

CLIENT OUTCOMES

1. Child will have consistent weight gain.
2. Child will have maximal level of developmental functioning.
3. Parents will verbalize understanding of child's condition, home care, and follow-up needs.

REFERENCES

American Academy of Pediatrics: Cytomegalovirus infection. In Pickering LK, editor: *2000 Red book: report of the Committee on Infectious Diseases,* ed 25, Elk Grove Village, Ill, 2000, The Academy.

Daley AJ, Gilbert GL: Cytomegalovirus infection in pregnancy, *J Paediatr Child Health* 37:589, 2001.

Damato EG, Winnen CW: Cytomegalovirus infection: perinatal implications, *J Obstet Gynecol Neonatal Nurs* 31(1):86, 2002.

Schleiss MR: Cytomegalovirus. In Rudolf CD, Rodolf AM, editors: *Rudolf's pediatrics,* ed 21, New York, 2003, McGraw-Hill.

21

◆

Developmental Dysplasia of the Hip

◆

PATHOPHYSIOLOGY

Developmental dysplasia of the hip (DDH), previously known as congenital hip dysplasia, is an abnormal development between the femoral head and the acetabulum. The hip is a ball (femoral head) and socket (acetabulum) joint that provides motion and hip stability. Three patterns are seen in DDH: (1) acetabular dysplasia (abnormal development)—delay in development of the acetabulum so that it is shallower than normal; the femoral head remains in the acetabulum; (2) subluxation—incomplete dislocation of the hip; the femoral head is not completely out of the acetabulum and can be partially dislocated; and (3) dislocation—the hip rests in a dislocated position, and the femoral head is not in contact with the acetabulum. DDH can eventually progress to either permanent reduction, complete dislocation, or dysplasia secondary to adaptive changes occurring in adjacent tissue and bone.

INCIDENCE

1. DDH occurs in 1 or 1.2 of 1000 live births.
2. In the United States, approximately 38,900 to 46,000 babies are affected each year.
3. Female/male ratio is 6:1.
4. Incidence increases with breech presentation.
5. Increased incidence is evident among siblings of affected children.
6. When only one hip is involved, the left hip is affected more often than the right hip.

7. There is frequent association with other musculoskeletal and congenital renal abnormalities.
8. Increased incidence is seen among cultures that tightly swaddle children or strap children in cradle boards during the first few months of life.
9. There is an association between DDH and the development of secondary hip arthritis in early adulthood.

CLINICAL MANIFESTATIONS
Infants
1. Possibly no symptoms evident because infant may have minimal displacement of femur
2. Unequal gluteal folds (prone position)
3. Shortening of limb on affected side
4. Restricted abduction of hip on affected side
5. Presence of Galeazzi's sign (Box 21-1)
6. Positive finding on Barlow's maneuver (see Box 21-1)
7. Positive finding on Ortolani's maneuver (see Box 21-1)

Toddlers and Older Children
1. Waddling gait (bilateral dislocation of the hip)
2. Increased lumbar lordosis (swayback) during standing (bilateral dislocation of hip)
3. Affected leg shorter than other
4. Positive finding on Trendelenburg's test (see Box 21-1)
5. Limping

COMPLICATIONS
1. Persistent acetabular dysplasia
2. Recurrent dislocation
3. Iatrogenic avascular necrosis of femoral head

LABORATORY AND DIAGNOSTIC TESTS
An anteroposterior and Lauenstein lateral pelvic radiographic study is obtained (assesses extent of femoral displacement or dislocation; not useful for infants younger than 1 month old). Ultrasonography, computed tomographic scan, and magnetic resonance imaging are also used.

BOX 21-1
Assessment Criteria

Ortolani's Maneuver

Used to reduce the dislocatable femoral head back into the acetabulum. The fingers are placed over the greater trochanter as the thigh is flexed and abducted, which results in lifting of the femoral head toward the acetabulum. A cluck (clicks are not pathologic) is heard in infants younger than 3 months of age, and a jerk is felt in older infants and children if a reduction of the dislocated hip is possible.

Barlow's Maneuver

Used to push unstable femoral head out of the acetabulum. Flex both hips and knees, then place hand over the knee. The leg is adducted past midline and outward. Positive sign is a sensation of abnormal movement.

Galeazzi's Sign

When both hips are flexed at 90-degree angle, one knee is below the level of the other (uneven knee levels).

Trendelenburg's Test

When the child stands on the leg of the affected side, the opposite hip slants downward instead of remaining level.

MEDICAL MANAGEMENT

Treatment varies with the severity of the clinical manifestations, child's age, and extent of the dysplasia. If the dislocation is corrected in the first few days to weeks of life, the chance is greater that a normal hip will develop. During the neonatal period, positioning and maintaining the hip in flexion and abduction is achieved with the use of a corrective device. Between the ages of 6 and 18 months, traction is used followed by cast immobilization. If soft tissue obstructs and complicates reduction and joint development, either closed or open reduction (depending on whether or not contracture of the adductor muscles and displacement of the femoral head have occurred) is performed and hip spica casting is applied.

NURSING ASSESSMENT

1. See the Musculoskeletal Assessment section in Appendix A.
2. See the assessment criteria in Box 21-1.
3. Assess for signs of skin irritation.
4. Assess child's response to traction and immobilization in spica cast.
5. Postoperatively, assess vital signs and signs of wound drainage.
6. Assess child's developmental level.
7. Assess parents' ability to manage home care for spica cast.

NURSING DIAGNOSES

- Mobility, Impaired physical
- Injury, Risk for
- Skin integrity, Risk for impaired
- Growth and development, Delayed
- Knowledge, Deficient

NURSING INTERVENTIONS

Instruct parents on maintenance and care of corrective device.

Pavlik Harness (Maintains Hip Flexion and Reduction of Unstable Hip)

1. Maintain harness (on continuously, including all aspects of normal care, for 3 to 6 months).
2. Perform skin care (lubricant and sponge bath).
3. Change diapers frequently.
4. Monitor for signs of skin irritation.

Abduction Brace (Maintains Hip in Abducted and Fixed Position)

1. Perform skin care.
2. Change diapers frequently (to prevent skin breakdown and to maintain clean brace).
3. Monitor for signs of skin irritation.

   If conservative treatment is unsuccessful or if condition is diagnosed after infant is 3 months of age, infant may be treated first with traction followed by closed or open reduction (as indicated) and then placement of a spica cast.

1. Monitor child's response to traction (2 to 3 weeks).
2. Monitor child's response to spica cast immobilization.

If open reduction is performed, do the following:

1. Prepare child and parents for surgery (see the Preparation for Procedures or Surgery section in Appendix J).
   a. Provide information about presurgical routine.
   b. Reinforce information given about surgery and open reduction.
2. Monitor child's response postoperatively.
   a. Monitor vital signs every 2 hours until stable, then every 4 hours and as needed.
   b. Monitor for signs of drainage on cast.
   c. Perform circulation checks every hour during the immediate postoperative period, then every 4 hours.
3. Provide both nonpharmacologic and pharmacologic pain relief measures as necessary (see Appendix H).
   a. Provide tactile comfort and holding.
   b. Administer analgesics.

Discharge Planning and Home Care

1. Instruct parents on applying and maintaining correction device (see the Nursing Interventions section in this chapter).
2. Instruct parents on care of spica cast.
   a. Apply waterproof material to cast edges (petal cast edges) in perineal area; change diaper often.
   b. Keep skin clean and dry under cast.
   c. Check for signs of infection and pressure sores (e.g., musty odor and reddened area).
   d. Monitor for small items placed in cast (e.g., food and small toys).
3. Instruct parents on appropriate feeding techniques.
   a. Feed infant in supine position.
   b. Child can be held in parent's arm or propped with pillows.
4. Instruct parents to provide age-appropriate stimulating activities (see the relevant section in Appendix B).

5. Instruct parents on car seat modifications.
6. Emphasize need for long-term follow-up.

CLIENT OUTCOMES

1. Infant's or child's hip will remain in desired position.
2. Infant or child will have intact skin without redness or breakdowns.
3. Parents will demonstrate care activities to accommodate infant's or child's corrective device or hip spica cast.

REFERENCES

Ashwill JW, Droske SC: *Nursing care of children—principles and practice,* Philadelphia, 1997, WB Saunders.

Butler J: Assessment and management of musculoskeletal dysfunction. In Kenner C et al, editors: *Comprehensive neonatal nursing: a physiologic perspective,* ed 2, Philadelphia, 1998, WB Saunders.

Eilert RE, Georgopoulos G: Orthopedics. In Hay WW Jr et al: *Current pediatric diagnosis and treatment,* ed 13, Stamford, Conn, 1997, Appleton & Lange.

Gillett C. Bernese periacetabular osteotomy for hip dysplasia in young adults, *AORN J* 75(4):736, 2002.

Kim HW, Weinstein SL: Intervening early in developmental hip dysplasia: early recognition avoids serious consequences later, *J Musculoskeletal Med* 15(2):70, 1998.

Omerogul H, Koporal S: The role of clinical exam risk factors in the diagnosis of developmental dysplasia of the hip: a prospective study of 188 referred young infants, *Arch Orthop Trauma Surg* 121(1-2):7, 2001.

Rudy C: Clinical insights. Developmental dysplasia of the hip: what's new in the 1990's? *J Pediatr Health Care* 10(2):85, 1996.

Thompson GH: Common orthopaedic problems of children. In Behrman RE, Kliegman RM: *Nelson essentials of pediatrics,* ed 3, Philadelphia, 1998, WB Saunders.

Wong DL et al: *Wong's essentials of pediatric nursing,* ed 6, St Louis, 2001, Mosby.

22

❖

Diabetes Mellitus: Insulin-Dependent

❖

PATHOPHYSIOLOGY

Insulin-dependent diabetes mellitus (IDDM), or juvenile-onset diabetes, is caused by a negligible or completely lacking secretory capacity of the beta cells of the pancreas, which results in insulin deficiency. Complete insulin deficiency necessitates the use of exogenous insulin to promote appropriate glucose use and to prevent complications related to elevated glucose levels, such as diabetic ketoacidosis and death.

Insulin is necessary for the following physiologic functions: (1) to promote the use and storage of glucose in the liver, muscles, and adipose tissue for energy; (2) to inhibit and stimulate glycogenolysis or gluconeogenesis, depending on the body's requirements; and (3) to promote the use of fatty acids and ketones in cardiac and skeletal muscles. Insulin deficiency results in unrestricted glucose production without appropriate use, which leads to hyperglycemia and increased lipolysis and production of ketones, and, in turn, to lipemia, ketonemia, and ketonuria. The insulin deficiency also heightens the effects of the counterregulatory hormones—epinephrine, glucagon, cortisol, and growth hormone (see Box 22-1 for these hormones' functions).

Diagnosis of IDDM is based on the individual's clinical history, laboratory work, and initial symptoms. The cause is unknown, although it is widely accepted that the presence of human lymphocyte antigens is associated with this disease. This presence suggests that the child may have a predisposition to a genetic defect in his or her immunologic response system,

BOX 22-1
Functions of Counterregulatory Hormones

Epinephrine
- Inhibits uptake of glucose by muscle
- Activates glycogenolysis and gluconeogenesis
- Activates lipolysis, causing release of fatty acids and glycerol

Glucagon
- Promotes production of glucose through glycogenolysis and gluconeogenesis

Cortisol
- Limits glucose use by inhibiting muscle uptake
- Increases glucose production by stimulating gluconeogenesis

Growth Hormones
- Impede glucose uptake

which results in the destruction of pancreatic beta cells. Other evidence suggests that infection (e.g., with coxsackievirus) serves as a trigger.

INCIDENCE

1. Fifteen percent of all diabetic individuals have IDDM.
2. Ninety-seven percent of newly diagnosed juvenile diabetic individuals have IDDM.
3. Mean age of onset is 11 years in girls and 13 years in boys.
4. Age ranges of peak incidence are 5 to 7 years and puberty.
5. Among preschool-aged children, the disease is more commonly diagnosed in boys.
6. Among children 5 to 10 years of age, the disease is more commonly diagnosed in girls.
7. The disease is diagnosed more often in winter than in summer.
8. Diabetic ketoacidosis is a frequent cause of morbidity and sometimes of death.

CLINICAL MANIFESTATIONS
Initial Effects

1. Polyuria
2. Polydipsia
3. Polyphagia
4. Recent weight loss (during a period of less than 3 weeks)
5. Fatigue
6. Headaches
7. Yeast infections in girls
8. Fruity breath odor
9. Dehydration (usually 10% dehydrated)
10. Diabetic ketoacidosis (Box 22-2)—hyperglycemia, ketonemia, ketonuria, metabolic acidosis, Kussmaul respirations
11. Abdominal pain

BOX 22-2
Signs of Diabetic Ketoacidosis

- Kussmaul respirations (deep sighing respirations)
- Hyperglycemia (serum glucose level higher than 300 mg/dl)
- Ketonuria (moderate to large amounts; positive Ketostix result)
- Metabolic acidosis (pH <7.3; increased partial pressure of carbon dioxide [Pco_2]; decreased partial pressure of oxygen [Po_2]; sodium bicarbonate [$NaHCO_3$] <15 mEq/L)
- Dehydration (as a result of polyuria and polydipsia)
- Fruity breath odor
- Electrolyte imbalance (falsely elevated potassium and sodium levels)
- Potential for life-threatening cardiac arrhythmias (as a result of electrolyte imbalance)
- Cerebral edema (caused by overzealous infusion of fluids)
- Coma (caused by electrolyte imbalance and acidosis)
- Death (infrequent)

Time Periods of Insulin Activity

- AM Regular works from breakfast to lunch
- AM Neutral protamine Hagedorn (NPH) works from breakfast to dinner
- PM Regular works from dinner to bedtime
- PM NPH works from bedtime to the next morning

12. Change in level of consciousness (due to progressive dehydration, acidosis, and hyperosmolality, which results in decreased cerebral oxygenation)

Diagnosis is confirmed by the presence of symptoms combined with an elevated blood glucose level (higher than 200 mg/dl) and glycosuria.

Long-Term Effects

1. Failure to grow at normal rate and delayed maturation
2. Neuropathy
3. Recurrent infection
4. Retinal and/or renal microvascular disease
5. Ischemic heart disease or arterial obstruction

COMPLICATIONS

1. Diabetic ketoacidosis
2. Coma
3. Hypokalemia and hyperkalemia
4. Hypocalcemia
5. Hypoglycemia
6. Osteopenia
7. Limited joint mobility
8. Microvascular changes resulting in retinopathy (maintaining a high degree of metabolic control is associated with delay in and possible prevention of microvascular changes)
9. Cardiovascular disease
10. Thromboemboli
11. Overwhelming infections

LABORATORY AND DIAGNOSTIC TESTS

For the individual newly diagnosed with diabetes:

1. Randomly determined plasma glucose level—200 mg/dl or higher
2. Fasting plasma glucose level—higher than or equal to 140 mg/dl
3. Glycosylated hemoglobin (hemoglobin A_{1c}) level— reflects percentage of hemoglobin to which glucose is attached

4. Blood urea nitrogen, creatinine levels—increased because of interference of ketones in measurement
5. Serum calcium, magnesium, phosphate levels—decreased as a result of diuresis
6. Serum electrolyte (potassium [K^+] and sodium [Na^+]) levels—may be falsely elevated as a result of hyperosmolarity
7. Complete blood count—white blood cells may be increased, with predominance of polymorphonuclear lymphocytes
8. Immunoassay—to measure level of C-peptides after glucose challenge (to verify endogenous insulin secretion)
9. Twenty-four-hour urine analysis for glucose—considered a more reliable measure of urine glucose level
10. Urinalysis and urine culture
11. Islet cell antibody testing

For diabetic ketoacidosis:

1. Plasma glucose level—higher than 300 mg/dl
2. Serum bicarbonate ($NaHCO_3$) level—less than 15 mEq/L
3. Arterial pH—less than 7.30
4. Electrocardiogram—increased T wave with hyperkalemia
5. Serum ketone level—higher than 3 mm/L

MEDICAL MANAGEMENT

Children with the initial diagnosis of IDDM are usually admitted to the hospital for stabilization and education but may be treated on an outpatient basis. The management of these children requires a multidisciplinary approach. Medical management includes the regulation of serum glucose, fluid, and electrolyte levels. This is accomplished through monitoring of laboratory results, administration of insulin, and intravenous (IV) administration of fluids containing the indicated additives. Secondary problems (i.e., infections) are also treated accordingly. Once glucose levels are stabilized, insulin doses are given to maintain serum glucose level. Regulation of nutrition and exercise is also a key factor in managing diabetes.

NURSING ASSESSMENT

1. See the Measurements section in Appendix A.
2. Assess hydration status.
3. Assess for hyperglycemia.
4. Assess for hypoglycemia.
5. Assess dietary patterns.
6. Assess activities and exercise patterns.
7. Assess self-administration of insulin and ability to monitor blood glucose levels.

NURSING DIAGNOSES

- Fluid volume, Deficient
- Infection, Risk for
- Nutrition: less than body requirements, Imbalanced
- Knowledge, Deficient (related to lack of information about the disease)
- Home maintenance, Impaired

NURSING INTERVENTIONS
Diabetic Ketoacidosis

1. Monitor and observe child for change in status of diabetic ketoacidosis (see Box 22-2).
2. Promote child's hydration status.
   a. Accurately record intake, output, and specific gravity.
   b. Monitor for dehydration.
      i. Dry or doughy skin
      ii. Increased specific gravity
      iii. Dry mucous membranes
      iv. Depressed fontanelles (infants)
   c. Monitor for fluid overload.
      i. Decreased specific gravity
      ii. Peripheral edema
   d. Administer and monitor IV solutions as ordered based on laboratory results and clinical appearance. (Saline bolus 10 to 20 ml/kg is usually given prior to maintenance IV.)
3. Monitor child's glucose level hourly.
   a. Blood glucose level should not fall below 250 mg/dl during the first 12 hours of treatment; glucose level

should not fall more than 100 mg/dl/hr because too rapid a decline in osmolarity predisposes child to cerebral edema.

  b. Regular insulin is preferably administered intravenously for treatment of diabetic ketoacidosis; typically, bolus dose (0.1 U/kg) is given, followed by continuous infusion (0.1 U/kg/hr).

    i. Prime tubing with insulin solution before starting infusion.

    ii. Insulin administration is switched to subcutaneous route once serum glucose level reaches 250 mg/dl, serum pH is 7.35, dehydration is corrected, and child is no longer on nothing-by-mouth status.

  c. Monitor urine for glucose and ketones with each voiding (dipstick).

4. Monitor child's neurologic status hourly until stable.
5. Monitor for signs of complications.

  a. Acidosis

  b. Coma

  c. Hyperkalemia and hypokalemia

  d. Hypocalcemia

  e. Cerebral edema

  f. Hyponatremia

Recovery and Maintenance

1. Monitor and observe for signs of hypoglycemia and hyperglycemia.
2. Promote glucose control.

  a. Monitor urine and blood glucose levels as needed to assess effectiveness of insulin.

  b. Insulin dose is given to maintain serum glucose level; typically, total insulin dose of two thirds neutral protamine Hagedorn (NPH) insulin and one third regular insulin is administered, two thirds of total dose before breakfast and one third before dinner (Box 22-3).

3. Promote adequate nutritional intake (see Box 22-3 for nutritional recommendations).
4. Monitor and establish appropriate relationship between insulin dose, dietary requirements, and exercise.

BOX 22-3
Nutritional Requirements in Diabetes

Purpose of Dietary Plan
- The dietary plan provides the necessary intake of calories for energy requirements and appropriate distribution of nutrients (carbohydrates, fats, and proteins).

Energy Requirements
- Carbohydrates: 40-60% of total calories
- Fats: 25-40% of total calories
- Proteins: 15-30% of total calories
- Ratio of polyunsaturated to saturated fat should be at least 2:1. Total daily fat intake should be 42 g.

Dietary Plans
- Two exchange systems are used by diabetic individuals: the American Diabetic Association (ADA) exchange group and the British Diabetic Association exchange system. The ADA exchange group has six exchange lists, which are for milk, fruit, vegetables, bread, meat, and fat. The exchange lists give the equivalent amounts of calories and nutrients.
- The British Diabetic Association exchange focuses on carbohydrate intake only. A liberal intake of protein is allowed and fats are less restricted. Many children and adolescents prefer carbohydrate counting because it allows for more flexibility in dietary management than the exchange system.

General Information
- Foods high in fiber retard carbohydrate absorption.
- Foods have different glycemic responses (glycemic index).
- Long delays between eating must be avoided.
- Extra food must be consumed for increased activity (10 to 15 g of carbohydrate for every 30 to 45 minutes of activity).
- Quantity of food needed between meals will vary according to increase or decrease in physical activity.

5. Provide emotional support to individual and family to promote psychosocial adaptation to diabetes.

🔺 Discharge Planning and Home Care

1. Instruct child and parents about management of diabetes.
   a. Insulin administration
   b. Dietary pattern
   c. Blood glucose monitoring at least four times per day
   d. Urine glucose monitoring
   e. Prevention of complications
   f. Care of hypoglycemic and hyperglycemic states
   g. Skin care
   h. Activity regimen
   i. Illness management
2. Initiate home care referral to assess adherence to diabetic regimen.
3. Promote resumption of normal activities.
4. Promote expression of concerns by child and parents about diabetes as a chronic illness and its long-term management.
5. Promote interest in support groups.

CLIENT OUTCOMES

1. Child will achieve normal growth and development.
2. Child will maintain normal serum glucose levels.
3. Child and family will demonstrate care required at home and have support system in place.

REFERENCES

Becker D, Ryan C: Hypoglycemia—a complication of diabetes therapy in children, *Trends Endocrinol Metab* 11(5):198, 2000.

Betschart J: Diabetes in the life cycle and research. In Franz M, editor: *A core curriculum for diabetes education,* Chicago, Ill, 2001, American Association of Diabetes Educators.

Jaffe M: Insulin dependent diabetes mellitus. In Sullivan M, editor: *Pediatric nursing care plans,* rev ed 2, Englewood, Colo, 1998, Skidmore-Roth.

Linder B: Improving diabetic control with a new insulin analog, *Contemp Pediatr* 14(10):52, 1997.

23

❖

Disseminated Intravascular Coagulation

❖

PATHOPHYSIOLOGY

Disseminated intravascular coagulation (DIC) is a defect in coagulation characterized by simultaneous hemorrhage and coagulation. DIC is the result of abnormal stimulation of the normal coagulation process with subsequent formation of widespread microvascular thrombi and depleted clotting factors. The syndrome is triggered by a variety of illnesses such as sepsis, multiple trauma, burns, and neoplasms. DIC can be described in terms of two precisely controlled coagulation processes that become accelerated and uncontrolled. Initially, the injury to tissue caused by the primary disorder (e.g., infection or trauma) activates a mechanism that releases thrombin, which is necessary for fibrin clot formation, into the circulation. Thrombin also activates the process that is necessary for the breakdown of fibrin and fibrinogen, which gives rise to fibrin and fibrinogen degradation products (FDPs). FDPs in the circulation act as anticoagulants. DIC is characterized by the following three major symptoms: (1) generalized hemorrhage; (2) ischemia caused by thrombi, hemodynamic changes, and metabolic derangements, which contributes to multiple organ failure; and (3) anemia. Prognosis is dependent on a variety of factors, including the severity of the primary and secondary conditions.

INCIDENCE

1. Exact incidence is unknown.
2. DIC occurs in both children and adults.

3. DIC results from an underlying injury or illness.
4. Stress and steroids are possible precipitating factors.
5. Mortality rate is high.

CLINICAL MANIFESTATIONS

1. Spontaneous bleeding
2. Hypoxia
3. Cutaneous oozing
4. Petechiae
5. Ecchymoses
6. Pain
7. Symptoms based on severity and extent of organic involvement
   a. Renal: oliguria, anuria
   b. Central nervous system: altered mental status
   c. Skin: mottled, necrotic lesions; cyanosis

COMPLICATIONS

1. Gangrenous extremities
2. Shock
3. Hypoxia
4. Multiple organ dysfunction syndrome

LABORATORY AND DIAGNOSTIC TESTS

1. Level of D-dimer (derived from fibrin)—elevated (indicative of thrombosis, procoagulant activation)
2. FDP level—elevated (fibrinolytic activation)
3. Level of antithrombin (AT; formerly antithrombin III)—decreased (evidence of inhibitor consumption)
4. Prothrombin time (PT)—prolonged
5. Partial thromboplastin time (PTT)—prolonged
6. Thrombin time (TT)—prolonged
7. Fibrinogen level—decreased
8. Complete blood count
   a. Platelet count—decreased
   b. Red blood cell morphology—presence of schistocytes
9. Clotting factor assays—usually decreased
10. Type and cross-match for blood product replacement therapy

The combination of elevated D-dimer and FDP levels is specific and sensitive in the diagnosis of DIC. AT is helpful in the assessment of the severity of the DIC. Prolonged PT and PTT and decreased fibrinogen levels are evidence of the late consumptive stage of DIC. PT, PTT, and TT may be altered by the use of anticoagulant therapy. Thrombocytopenia, an indirect indicator of fibrin clot formation, is a late sign of DIC and is nonspecific to the process. Clotting factor assays are not available in most standard laboratories.

MEDICAL MANAGEMENT

The major focus in the medical management of DIC is the correction of the primary illness or injury that initiated the coagulopathy. Correcting the underlying problem may control the DIC so that normal coagulation can be restored. Treatment of infection, shock, acidosis, and hypoxia must be priorities. Fluid replacement therapy with crystalloids is essential in the early stages of shock. Although blood replacement therapy with whole blood, cryoprecipitate, red blood cells, fresh frozen plasma, and platelet concentrates is often required, it is risky because these products enhance the clotting process. Heparin therapy has been advocated because it interferes with the coagulation cascade and antagonizes the production of thrombin. This therapy remains very controversial, however, and its use may increase bleeding. Overall, treatment must be tailored to the clinical and laboratory data available.

NURSING ASSESSMENT

1. See the Cardiovascular Assessment section in Appendix A.
2. Recognize conditions that predispose to DIC.
3. Assess for signs of bleeding.
4. Assess bleeding sites.
5. Assess oxygenation.
6. Assess for signs and symptoms of impaired tissue perfusion and organ failure.
7. Assess family coping skills.

NURSING DIAGNOSES

- Fluid volume, Risk for deficient
- Tissue perfusion, Ineffective

- Gas exchange, Impaired
- Pain
- Skin integrity, Risk for impaired
- Injury, Risk for
- Infection, Risk for
- Anxiety

NURSING INTERVENTIONS

1. Monitor child's clinical status; report any significant changes.
   a. Monitor for signs of hemorrhage—bleeding, petechiae, cutaneous oozing, dyspnea, lethargy, pallor, increased apical pulse, decreased blood pressure, headache, dizziness, muscle weakness, restlessness.
   b. Monitor for signs of ischemia—changes in level of consciousness, decreased urine output, electrocardiogram changes, gangrenous extremities, mottled skin, necrotic skin lesions, respiratory failure.
2. Control bleeding.
   a. Do not disturb clots.
   b. Use pressure to control bleeding when possible.
   c. Administer blood products safely.
   d. Monitor bleeding closely—inspect skin carefully.
   e. Measure blood loss.
   f. Monitor laboratory data.
   g. Test urine output for gross and occult blood.
3. Promote adequate oxygenation.
   a. Position child for effective ventilation.
   b. Administer oxygen and monitor response.
   c. Perform frequent respiratory assessments.
   d. Reduce oxygen needs.
   e. Control environmental stimuli.
4. Provide measures to alleviate or control pain.
   a. Immobilize joints.
   b. Apply hot or cold compresses.
   c. Use bed cradle.
   d. Use air mattress.
   e. Change child's position frequently.
   f. Provide mouth and skin care.

    g. Utilize pain scale to assess degree of pain.

    h. Administer pain medication.

5. Monitor child's therapeutic and untoward response to administration of blood products.

    a. Platelets—used to decrease bleeding, correct low platelet count

    b. Fresh frozen plasma—used to correct deficiencies of fibrinogen, prothrombin, factor II, factor VIII, and other factors

    c. Fresh whole blood and packed red blood cells—used to maintain hematocrit

6. Monitor child's therapeutic and untoward response to administration of heparin.

7. Provide support for individual and family.

    a. Identify knowledge deficits.

    b. Provide accurate information.

    c. Give honest answers in clear, concise terms.

    d. Provide consistent caregivers.

🔺 Discharge Planning and Home Care

1. Instruct parents to observe and report any signs of complications.

    a. Infection

    b. Organ dysfunction

    c. Abnormal bleeding

2. Instruct parents about follow-up appointments.

    a. Name and phone number of physician

    b. Date and time of follow-up appointment

CLIENT OUTCOMES

1. Child will have normal coagulation.

2. Child will have adequate perfusion.

3. Child will have minimal organ damage.

REFERENCES

James SR et al: *Nursing care of children: principles and practice,* ed 2, Philadelphia, 2002, WB Saunders.

Levi M, Cate HT: Disseminated intravascular coagulation, *N Engl J Med* 341(8):586, 1999.

Maxson JH: Management of disseminated intravascular coagulation, *Crit Care Nurs Clin North Am* 12(3):341, 2000.

Yu M et al: Screening tests of disseminated intravascular coagulation: guidelines for rapid and specific laboratory diagnosis, *Crit Care Med* 28(6):1777, 2000.

24

❖

Drowning and Near-Drowning

❖

PATHOPHYSIOLOGY

Each year between 4000 and 5000 people drown in the United States, and the number of near-drownings is estimated to be three to four times the number of drownings. Drowning is defined as death from asphyxia while submerged or within 24 hours of submersion. Near-drowning occurs when the child survives longer than 24 hours after submersion, regardless of the final outcome. Secondary drowning refers to cases in which the child is successfully resuscitated but then dies more than 24 hours after submersion because of progressive pulmonary dysfunction.

The physiologic events that occur after submersion are sequential. After the initial panic and struggle, victims will hold their breaths, and some will swallow a small amount of water, vomit, then aspirate the vomitus. Laryngospasm follows, which leads to hypoxia and death (dry drowning). In most children laryngospasm occurs initially; this leads to hypoxia, which causes cardiac arrest and relaxation of the airway, so that the lungs are permitted to fill with large amounts of water (wet drowning). Regardless of whether the child aspirates water, hypoxia is the most important physiologic consequence of submersion injuries and affects all organ systems.

Submersion also results in hypothermia. The child's relatively large surface area leads to a rapid decrease in body temperature when the child is in cold water. Severe hypothermia in young children may protect the brain when the diving reflex occurs, causing bradycardia and shunting of blood away from the periphery and thereby increasing the cerebral and coronary circulation.

Prognosis is affected by a variety of factors, such as duration of submersion, extent of hypothermia, physiologic response of the victim, and length of time until effective cardiopulmonary resuscitation is provided. Irreversible brain damage usually occurs after 4 to 6 minutes of submersion, but some children have experienced complete recovery after a much longer period (10 to 30 minutes) in very cold water. Morbidity and death are directly related to the degree of neuronal damage.

INCIDENCE

1. Drowning is the second leading cause of accidental death in children.
2. Preschool children and teenagers have the highest risk for drowning and near-drowning.
3. Forty percent of the victims are younger than 4 years of age.
4. Boys are five times more likely to drown than girls.
5. Peak incidence is during summer months, on weekends, and between 4 PM and 6 PM.
6. Most drownings occur in residential swimming pools.
7. Younger children most often drown in pools, bathtubs, hot tubs, toilets, and buckets.
8. Older children most often drown in lakes, rivers, and oceans while boating or diving, or with associated alcohol ingestion.

CLINICAL MANIFESTATIONS

Clinical manifestations are directly related to the extent of injury and level of consciousness following rescue and resuscitation.

1. Respiratory distress—ranging from rapid, shallow breathing to apnea
2. Cyanosis
3. Pink, frothy sputum
4. Pulmonary edema
5. Flaccidity
6. Decorticate or decerebrate posturing
7. Coma
8. Seizures

9. Shock
10. Arterial blood gas abnormalities
11. Abnormal chest radiographic studies
12. Dysrhythmias
13. Metabolic acidosis
14. Hyperkalemia
15. Hyperglycemia
16. Hypothermia

COMPLICATIONS

1. Hypoxic encephalopathy
2. Secondary drowning
3. Aspiration pneumonia
4. Pulmonary interstitial fibrosis
5. Ventricular dysrhythmias
6. Renal failure
7. Disseminated intravascular coagulation
8. Pancreatic necrosis
9. Infection

LABORATORY AND DIAGNOSTIC TESTS

1. Chest radiographic study—variable findings (from scattered parenchymal infiltrates to extensive pulmonary edema)
2. Arterial blood gas values—to detect respiratory and metabolic acidosis
3. Computed tomographic scan
4. Electroencephalogram—to assess seizure activity and document brain death
5. Complete blood count, hematocrit, hemoglobin—to determine extent of hemodilution or hemoconcentration and need for fluid resuscitation
6. Serum electrolyte levels—to determine need to correct any imbalances caused by submersion
7. Blood urea nitrogen level—to determine renal function
8. Creatinine clearance—to determine renal function
9. Blood culture and sensitivity—to detect superimposed respiratory infection

MEDICAL MANAGEMENT

Aggressive basic and advanced life support at the scene is essential because the full extent of the central nervous system injury cannot be accurately assessed at the time of rescue. Ensuring an adequate airway, breathing, and circulation is the top priority. Other injuries must be considered, and the need for hospitalization is determined by the severity of the event and clinical evaluation. Individuals with respiratory symptoms, decreased oxygen saturation, and altered level of consciousness must be admitted to the hospital. Ongoing attention to oxygenation, ventilation, and cardiac function is the priority. Protecting the central nervous system and reducing cerebral edema are of paramount importance and directly relate to outcome.

Treatments used include high-flow oxygen therapy and positive end-expiratory pressure for adequate oxygenation, and administration of crystalloid solution for fluid resuscitation, dopamine and dobutamine for cardiac therapy, furosemide (Lasix) for diuresis, and mannitol (Mannitor) for control of intracranial hypertension and for sedation.

NURSING ASSESSMENT

1. See the Respiratory Assessment section in Appendix A.
2. Assess for spontaneous respirations.
3. Assess cardiovascular status.
4. Assess core temperature.
5. Assess for level of consciousness.
6. See the Neurologic Assessment section in Appendix A.

NURSING DIAGNOSES

- Gas exchange, Impaired
- Altered cerebral tissue perfusion
- Cardiac output, Decreased
- Fluid volume, Excess
- Hypothermia
- Nutrition: less than body requirements, Imbalanced
- Family processes, Interrupted

NURSING INTERVENTIONS

1. Monitor respiratory system.
   a. Assess respiratory status, including breath sounds and work of breathing.
   b. Maintain patent airway.
   c. Suction airway as needed.
   d. Insert nasogastric tube to prevent aspiration.
   e. Monitor oxygen therapy.
   f. Monitor oxygen level.
2. Monitor cardiovascular system.
   a. Assess cardiovascular status, including vital signs, perfusion, skin temperature and color, and urine output.
   b. Monitor fluid lines and fluid resuscitation efforts.
3. Monitor and record child's level of neurologic functioning.
   a. Perform neurologic assessment (frequency depends on status).
   b. Observe and report signs of intracranial pressure (ICP) (lethargy, increased blood pressure, decreased respiratory rate, increased apical pulse, dilated pupils).
   c. Prevent ICP by positioning head at midline, elevating head of bed 30 degrees, and preventing or managing elevated body temperature.
4. Monitor and maintain fluid balance.
   a. Record intake and output.
   b. Maintain patency and care for Foley catheter.
   c. Maintain fluids as ordered.
   d. Observe for signs and symptoms of alteration in fluid balance, including performing laboratory testing.
5. Monitor and maintain homeostatic temperature regulation.
   a. Monitor temperature.
   b. Initiate and continue rewarming techniques, including use of warming lights, warm mattress, and warm intravenous fluids.
   c. Check skin perfusion.
6. Provide and maintain adequate nutritional intake.
   a. Assess nutritional status.

b. Assess child's capacity to tolerate nasogastric or oral feedings (monitor weight, check for residuals and vomiting).

c. If total parenteral nutrition is ordered, monitor infusion, side effects, and blood chemistry results.

7. Provide emotional and other support to family.

a. Provide calm reassurance and realistic progress reports of child's status, including hope.

b. Provide for physical needs of family such as privacy and access to bathroom and telephone, and identify a staff member to contact with questions.

c. Explain all treatments.

d. Allow parents and family members to be with child as appropriate.

Discharge Planning and Home Care

1. Instruct parents about instituting preventive measures: learning cardiopulmonary resuscitation; providing water safety and swimming lessons for child; accident-proofing backyard (e.g., pool cover, fence enclosures); and appropriately supervising children during pool use.

2. Instruct parents regarding developmental level of child and safety issues.

3. Instruct parents on follow-up care.

CLIENT OUTCOMES

1. Child will return to optimal level of neurologic function.
2. Respiratory distress will be reduced or eliminated.
3. Child will maintain adequate perfusion, and vital signs will be within normal ranges.

REFERENCES

Beyda DH: Childhood submersion injuries, *J Emerg Nurs* 24(2):140, 1998.

Hockenberry M: *Wong's nursing care of infants and children,* ed 7, St Louis, 2003, Mosby.

Laskowski-Jones L: Responding to summer emergencies, *Nursing* 30(5):34, 2000.

Lassman J: Injury prevention. Water safety, *J Emerg Nurs* 28(3):241, 2002.

Zuckerman GB, Conway EE Jr: Drowning and near drowning: a pediatric epidemic, *Pediatr Ann* 29(6):360, 2000.

25

❖

Epiglottitis

❖

PATHOPHYSIOLOGY

Epiglottitis is an acute bacterial infection of the epiglottis and the surrounding areas (the aryepiglottic folds and the supraglottic area) that causes airway obstruction. The infection is caused by *Haemophilus influenzae* type B or, on rare occasions, by staphylococci, streptococci, pneumococci, or *Candida albicans*. The use of *H. influenzae* type B vaccine in infants has resulted in a dramatic reduction in the incidence of epiglottitis. Onset is sudden and infection progresses rapidly, causing acute respiratory difficulty. This condition requires emergency airway stabilization and medical measures because a fatal outcome can occur. The child is extubated when the epiglottis appears normal and the child is able to breathe around the tube (usually 48 to 72 hours after antibiotic treatment is started).

INCIDENCE

1. Children aged 2 to 7 years are most often affected.
2. Incidence is highest in winter, but infection can occur anytime.
3. Epiglottitis may be preceded by upper respiratory tract infection.

CLINICAL MANIFESTATIONS

1. Respiratory difficulty, which can progress to severe respiratory distress in a matter of minutes or hours (dyspnea)
2. Dysphagia, constant drooling
3. Inspiratory stridor
4. Hoarse or brassy cough (may or may not be present)

5. Edematous, cherry-red epiglottis
6. Red and inflamed oral cavity
7. Breathing in upright position with head extended forward
8. Complaint of intense sore throat
9. Sudden increase in temperature
10. Muffled voice
11. Pale color
12. Decreased breath sounds
13. Substernal or suprasternal and intercostal retractions
14. Bilateral cervical adenitis
15. Lethargy

COMPLICATIONS
1. Airway obstruction
2. Laryngospasm
3. Death

LABORATORY AND DIAGNOSTIC TESTS
1. Oxygen saturation—decrease in the amount of oxygen
2. Arterial blood gas values—decreased pH, decreased partial pressure of oxygen (Po_2), increased partial pressure of carbon dioxide (Pco_2)
3. Lateral neck radiographic study—to confirm diagnosis. The epiglottis will be swollen and the hypopharynx will be dilated. This is known as the "thumb sign."
4. Throat culture—to rule out other bacterial infections
5. Blood culture—to rule out other bacterial infections
6. Direct laryngoscopy—to confirm diagnosis; performed in operating room to prevent complications

MEDICAL MANAGEMENT
Children suspected of having epiglottitis should be examined where personnel and equipment are available for an emergency tracheal intubation or tracheostomy. Visual examination of the throat is contraindicated until this requirement is met. Lateral neck radiographic studies may help confirm the diagnosis but should be performed in the least distressing manner possible, usually with the child being held in the parent's lap. Endotracheal intubation or tracheostomy is performed in the operating room

along with draws for laboratory testing, collection of throat culture specimen, and placement of intravenous lines. The child is observed in the intensive care area until swelling of the epiglottis decreases, usually by the third day. Antibiotics are given for a total of 7 to 10 days following extubation.

NURSING ASSESSMENT

Caution: Do not examine the throat if epiglottitis is suspected due to risk of reflex laryngospasm, which will result in complete airway obstruction.

1. See the Respiratory Assessment section in Appendix A.
2. Assess hydration status.
3. Assess anxiety level.

NURSING DIAGNOSES

- Suffocation, Risk for
- Airway clearance, Ineffective
- Breathing pattern, Ineffective
- Tissue perfusion, Ineffective
- Anxiety
- Family processes, Interrupted

NURSING INTERVENTIONS

1. Monitor respiratory status (including vital signs).
   a. Temperature, apical pulse, respiratory rate, blood pressure
   b. Presence of inspiratory stridor
   c. Presence of intercostal retractions
   d. Presence of circumoral cyanosis
   e. Use of accessory muscles
   f. Ability to handle oral secretions
   g. Oxygen saturation—noninvasive monitoring
   h. Arterial blood gas values—defer until child is in operating room
2. Observe and report signs of increased respiratory distress or changes in respiratory status.
3. Maintain position of comfort and security for child to facilitate breathing (usually upright in parent's lap). Never leave child unattended.

4. Prepare child preoperatively for airway insertion (endotracheal tube or tracheostomy) if condition allows.
5. Assist and support physician during emergency procedure.
   a. Ventilate through bag and mask if child experiences obstruction of breathing before reaching operating room.
   b. Observe and monitor respiratory status during intubation.
6. Maintain patency of airway and ventilator function.
7. Provide tracheostomy care (if tracheostomy is performed).
   a. Maintain patent airway.
   b. Monitor cardiopulmonary status.
   c. Use aseptic technique when suctioning.
   d. Clean tracheostomy site.
   e. Observe tracheostomy tube for incrustation.
8. Monitor action and side effects of prescribed medications.
   a. Sedate as needed.
   b. Restrain as needed.
9. Assess hydration status: monitor input and output and specific gravity.
10. Provide for child's developmental needs during hospitalization.
    a. Provide age-appropriate toys (see the relevant section in Appendix B).
    b. Incorporate home routines into hospital care (e.g., feeding practices and bedtime rituals).
    c. Encourage expression of feelings through age-appropriate means.
11. Provide consistent nursing care to promote trust and alleviate anxiety.

Discharge Planning and Home Care
1. If child is discharged on regimen of oral antibiotics, provide teaching regarding administration and side effects.
2. Educate family on value of *H. influenzae* type B vaccine.

CLIENT OUTCOMES

1. Child's respiratory status will return to normal.
2. Child and family will demonstrate understanding of home care and follow-up needs.

REFERENCES

Chernick V, Boat TF, editors: *Kendig's disorders of the respiratory tract in children,* ed 6, Philadelphia, 1998, WB Saunders.

Kearney K: Emergency epiglottitis, *Am J Nurs* 101(8):37, 2001.

Kelley S, editor: *Pediatric emergency nursing,* ed 2, East Norwalk, Conn, 1994, Appleton & Lange.

Stewart KB: Action stat: epiglottitis, *Nursing* 31(2):64, 2001.

Tintinalli JE, editor: *Emergency medicine: a comprehensive study guide,* ed 5, New York, 2000, McGraw-Hill.

26

◆

Foreign Body Aspiration

◆

PATHOPHYSIOLOGY

Foreign body aspiration refers to the lodgment of an object or substance in the airway. The foreign body tends to lodge most often in the cricopharyngeal area because of the strong propulsive pharyngeal muscles that move it to this location. Obstruction may be partial or complete. Complete airway obstruction usually occurs in the upper airway and is life threatening. Most objects aspirated by children are small enough to pass through the larynx and trachea and lodge in either of the main bronchi. The right main bronchus is a more common site because it is larger, receives greater airflow, and has a straighter line of entry than the left bronchus. The mechanisms of airway obstruction depend on the site of obstruction and whether the foreign body is partially or completely obstructing an airway. Atelectasis occurs distal to the area where air can no longer enter. Air trapping or hyperinflation occurs when air is inhaled but can be only partially exhaled.

In many cases foreign bodies are spontaneously expelled from the tracheobronchial tree, and symptoms that persist are from residual irritation and bronchial edema. When foreign body aspiration is diagnosed quickly and the object or substance is removed in a prompt manner, the condition follows a typically benign course. Aspiration of foreign bodies containing saturated fats, such as peanuts, is more problematic due to irritation and inflammation of mucosal tissue. The longer a foreign body remains lodged in place, the more complications can develop, related to increasing edema, inflammation, and threat of infection.

INCIDENCE

1. Foreign body aspiration most commonly occurs in children 6 months to 6 years of age; 90% of cases occur in children younger than 5 years of age; 65% of these are infants.
2. Foreign body aspiration is the leading cause of accidental death in children younger than 1 year of age.
3. Peanuts and other nuts account for about half of all aspirated foreign bodies; vegetable pieces, seeds, and raisins are also common culprits.
4. Large objects such as hot dogs, grapes, balloon fragments, and popcorn may obstruct the glottic inlet and lead to respiratory arrest.

CLINICAL MANIFESTATIONS

Clinical manifestations vary according to the site at which the foreign body lodges and the degree of obstruction that occurs.

1. Initial coughing, gagging, or choking episode, which may or may not be observed
2. Acute coughing or wheezing
3. Subtle chronic cough or wheeze
4. Dyspnea
5. Retractions
6. Cyanosis
7. Decreased breath sounds over affected side
8. Possible quiet period or symptomless phase
9. Fever
10. Hoarseness (larynx)
11. Stridor (larynx)
12. Aphonia (larynx)
13. Audible slap with coughing as foreign body moves (in trachea)
14. Difficulty swallowing, excessive drooling

COMPLICATIONS

Complications most often result from delayed diagnosis and removal.

1. Bronchospasm
2. Atelectasis

3. Bronchitis
4. Bronchiectasis
5. Pneumonia
6. Pneumothorax
7. Lung abscess
8. Bronchopulmonary fistula
9. Death

LABORATORY AND DIAGNOSTIC TESTS

1. Chest radiographic study—anterior, posterior, lateral, and oblique views, to evaluate for opaque foreign body location; for nonopaque foreign body, assess x-ray films for area of atelectasis or, with inspiratory and expiratory x-ray films, assess for air trapping
2. Laryngoscopy and bronchoscopy—performed with general anesthesia in the operating room; provide direct visualization of the upper trachea (a telescope can be used to locate the foreign body, and removal is accomplished by inserting optical forceps)
3. Fluoroscopy—provides a dynamic image of the structures under radiographic study; gives an advantage over radiographic study alone in showing trapped air distal to the foreign body site
4. Xeroradiography (a radiographic technique that uses specially coated x-ray film)—provides higher resolution of images such as nonmetallic foreign bodies
5. Pulse oximetry—to measure oxygen saturation

MEDICAL MANAGEMENT

Emergency management of foreign body aspiration may begin prior to hospitalization for a life-threatening obstruction when attempts at relief via the Heimlich maneuver or blow to the back cannot be delayed. Once foreign body aspiration is suspected, immediate attention is warranted, with aggressive diagnostic workup including bronchoscopy for identification and removal to prevent complications.

Medications that may be used are as follows:

1. Inhaled bronchodilators for laryngospasm or bronchospasm
2. Corticosteroids to decrease airway edema
3. Systemically acting antibiotics in cases in which fragment retention is suspected, purulent secretions are noted in the airway, or signs and symptoms of pneumonia are present

NURSING ASSESSMENT

1. See the Respiratory Assessment section in Appendix A.
2. Assess level of anxiety.

NURSING DIAGNOSES

- Airway clearance, Ineffective
- Anxiety
- Gas exchange, Impaired
- Knowledge, Deficient (related to child safety)

NURSING INTERVENTIONS
Emergency Measures

In cases of total airway obstruction or ineffective airway clearance, an airway must be established.

1. Deliver back blows followed by chest thrusts for infants 1 year and younger.
2. Perform Heimlich maneuver (abdominal thrusts) in children older than 1 year.

Preoperative Care

1. Provide continuous respiratory monitoring; be prepared to assist with emergency airway management if partial obstruction becomes complete.
2. Monitor vital signs and oxygen saturation.
3. Provide position (of comfort) to ensure adequate airway.
4. Provide nothing by mouth before surgery.
5. Prepare child for bronchoscopy and/or thoracotomy.
6. Provide consistent nursing care to promote trust and to alleviate anxiety.

Postoperative Care

1. Perform frequent respiratory assessments to detect signs and symptoms of respiratory distress from secondary airway edema.
2. Assess effects of administered medications.

Discharge Planning and Home Care

1. Instruct parents to observe for, and report immediately, signs of respiratory distress.
2. Provide list of resources for parents in case of emergency.
3. Instruct parents in foreign body airway obstruction removal and cardiopulmonary resuscitation.
4. Instruct in prevention of foreign body aspiration.
   a. Offer types and sizes or portions of food appropriate for age of child.
   b. Discourage child from eating during performance of other activities.
   c. Restrict access to toys or other objects small enough to fit through standard toilet paper roll, as they could cause choking in young children.
   d. Provide anticipatory guidance to parents regarding direct inspection of toys and reading of warning labels to assure that toys are age appropriate.
5. Make referral for home safety assessment if indicated.

CLIENT OUTCOMES

1. Child will achieve and maintain patent airway.
2. Child will return to safe home environment.

REFERENCES

Chernick V, Boat TF, editors: *Kendig's disorders of the respiratory tract in children,* ed 6, Philadelphia, 1998, WB Saunders.

Stoddard FG et al, editors: *Basic life support for healthcare providers,* Dallas, 2001, American Heart Association.

Tintinalli JE, editor: *Emergency medicine: a comprehensive study guide,* ed 5, New York, 2000, McGraw-Hill.

Zaritsky AL et al: *Pediatric advanced life support provider manual,* Dallas, 2002, American Heart Association.

27

◆

Fractures

◆

PATHOPHYSIOLOGY

Fractures can have a variety of causes, including (1) a direct force applied to the bone; (2) an underlying pathologic condition, such as rickets, that leads to spontaneous fracturing; (3) abrupt, intense muscle contractions; and (4) an indirect force (e.g., being hit by a flying object) applied from a distance. Other causes of fractures include child abuse, metastatic neuroblastoma, Ewing's sarcoma, osteogenic sarcoma, osteogenesis imperfecta, copper deficiency, osteomyelitis, overuse injuries, and immobilization resulting in osteoporosis.

There are a variety of fractures, which can be categorized using the Salter-Harris classification system (Box 27-1). The most common type seen in children younger than 3 years of age is the greenstick fracture. This type is characterized by an incomplete break of the cortex, which occurs because the bone is softer and more pliable than the bones of older children. Other fractures (and their related sites) include upper epiphyseal and supracondylar fractures, lateral condylar humeral fractures, and medial epicondylar fractures (humerus); proximal radial physis and radial neck fractures, and nursemaid's elbow (elbow); fractures of the shaft of the radius and ulna (forearm); and fractures of the femoral shaft and tibia (lower limb).

INCIDENCE

1. Upper extremity fractures account for 75% of all fractures sustained by children and frequently occur during a fall onto an outstretched hand.
2. Abuse should be considered in all children younger than 15 months of age with humeral fractures, including

BOX 27-1
Salter-Harris Classification

Type I
- Fracture passes through growth plate without involvement of metaphysis or epiphysis
- Occurs with mild traumatic injuries
- Seen most often in distal fibula

Type II
- Fracture extends through growth plate, involving metaphysis
- Occurs as a result of severe trauma such as car accident, fall from skateboard
- Seen most often in distal radius and proximal humerus

Type III
- Fracture extends through growth plate, involving epiphysis and joint
- Occurs during moderately severe trauma
- Seen most often in distal tibia

Type IV
- Fracture involves metaphysis, extending through growth plate into epiphysis
- Occurs as a result of falls, skateboard and bicycle accidents
- Seen most often in humerus
- Can result in serious damage

Type V (Rare)
- Growth plate is crushed
- Compression fracture, resulting from falling or projectile impact

supracondylar and spiral fractures. In one study of 215 children, 60% of femur fractures in children younger than 1 year of age were due to abuse. Child abuse can also be suspected with rib and skull fractures.
3. Pelvic fractures constitute a small portion of skeletal fractures in children; they rank second in terms of morbidity and mortality.
4. Most fractures occur to pedestrians.

5. Skull fracture ranks first in terms of morbidity and mortality.
6. Injuries to the growth plate occur in one third of skeletal traumas.

CLINICAL MANIFESTATIONS

1. Pain, relieved with rest
2. Tenderness
3. Swelling
4. Impaired function, limping
5. Limited motion
6. Ecchymosis surrounding site
7. Crepitus at site of fracture
8. Decreased neurovascular function distal to site of fracture
9. Distal atrophy

COMPLICATIONS

1. Deformity of limb
2. Limb length discrepancy
3. Potential for growth arrest
4. Joint incongruity
5. Limitation of movement
6. Nerve injury resulting in numbness and/or nerve palsy
7. Circulatory compromise
8. Volkmann's ischemic contracture
9. Gangrene
10. Compartment syndrome
11. Refracture

LABORATORY AND DIAGNOSTIC TESTS

1. Radiographic study of injury site
2. Bone scan—performed if radiographic studies are negative
3. Magnetic resonance imaging
4. Complete blood count
5. Erythrocyte sedimentation rate
6. Ultrasonography

MEDICAL MANAGEMENT

Management varies according to the type of fracture. Management modalities include open reduction, traction, casting, percutaneous pinning, and remodeling. Analgesics are used for pain relief. The dosage and type depend on the intensity of the child's pain.

NURSING ASSESSMENT

1. Assess site of injury for pain, swelling, change in skin color, and neurovascular impairment.
2. Assess for cause of injury.
3. Assess child's need for pain relief.
4. Assess for signs and symptoms of infection.
5. Assess for wound healing (if open reduction was performed).
6. Assess for skin irritation (if casted).
7. Assess for cast or traction integrity.
8. Assess for hydration status.
9. Assess for signs and symptoms of complications such as fat emboli, compartment syndrome.
10. Assess child's and family's ability to adhere to treatment regimen.
11. Assess child's ability to participate in self-care activities.
12. Assess child's need for diversional activities.

NURSING DIAGNOSES

- Injury, Risk for
- Mobility, Impaired physical
- Tissue integrity, Impaired
- Infection, Risk for
- Pain
- Self-care deficit syndrome
- Diversional activity, Deficient
- Knowledge, Deficient

NURSING INTERVENTIONS
Admission

1. Monitor and document condition and cause of injury.
   a. Amount of swelling
   b. Amount of pain
   c. Change in skin color
   d. Circulatory status of limb distal to injury (color, warmth, pulses)

    e. Neurologic status of limb distal to injury (tingling, numbness)

    f. Factors associated with injury

2. Apply splint or Jones dressing to affected limb to alleviate pain and prevent further injury (traction may be used).

    a. Apply to one side of affected limb.

    b. Immobilize fracture site and joints above and below it.

    c. Stabilize splints with bandages.

    d. Apply Jones dressing—wrap extremity with two or three layers of cotton and cover with Ace bandage; repeat process three or four times.

3. Maintain nothing-by-mouth status until after treatment; child may have to be anesthetized.

4. Prepare child and family for selected treatment modality.

Later Treatment

1. Observe and report status of limb distal to fracture site.

    a. Neurovascular status

       i. Upper limbs—radial and ulnar pulses

      ii. Lower limbs—dorsalis pedis and posterior tibial pulses

     iii. Motor function and sensation

    b. Edema and swelling

    c. Skin color and warmth

2. Alleviate edema and swelling of trauma site and area distal to it.

    a. Elevate limb for 24 to 48 hours.

    b. Apply ice if necessary.

    c. Monitor every hour immediately after treatment, then every 4 hours for 48 hours.

3. Promote skin integrity.

    a. Apply alcohol to reddened areas.

    b. Petal cast edges to prevent skin irritation.

    c. Reposition every 2 hours to alleviate increased pressure on bony prominences.

    d. Observe for reddened areas every 4 hours.

4. Observe and report signs of infection.

    a. Elevated temperature

   b. Offensive odors
   c. Drainage
5. Observe for and record bleeding; note and outline amount.
6. Provide cast care (as indicated).
7. Maintain traction (as indicated).
8. Provide age-appropriate diversional activities to alleviate or minimize effects of sensory deprivation and immobilization (see Appendix B).
9. Promote adequate fluid and nutritional intake.
   a. Encourage fluid intake; maintenance fluids—
      0 to 10 kg: 100 ml/kg; 11 to 20 kg: 50 ml/kg
      (plus 100 ml/kg for the first 10 kg); above 20 kg:
      20 ml/kg.
   b. Provide high-fiber and high-roughage diet to promote peristalsis.
   c. Provide well-balanced diet to promote healing.
10. Prevent complications of unaffected limb; provide daily exercises.
11. Refer case to child protective services if child abuse is suspected (see Chapter 13).

Discharge Planning and Home Care

1. Monitor child's and family's ability to keep follow-up appointments.
2. Instruct parents and child about care of cast, use of crutches, movement, weight bearing, return to school or home teaching.
3. Instruct parents and child to monitor and report signs of complications.
   a. Skin breakdown
   b. Signs of infection
   c. Signs of bleeding
   d. Contractures
4. Review home safety precautions to help prevent further injuries.
5. Review vehicular safety precautions such as proper use of seat belts and car seats.

CLIENT OUTCOMES

1. Child's fracture will heal without complications.
2. Child's pain will be minimized or alleviated.
3. Child will participate in self-care activities as fully as possible.

REFERENCES

Battaglia TC et al: Factors affecting forearm compartment pressures in children with supracondylar humeral fractures, *J Pediatr Orthop* 22(4):431, 2002.

Brunner R, Doderlein L: Pathological fractures in children with cerebral palsy, *J Pediatr Orthop* 5(4):232, 1996.

Davidson RS et al: Ultrasonic evaluation of the elbow in infants and young children after suspected trauma, *J Bone Joint Surg Am* 76(12):1804, 1994.

Farnsworth CL et al: Etiology of supracondylar humerus fractures, *J Pediatr Orthop* 18(1):38, 1998.

Gregory P et al: Early complications with external fixation of pediatric femoral shaft fractures, *J Orthop Trauma* 10(3):191, 1996.

Meadows LL: Pediatric management problems: femoral fracture due to child abuse, *Pediatr Nurse* 20(2):168, 1994.

Mintzer C, Waters PM: Acute open reduction of a displaced scaphoid fracture in a child, *J Hand Surg* 19(5):760, 1994.

Sofka CM, Potter HG: Imaging of elbow injuries in the child and adult athlete, *Radiol Clin North Am* 40(2):251, 2002.

Starling SP et al: Pelvic fractures in infants as a sign of physical abuse, *Child Abuse Negl* 26(5):475, 2002.

Strait RT et al: Humeral fractures without obvious etiologies in children less than 3 years of age: when is it abuse? *Pediatrics* 96(4 pt 1):667, 1995.

Townsend DJ, Bassett GS: Common elbow fractures in children, *Am Fam Physician* 53(6):2031, 1996.

Wiss D: What's new in orthopaedic trauma, *J Bone Joint Surg Am* 83(11):1762, 2001.

28

◈

Gastroenteritis

◈

PATHOPHYSIOLOGY

Gastroenteritis is defined as inflammation of the mucous membranes of the stomach and intestines. Acute gastroenteritis is characterized by diarrhea and, in some cases, vomiting, which results in fluid and electrolyte losses that lead to dehydration and electrolyte imbalances. The major causes of acute gastroenteritis include viruses (rotavirus, enteric adenovirus, Norwalk virus, and others), bacteria or their toxins (*Campylobacter, Salmonella, Shigella, Escherichia coli, Yersinia,* and others), and parasites *(Giardia lamblia, Cryptosporidium)* (Table 28-1). These pathogens cause illness by infecting the cells, producing enterotoxins or cytotoxins that damage the cells, or adhering to the walls of the intestines. In acute gastroenteritis, the small intestine is the most often affected.

Acute gastroenteritis is transmitted by the fecal-oral route from person to person or through contaminated water and food supplies. Spending time in day care facilities increases the risk for gastroenteritis, as does travel to developing countries. Most infections are self-limited, and prognosis is favorable with treatment. Malnourished children may have more severe infections and take longer to recover.

INCIDENCE

1. Acute gastroenteritis is the second most common condition affecting children (the cold is the first).
2. About half of all cases of gastroenteritis occur in a 3- to 4-month winter peak.
3. The highest rate of illness occurs in children between 3 months and 2 years of age.

TABLE 28-1
Characteristics of Acute Gastroenteritis

Pathogen	Vomiting	Diarrhea	Fever	Stool Characteristics	Abdominal Pain	Epidemiologic Features
Rotavirus	Very common	5-7 days; organism shed in stool even with mild or no symptoms	Common	Profuse, watery; green, yellow, or clear; no blood or pus	Some, with tenesmus	1-3 day incubation period
Enteric adenovirus	Occasionally	About 14 days	Occasionally, low grade	Watery		3-10 day incubation period
Norwalk virus	Very common	Less common, lasts 1-3 days	Common	Watery	Moderate to severe cramping	12-48 hour incubation period; outbreaks in school-aged children common
Salmonella	Sometimes, nausea common	2-7 days; 40% of cases excrete	Very common	Green, watery, and foul smelling;	Very common, with tenesmus	6-72 hour incubation period; 1-2%

(continued)	organisms in stool for 4 weeks; 45% of children 5 years continue to excrete organisms for 12 weeks or more	Uncommon	blood may or may not be present		become chronic carriers
Shigella	≥1 week; organisms shed for 7-30 days, rarely longer; if antibiotics are given shedding is reduced	Common	Mucoid, bloody, green with pus (dysentery form characterized by watery diarrhea, high fever, malaise followed by tenesmus and colitis in 24 hours)	Tenderness very common, cramps sometimes occur	1-7 day incubation period; easily transmitted; increased incidence in day care facilities—child should have negative stool culture results and no diarrhea before return to school or day care

Continued

TABLE 28-1
Characteristics of Acute Gastroenteritis—cont'd

Pathogen	Vomiting	Diarrhea	Fever	Stool Characteristics	Abdominal Pain	Epidemiologic Features
Campylobacter jejuni	Nausea but seldom vomiting	3 days to 1 week	Common	Starts as watery, frequently with blood or mucus; onset may be gradual or explosive	Cramping very common, tenderness common	2-4 day incubation period, sometimes as long as 7 days; breast-feeding may be protective
Escherichia coli—enterotoxigenic	None	5 days, sometimes as long as 10 days	Uncommon	Profuse watery stool, sometimes with mucus but no pus or blood	Cramping very common	10-hour to 6-day incubation period; seen in developing countries
Escherichia coli—enteroinvasive	Common	7-10 days	Common	Watery stool, may or may not be bloody (less volume than with enterotoxigenic strain)	Abdominal pain common	10-hour to 6-day incubation period

Escherichia coli—entero-pathogenic	Common	1 week in older child/adult; may last 2 weeks or longer in infants	Sometimes	Profuse watery stool, no blood or mucus	Cramping common	10-hour to 6-day incubation period
Yersinia entero-colitica	Not in children <4 years; common in older child	Few days to 6 weeks	Very common (up to 40° C)	Mucoid or watery, often with leukocytes or blood	Abdominal tenderness common	Typically has a 4-6 day incubation period; sometimes confused with appendicitis

4. Rotavirus is the causative agent in approximately 50% of hospital admissions for acute gastroenteritis; between 5% and 10% of admissions result from infection with enteric adenoviruses; and another 15% are due to bacterial causes.
5. Breast-fed infants contract gastroenteritis less often than formula-fed infants; maternal antibodies to some enteric pathogens are transferred in breast milk.

CLINICAL MANIFESTATIONS

1. Loose consistency of stools (diarrhea) with increased frequency
2. Vomiting (usually of short duration)
3. Fever (may or may not be present)
4. Abdominal cramping, tenesmus
5. Dry mucous membranes
6. Sunken fontanelle (infant)
7. Weight loss
8. Malaise

COMPLICATIONS

1. Severe dehydration, electrolyte imbalance
2. Decompensated hypovolemic shock (hypotension, metabolic acidosis, poor systemic perfusion)
3. Febrile seizures
4. Bacteremia

LABORATORY AND DIAGNOSTIC TESTS

1. Fecal occult blood test—to check for presence of blood (more common with bacterial origin)
2. Stool evaluation for volume, color, consistency, presence of mucus or pus
3. Complete blood count with differential
4. Enzyme immunoassay antigen tests—to confirm presence of rotavirus
5. Stool culture (if hospitalized, pus is present in stool, or course of diarrhea is prolonged)—to determine pathogen
6. Stool evaluation for ova and parasites
7. Duodenal aspiration (if *G. lamblia* is suspected)

8. Urinalysis and culture (specific gravity increases with dehydration; *Shigella* organisms are shed in urine)

MEDICAL MANAGEMENT

When the child is mildly dehydrated, rehydration may be accomplished orally on an outpatient basis with commercially available oral rehydration solutions (Pedialyte, Ricelyte). Oral rehydration fluids are given frequently, in small volumes (5 to 15 ml), even in the event of vomiting. Breast-fed infants can continue to be nursed during periods of diarrhea. In the case of severe dehydration, the child is admitted for intravenous (IV) therapy to correct dehydration. The amount of dehydration is calculated and fluid is replaced over 24 hours, at the same time that maintenance fluids are given.

When shock is present, fluid resuscitation commences immediately (20 ml/kg of normal saline solution or lactated Ringer's solution; repeat if needed). In these cases, when rapid peripheral IV access is unsuccessful, the intraosseous route may be used for emergency fluid administration in a child younger than 6 years of age. When systemic perfusion has been improved, correction of existing dehydration is begun.

Once rehydration is completed, the diet may be advanced to a regular diet of easily digested foods. Foods best tolerated are complex carbohydrates (rice, wheat, cereals, potatoes, and bread), yogurt, lean meats, fruits, and vegetables. The classic BRAT diet (bananas, rice, applesauce, and toast), although well tolerated, is low in protein, fat, and calories for energy. Juices, sports beverages, and soft drinks should be avoided.

Feeding and oral administration of rehydration fluids have reportedly decreased the duration of diarrhea. Early return to normal oral feedings is important, especially in cases of preexisting malnutrition.

Administration of antiemetics and antispasmodics is generally not recommended. Neither is the use of antibiotics indicated in most cases, because bacterial and viral gastroenteritis is self-limited. Antibiotics are used, however, in the treatment of diseases caused by *Shigella* organisms, *E. coli, Salmonella* organisms (when sepsis or localized infection is present), and

G. lamblia. Use of antibiotics may increase the duration of the carrier state in *Salmonella* infections.

NURSING ASSESSMENT
See the Gastrointestinal Assessment section in Appendix A.

NURSING DIAGNOSES
- Fluid volume, Risk for deficient
- Diarrhea
- Skin integrity, Risk for impaired
- Knowledge, Deficient

NURSING INTERVENTIONS
1. Promote and monitor child's fluid and electrolyte balance.
   a. Monitor IV fluids.
   b. Assess intake and output (weigh diapers).
   c. Assess hydration status.
   d. Monitor daily weight.
   e. Assess child's ability to rehydrate by mouth.
2. Prevent further gastrointestinal tract irritability.
   a. Assess child's ability to take nourishment by mouth (i.e., first provide oral rehydration fluids [Pedialyte, Ricelyte], then advance to regular diet of easily digested foods).
   b. Assess for signs of lactose intolerance when milk is introduced.
   c. Consult with dietitian about selection of foods.
3. Prevent skin irritation and breakdown.
   a. Change diapers frequently, assessing skin condition each time.
   b. Wash perineum with mild soap and water and expose perineum to air.
   c. Apply zinc oxide or lubricating ointment to perineum (acidic stools irritate skin).
4. Follow universal precautions and/or enteric precautions to prevent transmission of infection (refer to institution's policies and procedures).

5. Provide for child's developmental needs during hospitalization.
   a. Provide age-appropriate toys (see the relevant section in Appendix B).
   b. Incorporate home routine into hospital care (e.g., feeding practices, bedtime ritual).
   c. Encourage expression of feelings through age-appropriate means.
6. Provide emotional and other support to family.
   a. Encourage verbalization of concerns.
   b. Refer to social services as needed.
   c. Provide for physical comforts (e.g., place to sleep and bathe).

Discharge Planning and Home Care

1. Instruct parents and child about personal and environmental hygiene.
   a. Good hand washing
   b. Sanitary disposal of excreta
   c. Sanitary food preparation
   d. Good toileting practices
   e. Safe drinking water
2. Reinforce dietary information provided to parents about menu planning.
3. Instruct parents to observe for and report signs of dehydration or problems with oral rehydration and advancement of feedings.
4. Instruct parents about follow-up appointment.

CLIENT OUTCOMES

1. Child's gastrointestinal function will return to normal.
2. Child will be well hydrated.
3. Parents and child will understand home care and medical follow-up needed.

REFERENCES

American Academy of Pediatrics: Practice parameter: the management of acute gastroenteritis in young children, Provisional Committee on Quality

Improvement, Subcommittee on Acute Gastroenteritis, *Pediatrics* 97(3):424, 1996.

American Academy of Pediatrics, Pickering LK, editor: *2000 Red book: report of the Committee on Infectious Diseases,* 25th ed, Elk Grove Village, Ill, 2000, The Academy.

Dennehy PH: Transmission of rotavirus and other enteric pathogens in the home, *Pediatr Infect Dis J* 19(10):S103, 2000.

Larson CE: Safety and efficacy of oral rehydration therapy for the treatment of diarrhea and gastroenteritis in pediatrics, *Pediatr Nurs* 26(2):177, 2000.

Perlstein PH et al: Implementing an evidence-based acute gastroenteritis guideline at a children's hospital, *Jt Comm J Qual Improv* 28(1):20, 2002.

Wright AL et al: Increasing breastfeeding rates to reduce infant illness at the community level, *Pediatrics* 101(5):837, 1998.

29

❖

Gastroesophageal Reflux

❖

PATHOPHYSIOLOGY

Gastroesophageal reflux (GER) is the presence of abnormal amounts of gastric contents in the esophagus, upper airways, and tracheobronchial area. The reflux of gastric contents can lead to inflammation and stricture of the esophagus. Resulting effects include aspiration of gastric contents, recurrent pneumonia, pulmonary disease, esophagitis, and esophageal stricture. Factors that can predispose the infant or child to GER are (1) high lower esophageal sphincter (LES) pressure, (2) high volume of reflux material in the esophagus, (3) rate of gastric secretion, and (4) inability of the stomach to empty. Resolution of GER is often a maturational process. However, a child may require surgery if he or she does not respond to medical management.

INCIDENCE

1. Vomiting occurs in 18% to 40% of children with GER.
2. Failure to thrive occurs in 34% of these children.
3. Bleeding occurs in 28% of these children.
4. Pulmonary complications occur in 12% of these children.

CLINICAL MANIFESTATIONS

1. Chronic vomiting (most common)
2. Weight loss, failure to thrive
3. Apnea (in infants) due to aspiration or obstruction
4. Hematemesis or melena due to esophageal bleeding
5. Recurrent bronchitis and/or pneumonia
6. Irritability, loss of appetite

COMPLICATIONS

1. Aspiration pneumonia
2. Respiratory disease (asthma, cough, stridor)
3. Apnea and cyanosis
4. Esophagitis
5. Chest pain/heartburn
6. Gastric fistula
7. Herniation

LABORATORY AND DIAGNOSTIC TESTS

1. Esophageal pH measurement (less than 4.0 is diagnostic)
2. Electric impedance measurement
3. Endoscopy—to detect presence of gross and microscopic esophagitis
4. Barium esophagram—to detect anatomic abnormalities; often fails to detect intermittent reflux
5. Nuclear medicine scintiscan—to assess gastric emptying
6. Manometry—to assess esophageal motility and LES function

MEDICAL MANAGEMENT

The treatment of GER reflects the severity of symptoms. Conservative management consists of feeding thickened formula; feeding small, frequent meals; and positioning prone with the head of the bed elevated. Placement in an infant seat postprandially is contraindicated because such seats increase intraabdominal pressure. Acid suppression and neutralization and the use of prokinetic medications are frequently recommended. In infants continuous tube feedings may be used when conventional medical treatment has failed.

When medical management fails to control the symptoms and complications of GER disease, surgical intervention is indicated. A fundoplication is performed. The upper end of the stomach is wrapped around the lower portion of the esophagus, and the fundus is sutured in front of the esophagus to create a circular acute-angle valve mechanism. Placement of a gastrostomy tube ensures adequate nutrition and simplifies care.

NURSING ASSESSMENT

1. See the Gastrointestinal Assessment section in Appendix A.
2. Assess feeding history.
3. Assess hydration status.
4. Assess frequency and volume of emesis and length of time between feedings and emesis.
5. Assess weight gain.

NURSING DIAGNOSES

- Fluid volume, Deficient
- Pain
- Nutrition: less than body requirements, Imbalanced
- Gas exchange, Impaired
- Knowledge, Deficient
- Home maintenance, Impaired

NURSING INTERVENTIONS

1. Promote adequate nutritional and fluid intake.
   a. Maintain head of bed in 30- to 60-degree position for 30 to 40 minutes after feeding.
   b. Raise head of bed with 6-inch blocks.
   c. Provide small, frequent feedings every 2 to 3 hours.
   d. Thicken formula with cereal.
   e. Provide last meal of day several hours before bedtime.
   f. Weigh child daily.
   g. Monitor intake and output.
2. Observe, monitor, and report signs of respiratory distress; assess for changes in respiratory status.
3. Preoperatively, prepare child and family for surgery.
4. Monitor surgical site for intactness.
5. Prevent abdominal distention.
   a. Maintain patency of nasogastric (NG) or gastrostomy tube if placed.
   b. Check position of NG tube.
   c. Auscultate for bowel sounds.
6. Monitor for signs and symptoms of postoperative hemorrhage.
   a. Decreased blood pressure and increased apical pulse
   b. Gross blood in NG drainage

  c. Coffee-ground NG drainage expected for first
   24 hours
7. Assist parents in verbalization of feelings—may express
  anger, guilt, or frustration because they feel inadequate or
  responsible.
8. Provide developmentally appropriate stimulation activities
  (see Appendix B).

🏠 Discharge Planning and Home Care

1. Instruct parents about medication administration.
2. Instruct parents about feeding techniques.
3. Instruct parents to report any vomiting or presence of
  frank blood.

CLIENT OUTCOMES

1. Child will have consistent weight gain.
2. Child will have decreased frequency and volume of emesis.
3. Child will have decreased pain (heartburn).
4. Child will not aspirate.

REFERENCES

Ault DL, Schmidt D: Diagnosis and management of gastroesophageal reflux in infants and children, *Nurse Pract* 23(6):78, 1998.

Berube M: Gastroesophageal reflux, *J Soc Parenter Nutr* 2(1):43, 1997.

Hockenberry M: *Wong's nursing care of infants and children,* ed 7, St Louis, 2003, Mosby.

Marcon MA: Advances in the diagnosis and treatment of gastroesophageal reflux disease, *Curr Opin Pediatr* 9:490, 1997.

Tsou VM, Bishop PR: Gastroesophageal reflux in children, *Otolaryngol Clin North Am* 31:419, 1998.

30

❖

Glomerulonephritis

❖

PATHOPHYSIOLOGY

Glomerulonephritis is a term used for a collection of disorders that involve the renal glomeruli (the renal glomeruli are responsible for filtering body fluids and wastes). Two types of this disease are seen, acute and chronic, with chronic being the progressive form. Acute glomerulonephritis is the most common form of nephritis in children. It is an inflammation of the glomeruli that usually follows a streptococcal upper respiratory tract infection. It is considered an immune complex disease. The glomerular injury is induced by antigen-antibody complexes trapped in the glomerular filter. The glomeruli become edematous and are infiltrated with polymorphonuclear leukocytes, which occlude the capillary lumen. This condition results in decreased plasma filtration, causing excessive accumulation of water and retention of sodium. The resultant plasma and interstitial fluid volumes lead to circulatory congestion and edema. Hypertension is associated with glomerulonephritis.

INCIDENCE

1. Glomerulonephritis is most common in school-aged children.
2. Ages of peak incidence are from 2 to 6 years.
3. The disorder occurs predominantly in boys in childhood, but no male or female predilection is seen in adolescence.
4. Sixty percent to 80% of children with acute glomerulonephritis have a history of a preceding upper respiratory tract infection or otitis media (typically, the child was in good health before the infection).

181

CLINICAL MANIFESTATIONS

1. Nephritis tends to have an average latency period of approximately 10 days, with onset of symptoms 10 days after the initial infection.
2. Initial signs are puffiness of the face, periorbital edema, anorexia, and dark urine.
3. Edema tends to be more prominent in the face in the morning; then it spreads to the abdomen and the extremities during the day (moderate edema may not be recognized by someone who is unfamiliar with the child).
4. Urinary output is decreased.
5. Urine is cloudy, smoky, or described as having the color of tea or cola.
6. The child is pale, irritable, and lethargic.
7. Younger children may appear ill but seldom express specific complaints.
8. Older children may complain of headaches, abdominal discomfort, vomiting, and dysuria.
9. Mild to moderate hypertension may be present.

COMPLICATIONS

Once acute glomerulonephritis progresses to the chronic stage, the following complications may be seen:

1. Deteriorating renal function (generally reflected by clinical manifestations and laboratory findings)
2. Proteinuria
3. Edema
4. Hypertension
5. Hematuria
6. Anemia (manifestation of progressive disease)
7. Hypertensive encephalopathy (characterized by headache, vomiting, irritability, convulsions, and coma)—can result from the chronic hypertension
8. Cardiac failure, possibly a result of an increase in blood volume secondary to retention of sodium and water—associated with pulmonary congestion
9. End-stage renal disease

LABORATORY AND DIAGNOSTIC TESTS

No diagnostic tests are specifically indicated for the diagnosis of glomerulonephritis. However, the following are commonly performed:

1. Examination of urine—proteinuria (1+ to 4+), hematuria; presence of casts, red blood cells, and white blood cells; decreased creatine clearance rates
2. Blood tests—elevated blood urea nitrogen, serum creatinine, and uric acid levels; electrolyte alterations (metabolic acidosis; decreased sodium and calcium; increased potassium, phosphorus, serum albumin, and cholesterol); mild anemia and leukocytosis; elevated antibody titers (antistreptolysin, antihyaluronidase, or antideoxyribonuclease B) and erythrocyte sedimentation rate
3. Renal biopsy—may be indicated; if performed, possible findings are increased number of cells in each glomerulus and subepithelial "humps" containing immunoglobulin and complement

MEDICAL MANAGEMENT

Acute glomerulonephritis has no specific treatment; thus therapy is targeted at the symptoms. Marked hypertension may be treated with diuretics and/or antihypertensives. Appropriate antibiotics are used for acute infections. Some medicinal approaches for treatment of chronic glomerulonephritis have included administration of glucocorticoids and immunosuppressive agents.

NURSING ASSESSMENT

1. See the Renal Assessment section in Appendix A.
2. Assess nutritional intake.
3. Assess fluid status.

NURSING DIAGNOSES

- Fluid volume, Excess
- Nutrition: less than body requirements, Imbalanced
- Knowledge, Deficient

NURSING INTERVENTIONS

1. Maintain bed rest and keep child comfortable until diuresis occurs; after diuresis, encourage quiet activity.
2. Closely monitor vital signs (especially blood pressure).
3. When hypertension is present, limit sodium intake and administer ordered medications.
4. Monitor urine for protein and occult blood.
5. Promote adequate nutritional intake: encourage high-carbohydrate meals, serve preferred foods, and try small, frequent feedings.
6. Limit potassium intake if hyperkalemia occurs.
7. Record weight daily and accurately record intake and output.
8. Monitor for complications—significant changes in vital signs, change in appearance or volume of urine, excessive weight gain, visual disturbances, motor disturbances, seizure activity, severe pain, or any behavioral changes.

🪦 Discharge Planning and Home Care

1. Provide family with education about child's illness and treatment plan.
2. Instruct about any medications child will take at home.
3. Instruct parents and child to monitor blood pressure and weight, and to obtain urinalyses for several months; follow-up appointments should be arranged.
4. Instruct parents to contact physician if any change is seen in child's condition, such as signs of infection, edema, alteration in eating habits, abdominal pain, headaches, change in appearance or amount of urine, or lethargy.
5. Explain any dietary restrictions to parents.

CLIENT OUTCOMES

1. Child will have a return to normal renal function.
2. Child and family will understand home care and follow-up needs.

REFERENCES

Higgens PM: Acute poststreptococcal glomerulonephritis in general practice: the contribution of infection to its onset and course, *Epidemiol Infect* 116(2):193, 1996.

Kasahara T et al: Prognosis of acute poststreptococcal glomerulonephritis is excellent in children when adequately diagnosed, *Pediatr Int* 43(4):364, 2001.

Lang MM, Towers C: Identifying post streptococcal glomerulonephritis, *Nurse Pract* 26(8):34, 2001.

Pan GG: Glomerulonephritis in childhood, *Curr Opin Pediatr* 9(2):154, 2001.

31

❖

Hemolytic-Uremic Syndrome

❖

PATHOPHYSIOLOGY

Hemolytic-uremic syndrome is an intravascular coagulation condition that primarily affects the kidney. It consists of the following symptomatology: (1) renal failure, (2) hemolytic anemia with fragmented red blood cells and platelets, and (3) thrombocytopenia. The exact cause is unknown, although findings suggest that most cases of idiopathic hemolytic-uremic syndrome are associated with one or the other of the enteric pathogens *Escherichia coli* and *Shigella dysenteriae*. The clinical manifestations result from changes in the capillary endothelium caused by the etiologic agent. The endothelial changes result in the following pathologic responses: (1) mechanical trauma to erythrocytes and platelets, which shortens their life span and results in anemia and thrombocytopenia; and (2) decreased renal blood flow and glomerular filtration rate, which results in cortical necrosis and consequent renal failure and acquired hemolytic anemia in infants and children. The severity of the condition varies. The length of the oliguria phase correlates with the ultimate prognosis for recovery. In addition, the prognosis is related to the efficacy and promptness of treatment.

INCIDENCE

1. A seasonal variation exists, with an increased incidence during spring and fall.
2. Hemolytic-uremic syndrome is most commonly seen in children 6 months to 5 years of age.
3. The incidence of hypertension as a long-term complication varies from 10% to 50%.

4. Hemolytic-uremic syndrome affects males and females equally.
5. It is uncommon for a sibling to be affected.
6. Mortality is 10% to 25%.

CLINICAL MANIFESTATIONS
Prodromal Phase

1. Hemolytic-uremic syndrome usually follows gastroenteritis or viral illness.
2. Prodromal phase in older children resembles upper respiratory tract illness.
3. Prodromal symptoms may last 1 week, whereas other symptoms may recur in children who appear to have recovered; severity varies. (See Box 31-1 for four types of clinical manifestation.)

BOX 31-1
Clinical Manifestations

Mild
- No anemia
- Oliguria*
- Hypertension*
- Seizures*

Severe
- Anuria for longer than 24 hours

Deteriorating Renal Function
- Progressive oliguria
- Azotemia
- Complete renal failure—may not occur
- Severe hypertension
- Cardiac failure

Recurrent Hemolytic-Uremic Syndrome
- First occurrence—mild
- Recurrent occurrence—mild to severe

*Child may manifest one or more symptoms but not all three.

Acute Phase

1. Oliguria, amber urine
2. Renal failure (metabolic disturbance or acidosis; hypocalcemia or hyperkalemia)
3. Oliguria/anuria for longer than 1 week, then diuresis
4. Abdominal pain (caused by splenic enlargement or gastrointestinal [GI] involvement)
5. Edema
6. Hypertension
7. Mild icterus
8. Pallor
9. Systemic bleeding manifestations—purpura, petechiae
10. Alteration in neurologic status
11. Anemia associated with uremia
12. Anorexia
13. Seizures
14. Moderate to severe respiratory distress caused by congestive heart failure and circulatory overload

COMPLICATIONS

1. Neurologic—mortality rate in children with neurologic symptoms (seizures, coma) is 90%.
2. Disseminated intravascular coagulation—primarily affects vasculature of kidney, nervous system, and GI tract.

LABORATORY AND DIAGNOSTIC TESTS

1. Renal scan—to assess renal perfusion
2. Renal biopsy—to assess renal involvement
3. Serum protein level—increased
4. Complete blood count—decreased hemoglobin; increased white blood cell count; significant reticulocytosis; reticulocyte count higher than 2%
5. Platelet count—less than 140,000/mm^3; remains low for 7 to 14 days
6. Serum albumin level—decreased
7. Arterial blood gas values—decreased pH; acidosis with acute renal failure
8. Electrolyte levels—consistent with renal failure (hyponatremia, hyperkalemia)

9. Tests for hyperuricemia, hypocalcemia, hyperphosphatemia
10. Urinalysis—gross hematuria, proteinuria, casts
11. Blood urea nitrogen, creatinine levels—increased; reflect severity of renal failure

MEDICAL MANAGEMENT

Early diagnosis and aggressive treatment are the goals. Early intervention with peritoneal dialysis is the most effective treatment for children who have been anuric for 24 hours or who demonstrate oliguria with hypertension and seizures. Supportive care is directed toward vascular support and stabilization.

Drugs such as corticosteroids, anticoagulants, or antiplatelet agents have not been found to be effective.

NURSING ASSESSMENT

1. See the Renal Assessment section in Appendix A.
2. Assess hydration status.
3. Assess cardiovascular status.

NURSING DIAGNOSES

- Fluid volume, Excess
- Cardiac output, Decreased
- Infection, Risk for
- Tissue integrity, Impaired
- Knowledge, Deficient
- Anxiety

NURSING INTERVENTIONS

1. Monitor and maintain fluid and electrolyte balance.
   a. Monitor types of fluids and administration rate to avoid fluid overload and cerebral edema.
   b. Accurately record intake and output.
   c. Record daily weights (twice per day during acute phase).
   d. Monitor blood pressure and pulse pressure.
   e. Replace fluids from urinary loss with isotonic solution (normal saline or lactated Ringer's solution).
   f. Assess hydration status every 4 to 6 hours during acute phase.

    g. Perform arterial pressure and central venous pressure monitoring.

2. Monitor electrolytes and observe for signs of imbalance.
   a. Hyperkalemia—muscular instability, electrocardiogram changes (peaked T waves, wide QRS complex, prolonged PR interval), cardiac arrhythmias
   b. Hypocalcemia—coma, seizures
   c. Hyponatremia—seizures
   d. Hypoglycemia—seizures

3. Transfuse with blood products as indicated.
   a. Washed packed red blood cells—for low hemoglobin level; transfuse slowly; do not raise hemoglobin level higher than 7 to 8 g/dl
   b. Platelets—as needed for bleeding

4. Observe and report signs and symptoms of impending complications.
   a. Shock
   b. Infection
   c. Disseminated intravascular coagulation
   d. Heart failure
   e. Potassium intoxication
   f. Overhydration
   g. Seizures
   h. Neurologic disturbance—lethargy, coma, hyperactivity
   i. Pulmonary edema
   j. Hypertension

5. Monitor for nutritional status; nasogastric feedings or hyperalimentation may be needed.

6. Prepare child and family for peritoneal dialysis or hemodialysis if indicated; indications include the following:
   a. Anuria for 24 to 48 hours
   b. Central nervous system disturbance
   c. Congestive heart failure
   d. Bleeding (GI and cutaneous)
   e. Blood urea nitrogen level higher than 150 mg/100 ml
   f. Uncontrollable hyperkalemia
   g. Hyponatremia of less than 130 mEq/L
   h. Change in neurologic status—lethargy to coma or hyperactivity

    i. Hyperphosphatemia of higher than 8 mg/100 ml
    j. Uncontrollable acidosis
    k. Hypocalcemia of less than 8 mg/100 ml
7. Provide information about procedures before they are performed and reinforce data provided to parents.

🔺 Discharge Planning and Home Care

1. Instruct child and family regarding dietary restrictions.
2. Instruct child and family regarding medications.

CLIENT OUTCOMES

1. Child will have normal or near-normal renal function.
2. Child will have return to normal blood pressure or control of blood pressure.
3. Child will have return to normal neurologic function or control of central nervous system symptoms.

REFERENCES

Behrman RE, Kliegman R, Jenson HB: *Nelson textbook of pediatrics,* ed 16, Philadelphia, 2000, WB Saunders.

Corrigan JJ, Boineau FG: Hemolytic-uremic syndrome, *Pediatr Rev* 22(11):365, 2001.

Hazinski MF: *Manual of pediatric critical care,* St Louis, 1999, Mosby.

Hockenberry M: *Wong's nursing care of infants and children,* 7th ed, St Louis, 2003, Mosby.

32

◆

Hemophilia

◆

PATHOPHYSIOLOGY

Hemophilia is a congenital blood coagulation disorder in which the child is deficient in clotting factor VIII (hemophilia A) or factor IX (hemophilia B, or Christmas disease). It is an inherited disorder that is transmitted by an X-linked recessive gene from the maternal side. Factor VIII and factor IX are plasma proteins that are necessary components of blood coagulation; they are needed for the formation of fibrin clots at the site of vascular injury. Severe hemophilia results when plasma concentrations of factors VIII and IX are less than 1%. Moderate hemophilia occurs with plasma concentrations between 1% and 5%. In mild hemophilia (severe bleeding only after major trauma and surgery), plasma concentrations are between 6% and 50% of the normal level. The clinical manifestations depend on the child's age and the severity of the deficiency of factors VIII and IX. Severe hemophilia is characterized by recurrent hemorrhages, occurring either spontaneously or after relatively minor trauma (20 to 30 episodes per year). The most common sites of hemorrhage are the joints, muscles, and soft tissue. The most common joint sites are the knees, elbows, ankles, shoulders, and hips. The muscles most often affected are the forearm flexor, the gastrocnemius, and the iliopsoas. Bleeding into the joint or muscle can lead to pain, limited mobility, need for ongoing physical therapy, and some degree of impaired functioning. Life-threatening bleeding episodes can occur in the brain, gastrointestinal tract, and neck and throat. Because of improvements in treatment, almost all individuals with hemophilia are expected to live a normal life span. Preliminary data from experimental gene therapy are promising.

INCIDENCE

1. Incidence is 1 in 7500 male births.
2. Incidence of hemophilia A is 20.6 in 100,000.
3. Incidence of hemophilia B is 5.3 in 100,000.
4. Twenty-five thousand males are severely affected.
5. The family histories of two thirds of affected children reveal an X-linked recessive form of inheritance.
6. About 30% of cases are the result of new mutations.
7. Central nervous system bleeding occurs in 3% of affected children.
8. Spontaneous bleeding and posttraumatic intracranial bleeding are associated with a 34% mortality rate and a 50% rate of long-term morbidity.
9. Ten percent of individuals with hemophilia A and hemophilia B develop immunoglobulin G antibodies that inhibit the activity of factors VIII and IX.
10. Hemophilia is one of the eight most costly diseases to treat.
11. Eighty percent of individuals with hemophilia in developing countries receive no treatment.

CLINICAL MANIFESTATIONS

Infancy (for Diagnosis)

1. Prolonged bleeding after circumcision.
2. Subcutaneous ecchymoses over bony prominences (at 3 to 4 months of age)
3. Large hematoma after infections
4. Bleeding from oral mucosa
5. Soft-tissue hemorrhages

Bleeding Episodes (Throughout Life Span)

1. Initial symptom—pain
2. After pain—swelling, warmth, and decreased mobility

Long-Term Sequelae

Prolonged bleeding into muscle causes nerve compression and muscle fibrosis.

COMPLICATIONS

1. Progressive arthritis/arthropathy
2. Compartment syndrome
3. Muscle atrophy
4. Muscle contractures
5. Paralysis
6. Intracranial bleeding
7. Neurologic impairment
8. Hypertension
9. Renal impairment
10. Splenomegaly
11. Hepatitis
12. Cirrhosis
13. Human immunodeficiency virus (HIV) infection from exposure to contaminated blood products
14. Formation of antibodies as antagonists to factors VIII and IX
15. Allergic transfusion reaction to blood products
16. Hemolytic anemia
17. Thrombosis and/or thromboembolism
18. Chronic pain

LABORATORY AND DIAGNOSTIC TESTS

1. Screening tests for blood coagulation
   a. Platelet count—normal in mild to moderate hemophilia
   b. Prothrombin time—normal in mild to moderate hemophilia
   c. Partial thromboplastin time—normal in mild to moderate hemophilia; prolonged in moderately severe hemophilia measures adequacy of intrinsic coagulation cascade
   d. Bleeding time—normal in mild to moderate hemophilia; assesses formation of platelet plugs in capillaries
   e. Functional assays of factors VIII and IX—confirm diagnosis
   f. Thrombin clotting time normal in mild to moderate hemophilia
2. Liver biopsy (sometimes)—used to obtain tissue for pathologic examination and culture

3. Liver function tests (sometimes)—used to detect presence of liver disease (e.g., serum glutamic-pyruvic transaminase, serum glutamic-oxaloacetic transaminase, alkaline phosphatase, bilirubin levels)

MEDICAL MANAGEMENT

The management of hemophilia consists of the administration of factor VIII or IX on a prophylactic basis or to treat bleeding episodes. Prophylactic administration is performed two to three times a week to maintain levels of factor VIII or IX. The amount administered depends on the plasma level of the deficient factor needed to treat the specific bleeding episode, and it must be sufficient to allow for the distribution of the factor throughout the body and its clearance from plasma. Dose varies from 20 U/kg to more than 100 U/kg administered by intravenous push or continuous intravenous infusion. Other methods used to treat bleeding episodes are the infusion of frozen plasma and cryoprecipitate (factor VIII). Desmopressin (DDAVP) is also used to increase plasma levels of factor VIII and can be used for nontransfusional treatment of individuals with mild or moderate hemophilia. Before the introduction of hepatitis vaccinations and viral inactivation procedures, hepatitis A, B, and C and HIV infection were serious complications associated with treatment. Plasma-derived factors are now safer for use, and recombinant products are used in treating approximately 60% of individuals with severe hemophilia in the United States. Nationwide federally funded hemophilia treatment centers staffed by interdisciplinary teams composed of hematologists, orthopedic specialists, dentists, nurses, social workers, and physical therapists provide comprehensive and interdisciplinary care to individuals and their families.

NURSING ASSESSMENT

1. See the Neurologic Assessment section in Appendix A.
2. Assess child for verbal and nonverbal behaviors indicating pain.
3. Assess site of involvement for extent of bleeding and sensory, nerve, and motor impairment.

4. Assess child's or adolescent's ability to engage in self-care activities (i.e., brushing teeth).
5. Assess child's or adolescent's level of development.
6. Assess child's or adolescent's and family's readiness for discharge and ability to manage home treatment regimen.

NURSING DIAGNOSES

- Fluid volume, Risk for deficient
- Pain
- Injury, Risk for
- Knowledge, Deficient
- Growth and development, Delayed
- Family processes, Interrupted
- Therapeutic regimen management, Ineffective
- Mobility, Impaired physical
- Caregiver role strain

NURSING INTERVENTIONS

1. The following interventions relate to acute episodes:
   1. Monitor child's or adolescent's response to administration of plasma products. Record amount of factor received, time, and child's response to treatment.
   2. Monitor child's pain behaviors and response to administration of pain medication and to nonpharmacologic measures to relieve pain (refer to Appendix H).
      a. Acetaminophen (avoid aspirin)
      b. Narcotic analgesics
      c. Application of ice to affected joint
      d. Immobilization of affected limb
   3. Monitor child or adolescent for further bleeding episodes; observe for signs and symptoms of bleeding.
      a. Symptoms manifested depend on site of bleeding, such as muscles, joints, or brain.
   4. Protect child or adolescent from further injury.
      a. Pad child's crib or bed.
      b. Apply pressure after venipunctures.
      c. Apply fibrin or gelatin foam to bleeding sites.

5. Instruct and monitor child or adolescent regarding dental care.
   a. Use of soft-bristle toothbrush
   b. Good nutritional intake
   c. Avoidance of excessive amounts of sweets
   d. Chewing of sugarless gum
   e. Need for regular dental visits
   f. Use of factor replacement before dental work
6. Provide education on long-term management of hemophilia.
   a. Understanding of genetics and heredity
   b. Understanding of pathophysiology
   c. Recognition of signs and symptoms
   d. Instruction in monitoring for bleeding episodes and complications
   e. Knowledge about when to call for medical assistance
   f. Instruction in how to administer factor products and medication and monitor for side effects
   g. Avoidance of nonsteroidal antiinflammatory drugs
   h. Use of universal precautions
7. Encourage quiet age-appropriate play or diversional activities (see Appendix B).
8. Provide age-appropriate explanations before treatments and procedures (see the Preparation for Procedures or Surgery section in Appendix J).
9. Provide emotional support to family (see the Supportive Care section in Appendix J).

🏠 Discharge Planning and Home Care

1. Instruct child or adolescent and parents on assuming self-care responsibilities for long-term management of hemophilia.
   a. Administration of replacement for deficient factor
   b. Signs and symptoms of bleeding episodes
   c. Use of universal precautions
   d. Possible side effects and complications of treatment
   e. Knowledge of how to institute emergency measures

    f. Ordering, storage, and handling of factor products and medications

    g. Care of central venous device/infusion site

    h. Prevention of and monitoring for complications

2. Discuss options and plan lifestyle activities to support achievement of developmentally appropriate milestones related to schooling, social relationships, and leisure and recreational pursuits, and achievement of self-care skills in activities of daily living (Appendix L).

3. Learn safety measures to prevent further injuries (avoidance of contact sports and physical play).

4. Discuss with parents and child methods to encourage autonomy and self-determination.

5. Refer family to appropriate community-based resources (see Appendix L).

    a. Health insurance coverage

    b. Community services

    c. Counseling on psychosocial concerns related to raising child with disability

    d. Genetic screening and counseling for family members

6. Encourage parents and child to express feelings about hemophilia and limitations it imposes on activities.

    a. Feelings of inferiority associated with having disease

    b. Feelings of inadequacy associated with disease

    c. Feelings of parental guilt, overprotection

    d. Feelings of stress associated with uncertain disease course and daily management

CLIENT OUTCOMES

1. Child's or adolescent's bleeding episodes will be controlled.

2. Child or adolescent and family will adhere to long-term treatment regimen.

3. Child or adolescent will attain developmental milestones.

4. Child or adolescent will learn to become independent and self-sufficient.

REFERENCES

Carlisle I: Factors of life, *Nurs Times* 93(6):56, 1997.

DiMichele MD: Hemophilia 1996, new approach to an old disease, *Pediatr Clin North Am* 43(3):709, 1996.

Jarvinen O et al: Carrier testing of children for two X-linked diseases: a retrospective study of comprehension of the test results and social and psychological significance of the testing, *Pediatrics* 106(6):1460, 2000.

Mannucci P, Tuddenham E: Medical progress: the hemophilias—from royal genes to gene therapy, *N Engl J Med* 344(23):1773, 2001.

Nursing Working Group, National Hemophilia Foundation: The basics of hemophilia, New York, The Foundation, available at http://www.hemophilia.org/resources/nurses/hemophilia.ppt, accessed December 8, 2002.

Orto C: Joint bleeding in hemophilia: a common complication, *Nursing 97* 27(4):32L, 1997.

Stover B: Training the client in self-management of hemophilia, *J Intravenous Nurs* 23(5):304, 2000.

Witkoff L: Iliopsoas muscle hemorrhage, *Nursing 2002* 32(2):104, 2002.

33

◇

Hepatitis

◇

PATHOPHYSIOLOGY

Hepatitis, or inflammation of the liver, can be caused by a viral agent. Hepatitis viruses can be classified into six types: hepatitis A virus (HAV), hepatitis B virus (HBV), hepatitis C virus (HCV), hepatitis D virus (HDV), hepatitis E virus (HEV), and hepatitis G virus (HGV). The hepatocytes (epithelial cells of the liver) are damaged either directly by the virus or by the body's immune response to the virus; in either case, there is altered cellular function that leads to inflammation, necrosis, and autolysis of the liver. Regeneration of cells begins when damaged cells are removed by phagocytosis. Usually recovery is with minimal residual damage, although chronic hepatitis and cirrhosis may develop.

Hepatitis A

Hepatitis A is the most highly contagious form of hepatitis and characteristically is an acute self-limited illness. It is transmitted primarily through the fecal-oral route. It can also be transmitted by unsanitary food handlers, contaminated food supplies, and shellfish from sewage-contaminated waters. It is rarely transmitted through transfusions. Epidemics of hepatitis A have been reported in institutions housing or caring for large numbers of children, such as day care centers, schools, and homes for the mentally retarded. The incubation period is approximately 1 month. Jaundice appears 4 to 6 weeks after exposure. The disease is transmissible 2 weeks prior to the onset of jaundice due to the high concentration of virus in the stool before definitive symptoms are exhibited. The communicable state continues up to 1 week after the onset of jaundice. Hepatitis A manifests a wide spectrum of symptoms and does not lead to chronic hepatitis. Children may have minimal symptoms or be asymptomatic. The child is rarely hospitalized, and there is no known carrier state.

Hepatitis B and Hepatitis C

HBV and HCV are transmitted through blood or blood derivatives and body secretions (wound exudates, semen, saliva, breast milk, urine). Hepatitis B occurs most commonly in the following populations of children: (1) infants whose mothers are chronic carriers of the viral antigen HB_sAg, (2) children receiving frequent transfusions or hemodialysis (may also develop hepatitis C), (3) children involved in intravenous drug abuse (may also develop hepatitis C), (4) institutionalized children, and (5) children with person-to-person contact with infected individuals. The incubation period for hepatitis B averages 90 days, whereas that for hepatitis C averages 45 days. Children with hepatitis C are typically asymptomatic. In the United States more than 60% of the cases of hepatitis C are associated with transfusions of blood or blood products. However, an improved blood screening test has greatly reduced the number of new cases. A carrier state and the development of chronic liver disease are possible with hepatitis B and C.

Hepatitis D

HDV can cause infection and clinical manifestations only in association with hepatitis B infection. The virus acts as a parasite of HBV. Coinfection with HDV increases the severity of the HBV infection, creating a more fulminating course and enhancing the potential for chronic liver disease. Hepatitis D is most common in hemophiliac individuals and intravenous drug abusers.

Hepatitis E

Hepatitis E is epidemic or enterically transmitted non-A, non-B hepatitis. Transmission occurs via the fecal-oral route. It can also be transmitted via contaminated water and is often seen after natural disasters in the developing regions of the world. No diagnostic test is available, so other forms of hepatitis must be ruled out.

Hepatitis G

The primary cause of HGV infection is through transfusion and organ transplantation. Transmitted through blood, this virus has been detected in up to 2% of American blood donors. Infections may persist up to 20 years with only rare elevation of liver enzyme levels. This type of hepatitis is usually benign, but more research is needed to determine long-term effects.

INCIDENCE

1. Approximately 90% of young children and infants with hepatitis do not exhibit jaundice.
2. Up to 90% of children younger than 1 year of age, 30% of children 1 to 5 years of age, and 5% of children older than 5 years of age with hepatitis B develop chronic hepatitis.
3. Hepatitis A is the most common type of hepatitis in children.
4. Approximately 200,000 cases of hepatitis B are reported each year; the majority of these are in adolescents and young adults.
5. Tropical and developing nations have a higher incidence of hepatitis A than industrialized and temperate-zone nations.
6. Incidence of hepatitis D is difficult to measure because it occurs concurrently with hepatitis B and may not be readily diagnosed.

CLINICAL MANIFESTATIONS
Hepatitis A

1. Acute febrile illness
2. Jaundice (develops as fever drops)
3. Anorexia
4. Nausea and vomiting
5. Malaise
6. Dark urine (precedes jaundice)
7. Hepatomegaly
8. Splenomegaly
9. No symptoms in 70% of children under 7 years of age

Hepatitis B, C, D, E, and G

1. Insidious onset
2. Jaundice

3. Anorexia
4. Malaise
5. Nausea
6. Abnormalities in liver function test results
7. Prodromal symptoms—arthralgia, arthritis, erythematous maculopapular rash
8. Polyarteritis nodosa
9. Hepatitis D—intensifies symptoms of hepatitis B and increases possibility of a chronic condition
10. Hepatitis C—characterized by mild asymptomatic infection with insidious onset of jaundice and malaise

COMPLICATIONS
Hepatitis A
Progression to fulminating disease (rare)

Hepatitis B and C
1. Hepatocellular cancer
2. Liver failure
3. Immunodeficiency
4. Cirrhosis
5. Fulminating hepatitis
6. Massive hepatic necrosis
7. Carrier state (persistent viral infection without symptoms)
8. Chronic liver disease (in 50% of individuals with hepatitis C)

Hepatitis D
1. Fulminating hepatitis
2. Liver failure
3. Carrier state

LABORATORY AND DIAGNOSTIC TESTS
1. Serum glutamic-oxaloacetic transaminase (SGOT) level—increased
2. Serum glutamic-pyruvic transaminase (SGPT) level—increased
3. Bilirubin level—elevated

4. Immunoglobulin M (IgM) antibodies (HAV antibody and anti–hepatitis A IgM)—diagnostic for hepatitis A

5. IgM antibodies (hepatitis B core antigen [HB_cAg]; anti-HB_s, IgM)

6. Immunoglobulin G (IgG) antibodies (HAV antibody and anti–hepatitis A IgG)—indicates susceptibility or past exposure to HAV

7. HB_sAg titer—diagnostic for hepatitis B; if persists longer than 6 months, indicates acute chronic hepatitis B

8. Anti-HB_cAg titer—diagnostic for chronic hepatitis

9. Anti-HB_s—indicates recovery and immunity to hepatitis B

10. Anti–hepatitis B_e antigen—indicates low titers of hepatitis B and insufficient disease transmission

11. Anti-HCV (IgG, IgM)—diagnostic for hepatitis C; approximately two thirds of individuals with HCV infection will not develop antibodies until 5 to 12 months after infection

12. Recombinant immunoblot assay 2—supplemental test used to detect hepatitis C antibody

Hepatitis D

1. Anti-HDV (antibody to HDV)—indicates past or present infection with HDV; appears after symptoms develop and may be short-lived

2. Aspartate aminotransferase (AST) level—increase indicates acute hepatitis

3. Alanine aminotransferase (ALT) level—increased in acute hepatitis

MEDICAL MANAGEMENT

Treatment is mainly supportive and includes rest, hydration, and adequate dietary intake. Hospitalization is indicated for severe vomiting, dehydration, abnormal clotting factor levels, or signs of fulminating hepatic failure (restlessness, personality changes, lethargy, decreased level of consciousness, and bleeding). Intravenous therapy, frequent laboratory studies, and physical examinations for progression of disease are the mainstay of hospital management.

The following medications may be used:

1. Immunoglobulin (Ig)—used for prophylaxis before and after exposure to HAV (administered within 2 weeks of exposure)
2. Hepatitis B immunoglobulin (HBIG)—given as prophylaxis after exposure
3. Hepatitis B vaccine (Recombivax HB or Engerix-B)—used to prevent occurrence of hepatitis B. Both vaccines are administered in a three-dose schedule. Unvaccinated children 11 years of age and older follow a two-dose schedule. (Note that children undergoing long-term hemodialysis and children with Down syndrome should be routinely vaccinated because of increased risk for acquisition of hepatitis B infection.)

NURSING ASSESSMENT

1. See the Gastrointestinal Assessment section in Appendix A.
2. Assess for areas of jaundice—skin and sclera.
3. Assess nutritional status.

NURSING DIAGNOSES

- Fluid volume, Deficient
- Nutrition: less than body requirements, Imbalanced
- Pain
- Home maintenance, Impaired
- Knowledge, Deficient

NURSING INTERVENTIONS

1. Provide and maintain adequate fluid and food intake.
   a. Monitor for signs of dehydration.
   b. Monitor and record intake and output.
   c. Provide small, frequent meals; antiemetics may be needed.
   d. Offer child's favorite foods.
2. Prevent secondary infections.
   a. Avoid contact of child with infectious sources.
   b. Use and encourage appropriate hand-washing technique.

    c. Monitor for signs of infection.

    d. Provide for rest periods.

3. Prevent or control spread of hepatitis.

    a. Refer to institutional procedures for isolation techniques.

    b. Inoculate those people exposed to hepatitis during incubation period.

       i. Immunoglobulin

       ii HBIG vaccine

    c. Vaccinate all children and those individuals at high risk with hepatitis B vaccine.

4. Provide pain relief and comfort measures.

    a. Placement in position of comfort

    b. Avoidance of unnecessary palpation of abdomen (hepatomegaly and splenomegaly)

5. Monitor for bleeding.

    a. Monitor results of coagulation studies.

    b. Intramuscular vitamin K may be ordered.

6. Monitor child closely for progression into fulminating hepatitis.

    a. Behavioral changes

    b. Lethargy

    c. Coma

🔺 Discharge Planning and Home Care

1. Ensure that all family members and others exposed to child receive inoculation of Ig or HBIG.

2. Instruct parents and child about signs and symptoms of hepatitis so they can monitor for them in individuals exposed to child.

3. Provide instruction to parents about sanitary measures to institute in home.

4. Refer to public health nurse or community nurse for assessment of use of preventive measures for hepatitis.

CLIENT OUTCOMES

1. Child's gastrointestinal and hepatic function will return to normal.

2. Child will return to normal activity levels without recurrence of illness.
3. Child and family will understand home care instructions, disease process, instructions for preventing spread or recurrence of disease, and importance of follow-up.

REFERENCES

American Academy of Pediatrics, Pickering LK, editor: *2000 Red book: report of the Committee on Infectious Diseases,* ed 25, Elk Grove Village, Ill, 2000, The Academy.

Garza AL, Forshner L: Hepatitis update, *RN* 60(12):39, 1997.

Katz A et al: *Krugman's infectious diseases of children,* St Louis, 1998, Mosby.

Marz J: Understanding the varieties of viral hepatitis, *Nursing 98* 28(7):43, 1998.

Selekman J: Hepatitis update, *Pediatr Nurs* 25(5):542, 1999.

34

❖

Hernia (Inguinal) and Hernia Repair

❖

PATHOPHYSIOLOGY

Inguinal hernia is the prolapse of a portion of the intestine into the inguinal ring, caused by a congenital weakness or failure of closure. An incarcerated hernia occurs when the prolapsed intestine causes constriction of the blood supply to the scrotal sac. The infant then develops pain and symptoms of intestinal obstruction (abdominal distention, colicky abdominal pain, absence of flatus, absence of stool, vomiting). A communicating hydrocele is always associated with hernia. The child is initially seen with an intermittent lump or bulge in the groin, scrotum, or labia. It becomes prominent with intraabdominal pressure such as that resulting from crying or straining. Contents of the hernia sac usually can be reduced with gentle pressure. Surgical repair (herniorrhaphy) is usually performed on an outpatient basis. Unfortunately, there is no effective non-surgical means of treating this condition.

INCIDENCE

1. Of term infants, 3.5% to 5.0% have a hernia. Incidence of bilateral hernias approaches 50% in premature and low-birth-weight infants. The majority of infantile inguinal hernias are diagnosed in the first month of life.
2. The incidence is highest during infancy (more than 50%), with the remaining cases generally occurring before 5 years of age.
3. Incidence is higher in males than in females (4:1).

4. Sixty percent of hernias occur on the right side, 30% on the left side, and 10% bilaterally.

CLINICAL MANIFESTATIONS (IF HERNIA IS INCARCERATED)

1. Bulge or swelling (intermittent)
2. Pain
3. Continuous crying
4. Vomiting
5. Abdominal distention
6. Bloody stools
7. Scrotal color changes (redness)

COMPLICATIONS

1. Recurrence of hernia
2. Incarcerated hernia
3. Atrophy of gonad

LABORATORY AND DIAGNOSTIC TESTS

None indicated, unless warranted by coexisting conditions.

SURGICAL MANAGEMENT

Children with reducible hernias are scheduled for elective surgery on an outpatient basis. A 1- to 2-cm transverse incision is made in the area overlying the inguinal canal. Children with suspected incarcerated hernias are admitted to the hospital, with immediate surgical repair performed to avoid bowel necrosis and, in boys, testicular infarction. Postoperatively these children are observed for at least 24 hours to be assessed for adequate return of gastrointestinal function and to receive prophylactic intravenous antibiotics. Analgesic medications are used for pain management. Oral feedings are begun when adequate peristalsis is established. The wound is often covered with a protective sealant after surgery.

NURSING ASSESSMENT

1. See the Gastrointestinal Assessment section in Appendix A.
2. Assess for presence of lump in area of groin, scrotum, or labia.

NURSING DIAGNOSES

- Tissue integrity, Impaired
- Fluid volume, Deficient
- Pain
- Knowledge, Deficient

NURSING INTERVENTIONS

Preoperative Care

1. Assess child's clinical status before surgery.
   a. Signs of infection
   b. Hemoglobin level higher than 10 g/dl
2. Explain anticipated preoperative and postoperative events using age-appropriate means.

Postoperative Care

1. Monitor child's clinical status.
   a. Measure vital signs as often as every 2 hours for first 24 hours, then every 4 hours.
   b. Assess for signs and symptoms of infection.
   c. Check temperature and observe for drainage from site, redness, inflammation.
   d. Change diaper frequently.
2. Monitor for signs and symptoms of complications.
   a. Recurrence of hernia
   b. Development of wound infection
3. Promote nutritional and fluid intake.
   a. Record intake and output.
   b. Monitor for signs of dehydration.
   c. Advance diet as tolerated.
4. Promote and maintain respiratory function.
   a. Have child turn, cough, and deep breathe.
   b. Perform postural drainage and percussion.
   c. Change child's position every 2 hours.
   d. Keep head of bed in semi-Fowler position.
5. Alleviate child's pain as needed.
   a. Maintain position of comfort.
   b. Use recreational and diversional activities and toys.
   c. Administer analgesics.

6. Provide and reinforce information given to parents about child's condition.

🔺 Discharge Planning and Home Care

1. Instruct parents about care of dressing (if present).
   a. Keep incision covered with plastic-coated dressing.
   b. Bathe child with incision covered by dressing.
   c. Protect incision from fecal and urinary contamination.
2. Instruct parents about short- and long-term management.
   a. Allow no major physical activity for 1 week after surgery.
   b. Administer acetaminophen (Tylenol) or ibuprofen (Motrin, Advil) for pain as needed.
   c. Monitor for complications.
   d. Scrotal swelling and bruising are very common after surgery and may last 1 to 3 weeks.

CLIENT OUTCOMES

1. Child's gastrointestinal function will return to normal.
2. Pain will be eliminated.
3. Child and family will understand home care and follow-up needs.

REFERENCES

Behrman RE, Kliegman RM: *Nelson essentials of pediatrics,* ed 4, Philadelphia, 2002, Mosby.

Hoekelman R et al: *Primary pediatric care,* ed 4, St Louis, 2001, Mosby.

Kapur P et al: Pediatric hernias and hydroceles, *Pediatr Clin North Am* 45(4):773, 1998.

Mandleco BL, Potts NL: *Pediatric nursing: caring for children and their families,* Clifton Park, NY, 2002, Delmar.

35

❖

Hirschsprung's Disease

❖

PATHOPHYSIOLOGY

Hirschsprung's disease, or congenital aganglionic megacolon, is the absence of ganglion cells in the rectum or the rectosigmoid portion of the colon. This absence results in abnormal or absent peristalsis and the total absence of spontaneous bowel evacuation. Intestinal contents are propelled to an aganglionic segment; because of the lack of innervation, fecal material accumulates there, which results in dilation of the bowel (megacolon) proximal to this area. In addition, the rectal sphincter fails to relax, which prevents the normal passage of stool and thereby contributes to the obstruction. It is speculated that Hirschsprung's disease is caused by both genetic and environmental factors, but the exact etiology is unknown. Hirschsprung's disease may manifest itself at any age, although it is most commonly observed in neonates.

INCIDENCE

1. Hirschsprung's disease occurs in 1 in 5000 live births.
2. The disease is four times more common in males than in females.
3. Incidence increases in siblings and offspring of affected children.
4. It is more common in children with Down syndrome.
5. This disease accounts for 15% to 20% of neonatal intestinal obstructions.

CLINICAL MANIFESTATIONS
Neonatal Period

1. Failure to pass meconium within 24 to 48 hours of birth
2. Bilious vomiting

3. Abdominal distention
4. Reluctance to feed

Infancy and Childhood

1. Constipation
2. Recurrent diarrhea
3. Ribbonlike, foul-smelling stool
4. Abdominal distention
5. Failure to thrive

COMPLICATIONS

1. Enterocolitis (acute)
2. Leakage at anastomosis (postsurgical)
3. Anal strictures (postsurgical)
4. Incontinence (long term)

LABORATORY AND DIAGNOSTIC TESTS

1. Abdominal radiographic studies (supine, erect, prone, lateral decubitus)—diagnostic
2. Barium contrast studies—diagnostic
3. Anorectal manometry—to determine ability of internal sphincter to relax
4. Rectal biopsy—to detect absence of ganglion cells (provides definitive diagnosis)

SURGICAL MANAGEMENT

Surgical treatment of Hirschsprung's disease is a two-stage process. Initially, a temporary colostomy is performed (1) to decompress the bowel and divert the fecal contents, and (2) to allow the dilated and hypertrophied portion of the bowel to regain normal tone and size (takes approximately 3 to 4 months). When the infant is between 6 and 12 months of age (or when the infant weighs 8 to 10 kg), a rectal pull-through procedure is performed in which all aganglionic bowel is removed and the normal bowel is reconnected to the anus. The colostomy is also closed.

NURSING ASSESSMENT

See the Gastrointestinal Assessment section in Appendix A.

Preoperative

1. Assess child's clinical status (vital signs, intake and output).
2. Assess for signs of bowel perforation.
3. Assess for signs of enterocolitis.
4. Assess child's level of pain (see Appendix H).
5. Assess child's and family's ability to cope with upcoming surgery.

Postoperative

1. Assess child's postoperative status (vital signs, bowel sounds, abdominal distention).
2. Assess for signs of dehydration or fluid overload.
3. Assess for complications.
4. Assess for signs of infection.
5. Assess child's level of pain (see Appendix H).
6. Assess child's and family's ability to cope with hospital and surgical experience.
7. Assess parents' ability to manage treatment regimen and ongoing care.

NURSING DIAGNOSES

- Anxiety
- Infection, Risk for
- Pain
- Fluid volume, Deficient
- Skin integrity, Risk for impaired
- Knowledge, Deficient

NURSING INTERVENTIONS
Preoperative Care

1. Monitor nutritional status before surgery.
   a. Offer diet high in calories, protein, and residue.
   b. Use alternative route of intake if infant cannot take oral fluids.
   c. Assess intake and output accurately every 8 hours.
   d. Weigh infant every day.
2. Prepare infant and family emotionally for surgery (see Appendix J).

3. Monitor clinical status preoperatively.
   a. Monitor vital signs every 2 hours as needed.
   b. Monitor intake and output.
   c. Observe for signs and symptoms of bowel perforation.
      i. Vomiting
      ii. Increased tenderness
      iii. Abdominal distention
      iv. Irritability
      v. Respiratory distress (dyspnea)
   d. Monitor for signs of enterocolitis.
   e. Measure abdominal girth every 4 hours (to assess for abdominal distention).
4. Monitor infant's reactions to presurgical preparations.
   a. Enemas until fluid is clear (to sterilize bowel preoperatively)
   b. Intravenous (IV) tube insertion
   c. Foley catheter insertion
   d. Preoperative medication
   e. Diagnostic testing
   f. Decompression of stomach and bowel (nasogastric [NG] or rectal tube)
   g. Nothing by mouth for 12 hours before surgery

Postoperative Care

1. Monitor and report child's postoperative status.
   a. Auscultate for return of bowel sounds.
   b. Monitor vital signs every 2 hours until stable, then every 4 hours (depending on hospital protocol).
   c. Monitor for abdominal distention (maintain patency of NG tube).
2. Monitor child's hydration status (depending on child's status and hospital protocol).
   a. Assess for signs of dehydration or fluid overload.
   b. Measure and record NG drainage.
   c. Measure and record colostomy drainage.
   d. Measure and record Foley catheter drainage.
   e. Monitor IV infusion (amount, rate, infiltration).
   f. Observe for electrolyte imbalances (hyponatremia or hypokalemia).

3. Observe and report signs of complications.
   a. Intestinal obstruction caused by adhesions, volvulus, or intussusception
   b. Leakage from anastomosis
   c. Sepsis
   d. Fistula
   e. Enterocolitis
   f. Frequent stools
   g. Constipation
   h. Bleeding
   i. Recurrence of symptoms
4. Promote return of peristalsis.
   a. Maintain patency of NG tube.
   b. Irrigate with normal saline solution every 4 hours and as needed.
5. Promote and maintain fluid and electrolyte balance.
   a. Record intake per route (IV, oral).
   b. Record output per route (urine, stool, emesis, stoma).
   c. Consult with physician about disparities.
6. Alleviate or minimize pain and discomfort (see Appendix H).
   a. Assess pain.
   b. Provide nonpharmacologic and/or pharmacologic pain interventions.
   c. Monitor child's response to administration of medications.
7. Prevent infection.
   a. Monitor incision site.
   b. Provide Foley catheter care every shift (protocols vary according to institution).
   c. Change dressing as needed (perianal and colostomy).
   d. Refer to institutional procedures manual for care related to specific procedure.
   e. Change diaper frequently to avoid fecal contamination.
8. Promote skin integrity.
   a. Provide skin care per institutional procedures.
   b. Use appropriate ostomy supplies.
9. Provide emotional support to child and family (see the Preparation for Procedures or Surgery section in Appendix J).

🔺 Discharge Planning and Home Care

1. Instruct parents to monitor for signs and symptoms of the following long-term complications:
   a. Stenosis and constrictions
   b. Incontinence
   c. Inadequate emptying
2. Provide instructions to parents and child about colostomy care.
   a. Skin preparation
   b. Use of colostomy equipment
   c. Stomal complications (bleeding, failure to pass stool, increased diarrhea, prolapse, ribbonlike stools)
   d. Care and cleaning of colostomy equipment
   e. Irrigation of colostomy (refer to Chapter 45 for further information)
3. Provide and reinforce instructions about dietary management.
   a. Low-residue diet
   b. Unlimited fluid intake
   c. Signs of electrolyte imbalance or dehydration
4. Encourage parents' and child's expression of concerns related to colostomy (see Appendix K).
   a. Appearance
   b. Odor
   c. Discrepancy between parents' child and "ideal" child
5. Refer to specific institutional procedures for information to be distributed to parents about home care (see Appendix K).

CLIENT OUTCOMES

1. Child will remain without signs of infection.
2. Child will have adequate hydration.
3. Child's stoma site will not show tissue breakdown.

REFERENCES

Bueno J et al: Factors impacting the survival of children with intestinal failure referred for intestinal transplantation, *J Pediatr Surg* 34:27, 1999.

Hart M: Hirschsprung's disease. In Burg FD et al: *Gellis and Kagan's current pediatric therapy,* ed 16, Philadelphia, 1999, WB Saunders.

James S et al: *Nursing care of children—principles and practice,* ed 2, Philadelphia, 2002, WB Saunders.

McCollum LL, Thigpen JL: Assessment and management of gastrointestinal dysfunction. In Kenner C et al, editors: *Comprehensive neonatal nursing: a physiologic perspective,* ed 2, Philadelphia, 1998, WB Saunders.

Swenson O: Hirschsprung's disease: a review, *Pediatrics* 109(5):914, 2002.

Wong DL et al: *Wong's essentials of pediatric nursing,* ed 6, St Louis, 2001, Mosby.

36

❖

Hodgkin's Disease

❖

PATHOPHYSIOLOGY

Hodgkin's disease is a malignancy of the lymphoid system. The cause is unknown. It is characterized by a proliferation of Reed-Sternberg cells that are surrounded by a pleomorphic infiltrate of reactive cells, predominantly composed of helper T cells. Although no tissue is exempt from involvement, Hodgkin's disease primarily affects nonnodal or extralymphatic sites, particularly the liver, spleen, bone marrow, lungs, and mediastinum. Hodgkin's disease is classified according to the predominating cells and is characterized by four histologic states: (1) lymphocytic predominance, (2) nodular sclerosis, (3) mixed cellularity, and (4) lymphocytic depletion. High survival rates have been achieved in children with Hodgkin's disease as a result of improved staging procedures and various treatment strategies.

INCIDENCE

1. Hodgkin's disease accounts for 5% of malignancies in children in the United States.
2. Hodgkin's disease has been reported in infants and young children but is rare before the age of 5 years. It is primarily a disease of young adults; however, it also occurs in children.
3. Only 10% to 15% of cases occur in children younger than 16 years of age. The majority of cases in children occur in children aged 11 years and older.
4. Hodgkin's disease is more common in males.
5. The survival rate for stage I and II disease is approximately 90%; for stage III and IV disease, 65%.
6. If the disease is left untreated, a 5-year survival rate of less than 5% is expected.

CLINICAL MANIFESTATIONS

1. Nontender, firm lymphadenopathy, usually centripetal and axial with cervical, supraclavicular, and mediastinal presentation. Mediastinal presentation is common in adolescents and young adults.
2. Painless, movable lymph nodes in tissues surrounding involved area
3. Elevated leukocyte count
4. Elevated erythrocyte sedimentation rate (ESR)
5. Fever
6. Malaise
7. Weight loss

COMPLICATIONS (RELATED TO TREATMENT)

1. Hypothyroidism
2. Cardiac dysfunction, including pericardial effusion, valvular heart disease, coronary artery disease, and constrictive pericarditis with tamponade
3. Pulmonary dysfunction, including fibrosis or pneumonitis
4. Impaired immunity
5. Soft tissue and bone growth impairment
6. Ovarian dysfunction in females and sterility in males
7. Secondary malignancy, including thyroid carcinoma, basal cell carcinoma, osteosarcomas, breast and colon carcinomas, soft tissue sarcomas, non-Hodgkin's lymphoma, and leukemia
8. Human immunodeficiency virus infection
9. Sex or growth hormone deficiencies

LABORATORY AND DIAGNOSTIC TESTS

1. Complete blood count—diagnostic (anemia may indicate advanced disease)
2. ESR—elevated at diagnosis
3. Serum copper, iron, calcium, and alkaline phosphatase levels—elevated at diagnosis
4. Liver and renal function tests—to assess organ involvement
5. Urinalysis—to determine renal involvement

6. Chest radiographic study—to determine mediastinal or hilar node involvement
7. Computed tomography—to evaluate mediastinal, pulmonary, and upper abdominal disease
8. Radionuclide scan—to determine extent of involvement at site
9. Lymphangiogram—to evaluate retroperitoneal involvement and to visualize size, architecture, and filling defects of nodes
10. Excisional lymph node biopsy—essential to diagnosis and staging
11. Surgical staging laparotomy—for pathologic staging

MEDICAL MANAGEMENT

Staging is used to determine the anatomic extent of the disease at the time of diagnosis and to select the most appropriate therapy (Box 36-1). Staging includes biopsy, history, physical examination, and radiographic data collection. At the time of diagnosis, approximately 60% of children with Hodgkin's disease have pathologic stage I or II disease. Pathologic stage III

BOX 36-1

System for Hodgkin's Disease: Ann Arbor Staging

Stage	Description*
I	Involvement of a single lymph node region or a single extralymphatic organ or site
II	Involvement of two or more lymph node regions on the same side of the diaphragm or localized involvement of an extralymphatic organ or site and one or more lymph node regions on the same side of the diaphragm
III	Involvement of lymph node regions or extralymphatic organs or sites or spleen on both sides of the diaphragm
IV	Diffuse involvement of one or more extralymphatic organs or tissues with or without associated lymph node involvement

*Subdivision A has no defined symptoms; subdivision B symptoms include unexplained recent weight loss or fever or night sweats.

disease is diagnosed in approximately 30% of children, and 10% have pathologic stage IV disease.

The treatment approach is guided by the stage of the disease at diagnosis. The goal of treatment is cure of the disease with minimal treatment-related toxicities and sequelae. For stage I and IIA Hodgkin's disease, external-beam radiation therapy is used. For stage IIB and IIIB Hodgkin's disease, total nodal irradiation is the treatment approach of choice. Treatment for stage IIIA Hodgkin's disease consists of radiotherapy and combination chemotherapy, and stage IV Hodgkin's disease is treated with combination chemotherapy.

The following medication regimens may be used:

1. MOPP drug regimen
   a. Mechlorethamine (nitrogen mustard)—interferes with DNA replication and RNA protein synthesis; causes myelosuppression
   b. Oncovin (vincristine)—antineoplastic agent; inhibits cell division by arresting mitosis at metaphase
   c. Procarbazine (Matulane)—antineoplastic agent; inhibits cell division by suppressing mitosis at interphase
   d. Prednisone—corticosteroid used for its antiinflammatory effect; inhibits phagocytosis and suppresses other clinical symptoms of inflammation
2. ABVD drug regimen (for treatment of MOPP-resistant disease)
   a. Adriamycin (doxorubicin)—antitumor antibiotic
   b. Bleomycin—antitumor antibiotic
   c. Vinblastine—causes metaphase arrest and protein synthesis
   d. Dacarbazine—causes myelosuppression

NURSING ASSESSMENT

1. Assess child's physiologic status (see Appendix A).
   a. Signs and symptoms of Hodgkin's disease
   b. Involvement of other body systems (e.g., respiratory, gastrointestinal)
   c. Adverse effects of treatment

2. Assess family's psychosocial needs (see Appendix J).
   a. Knowledge
   b. Body image
   c. Family structure
   d. Family stressors
   e. Coping mechanisms
   f. Support systems
3. Assess child's developmental level (see Appendix B).
4. Assess family's ability to manage home care (see Appendix K).

NURSING DIAGNOSES

- Tissue integrity, Impaired
- Anxiety
- Fluid volume, Deficient
- Nutrition: less than body requirements, Imbalanced
- Skin integrity, Impaired
- Oral mucous membranes, Impaired
- Pain
- Fatigue
- Growth and development, Delayed
- Therapeutic regimen management, Ineffective

NURSING INTERVENTIONS
Staging Procedure

1. Provide preprocedural education to child and family (see Appendix J).
2. Prepare child for clinical staging procedures with age-appropriate approach (see Appendix J).
3. Assist and support child in collection of laboratory specimens.
4. Provide instruction, support, and family crisis intervention.

Radiation and/or Chemotherapy Phase

1. Provide sedation for radiation treatments.
2. Monitor cardiorespiratory status during treatments.
3. Prepare for treatment-induced emergencies.
   a. Metabolic disturbances
   b. Hematologic disturbances
   c. Space-occupying tumors

4. Assess for signs of extravasation.
   a. Cell lysis
   b. Tissue sloughing
5. Monitor for signs and symptoms of infection.
6. Assess skin integrity.
7. Minimize side effects of radiotherapy and/or chemotherapy.
   a. Bone marrow suppression
   b. Nausea and vomiting
   c. Anorexia and weight loss
   d. Oral mucositis
   e. Pain
8. Provide ongoing emotional support to child and family (see Appendix J).
9. Refer to child life specialist to assist with continued coping strategies.
10. Provide ongoing education about treatment and medications.
11. Refer family to social services for support and resource utilization (see Appendix K).

Discharge Planning and Home Care

Instruct child and parents about home care management, including the following:

1. Signs of infection and guidelines on when to seek medical attention
2. Care of child's central venous access device, including site care, dressing change, flushing, and emergency care
3. Medication administration (provide written information)
4. Adherence to treatment regimen and medical appointments
5. Proper nutrition for optimal weight gain and health maintenance
6. School attendance and/or activity restrictions
7. Potential behavioral changes in child and/or siblings

CLIENT OUTCOMES

1. Child and family will demonstrate ability to cope with life-threatening illness.
2. Child will be free of infection.
3. Child and family will understand home care and long-term follow-up needs.

REFERENCES

Boyle DA, Angert VJ: Lymphoma at the extremes of age, *Semin Oncol Nurs* 14(4):302, 1998.

Bryant R: Managing side effects of childhood cancer treatment, *J Pediatr Nurs* 18(2):113, 2003.

Donaldson SS et al: Hodgkin's disease—finding the balance between cure and late effects, *Cancer J Sci Am* 5(6):325, 1999.

Foley G et al, editors: *Nursing care of the child with cancer,* ed 2, Philadelphia, 1993, WB Saunders.

Garber TL: Quality improvement: treatment for Hodgkin disease in adolescent girls and young adult women, *Radiat Ther* 7(2):182, 1998.

Morrison C et al: Hodgkin's disease in primary care, *Nurse Pract* 25(7):44, 2000.

37

❖

HIV Infection and AIDS

❖

PATHOPHYSIOLOGY

The cause of acquired immunodeficiency syndrome (AIDS) is infection with the human immunodeficiency virus (HIV), which attaches to and enters helper T CD4$^+$ lymphocytes. The virus infects CD4$^+$ lymphocytes and other immunologic cells, and the person experiences a gradual destruction of CD4$^+$ cells. These cells, which amplify and replicate immunologic responses, are necessary to maintain good health, and when they are reduced in numbers and damaged, other immune functions begin to fail.

HIV can also infect macrophages, cells that the virus uses to cross the blood-brain barrier into the brain. B-lymphocyte function is also affected, with increased total immunoglobulin production associated with decreased specific antibody production. As the immune system progressively deteriorates, the body becomes increasingly vulnerable to opportunistic infections and is also less able to slow the process of HIV replication. HIV infection is manifested as a multisystem disease that may be dormant for years as it produces gradual immunodeficiency. The rate of disease progression and clinical manifestations vary from person to person.

The virus is transmitted only through direct contact with blood or blood products and body fluids, such as cerebrospinal fluid, pleural fluid, human milk, semen, saliva, tears, urine, and cervical secretions. In the United States intravenous drug use, sexual contact, perinatal transmission from mother to infant, and breast-feeding are established modes of transmission. There is no evidence that HIV infection is acquired through casual contact. Administration of zidovudine to pregnant

HIV-infected women significantly reduces transmission from mother to child.

Currently, the majority of reported cases of HIV infection and AIDS in the United States occur in gay and bisexual men. However, the highest rates of new transmission of HIV are among heterosexual individuals. Sixty-five percent of HIV-positive adolescents aged 13 to 19 were infected through sexual exposure or intravenous drug use. With recent advances in the screening of blood products for HIV, the incidence of new infections from blood transfusions has been greatly reduced in developed countries.

Four populations in the pediatric age group have been primarily affected:

1. Infants infected through perinatal transmission from infected mothers (also referred to as vertical transmission); this accounts for more than 90% of AIDS cases among children younger than 13 years of age
2. Children who have received blood products (especially children with hemophilia)
3. Adolescents infected after engaging in high-risk behavior
4. Infants who have been breast-fed by infected mothers (primarily in developing countries)

INCIDENCE

1. Children account for 2% of all reported cases of AIDS in the United States.
2. Ninety percent of infected children in the United States acquired the infection from their mothers.
3. The number of infants infected by perinatal transmission was 66% lower in 1998 than in 1993, reportedly due to diagnosis and treatment of pregnant women.
4. Among adolescents, more than 50% of cases are in girls.

CLINICAL MANIFESTATIONS
Infants and Children

The majority of children who are born to HIV-infected mothers become symptomatic during the first 6 months of life, with the development of lymphadenopathy as the initial finding

(Box 37-1). The most common clinical manifestations include the following:

1. Lymphadenopathy
2. Hepatomegaly
3. Splenomegaly
4. Failure to thrive
5. Hepatitis
6. Recurrent upper respiratory tract infections
7. Parotitis
8. Chronic or recurrent diarrhea
9. Recurrent bacterial and viral infections

BOX 37-1

Clinical Categories of HIV Infection for Children Under 13 Years of Age

Category N: Not Symptomatic or One Condition Listed in Category A

Children with no signs or symptoms thought to be the result of HIV infection

Category A: Mildly Symptomatic

Children who have two or more of the following:

- Dermatitis
- Hepatomegaly
- Lymphadenopathy
- Parotitis
- Recurrent/persistent upper respiratory tract infection, sinusitis, or otitis media
- Splenomegaly

Category B: Moderately Symptomatic

Children who have symptomatic conditions that are attributed to HIV infection:

- Anemia, neutropenia, thrombocytopenia persisting >30 days
- Bacterial meningitis, pneumonia, or sepsis
- Cardiomyopathy
- Cytomegalovirus infection with onset before 1 month of age
- Diarrhea, recurrent or chronic
- Hepatitis
- Herpes stomatitis, recurrent
- Herpes simplex virus bronchitis, pneumonitis, or esophagitis with onset before 1 month of age

BOX 37-1
Clinical Categories of HIV Infection for Children Under 13 Years of Age—cont'd

- Herpes zoster (shingles), two or more episodes
- Leiomyosarcoma
- Lymphoid interstitial pneumonia or pulmonary lymphoid hyperplasia complex
- Nephropathy
- Nocardiosis
- Persistent fever >1 month
- Thrush persisting for longer than 2 months in a child over 6 months of age
- Toxoplasmosis, onset before 1 month of age
- Varicella, disseminated (complicated chickenpox)

Category C: Severely Symptomatic
Children who have any of the following conditions:
- Bacterial infections, multiple or recurrent
- Candidiasis of the trachea, bronchi, lungs, or esophagus
- Chronic herpes simplex ulcer (>1 month duration) or bronchitis, pneumonitis, or esophagitis with onset >1 month of age
- Coccidioidomycosis, disseminated or extrapulmonary
- Cryptococcosis, extrapulmonary
- Cryptosporidiosis with diarrhea >1 month
- Cytomegalovirus disease (other than liver, spleen, nodes), onset at age >1 month
- Cytomegalovirus retinitis (with loss of vision)
- Histoplasmosis, disseminated or extrapulmonary
- HIV encephalopathy
- Isosporiasis, chronic intestinal (>1 month duration)
- Kaposi's sarcoma
- Lymphoma (Burkitt's or immunoblastic sarcoma)
- Lymphoma, primary in brain
- *Mycobacterium tuberculosis* infection, disseminated or extrapulmonary
- *Pneumocystis carinii* pneumonia
- Progressive multifocal leukoencephalopathy
- *Salmonella* septicemia, recurrent
- Toxoplasmosis of brain, onset at age >1 month
- Wasting syndrome caused by HIV

Modified from Centers for Disease Control and Prevention: 1994 Revised classification system for human immunodeficiency virus infection in children less than 13 years of age, *MMWR* 43(RR-12):1, 1994.

10. Persistent Epstein-Barr virus infection
11. Oropharyngeal thrush
12. Thrombocytopenia
13. Neuropathy
14. Lymphoid interstitial pneumonia

Fifty percent of children with HIV infection have neurologic involvement that primarily manifests itself as a progressive encephalopathy, developmental delay, or loss of motor milestones.

Adolescents

Most adolescents who are infected experience an extended period of asymptomatic illness that may last for years. This may be followed by signs and symptoms that begin weeks to months before the development of opportunistic infections and malignancies. The signs and symptoms include the following:

1. Fever
2. Malaise
3. Fatigue
4. Night sweats
5. Insidious onset of weight loss
6. Recurrent or chronic diarrhea
7. Generalized lymphadenopathy
8. Oral candidiasis
9. Arthralgias and myalgias

COMPLICATIONS

1. High risk for development of opportunistic infections
2. Severe wasting
3. Progressive encephalopathy

LABORATORY AND DIAGNOSTIC TESTS

1. Enzyme-linked immunosorbent assay (usual initial test)—detects antibody to HIV antigens (almost universally used to screen for HIV in persons older than 2 years of age)
2. Western blot test (usual confirmatory test)—detects antibody against several specific HIV proteins
3. HIV culture—viral culture requires up to 28 days for positive results

4. HIV DNA polymerase chain reaction (PCR) test—
   detects HIV DNA. Preferred test for children under
   18 months of age
5. HIV antigen test—detects HIV antigen

Infants born to HIV-positive mothers should have an HIV DNA
PCR test at 48 hours of life, at 1 to 2 months, and again at 3 to
6 months of age.

   The following laboratory findings are commonly seen in
HIV-infected infants and children:

1. Reduced absolute CD4$^+$ lymphocyte count
2. Reduced CD4$^+$ percentage
3. Reduced CD4$^+$/CD8$^+$ ratio
4. Lymphopenia
5. Anemia, thrombocytopenia
6. Hypergammaglobulinemia (immunoglobulin G,
   immunoglobulin A, immunoglobulin M)
7. Decreased response to skin tests (*Candida albicans,*
   tetanus)
8. Poor response to vaccines that have been given (diphtheria,
   tetanus, measles, *Haemophilus influenzae* type B)

An infant born to an HIV-positive mother who is younger than
18 months of age and who has tested positive on two separate
determinations from HIV culture, HIV PCR test, or HIV antigen test is termed "HIV infected." An infant born to an HIV-
positive mother who is younger than 18 months of age and who
has not tested positive to these three tests is categorized as "peri-
natally exposed." Infants born to HIV-infected mothers who
have been determined to be HIV-antibody negative and
who have no other laboratory evidence of infection are termed
"seroreverters."

MEDICAL MANAGEMENT

Currently no cure exists for HIV infection and AIDS.
Antiretroviral drugs are used to control disease progression.
Management begins with a staging evaluation to determine dis-
ease progression and the appropriate course of treatment.
Children are categorized according to Table 37-1 using three
parameters: immune status, infection status, and clinical status.
A child with mild signs and symptoms but with no evidence of

TABLE 37-1
Categorization of Children with HIV Infection and AIDS

Immune Categories	Clinical Categories		
	(N) No Signs or Symptoms	(A) Mild Signs or Symptoms	(B) Moderate Signs or Symptoms	(C) Severe Signs or Symptoms
(1) No evidence of suppression	N1	A1	B1	C1
(2) Evidence of moderate suppression	N2	A2	B2	C2
(3) Severe suppression	N3	A3	B3	C3

immune suppression is categorized as A2. The immune status is based on the CD4$^+$ count or CD4$^+$ percentage and the child's age, according to Table 37-2. Zidovudine (AZT, ZDV), didanosine (DDI), zalcitabine (DDC), and lamivudine (3TC) slow down multiplication of the virus. Combination drug treatment is used, and many children are enrolled in research drug protocols.

In addition to controlling disease progression, treatment is directed at preventing and managing opportunistic infections such as candidiasis and interstitial pneumonia. Trimethoprim sulfamethoxazole (Septra, Bactrim) and pentamidine are used for treatment and prophylaxis of *Pneumocystis carinii* pneumonia. Monthly intravenous administration of immunoglobulin has been useful in preventing serious bacterial infections, as well as hypogammaglobulinemia, in children.

Immunizations are recommended for children with HIV infection. Instead of the oral poliovirus vaccine, the inactivated poliovirus vaccine is given.

NURSING ASSESSMENT

1. See Appendix A.
2. Assess nutritional status.

TABLE 37-2
Determination of Immune Category Based on Age and CD4$^+$ Count

Immune Categories	Age Groups: CD4$^+$ Count and Percentage		
	0-11 Months	1-5 Years	6-12 Years
(1) No evidence of suppression	>1500 >25%	>1000 >25%	>500 >25%
(2) Evidence of moderate suppression	750-1499 15-25%	500-999 15-25%	200-499 15-25%
(3) Severe suppression	<750 <15%	<500 <15%	<200 <15%

Modified from Centers for Disease Control and Prevention: 1994 Revised classification system for human immunodeficiency virus infection in children less than 13 years of age, *MMWR* 43(RR-12):1, 1994.

3. Assess for opportunistic infections.
4. Assess for knowledge of transmission—safe sex, avoidance of needle sharing, and so on.

NURSING DIAGNOSES

- Infection, Risk for
- Growth and development, Delayed
- Nutrition: less than body requirements, Imbalanced
- Family processes, Interrupted
- Grieving, Anticipatory
- Noncompliance
- Social interaction, Impaired

NURSING INTERVENTIONS

1. Protect infant, child, or adolescent from infectious contacts (Box 37-2); although casual person-to-person contact does not transmit HIV, a number of recommendations have been made for children with HIV infection and AIDS.
   a. Care providers in foster homes should be educated on precautions regarding blood exposure, saliva contamination, and infection protection.

BOX 37-2
Preventive Measures

Preventive efforts are of vital importance in dealing with AIDS. Reducing the number of sexual partners, especially those in high-risk groups, would decrease the incidence of this disease in the adolescent population, as would involvement in drug rehabilitation programs and avoidance of nonsterile needles. Also, sexual abuse of adolescents contributes to AIDS risk.

Prevention of AIDS in the adult population would result in the greatest decrease of this disease in children. In addition, elimination of infected blood and blood products would decrease the likelihood of transmission to children. Blood and blood products are now screened for the antibody to HIV, so that 95% of infected blood is eliminated from the market.

Research indicates that hepatitis B vaccine is safe from AIDS virus contamination. An HIV-positive mother should not breastfeed because transmission via breast milk has been identified.

    b. Day care attendance should be evaluated on an individual basis.

    c. Child should attend school if health, neurologic development, behavior, and immune status are appropriate.

2. Prevent transmission of HIV infection.

    a. Clean spills of blood or other body fluids with bleach solution (10:1 ratio of water to bleach).

    b. Wear latex gloves when exposure to blood or body fluids is anticipated.

    c. Wear mask with protective eyewear if aerosolization or splashing with blood or body fluids with visible blood is anticipated.

    d. Wash hands after exposure to blood or body fluids and after removing gloves.

    e. Place uncapped needles attached to syringes (and other sharps) in closed, puncture-proof container labeled as biohazardous/infectious waste.

    f. Dispose of waste contaminated with visible blood in biohazard plastic bag.

3. Protect child from infectious contacts when he or she is immunocompromised.

    a. Screen for infections.

    b. Place child in room with noninfectious children.

    c. Restrict visitors with active illnesses.

4. Assess child's achievement of developmental milestones and nutritional status.

    a. Provide age-appropriate, stimulating activities (see Appendix B).

    b. Monitor growth pattern (height, weight, head circumference) and refer to dietitian for assistance with nutritional interventions (see Appendix I).

5. Involve social services, child life therapists, and other health team members to assist child and family with crisis and stresses of chronic and fatal illness.

    a. Encourage expression of feelings.

    b. Refer to clergy for spiritual support.

    c. Discuss likelihood of child's death with parents and child.

    d. Encourage family members to discuss likelihood of child's death with each other, relatives, and friends.

    e. Encourage family to discuss likelihood of parents' death (if applicable).

6. Assist family in identifying factors that impede compliance with treatment plan.

    a. Educate child and family about medical research protocols.

    b. Educate child and family about risks of noncompliance.

    c. Assist family in establishing schedule that optimizes therapeutic effect of medication and fits into family's lifestyle.

7. Encourage child to participate in activities with other children.

    a. Assist child and family in identifying personal strengths.

    b. Educate school or day care personnel and classmates about HIV infection and AIDS.

    c. Educate adolescent about sexual transmission, abstinence, use of condoms with nonoxynol 9, and dangers of promiscuity and other risky behaviors.

    d. Educate adolescent about relationship between substance abuse and practice of risky behaviors.

    e. Encourage use of support network of family and friends and refer to AIDS support group as needed.

    f. Collaborate with school nurse regarding child's condition.

Discharge Planning and Home Care

1. Instruct child and family to contact medical team in case of signs or symptoms of infection.

2. Instruct child and family to observe response to medications and notify physician of adverse reactions.

3. Instruct child and family about follow-up appointments.

    a. Name and phone number of physician and appropriate health care team members

    b. Date, time, and purpose of follow-up appointments

CLIENT OUTCOMES

1. Child will exhibit no signs or symptoms of infection.
2. Child and family will demonstrate understanding of home care and follow-up needs.
3. Child will participate in activities with family and peers.

REFERENCES

American Academy of Pediatrics, Pickering LK, editor: *2000 Red book: report of the Committee on Infectious Diseases,* ed 25, Elk Grove Village, Ill, 2000, The Academy.

Centers for Disease Control and Prevention: 1994 Revised classification system for human immunodeficiency virus infection in children less than 13 years of age, *MMWR* 43(RR-12):1, 1994.

Deatrick JA et al: Nutritional assessment for children who are HIV-infected, *Pediatr Nurs* 24(2):137, 1998.

Hockenberry M: *Wong's nursing care of infants and children,* ed 7, St Louis, 2003, Mosby.

Kattan M: Pulmonary disorders in pediatric HIV infection. In Chernick V, Boat TF, editors: *Kendig's disorders of the respiratory tract in children,* ed 6, Philadelphia, 1998, WB Saunders.

Pizzo PA, Wilfert CM: Pediatric AIDS: the challenge of HIV infection in infants, children and adolescents, ed 2, Baltimore, 1994, Williams & Wilkins.

38

◇

Hydrocephalus

◇

PATHOPHYSIOLOGY

Hydrocephalus results from (1) obstruction of cerebrospinal fluid (CSF) flow, (2) interference with absorption of CSF, and (3) overproduction of CSF. When the movement or flow of CSF is restricted, intracranial pressure (ICP) rises, the ventricular system dilates proximal to the obstruction of the flow, and hydrocephalus ensues. Several causative factors account for hydrocephalus. The most common cause is myelomeningocele; others include intrauterine infections, tumors, vascular malformations, abscesses, intraventricular cysts, intraventricular hemorrhage, meningitis, aqueductal stenosis, and cerebral trauma. There are two types of hydrocephalus: congenital and acquired.

INCIDENCE

Congenital hydrocephalus occurs in 3 or 4 of 1000 live births.

CLINICAL MANIFESTATIONS

Signs and symptoms are the results of increased ICP and vary with the child's age and the skull's ability to expand.

Infants

1. Vital sign changes (decreased heart rate, decreased respiratory rate, increased blood pressure, increased temperature)
2. Progressive head enlargement (above 95th percentile); enlarged, bulging, tense fontanelles (especially nonpulsatile); split sutures; distention of superficial scalp veins; prominence of frontal portions of skull
3. Irritability or lethargy

4. Poor feeding, vomiting
5. Seizure activity
6. Delay or regression in developmental milestones
7. Symmetrically increased transillumination over skull
8. Downturned eyes ("sunset eyes")

Older Children

1. Vital sign changes (decreased heart rate, decreased respiratory rate, increased blood pressure, increased temperature)
2. Frontal headache, nausea and vomiting
3. Anorexia and/or abdominal pain
4. Ataxia
5. Lower extremity spasticity
6. Visual changes (e.g., diplopia, sunset eyes, papilledema)
7. Change in mental status; behavioral changes
8. Deterioration in child's school performance or cognitive ability
9. Seizures

COMPLICATIONS

1. Increased ICP
2. Infection
3. Shunt malfunction
4. Delays in cognitive, psychosocial, and physical development
5. Decreased intelligence quotient

LABORATORY AND DIAGNOSTIC TESTS

1. Computed tomographic scan—most useful method of diagnosis
2. Ventricular tap—direct puncture into ventricle through anterior fontanelle to monitor CSF pressure or to temporarily remove CSF to decrease ICP
3. Magnetic resonance imaging—may be used for complex lesion

SURGICAL MANAGEMENT

The traditional management is surgical shunt insertion. The shunt removes the excessive CSF and decreases ICP. The proximal end of the shunt is inserted in the lateral ventricle; the distal end is extended to the peritoneal cavity or right atrium as a means of draining excessive fluid into another body cavity. The ventricular-peritoneal (VP) shunt is used most frequently because the atrioventricular shunt requires repeated revisions as a result of growth and the associated risk of bacterial endocarditis. The symptoms of increased ICP are relieved. After surgery the child is more alert, and vomiting, anorexia, and bulging of the fontanelle are decreased. Because seizure activity remains a possibility after shunt placement, anticonvulsants may be given. Antibiotics as indicated by the results of culture and sensitivity tests are used for shunt infections. VP shunt placement may be avoided in those children for whom an endoscopic third ventriculostomy, a laser-assisted ventriculostomy, or a ventriculocisternostomy can be accomplished. The advantage of these procedures is that a VP shunt is often unnecessary and therefore the shunt will not need to be revised every few years (nearly one half of all shunt procedures performed are for revision of an original shunt).

The following are possible complications of surgery:

1. Shunt malfunction (blockage)
2. Shunt infection, meningitis
3. Overdrainage of CSF, shunt disconnection
4. Progressive mental deterioration
5. Seizures

NURSING ASSESSMENT

1. See the Neurologic Assessment and Musculoskeletal Assessment sections in Appendix A.
2. Assess for increased ICP.

NURSING DIAGNOSES

- Tissue perfusion, Ineffective (cerebral)
- Infection, Risk for
- Skin integrity, Risk for impaired
- Nutrition: less than body requirements, Imbalanced
- Injury, Risk for
- Growth and development, Delayed
- Knowledge, Deficient
- Therapeutic regimen management, Ineffective

NURSING INTERVENTIONS
Preoperative Care

1. Monitor for, prevent, and intervene in case of increased ICP.
   a. Place child in position of comfort; raise head of bed to 30 degrees (to decrease congestion and increase drainage). Maintain head in neutral position.
   b. Monitor for signs of increased ICP.
      i. Decreased respiratory rate, decreased heart rate, increased blood pressure, and increased temperature
      ii. Decreased level of consciousness (LOC)
      iii. Seizure activity
      iv. Vomiting
      v. Alteration in pupil size, symmetry, and reactivity
      vi. Fullness of fontanelles—tense to bulging
   c. Decrease external stimuli.
   d. Maintain oxygen and suction at bedside.
2. Prepare child and parents for surgical procedure.
   a. Provide age-appropriate explanations (see the Preparation for Procedures or Surgery section in Appendix J).
   b. Provide and reinforce information given to parents about child's condition and treatment.

Postoperative Care

1. Monitor child's vital signs and neurologic status; report signs of increased ICP (decreased LOC, anorexia, poor/ineffective sucking, vomiting, convulsions, seizures, or sluggishness).
2. Monitor and report signs of site infection (fever, tachycardia, general malaise, tenderness, inflammation, nausea, and vomiting).
3. Monitor and maintain functioning of shunt.
   a. Report signs of shunt malfunction (irritability, decreased LOC, vomiting).
   b. Check shunt for fullness.
   c. Elevate head of bed 30 degrees (to increase drainage and decrease venous congestion). Some newer techniques require child to be flat initially after surgery.

    d. Position child on left side (nonoperative side), turn according to surgeon's orders. Use foam rubber or synthetic sheepskin pad and air, water, or alternating air mattress to relieve pressure points on head.

    e. If VP shunt was placed, then child will be on nothing-by-mouth status with nasogastric tube in place due to placement of abdominal catheter. Administer intravenous fluids as ordered. Assess intake and output closely. Check for return of bowel sounds.

    f. Monitor for seizure activity.

4. Support child and parents to help them deal with emotional stresses of hospitalization and surgery (refer to the Supportive Care section in Appendix J).

    a. Provide age-appropriate information before procedures (refer to the Preparation for Procedures or Surgery section in Appendix J).

    b. Encourage participation in recreational and diversional activities.

    c. Incorporate child's home routine into daily activities.

🔺 Discharge Planning and Home Care

1. Instruct parents to monitor for and report signs of shunt complications.

    a. Shunt malfunction

    b. Shunt infection

2. Provide parents with assistance in contacting community resources.

    a. Follow-up by home health nurse (see Appendix K)

    b. Support group for parents of children with hydrocephalus

    c. Referral to early intervention programs (see Appendix L)

    d. Selection of preschool and recreational programs

3. Encourage parents to increase fluid and roughage in child's diet to prevent constipation, because straining at passing stool causes increased ICP.

4. Assess cognitive, linguistic, adaptive, and social behaviors to determine development; use developmental history to

assess achievement of early milestones and refer to appropriate specialists as needed.

CLIENT OUTCOMES

1. Child will not have signs or symptoms of increased ICP.
2. Child's skin will remain clean, dry, and intact without signs of erythema or ulceration.
3. Child's weight will remain within 50th to 95th percentile; no vomiting will occur.
4. Child and parents will understand how to monitor for and report shunt complications.
5. Child will demonstrate regular observable growth and achieve age-appropriate developmental milestones.
6. Parents will be able to describe hydrocephalus and how it affects their child; identify measures used to treat the disorder; and state realistic expectations about their child's condition following shunt insertion.

REFERENCES

Bradley WG Jr: Diagnostic tools in hydrocephalus, *Neurosurg Clin North Am* 12:661, 2001.

Chumas P et al: Hydrocephalus—what's new? *Arch Dis Child Fetal Neonatal Ed* 85:F149, 2001.

Del Bigio MR: Pathophysiologic consequences of hydrocephalus, *Neurosurg Clin North Am* 12:639, 2001.

Elias ER, Hobbs N: Spina bifida: sorting out the complexities of care, *Contemp Pediatr* 15(4):156, 1998.

Fletcher JM et al: Behavioral adjustment of children with hydrocephalus: relationships with etiology, neurological, and family status, *J Pediatr Psychol* 20(1):109, 1995.

Gerzeny M: Advances in endoscopic neurosurgery, *AORN J* 67(5):957, 1998.

Lauton KH et al: Current practices and advances in pediatric neurosurgery, *Nurs Clin North Am* 32(1):73, 1997.

39

◆

Hyperbilirubinemia

◆

PATHOPHYSIOLOGY

Neonatal hyperbilirubinemia or physiologic jaundice, a total serum bilirubin level higher than 5 mg/dl, is due to the neonate's predisposition for bilirubin production and limited ability to excrete it. By definition, there is no other abnormality or pathologic process present to account for the jaundice. The yellow coloration of the skin and mucous membranes is due to the deposition of unconjugated bilirubin pigment. The primary source of bilirubin is the breakdown of hemoglobin in aging or hemolyzed red blood cells (RBCs). In the neonate, RBCs have a higher turnover and a shorter life span, which enhance the higher production rate of bilirubin. The immaturity of the neonatal liver is a limiting factor in bilirubin excretion.

Unconjugated or indirect bilirubin is lipid soluble and binds to plasma albumin. The bilirubin is then taken up by the liver, where it is conjugated. Conjugated or direct bilirubin is excreted in the bile into the intestines. In the intestines, bacteria convert the conjugated bilirubin into urobilogen. The majority of the highly soluble urobilinogen is reexcreted by the liver and is eliminated in the feces; the kidneys excrete 5% of the urobilogen. Not only do increased RBC destruction and liver immaturity promote increased bilirubin levels, but other intestinal bacteria can deconjugate bilirubin, which allows it to be reabsorbed into the circulation and further raises bilirubin levels.

INCIDENCE

1. Age of onset is 2 to 3 days.
2. Severity differs among different races, with Asian and Native American infants presenting higher bilirubin levels.
3. Infants from certain geographic areas, particularly areas around Greece, have an increased incidence of hyperbilirubinemia.

CLINICAL MANIFESTATIONS

1. Jaundice is first noted on head and trunk and progresses downward.
2. Jaundice is noted on sclera, skin, and mucous membranes.
3. Urine becomes dark gold to brown color.
4. Bilirubin levels decline by fifth day and are usually within normal limits by tenth day of life.

COMPLICATIONS

1. Dehydration
2. Lethargy
3. Poor feeding
4. Kernicterus or encephalopathy resulting from deposition of unconjugated bilirubin in brain cells

LABORATORY AND DIAGNOSTIC TESTS

1. Complete blood count, liver function tests, blood typing, and Coombs' test—to rule out other causes
2. Indirect bilirubin levels—elevated

MEDICAL MANAGEMENT

Medical management is largely supportive. Prevention of neonatal hyperbilirubinemia should always be attempted by initiating feedings as soon as possible after birth. Bilirubin levels should be monitored, and the infant will be placed under phototherapy as the blood level dictates. All other causes of hyperbilirubinemia should be ruled out at this time. Other causes include Rh incompatibility, hemolytic disease, and biliary atresia. Infants at high risk for developing hyperbilirubinemia, such as premature infants and those with hypoxia and acidosis, may be placed under phototherapy prior to developing a significant bilirubin level.

NURSING ASSESSMENT

1. Assess skin color for progression of jaundice by applying pressure over bony prominence, which causes blanching and allows yellow color to become more evident.
2. Assess hydration status.
3. Assess nutritional intake.
4. Assess temperature control when under phototherapy.
5. Assess bowel elimination pattern.

NURSING DIAGNOSES

- Fluid volume, Deficient
- Nutrition: less than body requirements, Imbalanced
- Constipation
- Parenting, Impaired

NURSING INTERVENTIONS

1. Introduce feedings as soon as possible after birth as preventive measure.
2. Monitor hydration status.
3. During phototherapy do the following:
   a. Shield infant's eyes with eye patches, which are removed every 3 to 4 hours and assessed for drainage or irritation.
   b. Place infant nude under light, but cover testes when positioning supine.
   c. Change body position frequently.
   d. Monitor body temperature.
   e. Turn down phototherapy lights during blood sampling, as they can produce falsely low bilirubin level.
4. Administer glycerin suppository as needed to facilitate elimination of direct bilirubin in stool.
5. Promote bonding by encouraging parent to hold and feed infant while under phototherapy.

Discharge Planning and Home Care

1. Provide parent education regarding nutritional and hydration needs.
2. Instruct family in use of home phototherapy system.

3. Instruct family to obtain follow-up bilirubin level measurements.

CLIENT OUTCOMES

1. Infant's jaundice and bilirubin levels will decrease.
2. Infant will not sustain injury from phototherapy lights.
3. Infant will remain well hydrated.

REFERENCES

Guyton AC, Hall JE: *Pocket companion to textbook of medical physiology,* ed 10, Philadelphia, 2001, WB Saunders.

James SR et al: *Nursing care of children: principles and practice,* ed 2, Philadelphia, 2002, WB Saunders.

Porter ML, Dennis RL: Hyperbilirubinemia in the term newborn, *Am Fam Physician* 64:599, 2002.

Wood AJ: Neonatal hyperbilirubinemia, *N Engl J Med* 344:581, 2001.

40

❖

Hypertension

❖

PATHOPHYSIOLOGY

Hypertension in the pediatric client is described as blood pressure that is persistently between the 90th and 95th percentiles. Table 40-1 identifies guidelines (based on age and sex) for suspect blood pressure values. A variety of mechanisms are associated with hypertension. The renin-angiotensin-aldosterone system maintains fluid volume and vascular tone through the production of angiotensin II (a vasoconstrictor) and the stimulation of aldosterone production (for sodium retention). The sympathetic nervous system affects peripheral vascular resistance, cardiac output, and renin release, influencing the regulation of blood pressure.

Hypertension is classified as primary or secondary. Primary hypertension can be ascribed to no identifiable cause, whereas secondary hypertension is attributable to a structural abnormality or to an underlying disease (renal, cardiovascular, endocrine, central nervous system, or collagenous). A variety of factors have been identified as contributing to hypertension, including diet (high in calories, saturated fats, and sodium), contraceptive use, positive family history, obesity, and minimal physical exercise. Children generally manifest no overt symptoms. If symptomatic, the disease may be quite severe. Prognosis is variable, depending on the age of onset and response to treatment.

Problems evident in adults may have originated during the first or second decade of life. The earlier the onset, the more severe the disease will be.

TABLE 40-1
Approximate Guidelines for Suspect Blood Pressure

	Age (years)	Blood Pressure (mm Hg)
Supine Position—Lowest of Three Readings		
Boys and girls	3-5	110/70
	6-9	>120/75
	10-14	>130/80
Seated Position—Average of Second and Third Readings		
Girls	14-18	>125/80
Boys	14	>130/75
	15	>130/80
	16-18	>135/85

Modified from Gilles S, Kagan B: *Current pediatric therapy,* ed 13, Philadelphia, 1990, WB Saunders.

INCIDENCE

1. Incidence is increased among children in lower socioeconomic groups.
2. Incidence is increased among black adolescents.
3. Incidence rates vary from 0.6% to 20.5% (depends on methodology used).
4. Noncompliance with treatment occurs among more than 50% of affected children; compliance improves when the child is dependent on the parent.
5. Males are affected more often than females.
6. Forty-five percent to 100% of cases of hypertension in individuals 2 to 18 years of age are attributed to primary hypertension.
7. Twenty-five percent of children with primary hypertension have a positive family history of the disorder.
8. One percent to 2% of children and 11% to 12% of adolescents are affected.

CLINICAL MANIFESTATIONS

1. Severe headaches
2. Blurred vision, symptoms of increased intracranial pressure

3. Marked irritability
4. Nosebleeds
5. Dizziness
6. Fatigue
7. Nervousness
8. Anorexia, failure to thrive, weight loss
9. Focal or generalized seizures
10. Severe back and/or abdominal pain
11. Papilledema
12. Retinal hemorrhage or exudate
13. Left ventricular hypertrophy
14. Altered renal function

COMPLICATIONS

1. Ischemic (coronary) heart disease
2. Side effects associated with use of antihypertensives (e.g., postexercise syncope, depression, and dizziness)
3. Altered renal function

LABORATORY AND DIAGNOSTIC TESTS

1. Urinalysis, urine culture—to assess for renal cause
2. Serum electrolyte levels—to assess for renal and metabolic status
3. Complete blood count—to assess for infection, fluid overload
4. Creatinine, blood urea nitrogen levels—to assess for renal cause
5. Serum cholesterol level—higher than 250 mg/100 ml
6. Serum triglyceride level—increased
7. Lipoprotein electrophoresis—elevated lipoprotein levels
8. Electrocardiogram—left ventricular hypertrophy
9. Chest radiographic study—left ventricular hypertrophy
10. Rapid-sequence intravenous pyelogram—to assess activation of renin-angiotensin system
11. Plasma renin activity study—to assess activation of renin-angiotensin system
12. Excretory venogram—to detect renal and renovascular abnormalities
13. Arteriogram—to detect renal and renovascular abnormalities

14. Radionuclide studies—to detect renal and renovascular abnormalities

MEDICAL MANAGEMENT

The aim of controlling hypertension is to reduce the associated risk of cardiovascular and renal complications. The step approach to treatment for the pediatric client is to educate the child and family on the importance of prevention. Nonpharmacologic interventions such as diet adjustment, exercise, and weight control should be the first approach when possible. The goal of antihypertensive therapy is to maintain pressure below the 90th percentile using the least amount and number of drugs. Medications should be started one at a time using a diuretic, beta-blocker, or calcium antagonist. Keeping the medication schedule as simple as possible helps to promote compliance.

NURSING ASSESSMENT

1. See the Renal Assessment section in Appendix A.
2. Assess neurologic status.
3. Assess nutritional history.

NURSING DIAGNOSES

- Tissue perfusion, Ineffective
- Cardiac output, Decreased
- Knowledge, Deficient

NURSING INTERVENTIONS

1. Monitor child's clinical status and assess for changes.
   a. Blood pressure (see Appendix D)
   b. Neurologic status
   c. Presence of bleeding
   d. Blurred vision
   e. Renal function
2. Monitor child's therapeutic and untoward response to administered medications.
3. Monitor and encourage child's nutritional intake.
   a. Administer diet restricted in sodium, fats, and calories.

   b. Reinforce dietary information and management plan
      provided by dietitian.
   c. Include family members in teaching.

🔺 Discharge Planning and Home Care

Instruct child and family about management of hypertension:
   1. Explanation of hypertension
   2. Medications
   3. Dietary restrictions and weight control
   4. Use of oral contraceptives
   5. Salt intake
   6. Exercise
   7. Smoking

CLIENT OUTCOMES

1. Child will remain normotensive.
2. Child and family will understand follow-up needs.
3. Child will remain compliant with medication regimen
   and diet.

REFERENCES

Flynn JJ: Pharmacologic management of childhood hypertension: current status,
   future challenges, *Am J Hypertens* 15(2 pt 2):30S, 2002.
Friedman AL: Approach to the treatment of hypertension in children, *Heart Dis*
   4(1):47, 2002.
Sorof J, Daniels S: Obesity hypertension in children: a problem of epidemic
   proportions, *Hypertension* 40(4):441, 2002.

41

❖

Hypertrophic Pyloric Stenosis

❖

PATHOPHYSIOLOGY

Hypertrophic pyloric stenosis is one of the more frequently occurring conditions requiring surgery. Hypertrophy (increased size) and hyperplasia (increased mass) of the circular muscle of the pylorus cause obstruction at the pyloric sphincter. The circular muscle increases to as much as twice the normal thickness, and the pylorus in lengthens, which results in severe narrowing of the lumen. In addition, the stomach dilates, and hypertrophy of the gastric antrum occurs. The cause is unknown, but multiple factors have been implicated, and evidence suggests that local innervation is involved. Hypertrophic pyloric stenosis may be associated with intestinal malrotation, esophageal or duodenal atresias, and anorectal anomalies. In addition, there is a genetic predisposition. In 2000, the Centers for Disease Control and Prevention (CDC) reported a possible link between the use of oral erythromycin and hypertrophic pyloric stenosis. The CDC does not recommend that physicians stop prescribing erythromycin, just that they be aware of the possible risk.

INCIDENCE

1. Hypertrophic pyloric stenosis occurs in 1.5 to 4 of 1000 live births, usually within the first 3 to 5 weeks of life.
2. Hypertrophic pyloric stenosis is less common in African Americans and is rare in Asian individuals.
3. Male/female ratio is 5:1.
4. The disorder is more common in firstborn children.

CLINICAL MANIFESTATIONS

1. Nonbilious vomitus; may be blood streaked (initial symptom)
2. Vomiting, usually occurring 30 to 60 minutes after feeding
3. Vomiting that becomes progressively more projectile
4. Hungry feeding, eagerness to be fed after vomiting
5. Vomiting of retained feeding with current feeding
6. Signs of dehydration (decreased tears, poor skin turgor, dark circles under eyes, sunken fontanelle)
7. Failure to gain weight or weight loss
8. Distended upper abdomen after feeding
9. Irritability, crying
10. Visible left-to-right gastric peristaltic waves
11. Palpable firm, movable, olive-shaped mass in right upper quadrant

COMPLICATIONS

1. Jaundice—caused by deficiency of hepatic glucuronide transferase
2. Hypochloremic metabolic alkalosis (acute)
3. Severe dehydration (acute), with increased blood urea nitrogen levels

LABORATORY AND DIAGNOSTIC TESTS

1. Complete blood count—elevated hemoglobin and hematocrit, due to hemoconcentration
2. Serum electrolyte levels—hypochloremia, hypernatremia, hypokalemia (may be masked by hemoconcentration from extracellular fluid depletion)
3. Arterial blood gas values—metabolic alkalosis
4. Upper gastrointestinal barium studies—diagnostic; show delayed gastric emptying, long narrow pyloric channel, persistent narrowing
5. Abdominal ultrasonography—first-line diagnostic study

MEDICAL AND SURGICAL MANAGEMENT

Prior to surgery, fluid and electrolyte abnormalities and acid-base imbalances are corrected with intravenous (IV) fluids and electrolyte replacement. A pyloromyotomy, a longitudinal incision down to the mucosa and fully across the pyloric length, is the standard surgical treatment for this disorder. Laparoscopy has been found to be safe and successful for the correction of hypertrophic pyloric stenosis, resulting in shorter surgical time, more rapid postoperative feeding, and quicker discharge.

NURSING ASSESSMENT

1. See the Gastrointestinal Assessment section in Appendix A.
2. Assess for signs and symptoms of dehydration.
3. Assess for signs and symptoms of electrolyte imbalances.
4. Assess child's response to oral intake.
5. Assess child's response to pain.
6. Assess wound for drainage and infection.
7. Assess child and family coping.

NURSING DIAGNOSES

- Fluid volume, Deficient
- Nutrition: less than body requirements, Imbalanced
- Pain
- Infection, Risk for
- Knowledge, Deficient

NURSING INTERVENTIONS
Preoperative Care

1. Promote and maintain fluid and electrolyte balance.
   a. Maintain patent IV route for administration of ordered fluids at specified rate.
   b. Maintain patent nasogastric (NG) tube, if present.
   c. Maintain nothing-by-mouth status.
   d. Connect NG tube to low continuous suction to prevent distention and vomiting and to decrease risk of aspiration.
   e. Replace NG output with IV fluids as ordered.
   f. Perform gastric lavage with normal saline through NG tube until fluid is clear (preoperative preparation).
   g. Strictly monitor input and output (including number and characteristics of stools, NG drainage, and amount of emesis).
   h. Record urine specific gravity every 8 hours.
   i. Record weight daily.

     j. Monitor for signs and symptoms of dehydration (vital signs, mucous membranes, fontanelle status).
2. Monitor and report child's response to fluid and electrolyte imbalance.
3. Monitor and report laboratory results.
4. Monitor for signs of fluid and electrolyte imbalances.
5. Prepare parents preoperatively for child's upcoming surgery (see the Preparation for Procedures or Surgery section in Appendix J).

Postoperative Care

1. Promote and maintain fluid and electrolyte balance.
   a. Maintain patent IV route for administration of ordered fluids at specified rate.
   b. Strictly monitor intake and output.
   c. Monitor for signs of dehydration (vital signs, mucous membranes, fontanelle status, urine output).
   d. Maintain patent NG tube, if present.
2. Monitor child's response to oral intake.
   a. Initiate fluids by mouth 4 to 6 hours postoperatively; assess response.
   b. Provide small, frequent feedings (15 to 20 ml per feeding) as tolerated.
   c. Begin with clear liquids (glucose and electrolytes); increase to full-strength formula as tolerated.
   d. Feed infant in upright position.
   e. Observe for signs of vomiting and hematemesis (may delay feedings by mouth for 48 hours).
   f. Monitor for weight gain.
3. Provide nonpharmacologic and pharmacologic pain relief measures as indicated (see Appendix H).
   a. Monitor for signs of pain—crying, irritability, stretching, back arching, increased motor activity.
   b. Assess child's therapeutic and untoward reactions to medications.
4. Monitor and maintain integrity of incisional site.
   a. Assess for signs of infection—redness, drainage, inflammation, warmth to touch.
   b. Perform incision site care per institution protocols.

5. Provide psychosocial support (see the Supportive Care section in Appendix J).

Discharge Planning and Home Care

1. Instruct parents to monitor child's response to feedings and observe for untoward symptoms.
   a. Persistent vomiting
   b. Signs of infection
   c. Weight gain
2. Instruct parents about care of incisional site.
3. Provide follow-up support and management for parents.
   a. Name and phone number of primary physician
   b. Phone number of clinic
   c. Name and phone number of clinical nurse specialist and primary nurse

CLIENT OUTCOMES

1. Child will retain feedings.
2. Child will be adequately hydrated.
3. Child will have appropriate weight gain.
4. Child will experience no complications, such as infection.
5. Parents will demonstrate understanding of infant's or child's condition, possible complications, and home care requirements.

REFERENCES

Dolgin SE: Pyloric stenosis. In Burg FD et al, editors: *Gellis and Kagan's current pediatric therapy,* ed 16, Philadelphia, 1999, WB Saunders.

Gollin G et al: Rapid advancement of feedings after pyloromyotomy for pyloric stenosis, *Clin Pediatr* 39(3):187, 2000.

Morash D: An interdisciplinary project that changed practice in feeding methods after pyloromyotomy, *Pediatr Nurs* 28(2):113, 2002.

More on erythromycin and pyloric stenosis . . . and erythromycin as a prokinetic agent, *Pediatr Alert* 27(4):23, 2002.

Scholz M: Erythromycin may cause IHPS in newborns, *RN,* June 2000, available online at http://www.nursepdr.com/members/news/m_jun00.html, accessed June 9, 2003.

Wong DL et al: *Wong's essentials of pediatric nursing,* ed 6, St Louis, 2001, Mosby.

42

◆

Idiopathic Thrombocytopenic Purpura

◆

PATHOPHYSIOLOGY

Idiopathic thrombocytopenic purpura (ITP) is one of the most common acquired bleeding disorders. ITP is a condition in which the number of circulating platelets is reduced in the presence of normal marrow. The thrombocytopenia results from antibody-mediated platelet destruction. Generally, ITP is preceded by a vaguely defined febrile illness 1 to 6 weeks before onset of symptoms. Clinical manifestations vary considerably. ITP can be classified into three types: acute, chronic, and recurrent (Box 42-1). Children are initially seen with the following symptoms: (1) fever, (2) bleeding, (3) petechiae, (4) purpura with thrombocytopenia, and (5) anemia. Prognosis is favorable, especially in children with the acute form.

INCIDENCE

1. The age range of peak incidence is 2 to 5 years.
2. Frequency is 4 to 8 cases in 100,000 children per year.
3. ITP affects males and females equally.
4. ITP occurs more commonly in white individuals.
5. Eighty percent of ITP in children is the acute type.
6. Incidence is seasonal—occurrence is more frequent in winter and spring.
7. Fifty percent to 85% of affected children have a viral illness before onset of ITP.
8. Ten percent to 25% of affected children develop the chronic form of ITP.

BOX 42-1
Types of Idiopathic Thrombocytopenic Purpura

Acute
- Child is initially seen with thrombocytopenia.
- Platelet count returns to normal within 6 months of diagnosis (spontaneous remission).
- Subsequent relapses are not seen.

Chronic
- Thrombocytopenia persists longer than 6 months after diagnosis.
- Onset is insidious.
- Platelet count remains below normal throughout disease.
- This form is seen primarily in adults.

Recurrent
- Individual is initially seen with thrombocytopenia.
- Repeated relapses occur.

CLINICAL MANIFESTATIONS
1. Prodromal phase—fatigue, fever, and abdominal pain
2. Spontaneous appearance on skin of petechiae and ecchymoses
3. Easy bruising
4. Epistaxis (initial symptom in one third of children)
5. Menorrhagia
6. Hematuria (infrequent)
7. Bleeding from oral cavity (infrequent)
8. Melena (infrequent)

COMPLICATIONS
1. Transfusion reaction
2. Relapse
3. Central nervous system hemorrhage (less than 1% of affected individuals)

LABORATORY AND DIAGNOSTIC TESTS
1. Platelet count—decreased to less than 40,000/mm^3 and often less than 20,000/mm^3

2. Complete blood count—anemia results from inability of red blood cells to use iron
3. Bone marrow aspiration—increased megakaryocytes
4. White blood cell count—mild to moderate leukocytosis; mild eosinophilia
5. Platelet antibody tests—done when diagnosis is questionable
6. Tissue biopsy of skin and gingiva—diagnostic
7. Antinuclear antibody test—to rule out systemic lupus erythematosus
8. Slit-lamp examinations—to screen for uveitis
9. Renal biopsy—to diagnose renal involvement
10. Chest radiographic study and pulmonary function test—diagnostic for pulmonary manifestations (effusion, interstitial pulmonary fibrosis)

MEDICAL MANAGEMENT

The goal of treatment in ITP is the reduction of antibody production and platelet destruction, and elevation and maintenance of the platelet count. Corticosteroids are often used as the initial therapy for ITP. If the child does not respond to the corticosteroid regimens, intravenous immune globulin (IVIG) is administered. IVIG stimulates a rapid rise in platelet count within 24 hours of administration. Immunosuppressants (vincristine and cyclophosphamide) may be used in difficult cases. A splenectomy may be performed if ITP lasts longer than 1 year or the child is older than 5 years of age.

NURSING ASSESSMENT

1. See the Hematologic Assessment section in Appendix A.
2. Determine location of purpuric areas.
3. Determine sites of bleeding.

NURSING DIAGNOSES

- Injury, Risk for
- Tissue integrity, Impaired
- Tissue perfusion, Ineffective
- Fluid volume, Deficient

- Fatigue
- Diversional activity, Deficient
- Knowledge, Deficient

NURSING INTERVENTIONS

1. Monitor child's clinical status.
   a. Vital signs—monitored every 2 hours (during acute phase)
   b. Bleeding sites
   c. Level of activity
   d. Purpuric area
   e. Areas susceptible to bruising
2. Monitor for and prevent infection.
   a. Screen contacts with child.
   b. Institute clean techniques when in contact with child.
   c. Monitor for signs of infection (pulmonary, systemic, localized).
   d. Administer medications.
3. Monitor child's response to blood product transfusions (whole blood, packed cells, platelets).
4. Monitor child's therapeutic and untoward response to administration of medications.
   a. Antibiotics
   b. Antipyretics (avoid aspirin)
   c. Iron preparations
   d. Immunosuppressives
5. Promote rest and conservation of child's energy.
   a. Maintain complete bed rest during acute stages.
   b. Assess child's response to activity as means of assessing tolerance and progression.
6. Provide diversional and age-appropriate activities for child during periods of limited activities (see Appendix B).
7. Provide age-appropriate explanations before procedures, treatments, and surgery, if splenectomy is indicated (see the Preparation for Procedures or Surgery section in Appendix J).

🛎 Discharge Planning and Home Care

1. Provide parents and child with instructions about administration of medications.
   a. Time and route of administration
   b. Monitoring for untoward effects
2. Instruct parents and child to monitor for signs and symptoms of thrombocytopenia and report immediately (i.e., petechiae, ecchymosis, blood in urine or stool, and headache).
3. Instruct parents to monitor child's activities.
   a. Encourage quiet activities; have child avoid contact sports until platelet level returns to normal.
   b. Balance rest and activity periods; increase activity as tolerated.
4. Instruct parents to avoid contact by child with persons who have infections, especially upper respiratory tract infections.
5. Instruct parents to avoid use of over-the-counter medications that may affect clotting (i.e., antihistamines, aspirin, other nonsteroidal antiinflammatory drugs).

CLIENT OUTCOMES

1. Child's platelet count will return to normal between relapses.
2. Child will be free of complications of the disease.
3. Child will not demonstrate signs and symptoms of infection.
4. Child and family will verbalize knowledge of treatment regimen.

REFERENCES

Modak SI, Bussel JB: Treatment of children with immune thrombocytopenia purpura: are we closer to resolving the dilemma? *J Pediatr* 133(3):313, 1998.

Noonan N: Immune thrombocytic purpura, *J Soc Pediatr Nurs* 3(2):82, 1998.

Nugent DJ: Immune thrombocytopenic purpura: why treat? *J Pediatr* 134(1):1, 1999.

43

❖

Imperforate Anus

❖

PATHOPHYSIOLOGY

The congenital malformation known as imperforate anus (anorectal agenesis) involves the anus, the rectum, or the junction between the two. There are two classifications of imperforate anus, related to the placement of the distal end of the colon (rectum). In high lesions, the rectum ends above the puborectalis sling, the main muscle complex responsible for sphincter control and fecal continence. In low lesions, the rectum has traversed the puborectalis sling, with an abnormal location in the perineum. Affected infants can be expected to have rectal continence after repair.

Along with the imperforate anus, the following may also occur:

1. In girls, a fistula may be present between the rectum and the vagina.
2. In boys, a fistula may be present between the rectum and the urinary tract at the scrotum.

The appearance of the defect varies, depending on its severity. A less-involved imperforate anus appears as a deep anal dimple and exhibits strong muscular reaction to pinprick, which indicates innervation of that area. More severe involvement is initially seen as a flat perineum with no dimple and poor muscular response to pinprick, a result of defective perineal innervation and muscle formation. A highly involved defect includes other anomalies as well (Table 43-1). The infant may initially be seen with poorly developed labia, undescended testicles, or ambiguous genitalia. Outcomes are favorable after definitive surgery is performed.

TABLE 43-1
Associated Anomalies

Type	Incidence (%)*
Esophageal atresia	13
Intestinal atresia	4
Intestinal malrotation	4
Cardiovascular defects	7
Skeletal deformities (spina bifida, agenesis of sacrum)	6
Genitourinary anomalies (renal agenesis, hypospadias, epispadias)	40

*Approximate percentages.

INCIDENCE

1. Imperforate anus occurs in 1 of every 4000 to 5000 live births.
2. Twenty percent to 75% of affected infants have an associated anomaly, with genitourinary tract malformations found most frequently (20% to 54%) and tracheo-esophageal fistula occurring in 10% of infants.
3. Imperforate anus affects boys and girls with equal frequency, and there is usually no family history of this abnormality.
4. The presence of associated anomalies is usually the cause of death.

CLINICAL MANIFESTATIONS

1. Physical examination showing absent external anal opening
2. Failure to pass meconium within first 24 hours after birth
3. Inability to take infant's rectal temperature
4. Passage of meconium through fistula or misplaced anus
5. Gradual distention and signs of bowel obstruction if no fistula present

COMPLICATIONS

1. Hyperchloremic acidosis
2. Continuing urinary tract infection

3. Urethral damage (result of surgical procedure)
4. Long-term complications
   a. Eversion of anal mucosa
   b. Stenosis (result of contraction of scar from anastomosis)
   c. Impactions and constipation (result of sigmoid dilation)
   d. Problems or delays associated with toilet training
   e. Incontinence (result of anal stenosis or impaction)
   f. Prolapse of anorectal mucosa (results in persistent seepage and incontinence)
   g. Recurrent fistulas (result of tension in surgical site and infection)

LABORATORY AND DIAGNOSTIC TESTS

1. Visual and digital rectal examination is generally diagnostic.
2. If a fistula is present, urine may be examined for meconium epithelial cells.
3. Inverted lateral radiographic study (Wangensteen-Rice technique) may demonstrate air collected in the blind-ending rectum at or near the perineum; may be misleading if the rectum is filled with meconium, which prevents air from reaching the end of the rectal pouch.
4. Ultrasonography may be helpful in locating the rectal pouch.
5. Needle aspiration for detecting the rectal pouch involves advancing the needle while attempting to aspirate; if no meconium has been obtained by the time the needle has been advanced 1.5 cm, the defect is assumed to be of a high type.

SURGICAL MANAGEMENT

Surgical therapy in the newborn varies with the severity of the defect. The higher the lesion, the more complicated the surgical correction procedure. For high anomalies, a colostomy is performed a few days after birth. The definitive surgery, a perineal anoplasty (an abdominal-perineal pull-through procedure), is generally delayed 3 to 12 months. This delay allows the pelvis to enlarge and the musculature to develop. It also enables the infant to gain weight and attain satisfactory nutritional status. Low lesions are corrected by pulling the rectal pouch through the sphincter to the opening on the anal skin. Fistulas, if present, are closed. Membranous defects require only minimal surgical treatment. The membrane is punctured with a hemostat or scalpel.

In most instances, correction of the imperforate anus requires a two-stage surgical approach. For mild to moderate defects, the prognosis is favorable. The defect can be repaired, and normal peristalsis and continence can be obtained. More serious defects are usually associated with other anomalies, which complicate the surgical outcomes.

NURSING ASSESSMENT

1. See the Gastrointestinal Assessment section in Appendix A.
2. Assess nutritional status.

NURSING DIAGNOSES

- Fluid volume, Risk for deficient
- Nutrition: less than body requirements, Imbalanced
- Tissue integrity, Impaired
- Infection, Risk for
- Pain
- Home maintenance, Impaired

NURSING INTERVENTIONS

Preoperative Care

1. Monitor infant's condition before surgery.
   a. Measure abdominal girth (assess for abdominal distention).
   b. Monitor vital signs every 4 hours.
   c. Monitor for bowel complications (perforation and enterocolitis).
   d. Monitor fluid and electrolyte balance (intake and output, nasogastric [NG] drainage).
2. Prepare infant for surgery.
   a. Monitor infant's response to evacuation of bowel.
   b. Using NG tube, decompress stomach.
   c. Using catheter, decompress bladder.
   d. Provide only clear liquids 24 to 48 hours before surgery.

    e. Monitor infant's response to antibiotics (e.g., neomycin) used to sterilize bowel.

3. Prepare infant for procedures and surgeries.

Postoperative Care

1. Monitor infant's response to surgery.
   a. Vital signs
   b. Intake and output—report discrepancies
   c. Surgical site—bleeding, intactness, signs of infection
2. Monitor for signs and symptoms of complications.
   a. Urinary tract infection
   b. Hyperchloremic acidosis
   c. Decreased urinary output
   d. Constipation
   e. Obstruction
   f. Bleeding
3. Promote and maintain fluid and electrolyte balance.
   a. Record intake per route (intravenous, NG, oral).
   b. Record output per route (urine and stool, NG drainage, emesis, Penrose drain).
   c. Assess hydration status (signs of dehydration, electrolyte imbalance).
4. Provide dressing care; maintain integrity of surgical site (depends on type of surgery).
   a. Monitor dilation of anus.
   b. Monitor endorectal pull-through incision (made over anal dimple and colon directly through to muscle cuff) for mucosal prolapse.
   c. Do not take rectal temperatures, give rectal medications, or perform rectal examinations.
   d. Keep anus clean and dry.
   e. Apply zinc oxide for skin lesions and irritation surrounding surgical site.
   f. Avoid tension on suture line; position infant on side or abdomen.
5. Promote adequate nutritional intake.
   a. Monitor bowel sounds; begin feeding fluids when bowel sounds are heard.
   b. Advance to full diet as tolerated.

6. Protect infant from infection.
   a. Provide Foley catheter care.
   b. Change dressing and note drainage.
   c. Monitor incisional site for drainage, redness, inflammation.
   d. Clean anal area frequently to prevent fecal contamination.
   e. Perform pulmonary toilet every 2 to 4 hours.
   f. Change infant's position every 2 hours.
   g. Monitor for signs of systemic infection or local abscess.
7. Promote functioning and maintain patency of colostomy.
8. Promote comfort and minimize pain.
   a. Provide sitz bath (initiate 1 week after surgery).
   b. Apply zinc oxide to excoriated and irritated areas of skin.
   c. Provide position of comfort.
   d. Use distractions (play activities).
   e. Monitor child's response to medication.

🔺 Discharge Planning and Home Care

1. Encourage parents to express concerns about outcomes of surgery.
2. Refer to specific institutional procedures for information distributed to parents about home care.
3. Instruct parents on signs of intestinal obstruction, poor tolerance of feedings, and impaired healing processes.
4. Instruct parents about follow-up techniques to promote optimal surgical outcomes.
   a. Colostomy care
   b. Dilation of anus
   c. Sitz baths
5. Instruct parents that, as children age, psychologic counseling should be part of follow-up care. Twenty nine percent of affected children experience some behavioral problems.

CLIENT OUTCOMES

1. Infant's gastrointestinal function will return to normal.
2. Infant will continue to grow at a steady pace.

3. Parents will verbalize understanding of home care and
   follow-up needs.

REFERENCES

Hartman GE et al: General surgery. In Avery GB et al, editors: *Neonatology: pathophysiology and management of the newborn*, ed 5, Philadelphia, 1999, Lippincott Williams & Wilkins.

Ludman L et al: Psychosocial adjustment of children treated for anorectal anomalies, *J Pediatr Surg* 30(3):495, 1995.

Pena A: Anorectal malformations. In Behrman RE et al, editors: *Nelson textbook of pediatrics*, ed 16, Philadelphia, 2000, WB Saunders.

Pena A: Imperforate anus and cloacal malformations. In Ashcraft KW, editor: *Pediatric surgery*, ed 3, Philadelphia, 2000, WB Saunders.

44

◆

Inborn Errors of Metabolism

◆

PATHOPHYSIOLOGY

Infants born with inborn errors of metabolism lack an enzyme essential in the body's biochemical reactions or have deficient amounts of it. All ingested food is broken down into fats, proteins, carbohydrates, vitamins, and minerals and then metabolized by enzymes. An enzyme deficiency, as seen with inborn errors of metabolism, prevents the usual chain of biochemical reactions, referred to as the metabolic pathway, from occurring properly. Instead, abnormal chains of metabolic substances are formed due to a deficiency in the key normal enzyme, which can cause a number of untoward outcomes, as observed with inborn errors of metabolism. Box 44-1 presents numerous genetic disorders that are enzyme deficiencies. Most of these enzyme deficiencies are inherited as autosomal recessive traits; others (rarely) are transmitted as sex-linked or mitochondrial disorders.

Metabolic disorders in the newborn are not necessarily identified in the hospital, because the clinical manifestations may not become evident until weeks or even months later. Clinical manifestations can be specific or general, depending on the disorder. Metabolic disorders have been categorized into three types: (1) those that are "silent" or slowly manifest symptoms, such as phenylketonuria, and that if not treated early can result in mental retardation; (2) those that present as an acute metabolic crisis in which shortly after birth (a few days) the infant demonstrates symptoms of respiratory distress, vomiting, and lethargy leading to coma, and that can be life threatening if not identified and treated, such as urea cycle disorders or organic acidemias; and (3) those that cause progressive neurologic disorders, such

BOX 44-1
Inborn Errors of Metabolism

Disorders of Carbohydrate Metabolism
Disorders of Galactose Metabolism
- Hereditary galactokinase deficiency
- Hereditary galactose-1-phosphate uridyltransferase deficiency
- Hereditary uridine diphosphate galactose 4-epimerase deficiency

Disorders of Fructose Metabolism
- Hereditary fructose intolerance
- Hereditary fructose-1,6-diphosphate deficiency

Carbohydrate Malabsorption in the Intestinal Brush Border
- Congenital lactase deficiency
- Sucrase-isomaltase deficiency
- Congenital glucose-galactose malabsorption

Glycogen Storage Diseases
- Von Gierke's disease (type Ia glycogen storage disease)
- Pompe's disease (type II glycogen storage disease)
- Cori's disease (type III glycogen storage disease)
- Andersen's disease (type IV glycogen storage disease)
- McArdle disease (type V glycogen storage disease)
- Hers' disease (type VI glycogen storage disease)
- Tarui's disease (type VII glycogen storage disease)
- Fanconi-Bickel disease (type XI glycogen storage disease)

Disorders of Amino Acid Metabolism
- Hyperphenylalaninemias
- Phenylketonuria and nonphenylkentonuric forms of hyperphenylalaninemia
- Hypertyrosinemias
- Hepatorenal tyrosinemia: fumarylacetoacetate hydrolase deficiency (type I tyrosinemia)
- Oculocutaneous tyrosinemia: tyrosine aminotransferase deficiency (type II tyrosinemia)
- Deficiency of 4-hydroxyphenylpyruvate dioxygenase (type III tyrosinemia)

Disorders of Histidine Metabolism
- Histidinuria
- Urocanicaciduria

Continued

BOX 44-1
Inborn Errors of Metabolism—cont'd

- Nonketotic hyperglycinemia
- Neonatal nonketotic hyperglycinemia
- Urea cycle enzymes and the congenital hyperammonemias

Amino Acid Transport Disorders

- Cystinuria type 1
- Cystinuria type 2
- Lysinuric protein intolerance (LPI)
- Hyperornithinemia-hyperammonemia-homocitrullinuria (HHH) syndrome
- Blue diaper syndrome
- Methioninuria
- Glycinuria
- Lysinuria

Urea Cycle Disorders

- Carbamyl phosphate synthetase (CPS) deficiency
- Ornithine transcarbamylase (OTC) deficiency
- Argininosuccinicaciduria (ASA)
- Argininemia
- Citrullinemia

Branched-Chain Amino Acid and Keto Acid Disorders

- Maple syrup urine diseases (MSUDs)
- Classic MSUD
- Intermediate MSUD
- Intermittent MSUD
- Thiamine-responsive MSUD
- Dihydrolipoyl dehydrogenase (E3)–deficient MSUD

Organic Acidemias: Disorders of Propionate and Methylmalonate Metabolism

- Propionicacidemia
- Methylmalonicacidemias

Disorders of Pyruvate Dehydrogenase Complex
Disorders of Pyruvate Carboxylase Complex
Pyruvate Kinase and Glucose-6-Phosphatase Deficiencies

- Pyruvate kinase deficiency
- Glucose-6-phosphate dehydrogenase deficiency

BOX 44-1
Inborn Errors of Metabolism—cont'd

Disorders of Lipid Metabolism
- Abetalipoproteinemia
- Familial combined hyperlipidemia
- Tangier disease

Familial Hyperlipoproteinemia: Familial Lipoprotein Lipase Deficiency
Familial Cholesterolemia
Disorders of Lysosomal Enzyme
Gangliosidoses
- G_{M1} Gangliosidosis
- G_{M2} Gangliosidoses
- Niemann-Pick disease type A
- Niemann-Pick disease type B
- Niemann-Pick disease type C

Disorders of Purine Metabolism
- Lesch-Nyhan syndrome
- Hereditary xanthinuria
- Pyrimidine metabolic disorders

Adapted from Theorell C, Degenhardt M: Assessment and management of metabolic dysfunction. In Kenner C et al, editors: *Comprehensive neonatal nursing: a physiologic perspective,* ed 2, Philadelphia, 1998, WB Saunders, pp 409-475; and Theorell C, Degenhardt M: Assessment and management of metabolic dysfunction. In Kenner C et al, editors: *Comprehensive neonatal nursing: a physiologic perspective,* ed 3, Philadelphia, 2003, WB Saunders, pp 486-530.

as Tay-Sachs disease. It is important that these disorders be detected and treated as soon as possible to prevent or minimize serious outcomes of developmental delays, learning disabilities, attention-deficit/hyperactivity disorder, or mental retardation. Widespread screening exists for the following inborn errors of metabolism: (1) phenylketonuria, (2) congenital hypothyroidism, (3) galactosemia, (4) maple syrup urine disease, and (5) congenital adrenal hyperplasia. In the future, gene-based therapy may offer promising options to correct the deficiency of the enzyme or substrate. Newborn screening guidelines are available from the Health Resources and Services

Administration of the U.S. Department of Health and Human Services, under the title "U.S. Newborn Screening System Guidelines II: Follow-Up of Children, Diagnosis, Management, and Evaluation: Statement of the Council of Regional Networks for Genetic Services (CORN)" (available from http://www.ask.hrsa.gov/detail.cfm?id=MCHN011). Risk factors associated with inborn errors of metabolism include past family history of unexplained neonatal and/or sibling deaths, consanguinity, multiple spontaneous abortions, psychomotor difficulties in family members, and symptoms associated with metabolic diseases, such as metabolic acidosis, ataxia, and hypoglycemia, in previous children.

INCIDENCE

1. Incidence is fewer than 1 in 10,000 births.
2. Sixty percent of pregnancy losses are caused by genetic problems.
3. Twenty percent to 30% of infant mortality is due to genetic defects, the leading cause of infant mortality.
4. Between 30% and 50% of postneonatal infant deaths are due to congenital anomalies.
5. Genetic defects are the fourth leading cause of diminished life span.
6. In most infants, autosomal recessive conditions will be identified by 1 month of age.
7. Incidence for certain disorders (e.g., sickle cell disease, Tay-Sachs disease, cystic fibrosis) is higher among specific ethnic groups.

CLINICAL MANIFESTATIONS

A number of presenting symptoms are linked with inborn errors of metabolism. Symptoms may be generalized or specific in manifestations. Examples of clinical manifestations associated with selected disorders are presented below.

1. Neuromuscular dysfunction
   a. Acute and progressive encephalopathies (disorders of histidine metabolism, disorders of lysosomal enzymes, classic maple syrup urine disease, disorders of amino acid metabolism)

    b. Hypotonia (disorders of histidine metabolism, classic maple syrup urine disease)

    c. Hypertonia (classic maple syrup urine disease)

    d. Abnormal eye movements (disorders of histidine metabolism)

    e. Seizures (Zellweger syndrome, Smith-Lemli-Opitz syndrome, classic maple syrup urine disease, intermittent maple syrup urine disease)

    f. Myoclonia

2. Cerebral/cognitive/developmental dysfunction

    a. Cycles of hyperexcitability and somnolence

    b. Lethargy (disorders of histidine metabolism, urea cycle defects, organic acidemias, disorders of amino acid metabolism)

    c. Hypothermia

    d. Changes in level of consciousness (disorders of lipid metabolism, urea cycle defects, organic acidemias, disorders of amino acid metabolism)

    e. Coma (disorders of histidine metabolism, classic maple syrup urine disease, intermittent maple syrup urine disease)

    f. Cataracts/blindness/retinal lesions (disorders of galactose metabolism, disorders of histidine metabolism, classic maple syrup urine disease, disorders of lysosomal enzymes)

    g. Irritability

    h. Temperature instability

    i. Developmental delay (disorders of galactose metabolism, Lesch-Nyhan syndrome)

    j. Mental retardation (disorders of amino acid metabolism, disorders of histidine metabolism [cystathionine β-synthase deficiency], classic maple syrup urine disease)

3. Respiratory dysfunction

    a. Tachypnea (urea cycle defects, organic acidemias, disorders of amino acid metabolism)

    b. Apnea (disorders of fructose metabolism, urea cycle defects, organic acidemias, disorders of amino acid metabolism)

     c. Respiratory distress (disorders of fructose metabolism, organic acidemias, Lesch-Nyhan syndrome)

     d. Respiratory alkalosis (urea cycle defects)

4. Cardiovascular dysfunction
   a. Cardiac failure
   b. Thromboembolism (disorders of histidine metabolism [cystathionine β-synthase deficiency])
   c. Cardiomyopathy

5. Immunologic or hematologic disturbances
   a. Infections (disorders of branched-chain amino and keto acids, disorders of fructose metabolism, glucose-6-phosphate dehydrogenase deficiency)
   b. Hydrops fetalis (lysosomal storage disorders)
   c. Organomegaly (lysosomal storage disorders)

6. Gastrointestinal/hepatic dysfunction
   a. Liver dysfunction (jaundice, hepatosplenomegaly, cholestasis) (disorders of fructose metabolism, disorders of galactose metabolism, pyruvate kinase deficiency, glucose-6-phosphate dehydrogenase deficiency, disorders of amino acid metabolism)
   b. Recurrent vomiting (disorders of carbohydrate metabolism, disorders of fructose metabolism, disorders of galactose metabolism, urea cycle defects, organic acidemias, disorders of amino acid metabolism, disorders of lipid metabolism)
   c. Diarrhea (disorders of carbohydrate metabolism)
   d. Problems with feeding (disorders of fructose metabolism, disorders of histidine metabolism, organic acidemias, disorders of amino acid metabolism)
   e. Weight loss (disorders of carbohydrate metabolism)
   f. Dehydration (disorders of carbohydrate metabolism)
   g. Failure to thrive (disorders of galactose metabolism)

7. Genitourinary disturbances
   a. Unusual urine odor or color (disorders of amino acid metabolism, disorders of branched-chain amino and keto acids [maple syrup urine disease])
   b. Varying renal involvement, including renal failure (disorders of amino acid metabolism)
   c. Unusual odor of breath or sweat
   d. Episode of Reye's-like symptoms
   e. Hypoglycemia (disorders of fructose metabolism, disorders of lipid metabolism, organic acidemias, disorders of amino acid metabolism)
8. Fluid-electrolyte imbalance
   a. Hyperammonemia (disorders of lipid metabolism, organic acidemias, disorders of amino acid metabolism)
   b. Metabolic acidosis (disorders of carbohydrate metabolism, organic acidemias, disorders of amino acid metabolism)
   c. Lactic acidosis (disorders of fructose metabolism)
   d. Ketonuria (maple syrup urine disease)
9. Integumentary system effects
   a. Pigmentation changes in skin, eyes, and hair (disorders of amino acid metabolism)
10. Musculoskeletal abnormalities
    a. Dysmorphism (pyruvate dehydrogenase deficiency)
    b. Skeletal malformations (disorders of histidine metabolism [cystathionine β-synthase deficiency], Lesch-Nyhan syndrome)
    c. Coarse facial features

COMPLICATIONS

Complications will vary depending on when the enzyme deficiency was identified and treated.

1. Developmental disabilities (the most common are movement or neuromuscular disorders and mental retardation)
2. Irreversible brain damage
3. Coma

4. Congenital heart defects
5. Hepatic failure

LABORATORY AND DIAGNOSTIC TESTS

Listed here are the laboratory tests most commonly used for the diagnosis of inborn errors of metabolism. Selection of tests will depend on the clinical presentation and severity of symptoms.

1. Serum glucose level
2. Blood gas values
3. Serum ammonia level
4. Complete blood count with differential
5. Coagulation studies
6. Serum electrolyte levels
7. Blood urea nitrogen assay
8. Serum creatinine level
9. Plasma ammonia level
10. Serum anion gap
11. Plasma and cerebrospinal fluid lactate levels
12. Urine test for glucose, ketones, phenylpyruvic acid, toxic substances
13. Urine level of reducing substances
14. Urine level of organic acids
15. Magnetic resonance imaging—used for diagnosis
16. Computed tomography—used for diagnosis
17. Electroencephalography—used for diagnosis
18. Nerve conduction velocity studies—used for diagnosis
19. Electromyography—used for diagnosis

In the event of infant death, the following tests should be performed:

1. Skin sample analysis for enzymes and culture of fibroblasts
2. Needle biopsy of kidney, liver, muscle, and brain

MEDICAL MANAGEMENT

The first priority of medical therapy is to treat the infant who has life-threatening symptoms such as acute metabolic encephalopathy with the goal of stabilizing the infant. Other acute episodes of illness the infant may experience are metabolic acidosis, electrolyte disturbances, respiratory distress, intractable seizures, and sepsis. These critical problems require aggressive medical treatment such as exchange transfusion, venovenous hemofiltration, peritoneal dialysis, hemodialysis, and assisted ventilation. The goal of this phase of critical care is stabilization of the infant and prevention of complications.

The goal of long-term treatment approaches to manage enzyme disorders can be described in the following general terms. Dietary substances creating the toxic substrate, such as phenylalanine, are restricted or excluded from the diet. An enzyme replacement can be given for enzyme deficiencies, similar to thyroid replacement for hypothyroidism. An alternate metabolic pathway can be stimulated that circumvents the blocked metabolic pathway. Clinical status can be improved with the administration of high doses of vitamins (e.g., pyridoxine, biotin, vitamin B_{12}). Enzyme therapy that involves replacing the deficient enzyme with a synthetic product is another treatment option. Depending on the diagnosis, a specific management plan for treatment will be instituted. Treatment plans will vary according to the particular syndrome and include nutritional therapy, such as administration of commercially prepared synthetic formulas; dietary supplementation; and, in some instances, invasive treatments such as splenectomy. Depending on the enzyme involved, bone marrow transplantation, liver transplantation, and gene therapy may be used to correct the metabolic disorder. Early detection and treatment are key to preventing or ameliorating the long-term effects of enzyme deficiencies.

NURSING ASSESSMENT

The purpose of nursing assessment of the child with an inborn error of metabolism varies depending on the circumstances. During the diagnostic period, nursing assessment is focused on stabilization of the infant's condition, diagnosis of the metabolic disorder, and initiation of the long-term treatment plan. Once the acute phase subsides, then nursing assessment is directed to monitoring the child's growth and development, response to treatment, long-terms effects, and family management of the child's ongoing and long-term treatment plan. The assessment information listed below addresses the long-term components of care. Assessment parameters for the acute phase can be found in other chapters pertaining to the infant's presenting symptoms, such as apnea or renal failure.

Ongoing nursing assessment of the child includes obtaining the nursing history and family pedigree (genogram); this includes gathering information on the family history of children with hypoglycemia, acute encephalopathy, metabolic acidosis, and psychomotor difficulties. Information is obtained on the mother's pregnancy history, such as spontaneous abortions, previous pregnancies, and unexplained neonatal deaths.

1. Assess for dysmorphic features, including evaluation of the following:
   a. Shape of head; presence of microcephaly (small for size), macrocephaly (large for size), or hydrocephaly (due to increase in cerebrospinal fluid)
   b. Shape and placement of ears
   c. Face—spacing of features, symmetry, signs of weakness or paralysis
   d. Eyes—level, spacing between eyes, color of iris, lens, epicanthal folds, cataracts, retinal changes
   e. Appearance of neck
   f. Shape of nose
   g. Shape and contour of lips, size of jaw, tongue size
   h. Hair distribution
2. Assess integumentary system.
   a. Skin pigmentation
   b. Ear tag
   c. Hairy patch at base of spine
3. Assess musculoskeletal system.
   a. Poor muscle tone
   b. Size of chest
   c. Extremities, including webbing of fingers, finger and toe length
4. Assess for neurologic signs and symptoms.
   a. Altered level of consciousness
   b. Lethargy
   c. Deficient motor skills
   d. Abnormal reflexes (hypotonia)

     e. Poor sucking

     f. Seizures

5. Assess for other anomalies (not listed earlier).
6. Assess for signs of infection (fever, increased white blood cell count, septic shock).
7. Assess for skin breakdown from pruritus, malnutrition, edema, and decreased ability to heal.
8. Assess for malnutrition (lethargy, weakness, poor feeding, decreased appetite, vomiting, failure to gain weight, inadequate caloric intake).
9. Assess child's comfort level (see Appendix H).
10. Assess coping responses and child's level of activity, and provide therapeutic environment for child.
    a. Encourage child and parents to express feelings of concern about child's condition.
    b. Provide developmentally appropriate information and reinforce data provided to child and parents (see the Preparation for Procedures or Surgery section in Appendix J).
11. Assess family's ability to manage child's long-term care and to access community-based services, and provide supportive measures as indicated (see Appendix L).
12. Assess for developmental delay, achievement of growth and development milestones, and age at which milestones are achieved (see Appendix B).

NURSING DIAGNOSES

- Injury, Risk for
- Body temperature, Risk for imbalanced
- Decreased intracranial adaptive capacity
- Imbalanced body temperature, Risk for
- Tissue perfusion, Ineffective
- Gas exchange, Impaired
- Respiratory function, Risk for Ineffective
- Excess fluid volume
- Nutrition: less than body requirements, Imbalanced
- Infection, Risk for
- Family processes, Interrupted
- Growth and development, Delayed

- Therapeutic regimen management, Ineffective
- Caregiver role strain

NURSING INTERVENTIONS
Care During Acute Phase

1. Monitor clinical status and immediately report any changes.
   a. Early signs of encephalopathy:
      i. Poor feeding
      ii. Vomiting
      iii. Lethargy
      iv. Irritability
      v. Abnormal muscle tone
   b. Other symptoms to report immediately:
      i. Apnea episodes
      ii. Drowsiness
      iii. Hiccups
      iv. Myoclonus
      v. Bulging fontanelles
      vi. Change in level of consciousness
2. Maintain cardiorespiratory stability.
   a. Establish infant's baseline respiratory and cardiac values and monitor for changes (see Appendix A).
      i. Monitor depth, symmetry, and rhythm of respirations.
      ii. Monitor rate and quality of heart sounds, murmurs.
   b. Monitor responsiveness to medical interventions.
   c. Monitor trends in oxygenation through oximetry and/or transcutaneous monitoring; monitor correlation between environment, positioning, and transcutaneous monitoring readings.
   d. Monitor arterial blood gas values and laboratory data.
   e. Monitor blood pressure and fluctuations with activity and treatments.
   f. Monitor action and side effects of medications.
   g. Coordinate delivery of routine care and procedures, and cluster care as appropriate.
   h. Suction as needed.
   i. Administer sedative and analgesics as needed.

3. Monitor neurologic status with serial measures.
    a. Report any deterioration or questionable findings; intervention may be required on emergency basis.
    b. Monitor level of consciousness.
        i. General appearance
        ii. Arousability
        iii. Orientation
        iv. Lethargy, reaction to sound, touch, and bright colors
    c. Monitor vital signs.
        i. Respiratory pattern
        ii. Blood pressure
        iii. Heart rate
        iv. Temperature
    d. Check pupils (pupils equal, react to light, accommodate).
    e. Monitor reaction to pain (see Appendix H).
    f. Check head circumference (check fontanelles).
    g. Use Glasgow Coma Scale (see the Neurologic Assessment section in Appendix A).
    h. Provide calm, quiet environment.
4. Monitor and maintain appropriate fluid, nutrient, and caloric intake.
    a. Maintain intravenous access as needed.
    b. Administer feedings via most appropriate route for medical status.
    c. Record weight daily and length and head circumference weekly.
    d. Monitor and record intake and output (including blood products, urine, and stool); check pH and specific gravity.
5. Assess for signs of infection and implement preventative measures.
    a. Practice good hand-washing and aseptic technique.
    b. Perform care for all invasive catheters and lines according to institutional procedures.
    c. Adhere to institutional policy for isolation procedures as indicated.

Ongoing and Long-Term Care

1. Monitor for adequate caloric intake and growth over time.
   a. Monitor for weight gain of approximately 20 to 30 g/day (see Appendix G).
   b. Monitor infant's ability to maintain adequate oral intake. (Infants who are tachypneic and have increased work of breathing may not be able to take food orally because of compromise of airway and risk of aspiration.)
   c. Monitor for increased oxygen requirements during and immediately after oral feedings; provide increased oxygen as needed.
   d. Provide supplementation to oral feedings through gavage or gastrostomy tube feedings.
      i. Ensure placement of gastrostomy/gavage feeding tubes.
      ii. Monitor for adverse response to feedings.
      iii. Provide oral stimulation with feedings.
2. Promote growth and development by integrating play and positive stimulation into care routine (see Appendix B).
   a. Provide opportunities for developmentally appropriate visual, auditory, tactile, and kinesthetic stimulation when infant is alert and stable.
   b. Integrate pattern and routine into care, including undisturbed night sleep and predictable daytime activities.
   c. Monitor infant's response to caregiving and developmental activities.
   d. Assess for increased oxygen requirements during and immediately following activity.
   e. Assess for patterns of response to activities and caregivers.
   f. Develop list of likes, dislikes, and comfort measures from assessed patterns of response.
   g. Decrease environmental and caregiver stimulation during periods of agitation and/or stress.
3. Facilitate integration of infant into his or her family.
   a. Assist parents in recognizing infant's responses to activity.

    b. Teach parents how they can best interact with and provide care for their child.

    c. Develop parents' confidence in caring for their child.

    d. Promote visitation and caregiving by other key family members, including siblings, as soon as appropriate.

4. Refer family to genetic specialists, because genetic counseling is advisable in view of genetic factor(s) associated with inborn errors of metabolism. If parents are planning for additional children, they may benefit from information about heritable nature of this child's condition.

    a. Carefully record family history, prior reproductive history of couple, and so on (may be very helpful to genetic specialists).

    b. Follow up with family after referral to genetic specialist.

    c. Answer any additional questions, clarify misconceptions.

    d. Reinforce information.

🔺 Discharge Planning and Home Care

1. Evaluate readiness for discharge. Factors to assess include the following:

    a. Stable cardiorespiratory and neurologic status

    b. Adequate nutritional intake and growth

    c. Stable medication needs

    d. Medical treatment plan that is realistic for home

       i. Parents or other caregivers can provide needed care.

       ii. Needed home equipment and monitoring are provided.

       iii. Parents have necessary social and/or financial support.

       iv. Provision is made for respite or home nursing needs.

2. Provide discharge instruction for parents covering the following:

    a. Explanation of genetic disorder

    b. Information on how to monitor for signs of respiratory distress and other medical problems

    c. Individualized feeding needs

    d. Well-baby needs

    e. Guidelines on when to call doctor

    f. Method of performing cardiopulmonary resuscitation

    g. Use of home equipment and monitoring devices

    h. Method of administering medications and monitoring for their effects

    i. Infection prevention

    j. Importance of smoke-free environment

    k. Appropriate developmental activities

    l. Recognition of infant's stress and interaction cues

    m. Available community resources and support services (e.g., early intervention) (see Appendix L)

3. Provide follow-up to monitor ongoing cardiorespiratory, neurologic, nutritional, developmental, and other specialized needs.

    a. Help parents make first follow-up appointments; provide written documentation of appointment times.

    b. Reinforce and reiterate information provided from genetic evaluation and counseling.

    c. Make referral for in-home nursing visits or care based on needs of infant and family (see Appendix K).

4. Refer as needed for counseling and other support resources.

    a. Refer to counseling professionals.

    b. Refer to parent support groups.

    c. Refer to community-based family resource centers (see Appendix L).

    d. Refer to internet resources, family support websites.

CLIENT OUTCOMES

1. Infant will have stable physiologic functioning.
2. Infant will reach maximum potential for growth and development.
3. Parents will be competent in care of their child.

REFERENCES

Bartlett K et al: New developments in neonatal screening, *Arch Dis Child Fetal Neonatal Ed* 77(2):151F, 1997.

Batshaw M: PKU and other inborn errors of metabolism. In Batshaw M, editor: *Children with disabilities,* ed 4, Baltimore, 1997, Paul H. Brookes.

Burton B: Inborn errors of metabolism in infancy: a guide to diagnosis, *Pediatrics* 12(6):e69, 1998 (electronic article).

Chakrapani A et al: Detection of inborn errors of metabolism in the newborn, *Arch Dis Child Fetal Neonatal Ed* 84(3):F205, 2001.

Fosberg S: Infant metabolic screening: a total quality management approach, *J Obstet Gynecol Neonatal Nurs* 26(3):257, 1997.

Gilbert-Barness E, Barness L: *Metabolic diseases: foundations of clinical management, genetics and pathology,* Natick, Mass, 2000, Eaton.

Hutchesson A et al: A comparison of disease and gene frequencies of inborn errors of metabolism among different ethnic groups in the West Midlands, *J Med Genet* 35(5):366, 1998.

Leonard J, Morris A. Inborn errors of metabolism around time of birth, *Lancet* 356(9229):583, 2000.

Theorell C, Degenhardt M: Assessment and management of the metabolic system. In Kenner C et al, editors: *Comprehensive neonatal nursing: a physiologic perspective,* ed 3, Philadelphia, 2003, WB Saunders.

45

❖

Inflammatory Bowel Disease

❖

PATHOPHYSIOLOGY

Inflammatory bowel disease refers to two gastrointestinal conditions: ulcerative colitis and Crohn's disease. Differentiating ulcerative colitis from Crohn's disease may be difficult; in 10% of cases, a differential diagnosis is not made. The etiologies of both diseases are unknown, although recent research has focused on genetic, immunologic, dietary, and infectious causes.

An association between ankylosing spondylitis and the histocompatibility of human leukocyte antigen (HLA-B27) and inflammatory bowel disease is a possibility. Ulcerative colitis and Crohn's disease have similar initial signs, including diarrhea, rectal bleeding, abdominal pain, fever, malaise, anorexia, weight loss, and anemia. Children may initially be seen with vague symptoms such as growth failure, anorexia, fever, and joint pains with or without gastrointestinal symptoms. Both conditions are characterized by remissions and exacerbations. Extracolonic manifestations such as joint problems, hepatobiliary conditions, skin rashes, and eye irritation can occur. Although the peak incidence of inflammatory bowel disease is between 15 and 25 years of age, 15% of all cases occur at age 15 years and younger. Prognosis is dependent on the following factors: (1) age at onset and rapidity of onset; (2) response to medical treatment; and (3) extent of involvement.

Ulcerative colitis is a recurrent inflammatory and ulcerative disease affecting primarily the large intestine. Lesions are continuous and involve the superficial mucosa, causing vascular congestion, capillary dilation, edema, hemorrhage, and ulceration. Muscular hypertrophy and deposition of fibrous tissue and fat result, which gives the bowel a "lead pipe" appearance because of narrowing of the bowel itself.

Crohn's disease is an inflammatory and ulcerative disease affecting any part of the alimentary tract from the mouth to the anus. The disease affects the deep walls of the bowel. The lesions are discontinuous, resulting in a "skipping" effect, with the diseased portions of the bowel separated by normal tissue. Fissures, fistulas, and thickened intestinal walls result. Granulomas occur in approximately 50% of cases.

INCIDENCE

1. Annual incidence of ulcerative colitis and Crohn's disease is 4 to 10 cases in 100,000 children.
2. Ulcerative colitis represents more than half of the 20,000 to 25,000 newly diagnosed cases of inflammatory bowel disease each year.
3. Age range of peak incidence is 15 to 25 years.
4. White individuals are affected more often than African American individuals.
5. A high preponderance of cases occur in American Jews.
6. Twenty-nine percent of those with ulcerative colitis have a family history of the disease.
7. Thirty-five percent of those with Crohn's disease have a family history of the disease.

CLINICAL MANIFESTATIONS
Ulcerative Colitis

1. Frequent, bloody stools (number of stools varies from 4 to 24)—major symptom
2. Pain relief after defecation
3. Rectal bleeding
4. Anorexia, pallor, and fatigue
5. Fever
6. Tachycardia
7. Peritoneal irritation
8. Electrolyte imbalance
9. Ten- to 20-pound weight loss over 2 months
10. Anemia, leukocytosis, increased erythrocyte sedimentation rate

11. Extraintestinal symptoms—skin rashes, arthritis
12. Flatulence
13. Severe pain, abdominal rigidity, distention
14. Growth retardation

Crohn's Disease

1. Diarrhea, occult blood
2. Cramping abdominal pain aggravated by eating
3. Pain in right lower quadrant of abdomen with or without palpable mass
4. Growth retardation
5. Weight loss
6. Abscess formation
7. Spiking fever
8. Leukocytosis
9. Perianal disease—fistula and fissures
10. Nutritional deficiencies—malnutrition, electrolyte imbalances
11. Amenorrhea, delay in sexual maturation
12. Cachexia
13. Finger clubbing
14. Arthritis

COMPLICATIONS
Ulcerative Colitis

1. Predisposition to cancer—20% increase in risk with each decade after first 10 years
2. Toxic megacolon
3. Hemorrhage
4. Sepsis

Crohn's Disease

1. Perforation
2. Toxic megacolon
3. Hemorrhage
4. Liver abscess and liver disease
5. Ureteral obstruction
6. Retroperitonitis
7. Erythema nodosum

8. Strictures
9. Fistulas

LABORATORY AND DIAGNOSTIC TESTS

1. Complete blood count—anemia
2. White blood cell count—increased with inflammation
3. Erythrocyte sedimentation rate—increased with inflammation
4. Hematocrit—decreased because of blood loss
5. Serum electrolyte levels—decreased potassium
6. Serum protein level—decreased proteins
7. Stool culture—for presence of infectious organisms
8. Hematest of stool—for presence of blood in stool
9. D-Xylulose absorption blood and urine test—to measure intestinal absorption when there are fatty stools
10. Sigmoidoscopy—to evaluate mucosa, rectum, sigmoid colon directly
11. Colonoscopy—to evaluate colon directly
12. Upper gastrointestinal tract radiographic series with small bowel follow-through—differential diagnosis
13. Barium enema—differential diagnosis
14. Biopsy—to determine type of inflammatory bowel disease; tissue specimens are taken from several sites

MEDICAL MANAGEMENT
Ulcerative Colitis

Medical management is the primary treatment of ulcerative colitis and centers around drug therapy and nutritional support. Antidiarrheal preparations may be used along with antiinflammatory agents to control or suppress the inflammatory process. Immunosuppressants are often used in advanced cases. Analgesics and narcotics may also be given for pain. Dietary modifications may be needed when diarrhea, fistulas, or lactose intolerance is present. Therapy depends on the severity of the illness. If the illness is severe, the child may require intravenous (IV) hyperalimentation, administration of corticosteroids, and close observation for electrolyte imbalances, acidosis, anemia, and intestinal perforation. Surgical intervention is eventually needed in 25% of cases and provides a cure.

Crohn's Disease

Pharmacologic interventions for Crohn's disease are similar to those for ulcerative colitis, with the addition of antibiotics to eradicate inflammatory bacterial agents. Because there is no known cure for this disease, the treatment goals are to reduce bowel inflammation, correct nutritional deficiencies, and provide relief of symptoms. Nutritional support may include dietary modifications, vitamins, oral supplements, or hyperalimentation. Up to 70% of children with Crohn's disease require surgery because of failure of medical management, intestinal fistulas or obstruction, and growth failure.

SURGICAL TREATMENT

Ileostomy

Ileostomy is performed to treat inflammatory bowel disease after medical therapeutic procedures have been unsuccessful. Ileostomy involves removal of the diseased portion of the bowel (small intestine), with the ileum used to form a stoma on the abdominal wall for bowel evacuation. A variety of surgical procedures may be used, depending on the extent and location of the affected portion of the bowel. An ileostomy with subtotal or total colectomy is performed on children who are malnourished and have moderate to severe rectal disease.

Colostomy

Permanent or temporary colostomies are performed for a variety of conditions. Permanent colostomies are performed for children with severe cases of Crohn's disease. The sigmoid colostomy is most frequently performed. Temporary colostomies (e.g., transverse loop and double-barrel colostomies) are performed in children most often. In all types of colostomy, an intact portion of the colon is brought through an abdominal incision and is sutured to the abdominal wall to form a stoma.

Clinical Manifestations

The surgery should result in amelioration of symptoms associated with the primary disease. The child is left with an abdominal stoma through which bowel contents are emptied into an attached appliance or into an abdominal pouch (Koch pouch).

Although the child does not live with a normally functioning bowel after surgery, most children do well. If the child, adolescent, or parent learns to care properly for the colostomy or ileostomy, a life filled with educational, social, and athletic activities can be expected.

Complications

1. Necrosis of colostomy (caused by inadequate blood supply)
2. Stricture formation
3. Retraction of stoma
4. Prolapsed stoma
5. Herniation
6. Bleeding
7. Intestinal obstruction
8. Wound infection
9. Peritonitis
10. Spillover of stool
11. Constipation bordering on obstruction
12. Nephrolithiasis
13. Fistula (if multiple fistulas or extensive undermining of subcutaneous tissue occurs, stoma must be excised and located elsewhere)

NURSING ASSESSMENT

1. See the Gastrointestinal Assessment section in Appendix A.
2. Assess for abdominal distention, bowel sounds, tenderness and pain, and abdominal girth.

NURSING DIAGNOSES

- Diarrhea
- Pain
- Tissue integrity, Impaired
- Nutrition: less than body requirements, Imbalanced
- Infection, Risk for
- Fluid volume, Risk for deficient
- Body image, Disturbed
- Knowledge, Deficient

- Home maintenance, Impaired
- Injury, Risk for

NURSING INTERVENTIONS

1. Promote and maintain proper hydration status.
   a. Record input and output.
   b. Record weight daily.
   c. Assess for signs of dehydration.
   d. Promote oral intake when appropriate.
   e. Monitor administration of elemental feedings or hyperalimentation.
2. Provide comfort and pain relief measures as indicated.
   a. Maintain bed rest during acute episode (decreased activity results in decreased peristalsis, diarrhea, pain).
   b. Provide diversional activities.
   c. Change child's position every 2 hours.
   d. Assess intensity, type, time, and pattern of occurrence of pain, and child's response to pain relief measures.
   e. Monitor child's response to analgesics and narcotics.
   f. Provide uninterrupted rest periods.
3. Promote skin integrity.
   a. For perineal care, apply A&D ointment or petroleum jelly to perineal area to prevent skin irritation or breakdown.
   b. Apply body moisturizers liberally.
   c. Provide sitz bath three times per day (for perianal or rectal fistulas or fissures).
   d. Provide foam mattress to prevent pressure sores.
   e. Change child's position every 2 hours.
4. Promote and support optimal nutritional status.
   a. Compile dietary history, including food allergies.
   b. Monitor tolerance to food, noting type and amount.
   c. Monitor response to elemental feedings.
   d. Monitor response to low-residue, bland, high-protein, high-calorie diet.
   e. Monitor for signs of electrolyte imbalances (hypotension, tachycardia, oliguria, atonic muscles, general sense of confusion).

   f. Restrict intake of greasy, spicy, and lactose-containing foods.

   g. Monitor administration of hyperalimentation; observe child's or adolescent's response.

      i. Maintain sterility of central line.

      ii. Accurately record input and output.

      iii. Obtain weight daily.

      iv. Monitor urinary specific gravity.

      v. Check urinary glucose and acetone.

      vi. Monitor electrolyte balance (especially blood glucose).

5. Monitor child's response to and untoward side effects of medications.

6. Monitor for, prevent, or report signs of potential or actual complications.

   a. Fistulas or fissures

   b. Hemorrhage

   c. Intestinal obstruction

   d. Liver abscess

   e. Ureteral obstruction

   f. Retroperitonitis

   g. Perforations

   h. Enterocolitis

Preoperative Care

Prepare infant, child, or adolescent physically for surgery.

1. Monitor infant's or child's response to enemas, laxatives, stool softeners (to evacuate bowel preoperatively).

2. Monitor infant's or child's response to decompression of stomach and bowel (nasogastric [NG] tube and rectal tube).

3. Provide nothing by mouth for 12 hours before surgery.

4. Insert Foley catheter to decompress bladder.

5. Administer antibiotics to sterilize bowel.

6. Monitor vital signs every 4 hours.

7. Monitor for bowel complications (perforation, toxic megacolon, or enterocolitis).

8. Demonstrate use of appliances.

Postoperative Care

1. Monitor child's response to surgery.
   a. Vital signs
   b. Intake and output (report any discrepancy)
   c. Dressing (amount of drainage, intactness)
2. Monitor for signs and symptoms of complications.
   a. Stoma complications (prolapse, bleeding, excessive diarrhea, ribbonlike stools, failure to pass stool, flatus)
   b. Intestinal obstruction or constipation
   c. Prolapse of proximal segment
   d. Bleeding
   e. Increased stooling
   f. Infection
3. Promote return of peristalsis.
   a. Maintain patency of NG tube.
   b. Check functioning of suction machine.
   c. Irrigate with normal saline solution every 4 hours and as needed.
   d. Check for placement of NG tube; auscultate and aspirate contents.
4. Promote and maintain fluid and electrolyte balance.
   a. Record intake per route (IV, NG, oral).
   b. Record output per route (urine, stool, NG drainage, emesis, stoma).
   c. Monitor for signs and symptoms of electrolyte imbalance.
   d. Consult with physician about disparities in input and output.
5. Alleviate or minimize pain and discomfort.
   a. Maintain position of comfort.
   b. Monitor child's response to administration of medications.
   c. Provide oral care (mouth can become dry with NG tube in place).
6. Provide stoma and skin care to promote healing and to prevent complications.
   a. Inspect stoma every 4 hours for retraction, prolapse, or protrusion greater than 2 cm.
   b. Check for bleeding at stoma site.

  c. Check for obstruction (enlarged, pale, and edematous stoma).

7. Provide ostomy care (refer to institutional manual for specific technical and institutional procedure).
  a. Care of appliance
  b. Skin care
  c. Prevention of complications
   i. Skin can become irritated by digestive enzymes.
   ii. Match adhesive to stoma size.
   iii. Apply protective cream to exposed area.

8. Protect child from infection.
  a. Provide Foley catheter care per hospital protocol.
  b. Change dressing as needed (perianal and colostomy).
  c. Monitor incision site.
  d. Refer to institutional procedure manual for care related to specific procedure.
  e. Perform pulmonary toilet every 2 to 4 hours.
  f. Change child's position every 2 hours (prevents atelectasis).
  g. Monitor for signs of systemic infection and local abscess.

9. Facilitate development of realistic adaptive body image.
  a. Encourage expression of feelings regarding stoma, outcome of surgery.
  b. Encourage socialization through peer support groups.
  c. Refer to community organizations.
  d. Provide active problem solving for concerns such as apparel and sexual activity.

10. Encourage socialization with peers as means to cope with impact of disease.

11. Modify chronic sick role behavior by promoting socialization and normal daily activities.

12. Encourage expression of fears of body mutilation.

🔺 Discharge Planning and Home Care

1. Instruct child, parents, and family about ostomy.
2. Instruct child or adolescent and parents to monitor for and report signs of complications.

   a. Mechanical obstruction
   b. Peritonitis or wound infection
3. Instruct child or adolescent and parents about administration of total parenteral nutrition or NG feedings.
4. Initiate referral to school nurse and teacher to promote continuity of care.
   a. Observations of child's response to condition
   b. Observations of untoward effects of medications and complications
   c. Observation of social interactions with peers and conduct in school
5. Refer to community organizations and other resources:
   a. Crohn's and Colitis Foundation of America
      386 Park Ave. S., 17th Floor
      New York, NY 10016-8804
      800-932-2423
      212-779-4098 (fax)
      http://www.ccfa.org
   b. United Ostomy Association, Inc.
      36 Executive Park
      Suite 120
      Irvine, CA 92714-6744
      949-660-8624
   c. *Managing Your Child's Crohn's Disease and Ulcerative Colitis*
      Keith J. Benkov and Harland S. Winter
      New York, 1996, Master Media

CLIENT OUTCOMES

1. Child will have stable gastrointestinal function.
2. Child will have positive adaptation to psychosocial aspects of disease and/or surgery.
3. Child and family will understand home care and follow-up needs.

REFERENCES

Baron M: Crohn's disease in children, *Am J Nurs* 102(10):26, 2002.
Behrman R, Kligman R: *Nelson essentials of pediatrics,* ed 16, Philadelphia, 2000, WB Saunders.

Botoman V et al: Management of inflammatory bowel disease, *Am Fam Physician* 57(1):57, 1998.

Hockenberry M: *Wong's nursing care of infants and children,* ed 7, St Louis, 2003, Mosby.

Moses P et al: Inflammatory bowel disease, *Postgrad Med* 103(5):77, 1998.

Robinson M: Optimizing therapy for inflammatory bowel disease, *Am J Gastroenterol* 92(12):12S, 1997.

46

❖

Iron Deficiency Anemia

❖

PATHOPHYSIOLOGY

Iron deficiency anemia is the most common anemia affecting children in North America. The full-term infant born of a well-nourished, nonanemic mother has sufficient iron stores until the birth weight is doubled, generally at 4 to 6 months. Iron deficiency anemia is generally not evident until 9 months of age. After that, iron must be available from the diet to meet the child's nutritional needs. If dietary iron intake is insufficient, iron deficiency anemia results. Most often, insufficient dietary iron intake results from inappropriately early introduction of solid foods (before age 4 to 6 months), discontinuation of iron-fortified infant formula or breast milk before age 1 year, and excessive consumption of cow's milk to the exclusion of iron-rich solids in the toddler. Also, the preterm infant, the infant with significant perinatal blood loss, and the infant born to a poorly nourished, iron-deficient mother may have inadequate iron stores. Such an infant would be at a significantly higher risk for iron deficiency anemia before age 6 months. Maternal iron deficiency may cause low birth weight and preterm delivery.

Iron deficiency anemia may also result from chronic blood loss. In the infant, this may be due to chronic intestinal bleeding caused by the heat-labile protein in cow's milk. In children of all ages, the loss of as little as 1 to 7 ml of blood through the gastrointestinal tract daily may lead to iron deficiency anemia. Other causes of iron deficiency anemia include nutritional deficiencies such as folate (vitamin B_{12}) deficiency, sickle cell anemia, thalassemia major, infections, and chronic inflammation. In teenaged girls, iron deficiency anemia may also be due to excessive menstrual flow.

INCIDENCE

1. Three percent of infants 12 to 36 months of age have iron deficiency anemia.
2. Nine percent of infants 12 to 36 months of age are iron deficient.
3. Incidence of iron deficiency and iron deficiency anemia among adolescent girls is 11% to 17%.
4. The age range of peak incidence for iron deficiency anemia is 12 to 18 months.
5. Prevalence rates of iron deficiency are higher among children living at or below the poverty level and among African American and Mexican American children.
6. Twenty percent to 40% of infants fed only non–iron-fortified formula or cow's milk are at higher risk for iron deficiency by age 9 to 12 months.
7. Fifteen percent to 25% of breast-fed infants are at higher risk for iron deficiency by age 9 to 12 months.
8. The leading cause of anemia in infants and children in the United States is iron deficiency. There was a significant increase in iron deficiency anemia in the United States in the 1990s.
9. Iron deficiency is the most common nutritional deficiency in the world.

CLINICAL MANIFESTATIONS

1. Conjunctival pallor (hemoglobin [Hb] 6 to 10 g/dl)
2. Palmar crease pallor (Hb below 8 g/dl)
3. Irritability and anorexia (Hb 5 g/dl or below)
4. Tachycardia, systolic murmur
5. Pica
6. Lethargy, increased need for sleep
7. Lack of interest in toys or play activities

COMPLICATIONS

1. Developmental delays (birth to 5 years of age)
2. Poor muscular development (long term)
3. Decreased attention span
4. Decreased social interactions
5. Decreased performance on developmental tests

6. Decreased ability to process information obtained through hearing
7. Contribution to lead poisoning (decreased iron enables gastrointestinal tract to absorb heavy metals more easily)
8. Increased incidence of cerebral vascular accident in infants and children

LABORATORY AND DIAGNOSTIC TESTS

No single test is acceptable for detecting or diagnosing iron deficiency.

1. Hb concentration (before treatment) (indicates concentration of iron-containing protein Hb in circulating red blood cells)—decreased (one of most common tests used)
2. Hematocrit (indicates proportion of whole blood occupied by red blood cells)—decreased (one of most common tests used)
3. Mean corpuscular volume and mean corpuscular hemoglobin concentration—decreased, yielding microcytic, hypochromic anemia or small, pale red blood cells
4. Red blood cell distribution width (cutoff: 14%)
5. Erythrocyte protoporphyrin concentration—1 to 2 years: 80 μg/dl of red blood cells
6. Transferrin saturation—younger than 6 months: 15 μg/L or less
7. Serum ferritin concentration—less than 16%
8. Reticulocyte count (during treatment)—increase within 3 to 5 days of initiating iron therapy indicates positive therapeutic response
9. Hb concentration (with treatment)—return to normal value within 4 to 8 weeks indicates adequate iron and nutritional support

MEDICAL MANAGEMENT

Treatment efforts are directed toward prevention and intervention. Prevention includes encouraging parents to feed the infant only breast milk until the infant is between 4 to 6 months of age, to eat foods that are iron rich, and to take iron-fortified prenatal vitamins (supplementation with approximately 1 mg/kg of iron per day). Iron supplementation should begin when infants are switched to regular milk. Therapy to treat iron deficiency anemia consists of a medication regimen.

1. By 6 months of age, breast-fed infants should receive 1 mg/kg of iron drops per day.
2. For breast-fed infants who were born prematurely or had low birth weight, 2 to 4 mg/kg (maximum of 15 mg) of iron drops daily is recommended starting at 1 month and continuing until 12 months of age.
3. Up to 12 months of age, only breast milk or iron-fortified infant formula should be used.
4. Between 1 and 5 years of age, children should not consume more than 24 ounces of soy, goat's, or cow's milk daily.
5. Between 4 and 6 months of age, infants should have two or more daily servings of iron-fortified cereal.
6. By 6 months of age, child should have daily feeding of foods rich in vitamin C to improve iron absorption.

Iron is administered by mouth. All iron forms are equally effective (ferrous sulfate, ferrous fumarate, ferrous succinate, ferrous gluconate). Vitamin C must be administered simultaneously with iron (ascorbic acid increases iron absorption). Iron is best absorbed when taken 1 hour before a meal. Iron therapy should continue for a minimum of 6 weeks after the anemia is corrected to replenish iron stores. Injectable iron is seldom used unless small bowel malabsorption disease is present.

Adolescent girls should be encouraged to eat foods rich in iron. Other prevention strategies include comprehensive screening for, diagnosis of, and treatment of iron deficiency.

NURSING ASSESSMENT

1. See the Cardiovascular Assessment section in Appendix A.
2. Assess child's response to iron therapy.
3. Assess child's activity level.
4. Assess child's developmental level (see Appendix B).

NURSING DIAGNOSES

- Activity intolerance
- Nutrition: less than body requirements, Imbalanced

- Fatigue
- Growth and development, Delayed

NURSING INTERVENTIONS

1. Monitor child's therapeutic and untoward effects from iron therapy.
   a. Side effects (e.g., tooth discoloration) are infrequent with oral therapy.
   b. Instruct about measures to prevent tooth discoloration.
      i. Take iron with fluids, preferably orange juice.
      ii. Rinse mouth after taking medication.
   c. Encourage increased fiber and water intake to minimize constipating effects of iron.
   d. For severe iron-induced constipation, consider lowering iron dose but extending length of treatment.
2. Instruct parents about appropriate nutritional intake (see Medical Management section in this chapter).
   a. Reduce child's milk intake.
   b. Increase intake of meat and appropriate protein substitutes.
   c. Encourage inclusion of whole grains and green leafy vegetables in diet.
3. Gather information about dietary history and eating behaviors.
   a. Assess for factors contributing to nutritional deficiency—psychosocial, behavioral, and nutritional.
   b. Plan with parents acceptable approach toward dietary habits.
   c. Refer to nutritionist for intensive evaluation and treatment.
4. Encourage breast-feeding because breast milk iron is well absorbed.

🔺 Discharge Planning and Home Care

1. Instruct about administering iron therapy (see item 1 under Nursing Interventions).
2. Instruct about meal planning and nutritional intake (see item 2 under Nursing Interventions).

3. Instruct about need for follow-up screenings and treatment approaches.

CLIENT OUTCOMES

1. Child's skin color will improve.
2. Child's pattern of growth will improve (as indicated on growth chart).
3. Child's activity level will be appropriate for age.
4. Parents will demonstrate understanding of home treatment regimen (i.e., medication administration, diet with appropriate iron-rich foods).

REFERENCES

Baptist EC, Castillo SF: Cow's milk–induced iron deficiency anemia as a cause of childhood stroke, *Clin Pediatr (Phila)* 41(7):533, 2002.

Centers for Disease Control and Prevention: Iron deficiency—United States, 1999-2000, *JAMA* 288(17):2114, 2002.

Centers for Disease Control and Prevention, US Department of Health and Human Services: Recommendations to prevent and control iron deficiency, *MMWR* 47(RR-3):1, 1998.

Eden AN: The prevention of toddler iron deficiency, *Arch Pediatr Adolesc Med* 156(5):519, 2002.

Saloojee H, Pettifor JM: Iron deficiency and impaired child development, *BMJ* 323(7326):1377, 2001.

47

❖

Juvenile Rheumatoid Arthritis

❖

PATHOPHYSIOLOGY

Juvenile rheumatoid arthritis (JRA) is a chronic inflammatory disease that begins before 16 years of age. It is the most common rheumatic disease in children and is a leading cause of disability. Although its etiology is unknown, possible causes include infection, autoimmunity, and genetic predisposition. JRA causes chronic inflammation of the synovium with joint effusion, which can result in eventual erosion and destruction of the articular cartilage. If the process persists long enough, adhesions between the joint surfaces and ankylosis of joints develop. The diagnosis is based on the following criteria:

1. The age at onset must be less than 16 years.
2. Objective evidence of arthritis must be present (defined as swelling or effusion, or presence of two or more of the following: limitation of range of motion, tenderness or pain on motion, and increased heat) in one or more joints.
3. The arthritis must persist for at least 6 weeks in a given joint.
4. Other specific diseases that may cause or be associated with arthritis must be excluded.

Common characteristics include morning stiffness, joint pain, limping gait, fatigue, anorexia, anemia, and weight loss. JRA diagnosed in children is classified into one of the following based on clinical signs present during the first 6 months of illness:

1. Systemic JRA
2. Polyarticular JRA
3. Pauciarticular JRA

INCIDENCE

1. JRA is twice as common in girls.
2. The incidence of JRA varies from 2 to 20 in 100,000.
3. Age ranges of peak incidence are 1 to 3 years and 8 to 11 years.
4. Rates of incidence are as follows: systemic, 10%; polyarticular, 30%; and pauciarticular, 60%.

CLINICAL MANIFESTATIONS

Systemic JRA

1. Systemic JRA is characterized by persistent, intermittent fever: daily or twice-daily temperature elevations to 102.2° F (39° C) or higher, with rapid return to normal temperature between fever spikes. This almost always occurs with the rheumatoid rash.
2. The rheumatoid rash is described as salmon-pink erythematous macules on the trunk and extremities. The rash is migratory and in 20% of cases is reported to be pruritic.
3. Arthritis may not occur until weeks or months after the onset of the symptoms.
4. Both large and small joints may be affected.
5. The arthritis pattern may be pauciarticular (one to four joints affected) or polyarticular (five or more joints affected). Those children with polyarthritis have a tendency for erosions and a poorer prognosis.
6. Extraarticular symptoms are present, including hepatosplenomegaly, lymphadenopathy, pericarditis, anemia, thrombocytosis, leukocytosis (as high as 45,000 to 60,000/mm^3), and pleuritis.

Polyarticular JRA

1. Arthritis is present in five or more joints in the first 6 months of disease.
2. Intermittent low-grade fever occurs.
3. Malaise and fatigue are present.
4. Anorexia and weight loss occur.
5. Morning stiffness, joint pain, and sluggishness with movement are characteristic.

6. Joint involvement is asymmetric.
7. The knees, wrists, elbows, and ankles are frequently involved.
8. The cervical region of the spine may be involved.
9. The temporomandibular joint may be involved, which may lead to impaired biting and shortness of the mandible.
10. Those with onset in late childhood or adolescence who are seropositive for rheumatoid factor have a pattern of development similar to that in adult rheumatoid arthritis (including clinical manifestations such as rheumatoid nodules, early onset of erosive synovitis, and a chronic disease course). They tend to have symmetric joint involvement and involvement of the small joints of the hands or feet.

Pauciarticular JRA

1. Arthritis is present in one to four joints in the first 6 months of disease.
2. Pauciarticular JRA primarily affects girls, aged 1 to 4 years.
3. The joints affected are the knees, ankles, and elbows. Shoulder and hip involvement are rare.
4. Painless swelling of joints is common.
5. Uveitis (15% to 20% of cases) is insidious and subacute.
6. Disease course is variable. After the first 6 months, 5% to 10% develop a polyarticular disease course.

COMPLICATIONS

1. Uveitis, found in 15% to 20% of children with pauciarticular-onset JRA, in 5% of those with polyarticular-onset JRA, and rarely in children with systemic-onset JRA. At increased risk for development of uveitis are girls with pauciarticular-onset disease. Those with positive antinuclear antibody test findings are at even higher risk. The onset is usually insidious and asymptomatic; however, approximately half of children have some symptoms (pain, redness, headache, photophobia, change in vision) later in the course of the disease. If not diagnosed early, the disease can result in

cataracts, glaucoma, visual loss, and blindness. If the disease is detected early, the prognosis is improved.
2. Flexion contractures
3. Limitation of movement
4. Growth disturbances, including leg length discrepancy and micrognathia
5. Cardiopulmonary complications and other systemic complications
6. Severe anemia and malnutrition
7. Renal, bone marrow, gastrointestinal, and liver toxicity to drugs
8. Microphage activation syndrome—a rare but acute complication of systemic JRA leading to severe morbidity and sometimes death. It causes rapid development of liver failure with encephalopathy, purpura, bruising, and mucosal bleeding.
9. Osteopenia

LABORATORY AND DIAGNOSTIC TESTS

1. Erythrocyte sedimentation rate and C-reactive protein level—increased with inflammation. These are useful in measuring disease activity and monitoring response to antiinflammatory medications. However, they are often normal in pauciarticular JRA.
2. Rheumatoid factor—present in only 15% of children with JRA (primarily those with polyarticular disease)
3. Antinuclear antibodies—primarily seen in pauciarticular JRA (in 40% of cases); reflect increased risk for uveitis
4. Complete blood count—systemic leukocytosis; 45,000 to 60,000/mm^3 white blood cell count with acute systemic JRA; thrombocytosis with normochromic or hypochromic anemia (thrombocytopenia is not seen in JRA)
5. Complement levels (C3)—often increased with disease activity
6. Immunoglobulin levels—correlate with disease activity
7. Synovial fluid analysis (cell count and culture)—to rule out other conditions
8. Urinalysis—mild proteinuria accompanies increased fever

9. Imaging studies (radiography, nuclear scan, magnetic resonance imaging, dual-energy x-ray absorptiometry [DEXA] scan, computed tomography, ultrasonography)—to monitor disease progression and to rule out other conditions

MEDICAL MANAGEMENT

Treatment goals for JRA are to reduce the inflammatory process; to maintain joint function and strength; to decrease pain; to minimize joint destruction, deformity, and complications; to promote optimal growth and development; to promote independence in activities of daily living; and to maintain the child or adolescent's self-esteem and self-image in the face of a chronic illness. Drug therapy is used to reduce inflammation. JRA is treated earlier and more aggressively to decrease disability. Physical and occupational therapy and a regular daily program of exercise are essential to promote mobility and function. Heat is used to relieve joint pain and stiffness. The treatment plan also includes frequent slit-lamp microscopy examinations by an ophthalmologist according to specified guidelines (Table 47-1).

1. Nonsteroidal antiinflammatory drugs (NSAIDs) are used to control inflammation, fever, and pain. Aspirin and salicylates are no longer used as the first-choice NSAIDs, because of the association with Reye's syndrome during influenza or varicella infection, and the availability of other NSAIDs. Naproxen (Naprosyn), ibuprofen, tolmetin (Tolectin), indomethacin (Indocin), and diclofenac sodium (Voltaren) are common NSAIDs used in JRA. Cyclooxygenase-2 inhibitors such as celecoxib (Celebrex) and rofecoxib (Vioxx) are also prescribed, although they have not been approved for use in children.

   To be effective as an antiinflammatory medication, NSAIDs must be taken on a routine basis. If adequate effectiveness is not achieved after 2 to 3 months, an alternative NSAID can be tried. Many children require a second-line medication in addition to an NSAID to control disease activity. The following second-line medications may be used.

TABLE 47-1
Slit-Lamp Examination Guidelines

Type of JRA	ANA Test	Age at Diagnosis	Recommended Frequency of Slit-Lamp Examination
Pauciarticular or polyarticular	Positive	<7 years	Every 3-4 months for 7 years; then yearly
Pauciarticular or polyarticular	Negative	<7 years of age	Every 6 months for 7 years; then yearly
Pauciarticular or polyarticular	—	≥7 years of age	Every 6 months for 4 years; then yearly
Systemic	—	—	Yearly

Modified from American Academy of Pediatrics, Section on Rheumatology and Section on Ophthalmology: Guidelines for ophthalmologic examinations in children with juvenile rheumatoid arthritis, *Pediatrics* 92(2):295, 1993.
ANA, Antinuclear antibodies; *JRA,* juvenile rheumatoid arthritis.

2. Methotrexate is the initial second-line medication for the treatment of JRA. Given orally once a week in small doses, it has been markedly effective in the treatment of arthritis in children. It is also given subcutaneously once a week for higher doses or in children with poor absorption or inadequate response.

3. Slower-acting antirheumatic drugs or disease-modifying antirheumatic drugs can be added to the medical treatment program for children who have an inadequate response to the NSAID and methotrexate combination. These include hydroxychloroquine (Plaquenil), sulfasalazine (Azulfidine), parenteral gold compounds, and penicillamine (Cuprimine).

4. Glucocorticosteroids are used for life-threatening complications of JRA. Oral steroid use should be limited as much as possible because of the potential side effects. Intravenous pulse steroids and intraarticular steroid injections (triamcinolone hexacetonide) are other methods of administration.

5. Tumor necrosis factor inhibitors have demonstrated much promise in the treatment of JRA. Etanercept (Enbrel) has been approved for pediatric use as a twice per week subcutaneous injection. Infliximab (Remicade), which is given as an infusion, is also being used for JRA treatment.

6. Intravenous immunoglobulin is sometimes used in severe, progressive systemic and polyarticular disease.

7. Cytotoxic agents (azathioprine, cyclophosphamide, and cyclosporin) are used occasionally in children with JRA who have life-threatening complications, major steroid toxicity, or severe progressive erosive disease. Cyclosporin has been found to be beneficial in treatment of the macrophage activation syndrome seen in systemic JRA.

NURSING ASSESSMENT

1. See the Musculoskeletal Assessment section in Appendix A.
2. Assess for pain.

3. Assess ability to perform activities of daily living.
4. Assess growth and development.

NURSING DIAGNOSES

- Pain
- Mobility, Impaired physical
- Self-care deficit, Bathing/hygiene
- Self-care deficit, Feeding
- Social interaction, Impaired
- Family processes, Interrupted

NURSING INTERVENTIONS

1. Provide pain relief measures as necessary.
   a. Tub bath or shower for joint stiffness
   b. Heating pad or ice packs applied to affected areas
   c. Whirlpool bath, paraffin bath, or hot packs for pain and stiffness
   d. Footed pajamas or sleeping bag
   e. Heated water bed or electric blanket
   f. Crutches, walker, or other device to avoid full weight bearing
2. Promote joint mobility, maintain strength, and prevent deformity of joints.
   a. Encourage compliance with physical therapy and occupational therapy exercises (range of motion/passive range of motion).
   b. Encourage participation in physical activity exercise.
   c. Avoid excessive strain on affected joints.
   d. Encourage participation in creative dance, bicycle riding, swimming, or walking.
   e. Counsel to avoid activities that place total body weight on affected non–weight-bearing joints (cartwheels, chin-ups, handstands, aerobics, contact sports, roller skating).
   f. Encourage use of splints to prevent flexion contractures.
   g. Encourage compliance with prone and active gluteal exercise with hip involvement.
   h. Provide cast with knee in severe flexion.
   i. Provide cervical collar for neck pain.

3. Collaborate with physical therapist and/or occupational therapist to devise methods that will promote independent functioning.
   a. Use splints as needed.
   b. Make modifications to utensils for easier grasp.
   c. Select clothes that are convenient to put on (Velcro fasteners).
   d. Elevate toilet seat.
4. Monitor growth and development pattern.
   a. Educate family about side effects of corticosteroid therapy and refer to dietitian as needed.
   b. Encourage age-appropriate activities that will conserve energy and promote development of perceptual skills and coordination.
5. Assist child with intervention strategies for common school problems.
   a. Instruct family to meet with school personnel to discuss child's diagnosis and make classroom modifications.
   b. Instruct child to change position or stretch every 20 minutes to prevent stiffness.
   c. Have child use "fat" pens or pencils, or felt-tip pens, for writing.
   d. Suggest obtaining extra set of schoolbooks to keep at home.
   e. Suggest use of computer for reports and tape recorder for note taking.
   f. Suggest allowance of extra time between classes.
   g. Encourage rest period after lunch.
   h. Plan schedule with less demanding subjects in the morning.
   i. Encourage participation in activities with other children.
   j. Assist family and school personnel in developing individualized education plan addressing modifications of school activities and special needs.
   k. Refer adolescent to vocational rehabilitation to assist with career planning (10th and 11th grades).

6. Provide education and support to child and family to maximize coping with a chronic and sometimes disabling disease.
   a. Encourage participation in support groups with other JRA-affected children and their families. Refer family to Arthritis Foundation and American Juvenile Arthritis Organization. Provide information to family about camps for children with arthritis.
   b. Assist family in identifying Internet websites that provide accurate and up-to-date information about JRA, such as http://www.arthritis.org.
   c. Monitor child's therapeutic response and adverse reactions to medications.
   d. Prepare child preoperatively for procedures and surgeries as indicated, which may include the following:
      i. Arthrocentesis
      ii. Arthroscopy (for intraarticular examination, synovial biopsy, or synovectomy)
      iii. Soft tissue release
      iv. Osteotomy
      v. Total joint or hip replacement
   e. Provide emotional support to child and family as indicated during hospitalization.
   f. Provide education and guidance to child and family regarding unconventional or unproven therapies.
   g. Assist adolescent/young adult with transition to adult medical providers, when applicable.

🔺 Discharge Planning and Home Care

1. Instruct child and family about follow-up appointments.
   a. Name and phone number of physician and appropriate health care team members
   b. Date, time, and purpose of follow-up appointments
2. Instruct child and family to observe response to medications and notify physician of adverse reactions.
3. Reinforce information given about JRA and encourage compliance with treatment plan.
4. Monitor compliance with consultation referrals.

CLIENT OUTCOMES

1. Child will exhibit no signs or symptoms of discomfort and will be able to move with minimal discomfort.
2. Child will be able to perform activities of daily living and participate in age-appropriate activities with minimal fatigue.
3. Child and family will demonstrate understanding of home treatment plan, including medications and home exercise program.

REFERENCES

American Academy of Pediatrics, Section on Rheumatology and Section on Ophthalmology: Guidelines for ophthalmologic examinations in children with juvenile rheumatoid arthritis, *Pediatrics* 92(2):295, 1993.

American Pain Society: *Guideline for the management of pain in osteoarthritis, rheumatoid arthritis, and juvenile chronic arthritis,* Glenview, Ill, 2002, The Society.

Cassidy JT, Petty RE: *Textbook of pediatric rheumatology,* ed 4, Philadelphia, 2001, WB Saunders.

Isenberg DA, Miller J II: *Adolescent rheumatology,* London, 1998, Martin Dunitz.

McIlvain-Simpson GR: Juvenile rheumatoid arthritis. In Jackson PK, Vessey JA, editors: *Primary care of the child with a chronic condition,* ed 3, St Louis, 2000, Mosby.

Purdy KS et al: You are what you eat: healthy food choices, nutrition, and the child with juvenile rheumatoid arthritis, *Pediatr Nurs* 22(5):391, 1996.

48

◆

Kawasaki Disease

◆

PATHOPHYSIOLOGY

Kawasaki disease is an acute febrile illness of young children that causes widespread systemic vasculitis. It is distinguished by marked immune system activation that contributes to the injury of small and medium-sized blood vessels. Also known as mucocutaneous lymph node syndrome, Kawasaki disease affects multiple body systems and can have life-threatening cardiovascular consequences. Although researchers speculate that Kawasaki disease has a viral or bacterial cause, the specific etiology is unknown. Typically, the disease occurs in three phases (acute febrile, subacute, and convalescent) and is self-limiting. Diagnosis, which is sometimes confusing, is based on strict adherence to clinical criteria. Initial treatment focuses on reducing the vascular inflammatory process, and prognosis is excellent with early recognition and treatment. The long-term prognosis for children with coronary artery abnormalities who survive the disease is not known.

INCIDENCE

1. Of all children with diagnosed Kawasaki disease, 80% are 4 years of age or younger, with toddlers most commonly affected.
2. Outbreaks of Kawasaki disease are more common in the winter and spring.
3. The incidence is higher in boys than in girls.
4. The disease occurs in all races, with a predominance in Japanese children.
5. Kawasaki disease occurs in siblings of affected children more frequently than in the general population.

6. No evidence exists to suggest that Kawasaki disease is spread by person-to-person contact.
7. Of untreated children with Kawasaki disease, 20% develop coronary artery abnormalities.
8. Of those treated with intravenous (IV) gamma globulin within the first week of illness, 5% develop coronary artery abnormalities.

CLINICAL MANIFESTATIONS
Acute Febrile Phase (7 to 14 Days)

For Kawasaki disease to be diagnosed in the child, five of the first six principal criteria must be met.

1. Fever—abrupt onset of high fever that lasts more than 5 days and is unresponsive to antibiotic and antipyretic therapy
2. Conjunctival injection lasting 1 to 2 weeks with no exudate or corneal scarring
3. Oropharyngeal manifestations, with red, dry, cracked lips; red, dry, "strawberry" tongue; and pharyngitis
4. Induration and edema of the extremities, with erythema of the palms and soles and swelling of digits
5. Erythematous body rash that is typically macular; it begins on the extremities, spreads to the trunk, and is often pruritic (no vesicles or petechiae)
6. Cervical lymphadenopathy, which is usually unilateral, is characterized by nodes larger than 1.5 cm, and "melts away" as the fever subsides
7. Acute myocarditis, decreased left ventricular function, and temporary arthritis

Subacute Phase (10 to 24 Days)

1. Thrombosis and hypercoagulability
2. Arthritis—most commonly in large joints (knees, hips, elbows)
3. Arthralgia caused by joint fluid
4. Desquamation of the extremities, beginning at the digits and followed by peeling off in sheets from the palms and soles

5. Panvasculitis of coronary arteries and formation of aneurysms; inflammation and thrombosis may lead to stenosis or obstruction

Convalescent Phase (6 to 8 Weeks)

1. Subsidence of signs of illness
2. Appearance of deep linear transverse grooves across the fingernails and toenails (Beau's lines)
3. Abnormal laboratory values—elevated sedimentation rate
4. Normalization of personality, appetite, and energy level

COMPLICATIONS

1. Congestive heart failure
2. Coronary artery aneurysms
3. Coronary thromboses
4. Myocardial infarction

LABORATORY AND DIAGNOSTIC TESTS

There are no specific diagnostic tests for Kawasaki disease; however, several abnormalities have been identified.

1. Electrocardiogram (ECG)
   a. Flat, depressed ST segment
   b. Flat, inverted T wave
   c. Conduction disturbances
2. Echocardiogram—used to assess cardiac enlargement, contractility of ventricles, and coronary aneurysms
3. Complete blood count—mild to moderate anemia, elevated white blood cell count (first phase) with predominance of neutrophils
4. Platelet count—usually elevated by third week of illness; elevation may persist for 3 months after onset
5. Erythrocyte sedimentation rate—elevated
6. C-reactive protein level—elevated
7. Serum glutamic-oxaloacetic transaminase level—elevated
8. Serum glutamic-pyruvic transaminase level—elevated
9. Serum albumin level—decreased
10. Serum lactic dehydrogenase level—elevated during acute febrile phase, decreased during convalescent phase

11. Immunoglobulin E and immunoglobulin M—elevated during acute febrile phase, decreased during convalescent phase
12. C3 level—increased in weeks 1 through 3 of illness then becomes normal

MEDICAL MANAGEMENT

Initial therapy is aimed at reducing the vascular inflammatory process and preventing thrombosis by inhibiting platelet aggregation. Surgical interventions may be required if obstructive cardiovascular disease results. Common medical therapy includes the following:

1. IV gamma globulin (IVGG) 2 g/kg given over 12 hours; decreases inflammation of the coronary arteries, speeds the resolution of fever and normalization of laboratory results.
2. Aspirin therapy
   a. Eighty to 100 mg/kg/day in four divided doses (until fever is controlled or until 14th day of illness) followed by dosage of 3 to 5 mg/kg/day in a single dose for 6 to 8 weeks.
   b. After 6 to 8 weeks, if echocardiogram is normal, child is afebrile, and erythrocyte sedimentation rate is normal, aspirin is stopped. If echocardiogram shows coronary artery abnormalities, low-dose aspirin therapy (3 to 5 mg/kg/day) is continued indefinitely.
3. Warfarin (Coumadin) is sometimes used in children with giant aneurysms.

NURSING ASSESSMENT

1. See the Cardiovascular Assessment section in Appendix A.
2. Assess for clinical criteria of Kawasaki disease.
3. Assess for febrile seizures.
4. Assess adequacy of hydration.

NURSING DIAGNOSES

- Fluid volume, Deficient
- Hyperthermia
- Decreased cardiac output

- Injury, Risk for
- Oral mucous membrane, Impaired
- Nutrition: less than body requirements, Imbalanced
- Pain
- Mobility, Impaired physical
- Fear

NURSING INTERVENTIONS

1. Monitor child's clinical status.
   a. Rectal temperature
   b. Skin turgor, mucous membranes, and anterior fontanelle
   c. Intake and output (should be strictly recorded)
   d. Specific gravity
   e. Stools (should be measured)
   f. Oral mucous membranes
   g. Erythematous body rash
   h. Blood pressure
2. Institute measures to lower fever.
   a. Medicate with antipyretics; monitor child's response to medications.
   b. Provide tepid sponge baths for temperatures higher than 102.2° F (39° C).
   c. Offer cool fluids.
   d. Assess which fluids (such as Popsicles and gelatin) child prefers.
   e. Maintain seizure precautions, because 3% to 5% of children between 6 months and 3 years of age may develop seizures when they have temperatures as low as 101.8° F (38.8° C).
   f. Explain unusual nature of fever to parents in terms of its intermittent pattern, duration, and resistance to antipyretics; anticipatory guidance will prevent parental anxiety about fever.
3. Monitor child for cardiac complications.
   a. Use cardiac monitor as ordered during acute and subacute phases; report arrhythmias to physician.
   b. Explain purpose of ECG and echocardiogram and aberrations caused by child's movement to parents and child.

    c. Allow child to change his or her own electrodes during daily bath.

4. Monitor for untoward signs and symptoms (hypotension, diaphoresis, nausea and vomiting, chills) during IVGG administrations and stop infusion until symptoms have subsided. Keep epinephrine available to treat anaphylaxis.

5. Monitor for signs of bleeding due to aspirin therapy.

6. Provide comfort measures for child.
   a. Perform oral hygiene frequently.
   b. Apply petroleum jelly to lips.
   c. Avoid soaps, ointments, and lotions on skin; keep skin clean, dry, and exposed to air.
   d. Cool, moist compresses may be applied to itching areas.
   e. Provide sheepskin for child to lie on.
   f. Discourage scratching through diversional activities; for young children, soft, loose mittens may be helpful.
   g. Encourage bed rest and elevation of extremities until swelling has subsided.
   h. Teach parents how to hold and comfort child who has IV line and electrodes in place.
   i. Keep stimulation to a minimum.
   j. Explain to parents that tactile stimulation may be irritating but soothing voice may provide security.
   k. Provide dim lights.
   l. Provide quiet music.

7. Provide for and promote child's nutrition.
   a. Provide comfort measures for mouth (see item 6).
   b. Begin with bland foods in small amounts.
   c. Encourage parents to bring in favorite foods from home and assess for favorite foods in hospital.
   d. Avoid hot, spicy foods.
   e. Offer high-calorie liquids.

8. Prevent contractions related to imposed restrictions and range-of-motion (ROM) limitations.
   a. Perform passive ROM exercises on edematous extremities during child's bed rest; teach parents how to do these exercises and explain their importance.
   b. When child is able, use active ROM exercises, making it into game for child.

    c. Place IV lines in position that allows maximal movement.

9. Alleviate anxiety caused by invasive procedures for diagnostic tests and by pain, new environment, strange people, knowledge deficit, and age-related fears.

    a. Provide play therapy during all phases of illness and for each new procedure (i.e., ECGs, needle play); base therapy on child's developmental level.

    b. Explain each procedure at child's and parents' cognitive levels.

    c. Suggest ways for parents to support their child during hospitalization and procedures (e.g., holding child after procedure).

    d. Consult parents and child about preferences among "quiet" toys and activities during acute phase of illness; encourage parents and volunteers to play with child, allowing for rest periods and then passive participation.

    e. Explain meaning of presence of swollen lymph nodes to parents.

🔺 Discharge Planning and Home Care

Instruct about long-term management.

1. Instruct parents and child, in developmentally appropriate manner, about importance of follow-up care, including ECGs, echocardiograms, and chest radiographic studies (two thirds of coronary aneurysms regress within 1 year).

2. Instruct parents verbally and with written reinforcement about signs and symptoms of cardiac complications (i.e., aneurysms and coronary thromboses); tell them to contact physician immediately if child has any of these signs and symptoms.

3. Instruct parents about importance of anticoagulant therapy such as aspirin and about side effects to watch for; explain to parents why some children with Kawasaki disease may need to undergo coronary artery bypass grafting.

4. Instruct parents about importance of good nutrition and adequate fluid intake.
5. Stress importance of adequate rest.
6. Educate parents about delaying administration of live virus vaccines (such as measles, mumps, rubella) for 5 months after child receives IVGG.

CLIENT OUTCOMES

1. Child's temperature will return to normal.
2. Changes in skin will resolve.
3. Child will walk without joint pain.

REFERENCES

Hockenberry M: *Wong's nursing care of infants and children,* ed 7, St Louis, 2003, Mosby.

Melish ME, Hotez P: Kawasaki disease. In Katz SL, editor: *Krugman's infectious diseases of children,* ed 10, St Louis, 1998, Mosby.

Rubin B, Cotton DM: Kawasaki disease: a dangerous acute childhood illness, *Nurse Pract* 23(2):34, 1998.

49

❖

Lead Poisoning

❖

PATHOPHYSIOLOGY

Lead poisoning is the excessive accumulation of lead in the blood. The majority of children with lead poisoning are asymptomatic. A lead level of less than 10 μg/dl indicates no lead poisoning; lead levels of 10 to 14 μg/dl are considered borderline; and lead levels equal to or higher than 15 μg/dl require some degree of intervention. Acute symptoms of lead poisoning are generally not evident until the lead level reaches 50 μg/dl or higher.

Younger children absorb a greater proportion of lead because of their greater intake of dietary fat and their decreased intake of calcium and iron. Excessive amounts of absorbed lead accumulate in the bones, soft tissue, and blood. Soft tissue absorption is of great concern because it can result in central nervous system (CNS) toxicity and reversible renal failure. Late signs of lead toxicity include coma, stupor, and seizures. Lead poisoning is considered chronic if the lead has been accumulated over a period longer than 3 months. Lead interferes with heme synthesis and has a toxic effect on the red blood cells; this results in a decrease in the number of red blood cells and the amount of hemoglobin in cells, which leads to anemia.

Lead is absorbed primarily through the gastrointestinal tract after ingestion of lead-contaminated substances. Lead-based paint is the most "high-dose" source of lead and is the most common and serious cause of lead poisoning. Children are exposed to lead-based paint when they ingest the fine dust particles from lead-based paint or paint chips from the walls of old homes. Other sources of lead include soil, ceramics and pottery, printed materials, and auto emissions. Lead is a component of several folk remedies used in Mexico (azarcón and greta for digestive problems), the Middle East (farouk rubbed on gums to help teething, bint al zahib used for colic), and Southeast Asia (pay-loo-ah for fever and rashes). Lead is no longer used to solder cans for food and beverages in the United States; however, soldering may still be a source of lead in imported containers of food and juices. A high incidence of lead poisoning is associated with pica.

INCIDENCE

1. Age range of peak incidence is 1 to 2 years.
2. Children between the ages of 6 months and 6 years who live in poorly maintained housing are at high risk.
3. The number of U.S. children between 1 and 5 years of age with blood lead levels of 10 µg/dl or more has declined to a current level of 4.4%. Declines are attributed to the elimination of lead from paint, gasoline, and food cans.

CLINICAL MANIFESTATIONS

Most children are asymptomatic, and lead poisoning is detected during routine screening. Symptoms that may be seen as lead levels rise include the following:

1. Anorexia
2. Constipation or diarrhea
3. Irritability
4. Nausea, vomiting
5. Abdominal pain or colic
6. Malaise

Symptoms of chronic lead poisoning are the following:

1. Increased incidence of learning disorders
2. Behavioral disorders
3. Perceptual deficits
4. Hyperactivity, decreased attention span

COMPLICATIONS

1. Renal toxicity
2. Cerebral edema
3. CNS toxicity—persistent vomiting, irritability, clumsiness, ataxia, loss of developmental skills
4. Severe and permanent brain damage—occurs in 80% of children who develop severe and acute encephalopathy

5. Late signs: stupor, coma, seizures, hypertension, and death

LABORATORY AND DIAGNOSTIC TESTS

1. Blood lead levels—equal to or higher than 10 μg/dl (venous specimen is preferred; if fingerstick specimen is obtained, careful cleansing of site is necessary to decrease contamination of specimen; venous specimen is obtained to confirm elevated level in capillary specimen)
2. Complete blood count—anemia and basophilic stippling
3. Serum iron level, total nonbinding capacity, and serum ferritin level—to assess for iron deficiency
4. Blood urea nitrogen level, creatinine clearance, and urinalysis—to assess for renal damage
5. Flat-plate radiographic study of abdomen—positive result indicates ingestion of lead
6. Edetate disodium calcium mobilization test—to obtain indication of potentially mobile amount of lead in body; indicates whether chelation therapy will be useful
7. δ-Aminolevulinic acid in urine—increased excretion in urine is abnormal
8. Coproporphyrin (coproporphyrin III) in urine—increased excretion associated with increased serum lead levels

MEDICAL MANAGEMENT

The primary focus of medical care is screening and decreasing primary exposure by removing lead sources from the child's environment. Screening includes assessing risk for lead poisoning at each physician's appointment. This assessment may be done by asking three risk-assessment questions: (1) Does your child live in or regularly visit a house or child care facility built before 1950? (2) Does your child live in or regularly visit a house or child care facility built before 1978 that is being remodeled or renovated or has been remodeled or renovated within the last 6 months? (3) Does your child have a sibling or playmate who has or did have lead poisoning?

In the past, blood lead level screening was recommended at 1 year of age for all children and was repeated at age 2 years. In 1997, the Centers for Disease Control and Prevention revised its guidelines related to screening children for blood lead levels and now recommends targeted screening of children at risk. Universal screening is recommended in communities where 27% or more of the housing was built before 1950 and also in communities where the percentage of 1- and 2-year-olds with blood lead levels of 10 µg/dl or higher is at least 12%. Universal screening may also be recommended when a community has inadequate data about the community's blood lead levels. Targeted screening is recommended in areas where fewer than 12% of the children have blood lead levels of 10 µg/dl or higher or where less than 27% of the housing was built before 1950. State public health officials determine appropriate screening using local data related to blood lead levels and housing data from the census. Table 49-1 summarizes screening frequency, environmental evaluation, education, and medical management based on blood lead level.

When blood lead levels rise above 45 µg/dl, chelation therapy is indicated to reduce lead burden in the body. All drugs used for chelation bind to the lead, which facilitates removal of the lead via urine (and, with some drugs, also via stool) and depletes the amount of lead in the tissues. Before outpatient therapy is begun, the lead must be removed from the child's environment to prevent possible increased absorption of lead by the chelating drug. Children hospitalized for chelation therapy are not discharged until environmental lead is removed or alternative housing is available. The major chelating agents used for children include succimer, edetate disodium calcium, dimercaprol, and D-penicillamine. Chelation therapy is also administered to children who are symptomatic who have blood lead levels lower than 45 µg/dl.

The child admitted to hospital with symptoms of encephalopathy receives immediate intravenous chelation therapy. Lumbar punctures are to be avoided in these children whenever possible. Fluids and electrolyte levels are closely monitored. Fluids may be restricted to basal requirements plus adjustments for fluid losses such as in vomiting. Mannitol is used to decrease cerebral edema and intracranial pressure. Seizures are managed initially with diazepam, followed by long-term anticonvulsant therapy. Iron deficiency anemia needs to be treated in all affected children. Prognosis and residual effects are related to how high lead levels were and how long they were elevated. Learning disorders and behavioral problems may result from even low levels of lead.

NURSING ASSESSMENT

1. See the Neurologic Assessment and Musculoskeletal Assessment sections in Appendix A.
2. Assess hydration status.
3. Assess nutritional status.
4. Assess home environment for lead source.

NURSING DIAGNOSES

- Poisoning, Risk for
- Home maintenance, Impaired
- Knowledge, Deficient
- Fluid volume, Deficient
- Nutrition: less than body requirements, Imbalanced

NURSING INTERVENTIONS

1. Monitor child's neurologic status and report the following:
   a. Changes in level of consciousness
   b. Twitching or seizure activity
   c. Complaint of headaches
   d. Projectile vomiting
   e. Abnormal pupillary response
   f. Bulging fontanelles
2. Monitor child's vital signs and report the following:
   a. Increased apical pulse
   b. Decreased or increased blood pressure
3. Monitor intake and output.
   a. Record urinary and stool output.
   b. Monitor fluid restrictions.
4. Monitor child's reaction to chelation therapy.
   a. Succimer
      i. Nausea, vomiting, diarrhea
      ii. Anorexia
      iii. Hypertension
      iv. Infection

TABLE 49-1
Lead Poisoning Screening and Intervention Guidelines

Blood Lead Level	Screening Frequency	Environmental Education	Inspection	Chelation Therapy
<10 µg/dl	Not lead poisoned	—	—	—
10-14 µg/dl	Borderline; confirm test results within 1 month and repeat in 3 months if still within range	Need to decrease lead exposure; importance of obtaining follow-up lead levels	—	—
15-19 µg/dl	Confirm test results within 1 month; repeat again in 2 months	Sources of lead exposure, symptoms of poisoning, and nutritional counseling	Obtain environmental history; intervene if appropriate	—
20-44 µg/dl	Confirm test within 1 week; if still within range a	Sources of lead exposure, symptoms of	Environment is evaluated; lead sources are	Considered when child is symptomatic, if

	complete medical history is taken, and nutritional assessment and physical examination are performed	poisoning, and nutritional counseling	identified and removed	lead level is >25 µg/dl in some cases
45-69 µg/dl	Confirm test results within 48 hours; closely monitor levels for response to chelation therapy	Sources of lead exposure, symptoms of poisoning, nutritional counseling, and chelation therapy	Environment is evaluated; lead sources are identified and removed	Initiated for both symptomatic and asymptomatic cases
≥70 µg/dl	Confirm test results immediately but do not wait for results to implement therapy	Sources of lead exposure, symptoms of poisoning, nutritional counseling, and chelation therapy	Environment is evaluated; child is not returned to environment until sources of lead are removed	A medical emergency; hospitalize for immediate intravenous chelation therapy

b. Edetate disodium calcium
   i. Decreased urine output
   ii. Decreased blood pressure (20 to 30 minutes after infusion)
   iii. Pain, erythema at infusion site
   iv. Symptoms of hypercalcemia
   v. Nausea, vomiting, anorexia
   vi. Numbness, tingling, myalgia, arthralgia
   vii. Maintain fluid restrictions if lead encephalopathy is present
c. Dimercaprol
   i. Fever (occurs in 30% of children)
   ii. Local pain, sterile abscess (if not given deep into muscle)
   iii. Increased blood pressure, tachycardia (may occur within minutes of administration and last for hours)
   iv. Decreased urinary output
   v. Garliclike odor to breath
   vi. Nausea, vomiting
   vii. Headache
   viii. Burning sensation of lips, mouth, and throat
d. D-Penicillamine
   i. Sensitivity reactions—rash, pruritus (common)
   ii. Anorexia, nausea, vomiting (infrequent)

5. Provide diet with regular meals rich in iron and calcium, low in fat.

🔺 Discharge Planning and Home Care

1. Instruct parents to identify and remove lead hazards from environment(s) in which child spends considerable time before discharge.
   a. Have lead-containing paint removed from surfaces by trained personnel.
   b. Regularly wet-mop and wash surfaces.
   c. Remove toys with lead-based paint and earthenware.
2. Instruct parents to supervise child with pica more closely and encourage frequent hand-washing.

3. Instruct and counsel parents about recommended follow-up services (see Table 49-1).
   a. Blood lead level is rechecked 7 to 21 days after chelation therapy to determine need to re-treat.
   b. Children who have had chelation therapy will be closely followed for a year or more.
      i. Those undergoing most types of chelation therapy will be seen every other week for 6 to 8 weeks, then monthly for 4 to 6 months.
      ii. Those who have had courses of edetate disodium calcium or dimercaprol will be seen weekly for 4 to 6 weeks, then monthly for 12 months.
4. Refer to community agencies for environmental evaluation and lead removal, if appropriate.
5. Provide education about lead poisoning.
   a. Symptoms of lead poisoning
   b. Sources of lead in environment
   c. Need to remove sources of lead to protect child
6. Encourage parent to take precautionary measures.
   a. Make sure child does not have access to peeling paint.
   b. Wash child's hands and face before he or she eats.
   c. Wash toys and pacifiers at least daily.

CLIENT OUTCOMES

1. Child will return to lead-free environment.
2. Child and family will understand home care and importance of follow-up.

REFERENCES

American Academy of Pediatrics, Committee on Environmental Health: Screening for elevated blood lead levels, *Pediatrics* 101(6):1072, 1998.

Campbell C, Osterhoudt KC: Prevention of childhood lead poisoning, *Curr Opin Pediatr* 12(5):428, 2000.

Centers for Disease Control and Prevention: *Screening young children for lead poisoning. Guidance for state and local public health officials,* Atlanta, 1997, US Department of Health and Human Services, Public Health Service.

Lane WG, Kemper AR: American College of Preventive Medicine practice policy statement: screening for elevated blood lead levels in children, *Am J Prev Med* 20(1):78, 2001.

Markowitz M: Lead poisoning, *Pediatr Rev* 21(10):327, 2000.

50

❖

Learning Disabilities

❖

PATHOPHYSIOLOGY

Learning disabilities are a group of neurologic disorders that affect an individual's ability to store, process, and produce information. Learning disabilities significantly interfere with educational achievement and performance, and create a gap between one's capabilities and performance. Impairment may be in the area of reading, writing, spelling, or mathematical functions. The most commonly identified learning disability is reading disability. Intelligence is generally average or above average in these children. However, academic achievement is markedly below what is expected, given the person's intellect, age, and educational opportunities.

Etiologic factors associated with learning disabilities include genetic predisposition; perinatal and birth injuries; and medical conditions occurring in infancy or childhood, such as head injury, malnutrition, or poisoning. Mental retardation, emotional or behavioral disorders, and autism are not learning disabilities. Environmental, socioeconomic, and cultural disadvantages do not produce learning disabilities. According to the *Diagnostic and Statistical Manual of Mental Disorders*, fourth edition, text revision, learning disabilities can be categorized into several types: reading disorder, mathematics disorder, disorder of written expression, and learning disorder not otherwise specified (Box 50-1). Learning difficulties become apparent in the early years of elementary school (kindergarten through third grade). It is estimated that between 25% and 50% of children with learning disabilities have other problems that interfere with their school performance. These associated conditions are attention-deficit/hyperactivity disorder (ADHD), memory problems,

BOX 50-1

Learning Disabilities: DSM-IV Criteria

Reading Disorder DSM-IV Criteria

A. Reading achievement, as measured by individually administered standardized tests of reading accuracy or comprehension, is substantially below that expected given the person's chronologic age, measured intelligence, and age-appropriate education.

B. The disturbance in criterion A significantly interferes with academic achievement or activities of daily living that require reading skills.

C. If a sensory deficit is present, the reading difficulties are in excess of those usually associated with it.

Mathematics Disorder DSM-IV Criteria

A. Mathematical ability, as measured by individually administered standardized tests, is substantially below that expected given the person's chronologic age, measured intelligence, and age-appropriate education.

B. The disturbance in criterion A significantly interferes with academic achievement or activities of daily living that require mathematical ability.

C. If a sensory deficit is present, the difficulties in mathematical ability are in excess of those usually associated with it.

Disorder of Written Expression DSM-IV Criteria

A. Writing skills, as measured by individually administered standardized tests (or functional assessments of writing skills), are substantially below those expected given the person's chronologic age, measured intelligence, and age-appropriate education.

B. The disturbance in criterion A significantly interferes with academic achievement or activities of daily living that require the composition of written texts (e.g., writing grammatically correct sentences and organized paragraphs).

C. If a sensory deficit is present, the difficulties in writing skills are in excess of those usually associated with it.

Learning Disorder Not Otherwise Specified

There are no specific criteria for this form of learning disability. The student's difficulties with academic achievement are associated with learning problems in the three areas of achievement: reading, mathematics, and written expression.

From American Psychiatric Association: *Diagnostic and statistical manual of mental disorders*, ed 4, text revision (DSM-IV-TR), Washington, DC, 2000, The Association.

emotional and behavioral problems, and problems with social skills.

INCIDENCE

1. Approximately 50% of students in special education have learning disabilities.
2. Approximately 17.5% of public school students are estimated to have problems learning to read.
3. The high school drop-out rate for students with learning disabilities is 1.5 times higher than that for students in general education.
4. Sixty percent to 80% of students with reading problems are male.
5. Male/female prevalence ratio for learning disorders is 4:1 to 5:1.
6. Reading disability accounts for approximately 80% of all learning disabilities.

CLINICAL MANIFESTATIONS

1. Difficulties with reading, writing, and/or mathematics
2. Deficits in school performance
3. School failure
4. Disruptive behaviors in classroom
5. Social skills deficits
6. Problems in relationships with peers and family members

COMPLICATIONS

1. Social skills deficits
2. Low self-esteem
3. Emotional and behavioral problems (e.g., conduct disorder, depression)
4. ADHD

LABORATORY AND DIAGNOSTIC TESTS

The more severe the learning disability, the earlier the disability will be detected.

1. Intelligence testing that is sensitive to child's ethnic and cultural background (Wechsler Intelligence Scale for

Children—Third Edition, Woodcock-Johnson
Psycho-Educational Battery—Revised Tests of Cognitive
Ability)
2. Tests of language and memory function (e.g., Test of
Awareness of Language Segments, Rapid Automatized
Naming Test)
3. Measurements of visual-perceptual skills (e.g., Bender
Visual Motor Gestalt Test, Goodenough-Harris Drawing
Test)
4. Standardized reading tests (e.g., Stanford Diagnostic
Reading Test, Gray Oral Reading Test—Revised)
5. Standardized math tests (e.g., Key Math—Revised)
6. Standardized written expression tests (e.g., Test of Written
Spelling—Second Edition)
7. Classroom observation and behavioral assessment

MEDICAL MANAGEMENT

The medical management of the child with a learning disability
involves coordination with a community-based interdisciplinary
team. Special education specialists, general education teachers and
counselors, transition specialists, school nurses, job developers,
and rehabilitation specialists, including the medical team (child
psychiatrists and pediatricians), work with the family to address
the child's long-term needs. Medications may be used to treat
associated problems such as ADHD and emotional problems that
affect the child's ability to learn.

NURSING ASSESSMENT

1. Assess child's need for instructional assistance in health
care settings and for adherence to treatment regimen.
2. Review interdisciplinary assessments and evaluations.
3. Assess visual and auditory acuity.

NURSING DIAGNOSES

- Thought processes, Disturbed
- Sensory perception, Disturbed
- Self-esteem, Chronic low
- Knowledge, Deficient
- Social interaction, Impaired

NURSING INTERVENTIONS

1. Consult with individualized education plan (IEP) specialists and educators in adapting strategies in health care settings.
2. Adapt instructional approaches, procedural explanations, and preprocedural preparations to be sensitive to child's learning disability.
3. Coordinate with special education members of child's team in formulating child's IEP pertaining to child's health care needs.
4. Facilitate coordination and implementation of child's IEP while hospitalized.

Discharge Planning and Home Care

1. Coordinate services with members of IEP team and integrate with health care instruction and development of instructional materials.
2. Develop individualized health care plan (IHP). IHP may be written separately by school nurse or integrated as part of IEP/individualized family service plan.
3. Integrate IEP objectives and strategies into child's health care plan in school setting (refer to Appendix L).
4. Refer to community-based services and support services (see Appendix L).
5. Refer to counseling/therapy services—individual, family, or group.
6. Refer to social skills training group.
7. Provide opportunities for social skills training.

CLIENT OUTCOMES

1. Child will achieve annual IEP goals and objectives.
2. Child will express positive comments about himself or herself.
3. Child will engage in positive social interactions with peers and family members.

REFERENCES

Adelman HLD: The next 25 years, *J Learn Disabil* 25:17, 1992.

American Psychological Association: *Diagnostic and statistical manual of mental disorders,* ed 4, text revision (DSM-IV-TR), Washington, DC, 2000, The Association.

Batshaw M: *Children with disabilities,* ed 4, Baltimore, 1997, Paul H. Brookes.

Haas M, editor: *The school nurse's source book of individualized healthcare plans,* North Branch, Minn, 1993, Sunrise River Press.

National Center for Learning Disabilities: Information for living and learning with a disability: LD basics, 1999, available at http://www.ncld.org, accessed December 10, 2002.

Swanson H: *Handbook on the assessment of learning disabilities: theory, research and practice,* Austin, Tex, 1991, Proed.

51

◆

Leukemia, Childhood

◆

PATHOPHYSIOLOGY

Acute lymphoid, or lymphocytic, leukemia (ALL) is a cancer of the tissues that produce white blood cells (leukocytes). Excessive amounts of immature or abnormal leukocytes are manufactured, and they invade various organs of the body. The leukemic cells infiltrate the bone marrow, displacing the normal cellular elements. As a consequence, anemia develops, and insufficient numbers of red blood cells are produced. Bleeding occurs as a result of the decreased number of circulating platelets. Infections arise more frequently because of the decreased number of normal leukocytes. Invasion of leukemic cells into the vital organs causes hepatomegaly, splenomegaly, and lymphadenopathy.

Acute nonlymphoid leukemia (ANLL) includes the following types of leukemia: acute myeloblastic leukemia, acute monoblastic leukemia, and acute myelocytic leukemia. Bone marrow dysfunction occurs, which results in decreased numbers of red blood cells, neutrophils, and platelets. Leukemic cells infiltrate lymph nodes, spleen, liver, bones, and the central nervous system (CNS), as well as the reproductive organs. Chloromas or granulocytic sarcomas are found in some affected children.

INCIDENCE
ALL

1. Leukemia is the most common type of childhood cancer; ALL accounts for about 80% of all cases of childhood leukemia.
2. Highest incidence is in children between the ages of 3 and 5 years.

3. Females have a better prognosis overall than males. At least 60% to 70% will achieve long-term survival or cure.
4. African Americans have less frequent remissions and a lower median survival rate.

ANLL

1. There is no age of peak incidence.
2. ANLL accounts for 15% to 25% of all cases of childhood leukemia.
3. Risk of the disease increases for children with congenital chromosome disorders such as Down syndrome.
4. It is more difficult to induce remission in children with ANLL than in those with ALL (70% remission rate). About 50% will survive.
5. Remission is briefer in children with ANLL than in children with ALL.
6. Fifty percent of children undergoing bone marrow transplantation have a prolonged remission.

CLINICAL MANIFESTATIONS
ALL

1. Evidence of anemia, bleeding, and/or infections
   a. Fever
   b. Fatigue
   c. Pallor
   d. Anorexia
   e. Petechiae and/or hemorrhage
   f. Bone and joint pain
   g. Vague abdominal pain
   h. Weight loss
   i. Enlargement and fibrosis of organs of reticuloendothelial system—liver, spleen, and lymph glands
2. Increased intracranial pressure resulting from infiltration of meninges
   a. Neck pain and stiffness
   b. Headache
   c. Irritability
   d. Lethargy

   e. Vomiting
   f. Papilledema
   g. Coma
3. CNS symptoms related to site of involvement
   a. Lower-extremity weakness
   b. Difficulty voiding
   c. Learning difficulties, especially with math and memorization (late side effect of therapy)

ANLL

1. Gingival hypertrophy
2. Chloroma of spine (mass lesion)
3. Perirectal necrotic or ulcerous lesions
4. Hepatomegaly and splenomegaly (in fewer than 50% of children)
5. Same clinical manifestations as in children with ALL (see section on ALL)

COMPLICATIONS
ALL

1. Bone marrow failure
2. Infections
3. Hepatomegaly
4. Splenomegaly
5. Lymphadenopathy

ANLL

1. Bone marrow failure
2. Infections
3. Disseminated intravascular coagulation
4. Splenomegaly
5. Hepatomegaly

LABORATORY AND DIAGNOSTIC TESTS

1. Complete blood count—children with white blood cell count (WBC) of less than 10,000/mm^3 at time of diagnosis have best prognosis; WBC of more than 50,000/mm^3 is an unfavorable prognostic sign in child of any age. Low hemoglobin level and hematocrit indicate

anemia. Low platelet count indicates potential for bleeding.
2. Lumbar puncture—assesses CNS involvement
3. Chest radiographic study—detects mediastinal involvement
4. Bone marrow aspiration study—finding of 25% blast cells confirms diagnosis
5. Bone scan or skeletal survey—assesses bone involvement
6. Renal, liver, and spleen scans—assesses leukemic infiltrates
7. Platelet count—indicates clotting capacity

MEDICAL MANAGEMENT

Drug protocols vary according to the type of leukemia and the type of drug regimen to which the child is assigned. The process of inducing remission in the child consists of three phases: induction, consolidation, and maintenance. During the induction phase (for approximately 3 to 6 weeks) the child receives a variety of chemotherapeutic agents to induce remission. The intensive therapy is extended for 2 to 3 weeks during the phase of consolidation to combat involvement of the CNS and other vital organs. Treatment to prevent CNS disease is essential. Maintenance therapy is administered for several years after diagnosis to sustain remission. Some medications used to treat childhood leukemias are prednisone, vincristine, asparaginase, methotrexate, mercaptopurine, cytarabine, allopurinol, cyclophosphamide, and daunorubicin.

Prednisone

Prednisone is primarily used for its potent antiinflammatory effects in disorders involving many organ systems. It is used for treatment of acute childhood leukemias. Possible side effects are the following:
1. Fluid and electrolyte disturbances—sodium retention, fluid retention, congestive heart failure in susceptible clients, potassium loss, hypertension
2. Musculoskeletal effects—muscle weakness, osteoporosis, pathologic fracture of long bones
3. Gastrointestinal effects—peptic ulcer with possible hemorrhage, pancreatitis, abdominal distention, increased appetite, weight gain

4. Dermatologic effects—impaired wound healing, petechiae and ecchymoses, facial erythema, hirsutism, hypopigmentation/hyperpigmentation
5. Neurologic effects—increased intracranial pressure with papilledema, convulsions, vertigo, and headache; irritability, mood swings
6. Endocrine effects—development of cushingoid state, manifestations of latent diabetes mellitus
7. Ophthalmic effects—posterior subcapsular cataracts
8. Metabolic effects—negative nitrogen balance resulting from protein catabolism

Dosage should be individualized according to the severity of the disease and the response of the child, rather than being determined by strict adherence to the level indicated by age or body weight. The drug is administered by mouth (PO).

Vincristine (Oncovin)

Vincristine is an antineoplastic agent that inhibits cell division during metaphase. It is used with cyclophosphamide (Cytoxan) in treatment of ALL. Possible side effects are the following:

1. Neuromuscular effects—peripheral neuropathy, nerve pain, paresthesias of hands and feet, loss of deep tendon reflexes, jaw pain, foot drop
2. Hematologic effects—thrombocytopenia, anemia, leukopenia
3. Gastrointestinal effects—stomatitis, anorexia, nausea, vomiting, diarrhea, constipation, paralytic ileus
4. Other effects—convulsions, hyperkalemia, hyperuricemia

Refer to treatment protocol for dosage. Administered by intravenous (IV) push. Avoid extravasation.

Asparaginase

Asparaginase decreases the level of asparagine (an amino acid necessary for tumor growth). It is used in the treatment of ALL. Possible side effects are the following:

1. Allergic manifestations—most serious side effects of asparaginase; are lessened by the addition of

mercaptopurine, cytosine arabinoside, and other immunosuppressants
   a. Chills and fever within 1 minute of administration
   b. Skin reactions
   c. Respiratory distress
   d. Hypotension
   e. Substernal pain
   f. Nausea and vomiting
   g. Anaphylaxis
2. Liver toxicity with attendant jaundice, hypoalbuminemia, and occasional depression of clotting factor levels
3. Pancreatitis
4. Diabetes mellitus
5. Disturbances of calcium metabolism

The dosage of asparaginase is highly individualized. It is administered intramuscularly (IM).

Methotrexate (Amethopterin)

Methotrexate is classified as an antimetabolite. It interferes with folic acid metabolism. Folic acid is essential to the synthesis of the nucleoproteins required by rapidly multiplying cells. Methotrexate is used in the treatment of ALL.

In the presence of infection, methotrexate should be used with caution. Therapy with other bone marrow depressants should also be avoided unless the condition of the child warrants their use. Methotrexate can be given by the oral, IM, IV, or intrathecal route. Avoid giving vitamins with folic acid when the child is receiving methotrexate. Possible side effects are the following:
1. Skin reactions—generalized erythematous rash, urticaria, acne, pruritus
2. Occasional alopecia
3. Oral and gastrointestinal tract ulcerations
4. Chills
5. Fever
6. Vomiting
7. Diarrhea
8. Cystitis

9. Bone marrow depression (with occasional hemorrhage or septicemia)
10. Liver toxicity
11. Pneumonitis

Mercaptopurine (Purinethol)

Mercaptopurine interferes with the synthesis of nucleic acid, which is especially needed when the cells are growing and multiplying rapidly.

The primary effects of mercaptopurine occur in tissues with rapid cellular growth and a high rate of nucleic metabolism (e.g., bone marrow and gastric epithelium). Leukocyte, thrombocyte, and reticulocyte formation is reduced. The drug is used in the treatment of ALL. Possible side effects are the following:

1. Anorexia
2. Nausea and vomiting
3. Diarrhea (sometimes bloody) caused by injury to gastrointestinal epithelium
4. Degenerative liver changes with jaundice at very large doses
5. Bone marrow depression

Mercaptopurine is administered PO only. Refer to treatment protocol for dosage.

Cytarabine (Cytosine Arabinoside; Cytosar)

Cytarabine is currently indicated for induction of remission in individuals with acute granulocytic leukemia. Cytarabine is a potent bone marrow suppressant. Individuals receiving this drug must be under close medical supervision and, during induction therapy, should have leukocyte and platelet counts performed frequently. The treatment is modified or suspended when the drug-induced depression has resulted in a platelet count lower than 50,000/mm^3 or a polymorphonuclear granulocyte count lower than 1000/mm^3. Possible side effects are the following:

1. Nausea and vomiting
2. Leukopenia, thrombocytopenia, bone marrow suppression
3. Anemia

4. Rash
5. Anorexia
6. Bleeding (all sites)
7. Diarrhea
8. Oral inflammation or ulceration
9. Megaloblastosis
10. Hepatic dysfunction
11. Anaphylaxis
12. Headaches

Cytarabine is not active when delivered orally. It may be given by IV infusion or injection. It must be stored in a refrigerator until reconstituted.

Allopurinol (Zyloprim)

Allopurinol inhibits the production of uric acid by blocking the biochemical reactions that immediately precede uric acid formation. The result is a lowering of blood and urinary uric acid levels. The drug is given prophylactically to prevent tissue urate deposits or renal calculi in those with leukemia who are receiving chemotherapy that results in the elevation of serum uric acid levels. Allopurinol also inhibits the oxidation of mercaptopurine, so that smaller doses of mercaptopurine are required (one fourth to one third of the regular dose). Possible side effects are the following:

1. Occasional liver toxicity
2. Asymptomatic increase in serum glutamic-oxaloacetic transaminase (SGOT) and serum glutamic-pyruvic transaminase (SGPT) levels

Allopurinol is administered PO. Increase hydration to at least twice maintenance level. Refer to treatment protocol for dosage.

Cyclophosphamide (Cytoxan)

Cyclophosphamide is a potent antitumor agent of the nitrogen mustard group and an alkylating agent, the exact mechanism of action of which has not been determined. In contrast to other mustard compounds, it is inert when placed in direct contact with bacteria, leukocytes, and most tumor cells in culture. Cyclophosphamide is used in the treatment of ALL and acute monocytic leukemia. Possible side effects are the following:

1. Nausea and vomiting
2. Anorexia
3. Alopecia (occurs in at least 50% of individuals)
4. Leukopenia (decreased WBC)
   a. Expected effect
   b. Ordinarily serves as guide to therapy
   c. Leaves child susceptible to bacterial infection
5. Sterile hemorrhagic cystitis (bladder mucosa may be injured by some active mustard derivatives that are excreted in the urine)
6. Liver dysfunction
7. Cardiotoxicity

Cyclophosphamide is administered IV, by IV fast drip, PO, or IM.

Daunorubicin (Daunomycin)

Daunorubicin binds to DNA. It is used to inhibit cell division during the treatment of acute leukemia. Possible side effects are the following:

1. Sclerosing of vein (use two-needle technique: mix with one needle and dispose of that needle; administer with new needle)
2. Nausea and vomiting (soon after administration)
3. Bone marrow depression
4. Cardiac dysrhythmia and death (rare; occurs at total dose greater than 650 mg/m^2)
5. Elevated liver enzyme levels (elevated SGPT, elevated SGOT)
6. Change in urine color to red

Daunorubicin is administered via IV push; refer to treatment protocol.

NURSING ASSESSMENT

1. See the Cardiovascular Assessment, Respiratory Assessment, and Neurologic Assessment sections in Appendix A.
2. Assess child's reaction to chemotherapy.
3. Assess for signs and symptoms of infection.

4. Assess for signs and symptoms of hemorrhaging.
5. Assess for signs and symptoms of complications: radiation somnolence, CNS symptoms, cell lysis.
6. Assess child and family coping.

NURSING DIAGNOSES

- Activity intolerance
- Infection, Risk for
- Fluid volume, Excess
- Tissue integrity, Impaired
- Nutrition, Imbalanced: less than body requirements
- Injury, Risk for
- Body image, Disturbed
- Anxiety
- Cardiac output, Decreased
- Respiratory function, Risk for ineffective
- Fatigue
- Growth and development, Delayed
- Family processes, Interrupted
- Therapeutic regimen management, Ineffective

NURSING INTERVENTIONS

1. Monitor child for reactions to medications (Table 51-1).
2. Monitor for signs and symptoms of infection.
   a. Be aware that fever is most important sign of infection.
   b. Treat all children as if they are neutropenic until test results are obtained. Isolate them from other clinic clients, especially children with infectious diseases and particularly those with chickenpox.
   c. Have child wear mask if he or she is around other people and is severely neutropenic (WBC lower than 1000/mm^3).
   d. Be aware that if child is neutropenic, he or she may not receive chemotherapy. Child may receive IV antibiotics if fever is also present. (More children with leukemia die from infection than from their disease.)
3. Monitor for signs and symptoms of hemorrhaging.
   a. Check skin for bruising and petechiae.
   b. Check for nosebleeds and bleeding gums.

   c. If injection is given, apply pressure to site for longer than usual (approximately 3 to 5 minutes) to ensure that bleeding has stopped. Check again later to be sure bleeding has not restarted.

4. Monitor for signs and symptoms of complications.

   a. Radiation somnolence: beginning 6 weeks after receiving craniospinal radiation, children exhibit great fatigue and anorexia for approximately 1 to 3 weeks. Parents often worry about relapse at this time and need to be reassured.

   b. CNS symptoms: these symptoms—headache, blurred or double vision, vomiting—can indicate CNS leukemic involvement.

   c. Respiratory symptoms: these symptoms—coughing, lung congestion, dyspnea—may indicate *Pneumocystis* or other respiratory infection.

   d. Cell lysis: rapid cell lysis after chemotherapy can affect blood chemistry results, causing increased calcium and potassium.

5. Monitor for concerns and anxiety about diagnosis of cancer and its related treatments; monitor for emotional responses such as anger, denial, and grief (see the Supportive Care section in Appendix J).

6. Monitor disruptions in family functioning.

   a. Base all interventions on family's cultural, religious, educational, and socioeconomic background.

   b. Involve siblings as much as possible because they have many concerns and feelings about changes in child and in family's functioning.

   c. Consider possibility that siblings feel self-blame and guilt.

   d. Encourage family unity by allowing 24-hour visitation privileges for all family members.

Discharge Planning and Home Care

The interventions identified for acute care management apply for long-term care as well.

TABLE 51-1
Nursing Interventions Related to the Child Undergoing Chemotherapy and Radiotherapy

Responses	Nursing Interventions
Diarrhea	Offer fluids PO.
	Perform skin care to buttocks and perineal area.
	Monitor effectiveness of antidiarrheal medications.
	Avoid high-cellulose foods and fruit.
	Offer small, frequent feedings; include child's favorite foods if possible.
	Decrease or eliminate meat.
	Observe for signs of dehydration.
	Monitor IV infusions.
Anorexia	Monitor intake and output.
Nausea and vomiting	Offer small, frequent feedings of any bland foods high in nutrients and calories.
	Consult with child and parents to develop meal plan that incorporates child's likes and dislikes.
	Maintain adequate fluid intake, using Popsicles, ice cream, gelatin, and noncarbonated beverages.
	Obtain weight daily.
	Observe for dehydration.

Continued

TABLE 51-1
Nursing Interventions Related to the Child Undergoing Chemotherapy and Radiotherapy—cont'd

Responses	Nursing Interventions
	Monitor side effects of antiemetics (e.g., chlorpromazine [Thorazine], promethazine HCl [Phenergan], hydroxyzine pamoate HCl [Vistaril], diphenhydramine HCl [Benadryl]).
Fluid retention	Monitor intake and output.
	Obtain weight daily.
	Evaluate for respiratory distress and edema.
	Provide frequent changes of position.
	Monitor side effects of diuretics.
Hyperuremia	Monitor intake and output.
	Encourage fluid intake.
	Provide skin care to decrease itching.
	Monitor serum creatinine and uric acid levels.
	Monitor side effects of allopurinol.
Chills and fever	Monitor vital signs and frequency of symptoms.
	Evaluate source of symptoms (e.g., tumor or infection).
	Monitor side effects of antipyretics.
	Provide comfort measures such as blankets and tepid sponge baths.
Stomatitis and mouth ulcers	Provide comfort measures such as frequent mouth rinses, use of mouth swabs, and hard candy.

	Avoid hard-bristle toothbrush.
	Avoid glycerin swabs.
	Avoid hard foods that require excessive chewing and foods that are acidic or spicy.
	Avoid hot foods.
Cardiotoxicity (doxorubicin and daunorubicin)	Monitor changes in electrocardiogram and vital signs.
	Observe for signs and symptoms of congestive heart failure.
Hemorrhagic cystitis (cyclophosphamide)	Encourage frequent voiding after drug administration.
	Offer oral fluids in large amounts.
	Monitor IV fluids.
	Encourage voiding before sleep.
Alopecia	Prepare child and family for hair loss.
	Reassure child and family that hair loss is temporary.
	Prepare child and family for hair regrowth that differs in color and texture from former hair.
	Arrange for another child in same developmental stage to visit child and talk about the experience.
	Suggest use of scarf, hat, or wig before hair loss as transition measure.
	Wash scalp frequently to prevent cradle cap.
Pain	Evaluate child's verbal and nonverbal behavior for evidence of pain.
	Note cultural factors affecting pain behavior.
	Use age-appropriate terminology when asking child about pain experience.

Continued

TABLE 51-1
Nursing Interventions Related to the Child Undergoing Chemotherapy and Radiotherapy—cont'd

Responses	Nursing Interventions
	Monitor vital signs.
	Evaluate sleep patterns that may be altered by pain.
	Monitor side effects of analgesics and narcotics.
	Offer approaches to deal with pain such as hypnosis, biofeedback, relaxation techniques, imagery, distraction, cutaneous stimulation, and desensitization.
Leukopenia	Observe for signs and symptoms of infection and inflammation.
	Monitor vital signs.
	Screen visitors for contagious diseases and infections.
	Monitor white blood cell count and differential.
	Ensure that good hygienic measures are maintained.
	Prevent breaks in skin integrity (e.g., keep nails short and prevent injuries).
Thrombocytopenia	Observe for signs and symptoms of bleeding (petechiae and/or hemorrhage).
	Monitor vital signs.
	Monitor platelet count.
	Prevent injury or trauma to body.
	Avoid taking temperature rectally.
	Avoid giving injections.
	Monitor platelet transfusions.
	Provide pressure on bleeding sites.

Anemia and/or fatigue	Evaluate signs and symptoms of anemia. Monitor complete blood count and differential. Provide for periods of rest and sleep. Encourage quiet play activities.
Increased risk of fractures	Avoid weight bearing on affected limb. Prevent accidents and injuries. Encourage nonambulatory play activities.
Delayed physical and sexual development	Provide anticipatory guidance to parents about child's growth retardation, skeletal deformities, and delayed sexual development. Discuss possibility of sterility with child and family.
Chromosomal damage	Instruct client and family about effects of radiation and chemotherapy on cells. Provide genetic counseling.
Hypersensitivity to the medication, resulting in anaphylactic shock	Have available the following medications: hydrocortisone, epinephrine, and diphenhydramine (Benadryl). Observe for dyspnea, restlessness, and urticaria.
Phlebitis and necrosis of tissue, resulting from infiltration of IV infusion	Avoid administration of vesicant agents near a joint. Stop IV flow if infiltration is suspected. Tissue may be treated with drug-specific antidote and hydrocortisone. Apply cold compress to site. Continue to observe site for signs of inflammation and necrosis. Grafting and surgical excision may be indicated if necrosis results.

IV, Intravenous; *PO,* by mouth.

CLIENT OUTCOMES

1. Child will achieve remission.
2. Child will be free of disease complications (such as infections, anemia, and CNS manifestations) and long-term complications of therapy.
3. Child and family will learn to cope effectively with living with and management of the disease.

REFERENCES

Barbour V: Long-term safety now priority in leukaemia therapy, *Lancet* 355(9211):1247, 2000.

Bryant R: Managing side effects of childhood cancer treatment, *J Pediatr Nurs* 18(1):87, 2003.

Chessells JM: Recent advances in management of acute leukaemia, *Arch Dis Child* 82(6):438, 2000.

Cohen D: Acute lymphocytic leukemia. In Foley GV et al, editors: *Nursing care of the child with cancer,* ed 2, Philadelphia, 1993, WB Saunders.

Colby-Graham MF, Chordas C: The childhood leukemias, *J Pediatr Nurs* 18(1):87, 2003.

Friebert SE, Shurin SB: Acute lymphocytic leukemia. Part 1. ALL: diagnosis and outlook, *Contemp Pediatr* 15(2):118, 1998.

Friebert SE, Shurin SB: Acute lymphocytic leukemia. Part 2. ALL: treatment and beyond, *Contemp Pediatr* 15(3):39, 1998.

Greaves M: Childhood leukaemia, *BMJ* 324(7332):283, 2002.

Kanarek RC: Facing the challenge of childhood leukemia, *Am J Nurs* 98(7):42, 1998.

Yeh CH: Adaptation in children with cancer: research with Roy's model, *Nurs Sci Q* 14(2):141, 2001.

52

❖

Meconium Aspiration Syndrome

❖

PATHOPHYSIOLOGY

Meconium, the first stool an infant passes, is a combination of fetal hair, swallowed amniotic fluid, bile salts, pancreatic enzymes, and sloughed mucosal cells from the infant's intestinal wall. When the fetus, in response to some uterine stressor, experiences vagal stimulation and relaxes the internal and external anal sphincters, meconium is passed into the amniotic fluid, which creates a condition that complicates about 8% to 20% of all deliveries. The fetus demonstrates normal or irregular respiratory movements, which can result in the accumulation of meconium in the mouth and pharynx before delivery. Once inhaled, thick particles of meconium can block the infant's airways, causing chemical pneumonitis. The degree of meconium staining is categorized as thick ("pea soup") or thin/watery. Meconium aspiration syndrome (MAS) usually occurs in infants who are term, postterm, or small for gestational age.

Meconium aspiration can cause severe respiratory distress in three ways: by creating inflammation of the bronchioles because it is a foreign substance, by blocking small bronchioles through mechanical plugging, and by increasing surfactant degradation due to lung cell trauma. The risk for MAS is increased with prolonged labor, fetal bradycardia or distress, breech presentation, intrauterine growth retardation, pregnancy-induced hypertension leading to placental dysfunction, prolapsed cord, and abruptio placentae.

INCIDENCE

1. In more than 500,000 births/year representing 8% to 20% of all births, meconium is present in the amniotic fluid. The incidence rises as the infant's gestational age increases. The incidence is higher in African American infants (1.5 times higher than in whites).
2. Meconium is found below the vocal cords in 20% to 30% of cases despite suctioning and in the absence of spontaneous respirations at birth.
3. Between 3% and 33% of infants develop MAS. The risk of MAS increases in the presence of thick meconium and depressed respirations at birth.
4. Death occurs in 4% to 19% of infants with MAS.

CLINICAL MANIFESTATIONS

1. Meconium staining of skin, umbilical cord, and nails
2. Barrel chest or chest hyperexpansion
3. Grunting
4. Retractions
5. Nasal flaring
6. Tachypnea
7. Cyanosis, generalized
8. Irregular or gasping respirations
9. Coarse bronchial breath sounds with audible rales

COMPLICATIONS

1. Air leak syndrome (approximately 20% to 30% of cases)
2. Pulmonary interstitial emphysema
3. Pulmonary hemorrhage
4. Pulmonary edema
5. Persistent pulmonary hypertension
6. Pneumonia
7. Asphyxia, severe
8. Infection (meconium is excellent growth medium for bacteria)
9. Thrombocytopenia
10. Anemia
11. Congestive heart failure
12. Hypotension

13. Metabolic acidosis
14. Mental retardation
15. Cerebral palsy
16. Seizures
17. Altered infant development and parenting behaviors

LABORATORY AND DIAGNOSTIC TESTS

1. Chest radiographic studies—diagnostic; used to visualize lungs to ascertain pulmonary status
2. Pulse oximetry—noninvasive technique to measure oxygen saturation, which usually corresponds to arterial partial pressure of oxygen (PaO_2).
3. Blood gas values—to evaluate cardiopulmonary status with respect to oxygenation

MEDICAL MANAGEMENT

Appropriate delivery room care consists of oropharyngeal suctioning before delivery of the infant's shoulders. If the infant is not vigorous at birth, this should be followed by visualization and suctioning of vocal cords and deep suctioning of the trachea to remove particulate meconium from the airway, ideally before the infant can take a first breath and aspirate meconium into the lungs.

Apgar scoring is not helpful in determining the need for resuscitation because the first score is assigned at 1 minute of age, but it is helpful in evaluating the effectiveness of resuscitative efforts.

Use of exogenous surfactant has been found to be somewhat helpful in treating MAS. MAS is frequently associated with an asphyxial event that may lead to an acute respiratory distress syndrome type of injury, and meconium contains a variety of substances that inactivate surfactant. Clinical trials have demonstrated that using natural surfactants to treat MAS has resulted in improved oxygenation, less requirement for assisted ventilation, and/or shorter hospitalization. Surfactant may become a routine treatment for MAS, along with alkalinization, nitric oxide (NO), high-frequency ventilation (HFV), and extracorporeal membrane oxygenation (ECMO).

NURSING ASSESSMENT

1. See the Respiratory Assessment section in Appendix A.
2. Assess for signs of respiratory distress and response to oxygen therapy. Monitor oxygen saturation levels.
3. Assess child's response to treatments.

NURSING DIAGNOSES

- Infection, Risk for
- Airway clearance, Ineffective
- Anxiety
- Attachment, Risk for impaired parent/infant/child

NURSING INTERVENTIONS

1. Suction infant's nose and throat, preferably before first breath is taken, to avoid meconium aspiration.
2. Prepare to intubate infant and suction meconium from trachea and bronchi immediately after birth.
3. Obtain specimens for blood gas analysis.
4. Obtain chest radiographic study as prescribed.
5. Monitor use of oxygen equipment.
6. Monitor for signs of respiratory distress and response to oxygen therapy.
7. Monitor and maintain body temperature to prevent cold stress.
8. Administer antibiotics to infant as prescribed.
9. Monitor for signs of complications.
10. Be prepared to institute NO, HFV, or ECMO, therapy as prescribed.
11. Perform postural drainage and vibration to help encourage removal of remaining meconium from lungs.
12. Provide support to infant's parents and explain treatment measures to alleviate their fears and anxieties (see Appendix J).

Discharge Planning and Home Care

1. Monitor readiness for discharge.
2. Provide appropriate discharge instructions for parents.

3. Assess cognitive, linguistic, adaptive, and social behaviors to determine development; use developmental history to assess attainment of early milestones and refer to appropriate specialists as needed (see Appendix B).
4. Refer to early intervention programs as appropriate (see Appendix L).

CLIENT OUTCOMES

1. Infant will be free from nosocomial infectious processes during hospitalization.
2. Infant will demonstrate improved respiratory function as evidenced by resolution of respiratory distress, improvement in arterial blood gas levels, and stabilization of vital signs within normal limits without supplemental oxygen.
3. Parents will express their fears and concerns.
4. Parents will demonstrate increased attachment behaviors and verbalize positive feelings regarding infant.

REFERENCES

American Academy of Pediatrics, Committee on Fetus and Newborn: Surfactant replacement therapy for respiratory distress syndrome, *Pediatrics* 103(3):684, 1999.

Bloom RS, Cropley C: *AAP/AHA textbook of neonatal resuscitation*, ed 4, Elk Grove Village, Ill, 2000, American Academy of Pediatrics.

Cleary GM, Wiswell TE: Meconium-stained amniotic fluid and the meconium aspiration syndrome, *Pediatr Clin North Am* 45(3):511, 1998.

Fuloria M, Wiswell TE: Managing meconium aspiration, *Contemp Pediatr* 17(4):125, 2000.

Kattwinkel J: Surfactant: evolving issues, *Clin Perinatol* 25(1):17, 1998.

53

❖

Meningitis

❖

PATHOPHYSIOLOGY

Meningitis is an acute inflammation of the meninges. The organisms responsible for bacterial meningitis invade the area either directly as a result of a traumatic injury or indirectly when they are transported from other sites in the body to the cerebrospinal fluid (CSF). A variety of agents can produce an inflammation of the meninges including bacteria, viruses, fungi, and chemical substances.

Since the introduction and widespread use of the *Haemophilus influenzae* type B vaccine, this organism has been largely controlled in the developed world. The principal bacterial pathogen in children and adults is *Streptococcus pneumoniae*, followed by *Neisseria meningitidis*. In infants 0 to 3 months of age, the most common causes are group B *Streptococcus, Escherichia coli,* and *Listeria monocytogenes.*

Aseptic meningitis is usually caused by enteroviruses and affects young adults more often than children. Older children usually manifest a variety of nonspecific prodromal signs and flulike symptoms that last for 1 to 2 weeks. Although fatigue and weakness may persist for a number of weeks, sequelae are uncommon. The child is evaluated and treated until bacterial meningitis is ruled out. Viral meningitis usually requires only a brief hospitalization; supportive care at home is the primary intervention.

Otitis media, sinusitis, or respiratory tract infections may be the initial stage of infection. In addition, a predisposition resulting from an immune deficiency increases the likelihood of occurrence of this disorder. Once the meninges are infected, the organisms are spread through the CSF to the brain and adjacent tissues. Prognosis varies, depending on the individual's age, the infecting organism, the speed with which antibiotic therapy is initiated, and the presence of complicating factors. Neonatal meningitis is associated with a high mortality rate and an increased incidence of neurologic sequelae. In many affected individuals, bacterial meningitis results in behavioral changes, motor dysfunction, and cognitive changes such as perceptual deficits.

INCIDENCE

1. Ninety percent of all bacterial meningitis cases are in children younger than 5 years of age.
2. More males than females contract meningitis.
3. Age range of peak incidence is 6 to 12 months.
4. The age range with the highest rate of morbidity is birth to 4 years.

CLINICAL MANIFESTATIONS
Neonates

1. Subnormal temperature
2. Fever—usually low grade
3. Pallor
4. Lethargy or somnolence
5. Irritability or fussiness
6. Poor feeding and/or sucking
7. Vomiting
8. Seizures
9. Poor tone
10. Diarrhea and/or vomiting
11. Bulging fontanelles
12. Opisthotonus

Infants and Young Children

1. Lethargy
2. Irritability
3. Pallor
4. Anorexia or poor feeding
5. Nausea and vomiting
6. Increased crying

7. Insistence on being held
8. Increased intracranial pressure
9. Increased head circumference
10. Bulging fontanelles
11. Seizures
12. "Sunset eyes"

Older Children

1. Headache
2. Fever
3. Vomiting
4. Irritability
5. Photophobia
6. Spinal and nuchal rigidity
7. Positive Kernig's sign
8. Positive Brudzinski's sign
9. Opisthotonic posturing
10. Petechiae (*H. influenzae* and meningococcal meningitis)
11. Septicemia
12. Shock
13. Disseminated intravascular coagulation
14. Confusion
15. Seizures

COMPLICATIONS

1. Deafness
2. Blindness
3. Subdural effusions (20% to 30% of cases)
4. Increased secretion of antidiuretic hormone
5. Developmental delay or intellectual impairments
6. Hydrocephalus
7. Cerebral edema
8. Chronic seizure disorder
9. Paresis of facial muscles

LABORATORY AND DIAGNOSTIC TESTS

1. Lumbar puncture and culture of CSF with the following results:
   a. White blood cell count—increased to more than 100/mm^3

b. Gram stain of CSF
c. Glucose level—decreased (bacterial); normal (viral)
d. Protein—high (bacterial, tubercular, congenital infections); slightly elevated (viral infections)
e. Pressure—increased, higher than 50 mm Hg in noncrying infant and higher than 85 mm Hg in child
f. Testing to identify causative organism—*Neisseria meningitidis,* gram-positive organisms (streptococci, staphylococci, pneumococci, *H. influenzae*), or viral agents (coxsackievirus, echovirus)
g. Lactic acid level—elevated (bacterial)

2. Serum glucose level—elevated
3. Complete blood count with differential, platelet count
4. Blood culture—to identify causative organism
5. Urine culture/urinalysis—to identify causative organism
6. Nasopharyngeal culture—to identify causative organism
7. Serum electrolyte levels—elevated if child is dehydrated; increased serum sodium (Na^+); decreased serum potassium (K^+)
8. Urine osmolarity—increased with increased secretion of antidiuretic hormone

MEDICAL MANAGEMENT

Meningitis is considered a medical emergency requiring early recognition and treatment to prevent neurologic damage. The child is placed in respiratory isolation for at least 24 hours after the initiation of therapy with intravenous (IV) antibiotics to which the causative organism is sensitive. Steroids may be administered as an adjunct to decrease the inflammatory process. Intravenous hydration therapy is instituted to correct electrolyte imbalances, in addition to providing hydration. With this fluid administration, the infused volume must be assessed frequently to prevent fluid overload complications such as cerebral edema. Treatment is then directed toward the identification and management of complications of the disease process. The most common complications are subdural effusion, disseminated intravascular coagulation, and shock.

NURSING ASSESSMENT

1. See the section on Neurologic Assessment in Appendix A.
2. Assess hydration status; strictly record intake and output.
3. Assess for pain.
4. Assess for sensory deficits.

NURSING DIAGNOSES

- Sensory perception, Disturbed
- Fluid volume, Deficient
- Pain
- Injury, Risk for
- Knowledge, Deficient

NURSING INTERVENTIONS

1. Monitor infant's or child's vital signs and neurologic status as often as every hour.
   a. Temperature, respiratory rate, apical pulse
   b. Level of consciousness
   c. Equality of pupil size, pupil reaction to light
2. Monitor child's hydration status.
   a. Skin turgor
   b. Urinary output
   c. Urinary osmolarity
   d. Signs and symptoms of hyponatremia
   e. Urine specific gravity
   f. Intake and output
   g. Weight (daily measurement)
3. Monitor child for seizure activity (see Chapter 74, Seizure Disorders).
4. Institute isolation procedures with respiratory precautions to protect others from infectious contact; keep child in isolation for 24 hours after antibiotic therapy is started.
5. Monitor IV infusion and side effects of medications.
   a. Antibiotics
   b. Anticonvulsants
   c. Steroids
6. Provide comfort measures in environment that is quiet and has minimal stressful stimuli.

   a. Avoid bright lights and noise.
   b. Avoid excessive manipulation of child.
 7. Position child with head of bed slightly elevated to decrease cerebral edema; monitor administration of fluids.
 8. Reduce temperature through use of tepid sponge baths or antipyogenic agents (acetaminophen, ibuprofen).
 9. Provide emotional support when child undergoes lumbar puncture and other tests.
   a. Provide age-appropriate explanations before procedures.
   b. Restrain child to prevent occurrence of injury.
10. Provide emotional and other support to family.
   a. Provide and reinforce information about condition and hospitalization.
   b. Encourage expression of feelings of guilt and self-blame.
   c. Encourage use of preexisting support sources.
   d. Provide for physical comforts (e.g., sleeping arrangements, hygiene needs).
11. Provide age-appropriate diversional activities (see relevant section in Appendix B).

Discharge Planning and Home Care

1. Instruct parents about administration of medications and monitoring for side effects.
2. Instruct parents in monitoring for long-term complications and their signs and symptoms.

CLIENT OUTCOMES

1. Child will return to normal or control central nervous system symptoms.
2. Child will not experience neck and/or head pain.

REFERENCES

Bedford H: Prevention, treatment, and outcomes of bacterial meningitis in childhood, *Prof Nurs* 17(2):100, 2001.

Kroll B: Bacterial meningitis and meningococcal infection, *Curr Opin Pediatr* 10(1):13, 1998.

Mandleco BL, Potts NL: Neurological alterations. In Potts NL, Mandleco BL, editors: *Pediatric nursing: caring for children and their families*, Clifton Park, NY, 2002, Delmar.

Simon P: Bacterial meningitis in children and adults: changes in community-acquired disease may affect patient care, *Postgrad Med* 103(3):102, 1998.

Wubbel L, McCracken G: Management of bacterial meningitis, 1998, *Pediatr Rev* 19(3):78, 1998.

54

❖

Mental Retardation

❖

PATHOPHYSIOLOGY

The term *mental retardation* refers to significant limitations in cognitive and adaptive functioning. This is a cognitive disability manifested during childhood (before age 18 years) that is characterized by below-normal intellectual functioning (intelligence quotient [IQ] is approximately 2 standard deviations below the norm, in the range of 65 to 75 or below) with other limitations in at least two adaptive areas of functioning: speech and language, self-care skills, home living, social skills, use of community resources, self-direction, health and safety, functional academics, leisure, and work. Newer definitions of mental retardation adopt a functional or ecologic approach rather than applying the terminology formerly used to describe levels of mental retardation, such as mild, moderate, severe, and profound. Refer to Box 54-1 and Box 54-2 for diagnostic criteria for mental retardation. Many advocates promote the use of newer designations—*cognitive disability, intellectual disability,* and *learning disability*—rather than the term *mental retardation.*

Causes of mental retardation can be classified as prenatal, perinatal, and postnatal. Prenatal causes include chromosomal disorders (trisomy 21 [Down syndrome], fragile X syndrome), syndrome disorders (Duchenne's muscular dystrophy, neurofibromatosis [type 1]), and inborn errors of metabolism (phenylketonuria). Perinatal causes can be categorized as those related to intrauterine problems such as abruptio placentae, maternal diabetes, and premature labor, and those related to neonatal conditions, including meningitis and intracranial hemorrhage. Postnatal causes include conditions resulting from head injuries, infections, and demyelinating and degenerative

BOX 54-1
Diagnostic Criteria for Mental Retardation

1. Significantly subaverage intellectual functioning: an intelligence quotient (IQ) of approximately 70 or below on an individually administered IQ test (for infants, a clinical judgment of significantly subaverage intellectual functioning).
2. Concurrent deficits or impairments in present adaptive functioning (i.e., the person's effectiveness in meeting the standards expected for his or her age by his or her cultural group) in at least two of the following areas: communication, self-care, home living, social and interpersonal skills, use of community resources, self-direction, functional academic skills, work, leisure, health, and safety.
3. The onset is before age 18 years.
   - **Code** based on degree of severity reflecting level of intellectual impairment:
   - **317** Mild mental retardation: IQ level 50-55 to approximately 70
   - **318.0** Moderate mental retardation: IQ level 35-40 to 50-55
   - **318.1** Severe mental retardation: IQ level 20-25 to 35-40
   - **318.2** Profound mental retardation: IQ level below 20 or 25
   - **319** Mental retardation, severity unspecified: when there is strong presumption of mental retardation but the person's intelligence is untestable by standard tests

From American Psychiatric Association: *Diagnostic and statistical manual of mental disorders,* ed 4, text revision (DSM-IV-TR), Washington, DC, 2000, The Association.

disorders. Fragile X syndrome, Down syndrome, and fetal alcohol syndrome (FAS) account for one third of the cases of mental retardation. The occurrence of associated problems such as cerebral palsy, sensory impairments, psychiatric disorders, and seizure disorders is more likely correlated with the more severe levels of mental retardation. Diagnosis is established early in childhood. Long-term prognosis is determined ultimately by the extent to which the individual can function independently in the community (i.e., employment, independent living, social skills).

INCIDENCE

1. More than 85% of persons with mental retardation have an IQ that classifies them in the mild level (IQ between 50 and 70).

BOX 54-2
Operational Definition of Mental Retardation

Mental retardation is a disability characterized by significant limitations both in intellectual functioning and in adaptive behavior as expressed in conceptual, social, and practical adaptive skills. This disability originates before age 18 years.

The following five principles are essential to the application of this definition:

1. Limitations in present functioning must be considered within the context of community environments typical of the individual's age peers and culture.
2. Valid assessment considers cultural and linguistic diversity as well as differences in communication, sensory, motor, and behavioral factors.
3. Within an individual, limitations often coexist with strengths.
4. An important purpose of describing limitations is to develop a profile of supports needed.
5. With appropriate personalized supports over a sustained period, the life functioning of the person with mental retardation generally will improve.

American Association on Mental Retardation: *Mental retardation: definition, classification, and systems of supports,* ed 10, Washington, DC, 2002, The Association.

2. Male/female ratio is 1.6:1.3. Incidence is higher in lower socioeconomic groups.
3. Risk of recurrence in families is as follows:
   a. Child with moderate to severe mental retardation of unknown origin: 3% to 9%
   b. Child with FAS and mother who continues to drink: 30% to 50%
   c. Child with Down syndrome (trisomy): less than 1%
   d. Child with Down syndrome (translocation): higher than 10%
4. Nearly 18% of infants with very low birth weight have severe disabilities.
5. Approximately 500,000 youths have mental retardation.
6. The dropout rate for students with disabilities is 25% to 30%.
7. The unemployment rate for persons with mental retardation is estimated to be between 66% and 75%.

CLINICAL MANIFESTATIONS

1. Cognitive impairments
2. Delayed expressive and receptive language skills
3. Failure to achieve major developmental milestones
4. Head circumference above or below normal range
5. Possible delayed growth
6. Possible abnormal muscle tone
7. Possible dysmorphic features
8. Delayed gross and fine motor development

COMPLICATIONS

1. Cerebral palsy
2. Seizure disorder
3. Behavioral/psychiatric problems
4. Communication deficits
5. Constipation (caused by decreased intestinal motility secondary to anticonvulsant medications, insufficient intake of fiber and fluids)
6. Associated congenital anomalies such as esophageal malformation, small bowel obstruction, and cardiac defects
7. Thyroid dysfunction
8. Sensory impairments
9. Orthopedic problems such as foot deformities, scoliosis
10. Feeding difficulties

LABORATORY AND DIAGNOSTIC TESTS

1. Standardized intelligence tests, including the following:
   a. Stanford-Binet IV for individuals aged 2 years to adulthood
   b. Wechsler Preschool and Primary Scale of Intelligence–Revised (WPPSI-R)
   c. Wechsler Intelligence Scale for Children—Third Edition (WISC-III) for children aged 6 years to 16 years, 11 months
   d. Wechsler Adult Intelligence Scale–Revised (WAIS-R) for youth and adults aged 16 years to 89 years
   e. Cognitive Assessment System for children aged 5 years to 17 years

    f. Kaufman Assessment Battery for Children (K-ABC) for children aged 2.5 years to 12.5 years

    g. Bayley Scales of Infant Development for infants aged 2 months to 30 months

    h. Leiter International Performance Scale—Revised (Leiter-R) for nonverbal individuals aged 2 years to 21 years

    i. Universal Nonverbal Intelligence Test (UNIT) for children aged 5 years to 17 years, 11 months

2. Measurements of adaptive behaviors

    a. Vineland Adaptive Behavior Scales for children from birth to 18 years, 11 months

    b. Adaptive Behavior Assessment System for children 5 years and older, adults

    c. American Association of Mental Retardation (AAMR) Adaptive Behavior Scales (ABS) for children aged 3 years to 21 years. Two versions exist:

       i. School and Community (ABS-S:2)

       ii. Residential and Community (ABS-RC:2)

3. Other laboratory and diagnostic tests (see Table 54-1)

MEDICAL MANAGEMENT

The following medications may be used:

1. Psychotropic medications (e.g., thioridazine [Mellaril], haloperidol [Haldol]) for youth with self-injurious behaviors

2. Psychostimulants for youth who demonstrate attention-deficit/hyperactivity disorder (e.g., methylphenidate [Ritalin])

3. Antidepressants (e.g., fluoxetine [Prozac])

4. Medications for aggressive behaviors (e.g., carbamazepine [Tegretol])

NURSING ASSESSMENT

The assessment process is comprehensive in scope based on the dimensions of biophysical, psychosocial, behavioral and educational needs. Assessment consists of comprehensive evaluation of deficits and strengths related to the following adaptive skills: communication, self-care, social interactions, use of

TABLE 54-1
Hypotheses and Strategies for Assessing Etiologic Risk Factors

Hypothesis	Possible Evaluation Strategies
Prenatal Onset	
Chromosomal disorder	Extended physical examination
	Referral to clinical geneticist
	Chromosomal and DNA analysis
Syndrome disorder	Extended family history and examination of relatives
	Extended physical examination
	Referral to clinical geneticist
Inborn error of metabolism	Newborn screening using tandem mass spectrometry
	Analysis of amino acids in blood, urine, and/or cerebrospinal fluid
	Analysis of organic acids in urine
	Measurement of blood levels of lactate, pyruvate, very long chain fatty acids, free and total carnitine, and acylcarnitines
	Measurement of arterial ammonia and gases
	Assays of specific enzymes in cultured skin fibroblasts
	Biopsies of specific tissue for light and electron microscopy and biochemical analysis
Cerebral dysgenesis	Neuroimaging (computed tomography or magnetic resonance imaging)
Social, behavioral, and environmental risk factors	Intrauterine and postnatal growth assessment
	Placental pathologic analysis
	Detailed social history of parents

Medical history and examination of mother
Toxicologic screening of mother at prenatal visits and of child at birth
Referral to clinical geneticist

Perinatal Onset

Intrapartum and
neonatal disorders
Review of maternal records (prenatal care, labor, and delivery)
Review of birth and neonatal records

Postnatal Onset

Head injury
Detailed medical history
Skull radiography and neuroimaging

Brain infection
Detailed medical history
Cerebrospinal fluid analysis
Neuroimaging

Demyelinating
disorders
Cerebrospinal fluid analysis
Neuroimaging

Degenerative
disorders
Specific DNA studies for genetic disorders
Assays of specific enzymes in blood or cultured skin fibroblasts
Biopsies of specific tissue for light and electron microscopy and biochemical analysis
Referral to clinical geneticist or neurologist

Continued

TABLE 54-1
Hypotheses and Strategies for Assessing Etiologic Risk Factors—cont'd

Hypothesis	Possible Evaluation Strategies
Seizure disorders	Electroencephalography
	Referral to clinical neurologist
Toxic-metabolic disorders	See "Inborn error of metabolism" in Prenatal Onset category
	Toxicologic studies
	Lead and heavy metal assays
Malnutrition	Body measurements
	Detailed nutritional history
Environmental and social disadvantage	Detailed social history
	History of abuse or neglect
	Psychologic evaluation
	Observation in new environment
Educational inadequacy	Early referral and intervention records
	Review of educational records

From American Association on Mental Retardation: *Mental retardation: definition, classification, and systems of supports*, ed 10, Washington, DC, 2002, The Association.

community resources, self-direction, maintenance of health and safety, functional academics, development of leisure and recreational skills, and work. Assessment considers the influence of the child's cultural and linguistic background, interests, and preferences.

Physical assessment includes measurement of growth (height and weight identified on growth charts) and evaluation for current infections, current status of congenital problems, thyroid functioning, dental care, auditory and visual acuity, nutritional and feeding problems, and orthopedic problems. Physical assessment also involves monitoring for secondary conditions associated with specific diagnoses, such as monitoring for hypothyroidism and depression in those with Down syndrome.

NURSING DIAGNOSES

- Self-care deficit syndrome
- Therapeutic regimen management, Ineffective
- Communication, Impaired verbal
- Nutrition: less than body requirements, Imbalanced
- Grieving, Anticipatory
- Family processes, Interrupted
- Bowel incontinence
- Urinary elimination, Impaired
- Caregiver role strain

NURSING INTERVENTIONS
Infants, Toddlers, and Preschoolers

1. Refer to early intervention program for development of individualized family service plan (IFSP) and interdisciplinary treatment plan or, if child, to community service coordinator/individualized education plan (IEP) coordinator (see Appendix L) providing opportunities for developmental learning (Appendix B).
   a. Fine motor development
   b. Gross motor development
   c. Sensory development
   d. Cognitive development
   e. Language development

    f. Psychosocial development

    g. Moral and faith development

2. Refer family to family resource centers and parent information centers that serve parents of children from birth to age 3 who are enrolled in early intervention programs to assist with family support needs, respite care, and sibling needs.

3. Collaborate with other professionals and disability specialists to formulate interdisciplinary plan of care that incorporates life-span approach with periodic evaluations and assessments of current needs.

4. Serve as health care resource/consultant to child's disability service coordinator/care manager.

5. Assist family in obtaining access to care services such as assistive technology, health insurance coverage, dental care, therapy services, income assistance, employment training, and job placement.

6. Refer to other sections in text for specific plans of care for associated special health care needs and health problems.

7. See the Discharge Planning and Home Care section in this chapter for long-term care.

8. Refer to Box 54-3 for support areas and representative support activities for nursing care needs of children and their families.

School-Aged Children

1. Collaborate with other professionals and disability specialists to formulate interdisciplinary plan of care that incorporates life-span approach with periodic evaluations and assessments of current needs.

2. Refer to other sections in text for special health care needs and health problems.

3. Collaborate with educational specialist in IEP development on identification of health-related needs that affect academic performance and adaptive functioning.

4. Collaborate with disability service coordinator/case manager to ensure that ongoing health-related needs

BOX 54-3

Support Areas and Representative Support Activities

Human Development Activities

- Providing physical development opportunities related to eye-hand coordination, fine motor skills, and gross motor activities
- Providing cognitive development opportunities related to coordinating sensory experiences, representing the world with words and images, reasoning logically about concrete events, and reasoning in more realistic and logical ways
- Providing social-emotional developmental activities related to trust, autonomy, initiative, mastery, and identity

Teaching and Education Activities

- Interacting with trainers or teachers and fellow trainees or students
- Participating in training or educational decisions
- Learning and using problems-solving strategies
- Operating technology for learning
- Accessing training or educational settings
- Learning and using functional academics (e.g., reading signs, counting change)
- Learning and using health and physical education skills
- Learning and using self-determination skills
- Receiving transitional services

Home Living Activities

- Using the restroom/toilet
- Laundering and taking care of clothes
- Preparing and eating food
- Housekeeping and cleaning
- Dressing
- Bathing and taking care of personal hygiene and grooming needs
- Operating home appliances and technology
- Participating in leisure activities within the home

Community Living Activities

- Using transportation
- Participating in recreation or leisure activities in the community
- Using services in the community
- Going to visit friends and family

Continued

BOX 54-3

Support Areas and Representative Support Activities—cont'd

- Participating in preferred community activities (e.g., church, volunteer work)
- Shopping and purchasing goods

Employment Activities

- Accessing or receiving job or task accommodations
- Learning and using specific job skills
- Interacting with coworkers
- Interacting with supervisors or coaches
- Completing work-related tasks with acceptable speed and quality
- Changing job assignments
- Accessing and obtaining crisis intervention and assistance
- Accessing employee assistance services

Health and Safety Activities

- Accessing and obtaining therapy services
- Taking medications
- Avoiding health and safety hazards
- Receiving home health care
- Ambulating and moving about
- Communicating with health-care providers
- Accessing emergency services
- Maintaining a nutritious diet
- Maintaining physical health
- Maintaining mental health and emotional well-being
- Following rules and laws
- Receiving respiratory care, feeding, skin care, seizure management, ostomy care, and other services for exceptional medical needs

Behavioral Activities

- Learning specific skills or behaviors
- Learning or making appropriate decisions
- Accessing and obtaining mental health treatments
- Making choices and taking initiatives
- Incorporating personal preferences into daily activities
- Learning or using self-management strategies
- Controlling anger and aggression
- Increasing adaptive skills and behaviors

BOX 54-3

Support Areas and Representative Support Activities—cont'd

Social Activities

- Socializing within the family
- Participating in recreation or leisure activities
- Making appropriate sexuality decisions
- Socializing outside the family
- Making and keeping friends
- Associating and disassociating from people
- Communicating with others about personal needs
- Using appropriate social skills
- Engaging in loving and intimate relationships
- Offering assistance and assisting others

Protection and Advocacy Activities

- Advocating for self and others
- Managing money and personal finances
- Protecting self from exploitation
- Exercising legal rights and responsibilities
- Belonging to and participating in self-advocacy or support organizations
- Obtaining legal services
- Making suitable choices and decisions
- Using banks and cashing checks

From American Association on Mental Retardation: *Mental retardation: definition, classification, and systems of supports,* ed 10, Washington, DC, 2002, The Association.

associated with long-term disability management and primary care needs are addressed.

5. Assist family in obtaining access to care services such as health insurance coverage, dental care, therapy services, after-school programs, recreational programs, and social skills and mobility training.

6. Refer to the Discharge Planning and Home Care section in this chapter.

7. Refer to Box 54-3 for support areas and representative support activities for nursing care needs of school-aged children and their families.

Adolescents

1. Collaborate with other professionals and disability specialists to formulate interdisciplinary plan of care that incorporates life-span approach with periodic evaluations and assessments of current needs.
2. Refer to other sections in text for special health care needs and health problems.
3. Collaborate with educational specialist in IEP transition planning to identify health-related needs that affect academic performance and adaptive functioning, acquisition of community living skills, and work-based instruction and on-the-job training.
4. Coordinate with health care transition specialist to ensure that health insurance coverage continues when pediatric eligibility terminates, to transfer individual from pediatric to adult health care specialty and primary care professionals, and to ensure learning of health self-care skills.
5. Collaborate with disability service coordinator/case manager to ensure that ongoing health-related needs associated with long-term disability management and primary care needs are addressed.
6. Assist youth and family with transition access to care services such as health insurance coverage, dental care, therapy services, employment training and placement, income assistance, rehabilitation services, recreational and leisure services, social and advocacy groups, and community living and mobility training (use of transportation).
7. Refer to the Discharge Planning and Home Care section in this chapter.
8. Refer to Box 54-3 for support areas and representative support activities for nursing care needs of youth and young adults.

🔺 Discharge Planning and Home Care

1. Refer child and family to agencies and professionals who can provide specialized services related to well-child care and dental care and hygiene.

2. Refer family to community resources for genetic counseling, financial assistance, adaptive equipment supply, and family support services.
3. Collaborate with families as needed in developing and implementing behavior treatment plan.
4. Facilitate learning of appropriate social, community, communication, community safety, and stranger avoidance skills, and development of peer relationships and leisure and recreational interests.
5. Facilitate child's inclusion into school programs, recreational programs, and community settings.
6. Coordinate services with members of infant's/child's/youth's interdisciplinary team in early intervention (IFSP) or educational (IEP) settings. Refer to Appendix L.

CLIENT OUTCOMES

1. Child/youth and family will express overall satisfaction as measured by quality-of-life indicators.
2. Family and child/youth will cope with challenges of living with disability.
3. Family will be adept in accessing community resources.
4. Child/youth will demonstrate autonomy, self-determination, and self-advocacy behaviors.
5. Youth will graduate from high school or obtain high school certificate.
6. Youth will have acquired school-based work experience as precursor for adult employment.
7. Child/youth will have participated in inclusive school and community-based activities.
8. Child/youth will have age-appropriate social relationships.

REFERENCES

American Association on Mental Retardation: *Mental retardation: definition, classification, and systems of supports,* ed 10, Washington, DC, 2002, The Association.

American Psychiatric Association: *Diagnostic and statistical manual of mental disorders,* ed 4, text revision (DSM-IV-TR), Washington, DC, 2000, The Association.

Batshaw M: *Children with disabilities,* Baltimore, 1994, Paul H. Brookes.

Batshaw M: Mental retardation, *Pediatr Clin North Am* 40(3):507, 1993.

Betz C: Adolescent transitions: a nursing concern, *Pediatr Nurs* 24(1):23, 1998.

Betz C: Nurse's role in promoting health transitions for adolescents and young adults with developmental disabilities, *Nurs Clin North Am* 18:1, 2003.

Haas M, editor: *The school nurse's source book of individualized healthcare plans,* vol 1, North Branch, Minn, 1993, Sunrise River Press.

Rauth J: Mentally retarded youth. In McArnarney E et al, editors: *Textbook of adolescent medicine,* Philadelphia, 1992, WB Saunders.

Roth S, Morse J: *A life-span approach to nursing care for individuals with developmental disabilities,* Baltimore, 1994, Paul H. Brookes.

55

◊

Muscular Dystrophy

◊

PATHOPHYSIOLOGY

Muscular dystrophy is a disorder that results in bilateral and symmetric wasting of the voluntary muscles. The muscles pseudohypertrophy, and the muscle tissue is replaced with both connective tissue and fatty deposits. Types of muscular dystrophy include Duchenne's, Becker's, limb-girdle, congenital, ocular, and facioscapulohumeral. The onset of sex-linked recessive types (Duchenne's, Becker's, limb-girdle, congenital) is earlier than that of dominant types (facioscapulohumeral, ocular). Duchenne's and Becker's muscular dystrophies are caused by mutations in the dystrophin gene. Dystrophin is a skeletal muscle protein that is absent in Duchenne's and altered in Becker's muscular dystrophy. Symptoms seen initially include gait abnormality and clumsiness. Muscles of sphincters, hands, feet, tongue, palate, and mastication are rarely affected. Mild to moderate retardation is not unusual. Learning differences are also common. Children affected with Duchenne's muscular dystrophy rarely live beyond 20 years of age unless they have long-term mechanical ventilatory support. Other characteristics of Duchenne's muscular dystrophy are the following:

1. It is transmitted as a sex-linked (X-linked) recessive gene.
2. It is characterized by progressive involvement of voluntary muscles.
3. It runs a rapid course.
4. Onset of symptoms occurs between 3 and 5 years of age.
5. Death occurs approximately 10 to 15 years after onset.

INCIDENCE

1. Duchenne's muscular dystrophy affects 1 of every 3000 boys (X-linked recessive). Rarely, girls can be affected.
2. Duchenne's muscular dystrophy accounts for approximately 50% of all cases.
3. Becker's muscular dystrophy affects boys and occurs in approximately 1 in 30,000 to 40,000 male births. Limb-girdle muscular dystrophy has approximately the same incidence.
4. Facioscapulohumeral muscular dystrophy affects both sexes equally.
5. Limb-girdle and ocular muscular dystrophies can affect either sex (autosomal recessive).
6. Approximately 50% of the sisters of boys with muscular dystrophy will be carriers, and one half of their male offspring will inherit the disease.
7. Approximately 50% of children with muscular dystrophy can be characterized as having normal personalities.
8. Learning differences and/or diminished intelligence quotient are not uncommon.

CLINICAL MANIFESTATIONS

Symptoms are related to the voluntary muscles that are affected. The most frequently occurring symptoms are the following:

1. Poor balance
2. Difficulty climbing stairs
3. Waddling gait or toe walking
4. Gowers' sign (hands "climbing" up legs when arising from sitting position) indicates hip girdle weakness
5. Difficulty running
6. Difficulty lifting arms above head due to involvement of shoulder girdle muscles
7. Often, loss of ambulation by 10 years of age
8. Pseudohypertrophy, particularly of calf muscles, but also of quadriceps, shoulder girdle, and hip girdle
9. Occurrence of scoliosis 2 years after child is wheelchair dependent

COMPLICATIONS

1. Cardiac decompensation and cardiomyopathy
2. Pulmonary infections
3. Osteoporosis
4. Obesity
5. Contractures
6. Scoliosis
7. Depression

LABORATORY AND DIAGNOSTIC TESTS

1. Electromyogram—demonstrates lower electric activity in affected muscles
2. Muscle biopsy—diagnostic; indicates presence of fat
3. Creatine phosphokinase level—marked increase in early stages of disease
4. Genetic and protein studies, such as dystrophin deletion studies
5. Nerve conduction studies—measure electrical activity of muscles

MEDICAL MANAGEMENT

A comprehensive, interdisciplinary team approach is used in the long-term management of muscular dystrophy in children. Generally, an interdisciplinary approach with participation of specialists in neurology, orthopedics, physical and occupational therapy, psychology and/or social work, and nursing is used. In those with Duchenne's muscular dystrophy, spinal fusion is usually performed between the ages of 11 and 13 years to avoid increasingly severe scoliosis and pulmonary compromise. Lower limb musculotendinous releases and bracing can help prevent contractures after ambulation becomes difficult. Intermittent positive pressure ventilation and nocturnal nasal bilevel positive airway pressure can help delay pulmonary complications. Young adults with Duchenne's muscular dystrophy may choose to use long-term mechanical support to survive to their late twenties. Ongoing research supports the use of gene and cell therapy, but these treatments are not considered ready for clinical practice as yet.

NURSING ASSESSMENT

1. See the Musculoskeletal Assessment section in Appendix A.
2. Assess child's adherence to physical therapy regimen.
3. Assess child's and family's adherence to pulmonary regimen.
4. Assess child's level of self-care functioning.
5. Assess child's and family's level of coping.
6. Assess child's and family's management of home treatment regimen. Assess home equipment needs.
7. Assess child's and family's need for information.
8. Consult with school nurse to assess for special accommodations needed at school (see Appendix L).

NURSING DIAGNOSES

- Mobility, Impaired physical
- Growth and development, Delayed
- Constipation (related to decreased mobility)
- Home maintenance, Impaired
- Gas exchange, Impaired
- Nutrition: more than body requirements, Risk for imbalanced
- Family processes, Interrupted
- Diversional activity, Deficient
- Self-care deficit syndrome
- Self-esteem, Chronic low
- Grieving, Dysfunctional
- Knowledge, Deficient
- Therapeutic regimen management, Ineffective
- Caregiver role strain

NURSING INTERVENTIONS

1. Advise consumption of high-fiber, low-fat diet with adequate water intake.
2. Advise use of braces and splints as indicated to avoid contractures.
3. Advise use of breathing aids to assist in gas exchange.
4. Assist parents in expressing and working through feelings of guilt, resentment, and anger.
5. Encourage and support parents seeking genetic counseling.
6. Encourage parents and siblings to mourn (loss of "perfect" child) and to learn to cope.

7. Encourage participation in academic support groups.
8. Consult with educational agencies (school transition team) about meaningful educator's career preparation.

🔺 Discharge Planning and Home Care

1. Promote optimal muscular functioning.
   a. Reinforce physical therapy exercise regimen.
   b. Discourage inactivity and encourage rest periods between activities for stamina (inactivity promotes progression of disease).
2. Promote self-care activities as means of enhancing child's sense of independence and self-sufficiency.
   a. Investigate and recommend use of adaptive devices as appropriate.
   b. Provide recommendations for home adaptations (e.g., grab bars, overhead slings, raised toilets, ramps, alternating pressure mattresses).
   c. Recommend use of adaptive equipment as necessary (e.g., braces to prevent slumping and to facilitate standing).
3. Encourage parents, in collaboration with child, to select realistic goals for achievement and living.
4. Provide support for child and family as they cope with disease.
   a. Refer to social worker or psychologist.
   b. Refer to Muscular Dystrophy Association.
   c. Refer to parent support group.
   d. Refer to peer support group.
5. Provide information about and make referrals to available educational resources (see Appendix L).
   a. Refer parents to educational specialist.
   b. Promote child's full inclusion in school.
6. Provide information and assess long-term care needs pertaining to the following:
   a. Scoliosis
   b. Pulmonary and cardiac problems
   c. Contractures, especially of hips, knees, and ankles
   d. Genetic transmission

CLIENT OUTCOMES

1. Child will maintain optimal physical mobility.
2. Child will maintain optimal cardiopulmonary function.
3. Child will maintain inclusion in social, educational, and recreational activities as able.
4. Child and family will make informed decisions about treatment and management of the disease.
5. Child and family will express feelings as disease progresses.

REFERENCES

Ahlstrom G, Sjoden PO: Assessment of coping with muscular dystrophy: a methodological evaluation, *J Adv Nurs* 20(2):314, 1994.

Bach JR: Therapeutic interventions and habilitation considerations—a historical perspective from Tamplin to robotics for pseudohypertrophic muscular dystrophy, *Semin Neurol* 15(1):38, 1995.

Bach JR, Chaudhry SS: Standards of care in MDA clinics, *Am J Phys Med Rehabil* 70(2):193, 2000.

Betz CL: Adolescents with chronic conditions: linkages to adult service systems, *Pediatr Nurs* 25(5):473, 1999.

Cossu G, Mavilio F: Myogenic stem cells for the therapy of primary myopathies: wishful thinking or hope for the future, *J Clin Invest* 105(12):1669, 2000.

Emery AEH: Fortnightly review: the muscular dystrophies, *BMJ* 317(7164):991, 1998.

Fenton-May J et al: Screening for Duchenne muscular dystrophy, *Arch Dis Child* 70(6):551, 1994.

Gomez-Merino E, Bach JR: Duchenne muscular dystrophy: prolongation of life by noninvasive ventilation and mechanically assisted coughing, *Am J Phys Med Rehabil* 81(6):411, 2002.

Harrigan J: Nursing practice management: muscular dystrophy, *J School Nurs* 12(2):38, 1996.

Natterlund B, Ahlstrom G: Experience of social support in rehabilitation—a phenomenological study, *J Adv Nurs* 30(6):1332, 1999.

Parker D et al: The role of palliative care in advanced muscular dystrophy and spinal muscular atrophy, *J Paediatr Child Health* 35(3):245, 1999.

Willig TN et al: Nutritional assessment in Duchenne muscular dystrophy, *Dev Med Child Neurol* 35(12):1074, 1993.

56

❖

Necrotizing Enterocolitis

❖

PATHOPHYSIOLOGY

Necrotizing enterocolitis (NEC) is the most common acquired gastrointestinal disease among sick newborns and is the single most common surgical emergency among newborns. It is a spectrum of illness that varies from a mild self-limiting process to a severe disorder characterized by inflammation and diffuse or patchy necrosis in the mucosal and submucosal layers of the intestine. The cause of NEC has been the focus of research for over 30 years, but although many theories have been proposed, the pathogenesis remains elusive and controversial. Most researchers agree that, regardless of the initiating event(s), the pathogenesis of NEC is multifactorial. Presently, the etiology is thought to involve three major pathologic mechanisms occurring in combination to create a favorable disease environment: ischemic injury to the bowel, bacterial colonization of the bowel, and the presence of a substrate such as formula.

The hypoxic/ischemic injury causes a reduced blood flow to the bowel. Birth asphyxia, umbilical artery cannulation, persistence of a patent ductus arteriosus, respiratory distress syndrome, maternal cocaine abuse, and/or exchange transfusion may be the initiating factor(s). Intestinal hypoperfusion damages the intestinal mucosa, and the mucosal cells lining the bowel stop secreting protective enzymes. Bacteria, whose proliferation is aided by enteral feedings (substrate), invade the damaged intestinal mucosa. Bacterial invasion results in further intestinal damage because of the release of bacterial toxins and hydrogen gas. The gas initially dissects beneath the serosal and submucosal layers of the bowel (pneumatosis intestinalis). The gas may also rupture into the mesenteric vascular bed, where it can be distributed to the venous system of the liver (portal venous air). The bacterial toxins in combination with ischemia result in necrosis. Full-thickness bowel necrosis results in perforation with the release of free air into the peritoneal cavity (pneumoperitoneum) and peritonitis. This chain of events is considered a surgical emergency.

INCIDENCE

The incidence of NEC varies considerably from nursery to nursery, both within a given geographic region and from region to region. These estimates may not accurately reflect the true incidence because of inconsistencies in definitions and in reporting of cases that are complicated by other confounding variables such as prematurity.

1. NEC occurs in 2% to 7% of all infants admitted to neonatal intensive care units.
2. NEC occurs in approximately 12% of neonates with birth weights of less than 1500 g.
3. Sixty-two percent to 94% of infants affected are premature.
4. Seven percent to 13% of infants in whom NEC develops are full-term infants. Many of these infants are being treated for congenital heart disease, anatomic gastrointestinal malformations, polycythemia, or other medical problems.
5. Mortality rate from NEC is inversely proportional to weight at birth and is higher than 50% for infants weighing less than 1000 g at birth.
6. NEC is the third leading cause of neonatal death, with an overall mortality rate of 10% to 50%.

CLINICAL MANIFESTATIONS

The onset of NEC occurs most commonly between day 3 and day 12 of life but can occur as early as the first 24 hours of life or as late as 90 days of age. The disease is characterized by a broad range of signs and symptoms that reflect the differences in severity, complications, and mortality of the disease. Typically, suspected NEC (stage I) consists of nonspecific clinical findings that represent physiologic instability and may resemble other common conditions in premature infants. These include the following:

1. Temperature instability
2. Lethargy
3. Recurrent apnea and bradycardia
4. Hypoglycemia
5. Poor peripheral perfusion
6. Increased pregavage gastric residuals
7. Feeding intolerance
8. Emesis (that may or may not be bilious)
9. Mild abdominal distention
10. Positive result on Hematest

Definite NEC (stage II) consists of the aforementioned nonspecific clinical findings plus the following:

1. Severe abdominal distention
2. Abdominal tenderness
3. Grossly bloody stools
4. Palpable bowel loops
5. Edema of abdominal wall
6. Possible absence of bowel sounds

Advanced NEC (stage III) occurs when the infant becomes acutely ill. Associated signs and symptoms include the following:

1. Deterioration of vital signs
2. Evidence of septic shock
3. Edema and erythema of abdominal wall
4. Right lower quadrant mass
5. Acidosis (metabolic and/or respiratory)
6. Disseminated intravascular coagulation

COMPLICATIONS

1. Immediate complications include the following:
   a. Sepsis (9% to 23%)
   b. Respiratory failure (91%)
   c. Renal failure (85%)
   d. Shock
   e. Patent ductus arteriosus
   f. Anemia
   g. Disseminated intravascular coagulation

    h. Thrombocytopenia

    i. Perforation

2. Long-term complications include the following:

    a. Stricture (25% to 35%)

    b. Short bowel syndrome (9% to 23%)

    c. Recurrent NEC (4% to 6%)

    d. Complications from total parenteral nutrition (TPN) (15%)

    e. Malabsorption

    f. Anastomotic leak

    g. Cholestasis

    h. Enterocolic fistula (2%)

    i. Atresia

    j. Failure to thrive

    k. Neurodevelopmental sequelae (15% to 33%)

LABORATORY AND DIAGNOSTIC TESTS

1. Laboratory results that reflect signs of sepsis include the following:

    a. Leukopenia (total white blood cell count [WBC] below $6000/mm^3$) or elevated WBC with increased band count

    b. Thrombocytopenia (platelet count above $50,000/mm^3$ before surgery)

    c. Electrolyte imbalance

    d. Acidosis (metabolic and/or respiratory)

    e. Hypoxia

    f. Hypercapnia

    g. Positive results of blood, stool, or urine cultures

2. Radiologic findings are the cornerstone for confirming the diagnosis of NEC. The standard anteroposterior and left lateral decubitus (or cross-table lateral) radiographs may show any or all of the following:

    a. Focal, nonspecific gaseous distension of bowel loops

    b. Thickening of bowel wall from edema

    c. Pneumatosis intestinalis (bubbles of subserosal air in bowel wall)

    d. Persistently dilated bowel loop

    e. Portal venous air

    f. Pneumoperitoneum (free abdominal air)

3. Other diagnostic studies are emerging that may be of diagnostic benefit, particularly in the early stages of NEC. These include the following:
   a. Portal vein ultrasonography—detects microbubbles in the portal vein before they can be identified on plain radiograph
   b. Assays of hydrogen in expired air—hydrogen level may be increased, indicating bacterial fermentation
   c. Upper gastrointestinal (GI) series with metrizamide contrast—detects pneumatosis before it is identified on plain radiograph

MEDICAL MANAGEMENT

In the absence of intestinal necrosis or perforation, aggressive medical management is the treatment of choice. Medical management is based on three general principles: (1) rest the bowel, (2) prevent continuing injury, and (3) correct or modify the systemic responses. Enteral feedings are discontinued, the GI tract is decompressed by low intermittent suction, and fluid and electrolyte imbalances are corrected. Intravenous antibiotic therapy directed against enteric flora is started; respiratory support, including intubation and ventilation, is often required; and efforts to support blood pressure and adequate perfusion to the bowel prevent continuing injury and help to correct systemic responses. Abdominal radiographs are obtained every 6 to 8 hours to monitor progression of the disease or detect perforation.

Although many infants can be treated successfully with medication and bowel rest, 25% to 50% require surgery. Indications for surgical intervention differ from institution to institution. A hallmark of successful surgical therapy is the anticipation of impending intestinal necrosis before perforation occurs to prevent gross peritoneal contamination. Evidence of progressive deterioration and ongoing necrosis is noted in worsening metabolic acidosis, respiratory failure, thrombocytopenia, oliguria, shock, and increasing abdominal wall distention. Indications for immediate surgical intervention are (1) pneumoperitoneum, (2) presence of portal venous air, (3) abdominal wall erythema or edema, and (4) intestinal gangrene (positive results on test of abdominal paracentesis specimen).

The principles of surgical management include (1) intestinal decompression, (2) careful examination of bowel with resection of perforated or unquestionably necrotic tissue, (3) preservation of as much bowel as possible, (4) preservation of the ileocecal valve if possible, and (5) preservation of bowel of questionable viability, with creation of a stoma proximal to this bowel. Marginally viable bowel may not be removed during the initial procedure; rather, resection may be deferred, with a follow-up second-look operation carried out in 24 to 48 hours to reassess bowel viability.

The type of surgical procedure required depends on the extent of bowel necrosis. If a short segment of necrotic bowel is present, a primary anastomosis may be adequate. Extensive necrosis or necrosis in a variety of areas may require resection and placement of an enterostomy. If an extensive amount of necrotic bowel is resected, the infant may be left with an insufficient length of bowel for digestion, which causes malabsorption, failure to thrive, and short bowel syndrome.

The timing of stoma closure is somewhat arbitrary. If the infant is thriving on enteral feedings and gaining weight, the stoma is usually closed at 3 to 5 months. A very proximal stoma that necessitates TPN or one that causes serious fluid and electrolyte problems should be closed sooner, usually after 4 to 6 weeks. If a stricture is found, it is resected during the procedure to close the stoma, and complete intestinal continuity is reestablished.

NURSING ASSESSMENT

1. See the Cardiovascular Assessment, Respiratory Assessment, and Gastrointestinal Assessment sections in Appendix A.
2. Assess hydration status.
3. Assess infant's temperature.
4. Assess postoperative pain.
5. Assess family coping strategies.

NURSING DIAGNOSES

- Infection, Risk for
- Fluid volume, Risk for deficient
- Nutrition: less than body requirements, Imbalanced

- Tissue perfusion, Ineffective
- Pain
- Parenting, Risk for impaired

NURSING INTERVENTIONS

1. Monitor cardiac and respiratory status (may need to monitor as often as every hour during acute phase of disease).
2. Observe and report signs of change in cardiac status.
3. Observe and report signs of change in respiratory status.
4. Assess and maintain optimal hydration status.
   a. Ensure adequate intake of fluids (100% to 150% of maintenance level).
   b. Monitor urine output (1 to 2 ml/kg/hr).
   c. Monitor orogastric tube drainage.
   d. Maintain nothing-by-mouth status.
5. Promote and maintain adequate body temperature.
6. Administer antibiotics as ordered.
7. Promote process of attachment between parents and infant.
8. Provide developmentally appropriate stimulation activities (see relevant section in Appendix B).

Preoperative Care

1. Monitor infant's condition before surgery.
   a. Measure abdominal girth (assess for increasing abdominal distention).
   b. Monitor vital signs every 1 to 2 hours.
   c. Monitor for GI complications (perforation).
   d. Monitor fluid and electrolyte status (intake and output, orogastric tube drainage).
   e. Arrange for radiologic examination every 6 to 8 hours.
2. Prepare infant for surgery by obtaining assessment data.
   a. Complete blood count, urinalysis, serum glucose level, blood urea nitrogen level
   b. Baseline electrolyte levels
   c. Blood coagulation testing
   d. Type and cross-match of blood
3. Prepare parents for infant's surgery.
   a. Provide information regarding disease process.

   b. Allow parents to express feelings.

   c. Emphasize that surgery will not immediately cure infant and that critical postoperative period is not unusual.

Postoperative Care

1. Monitor infant's response to surgery.
   a. Vital signs
   b. Intake and output—report discrepancies
   c. Surgical site—bleeding, intactness, signs of infection
2. Monitor for and report signs and symptoms of complications.
   a. Increased need for respiratory support
   b. Decreased urinary output
   c. Bleeding
3. Promote and maintain fluid and electrolyte balance.
   a. Record parenteral intake accurately.
   b. Record output per route (urine, orogastric tube drainage, stoma drainage).
   c. Assess hydration status (signs of dehydration, electrolyte imbalance).
4. Provide dressing care; maintain integrity of surgical site and stoma area.
5. Protect infant from infection.
   a. Monitor incision for drainage, redness, and inflammation.
   b. Administer antibiotics as ordered.
6. Promote comfort and minimize pain.
   a. Provide position of comfort using blanket rolls or positioning mattress.
   b. Cluster care.
   c. Monitor infant's response to nonpharmacologic comfort measures (swaddling, containment).
   d. Monitor infant's response to pain medications.
7. Provide emotional support to parents during infant's hospitalization.
   a. Encourage parental expression of feelings.
   b. Provide reinforcement of parents' caregiving activities.
   c. Encourage parents to call and visit as often as possible.

🔺 Discharge Planning and Home Care

1. Encourage parents to express concerns about outcomes of surgery.
2. Refer to specific institutional procedures for information to be distributed to parents about home care.
3. Instruct parents regarding signs of intestinal obstruction, strictures, poor tolerance of feedings, and impaired healing processes.
4. Instruct parents about follow-up techniques to promote optimal surgical outcomes.
   a. Ostomy care
   b. Central line care (if on long-term TPN)
5. Provide family with name of physician to contact for medical or health care follow-up.

CLIENT OUTCOMES

1. Infant will return to normal gastrointestinal function.
2. Infant's growth will continue at steady pace following growth chart parameters.
3. Parents will verbalize understanding of home care and follow-up needs.

REFERENCES

Caplan MS, Jilling T: New concepts in necrotizing enterocolitis, *Curr Opin Pediatr* 13(2):111, 2001.

Caty MG, Azizkhan RG: Necrotizing enterocolitis. In Ashcraft KW, editor: *Pediatric surgery,* ed 3, Philadelphia, 2000, WB Saunders.

Kitterman JA: Necrotizing enterocolitis. In Rudolf CD, Rudolf AM, editors: *Rudolf's pediatrics,* ed 21, New York, 2003, McGraw-Hill.

Ledbetter DJ, Juul SE: Necrotizing enterocolitis and hematopoietic cytokines, *Clin Perinatol* 27(3):697, 2000.

McCollum L et al: Assessment and management of gastrointestinal dysfunction. In Kenner C et al, editors: *Comprehensive neonatal nursing,* ed 2, Philadelphia, 1998, WB Saunders.

57

❖

Nephrotic Syndrome

❖

PATHOPHYSIOLOGY

Nephrotic syndrome is the clinical state caused by glomerular damage. Increased glomerular membrane permeability to plasma proteins results in (1) proteinuria, (2) hypoalbuminemia, (3) hyperlipidemia, and (4) edema. The loss of protein from the vascular space causes decreased plasma osmotic pressure and increased hydrostatic pressure, which result in the accumulation of fluids in interstitial spaces and abdominal cavities. The decrease in vascular fluid volume stimulates the renin-angiotensin system, which leads to secretion of antidiuretic hormone and aldosterone. Tubular reabsorption of sodium (Na^+) and water is increased, expanding the intravascular volume. This fluid retention leads to increased edema. Coagulation and venous thrombosis may occur because decreased vascular volume causes hemoconcentration and urinary loss of coagulation proteins. Loss of immunoglobulins in the urine can lead to increased susceptibility to infection.

Nephrotic syndrome is the pathologic outcome of various factors that alter glomerular permeability. Nephrotic syndrome can be categorized into primary and secondary types (Box 57-1). Nephrotic syndrome is classified according to the clinical findings and results of microscopic examination of renal tissue. Based on clinical classification, the syndrome types differ in disease course, treatment, and prognosis. Symptoms may become chronic. Some children experience relapses that gradually decrease with age. Prognosis is poor in children who do not respond to treatment.

BOX 57-1
Types of Nephrotic Syndrome

Primary
- Congenital disease
- Finnish-type nephrotic syndrome (inherited)
- Minimal-change nephrotic syndrome (most common type)

Secondary
- After infectious disease
- Drug toxicity (aminoglycosides, amphotericin B)
- Radiocontrast dye toxicity
- Glomerulonephritis
- Systemic bacterial infection
- Hepatitis B
- Human immunodeficiency virus infection
- Subacute bacterial endocarditis
- Vascular disease
- Hemolytic-uremic syndrome
- Renal vein thrombosis
- Systemic lupus erythematosus
- Henoch-Schönlein purpura
- Goodpasture's syndrome
- Familial disease
- Alport's syndrome
- Diabetes mellitus
- Drug and heavy metal exposure
- Allergic nephrosis

INCIDENCE

1. Incidence is slightly higher in boys than in girls.
2. The mortality rate and prognosis of nephrotic syndrome in children vary with the cause, severity, extent of renal damage, child's age, underlying condition, and response to treatment.
3. Nephrotic syndrome primarily affects children of preschool age. It occurs most frequently in children between 1 and 8 years of age.
4. Minimal-change nephrotic syndrome accounts for approximately 80% of all cases of nephrotic syndrome in children.

CLINICAL MANIFESTATIONS

Although the child's symptoms will vary with different disease processes, the most common symptoms associated with nephrotic syndrome are the following:

1. Decreased urine output with dark, frothy urine
2. Fluid retention with severe edema (face, abdomen, genital area, and extremities)
3. Abdominal distension due to edema and bowel edema leading to respiratory difficulty, abdominal pain, anorexia, and diarrhea
4. Pallor
5. Fatigue and activity intolerance
6. Abnormal laboratory test values

COMPLICATIONS

1. Intravascular volume depletion (hypovolemic shock)
2. Hypercoagulability (venous thrombosis)
3. Respiratory compromise (related to fluid retention and abdominal distension)
4. Skin breakdown (from severe edema, poor healing)
5. Infection (especially cellulitis, peritonitis, pneumonia, and septicemia)
6. Untoward side effects of steroid therapy
7. Growth failure and muscle wasting (long term)

LABORATORY AND DIAGNOSTIC TESTS

Urine Tests

1. Urinalysis
   a. Proteinuria (can reach more than 2 g/m^2/day)
   b. Hyaline and granular casts
   c. Hematuria
2. Urine dipstick test—positive results for protein and blood
3. Urine specific gravity—falsely elevated due to proteinuria
4. Urine osmolality— increased

Blood Tests

1. Serum albumin level—decreased (less than 2 g/dl)
2. Serum cholesterol level—increased (may be up to 450 to 1000 mg/dl)

3. Serum triglyceride levels—increased
4. Hemoglobin level and hematocrit—increased
   (hemoconcentration)
5. Platelet count—increased (up to 500,000 to 1,000,000/μl)
6. Serum electrolyte levels—vary with individual disease states

Diagnostic Tests

Renal biopsy (not routinely done) indicates glomerular status, type of nephrotic syndrome, response to medical management, and disease course. Microscopic evaluation shows abnormal appearance of basement membranes.

MEDICAL MANAGEMENT

Medical management may include the following:

1. Corticosteroid administration (prednisone or prednisolone) to induce remission. Dose will be tapered after 4 to 8 weeks of therapy. Relapses are treated with high doses for several days.
2. Protein replacement (dietary or intravenous albumin)
3. Reduction of edema
   a. Diuretic therapy (use with caution to prevent intravascular volume depletion, thrombus formation, and/or electrolyte imbalances)
   b. Sodium restriction (reduces edema)
4. Maintenance of electrolyte balance
5. Pain medication (for discomfort related to edema and invasive therapy) (see Appendix H)
6. Antibiotic administration (prophylactic oral penicillin or other agent)
7. Immunosuppressive therapy (cyclophosphamide, chlorambucil, or cyclosporin)—for children who fail to respond to steroids

NURSING ASSESSMENT

1. See the Renal Assessment section in Appendix A.
2. Assess for signs and symptoms of fluid volume excess.
   a. Local edema (periorbital, facial, external genitalia, abdominal)

    b. Ascites with taut and shiny skin over abdomen (assess abdominal girth)

    c. Weight gain

    d. Decreased urine output

    e. Dark, frothy urine

    f. Anasarca (severe, generalized edema)

    g. Pulmonary congestion, increased respiratory effort, pleural effusions, pulmonary edema

3. Assess for signs of electrolyte imbalance.

    a. Assess for signs of hypokalemia.

        i. Cardiovascular: arrhythmias, flattened T waves, decreased ST segment, widened QRS, increased PR interval, gallop rhythm, increased or decreased heart rate, hypotension

        ii. Central nervous system (CNS) and musculoskeletal: apathy, drowsiness, muscle weakness, muscle cramping, hyporeflexia

    b. Assess for signs of hyponatremia from diuretic use.

        i. CNS: apathy, weakness, dizziness, lethargy, encephalopathy, seizures

        ii. Cardiovascular: hypotension

        iii. Gastrointestinal (GI): nausea, abdominal cramping

    c. Assess for signs of hypernatremia from hemoconcentration.

        i. CNS: disorientation, muscle twitching, lethargy, irritability

        ii. GI: intense thirst, dry membranes, nausea and vomiting

        iii. Other: dry, flushed skin, increased temperature, oliguria

4. Assess protein loss and nutritional status.

    a. Monitor serum protein and urine protein excretion.

    b. Assess appetite and nutritional intake.

    c. Assess nails for signs of prolonged hypoalbuminemia: white (Muehrcke) lines parallel to lunula.

    d. Assess for pallor.

    e. Assess for nonspecific irritability, weakness, fatigue.

5. Assess for side effects from medication administration.
   a. Steroids (cushingoid features, hyperglycemia, infection, hypertension, obesity, GI bleeding, growth retardation, bone demineralization, cataracts)
   b. Alkylating agents (leukopenia, gonadal dysfunction, sterility)
   c. Diuretics (intravascular volume depletion, thrombus formation, electrolyte imbalance)
6. Assess for signs of decreased cardiovascular functioning (hypotension, hypertension, shock, congestive heart failure, cardiac dysrhythmias, fluid volume deficit).
   a. Blood pressure (hypotension or hypertension)
   b. Heart rate and rhythm (tachycardia, arrhythmias)
   c. Distal perfusion (pulses, capillary refill, temperature, color)
   d. Left ventricular hypertrophy (arrhythmias, increased heart size, decreased output)
7. Assess for signs of ineffective breathing pattern and pulmonary infection.
   a. Respiratory rate and pattern (tachypnea, irregular pattern)
   b. Use of accessory muscles (retractions, shoulder shrugging) and nasal flaring
   c. Need to sit upright or to have head of bed elevated
   d. Abnormal breath sounds (rales, rhonchi, decreased breath sounds in lower lobes)
   e. Abnormal chest radiograph
   f. Cyanosis, decreased oxygen saturation
   g. Respiratory acidosis
8. Assess for signs of infection.
   a. Fever
   b. Increased white blood cell count
   c. Positive culture results (pulmonary secretions, urine, blood, other body fluids)
   d. Signs of cellulitis: local swelling, redness, tenderness
   e. Signs of pneumonia
   f. Signs of peritonitis: red, tender abdomen
   g. Septicemia/septic shock

9. Assess for skin breakdown from severe edema.
10. Assess child's comfort level and ability to tolerate activity. Address child's and family's concerns and fears related to disease and altered body image.
11. Assess child's and family's coping response to illness.
    a. Assess family functioning related to child's irritability and mood swings.
    b. Assess coping related to altered body image from severe edema and pallor.
    c. Assess child's and family's response to bed rest and activity limitation.

NURSING DIAGNOSES

- Urinary elimination, Impaired
- Fluid volume, Excess
- Fluid volume, Risk for deficient
- Nutrition: less than body requirements, Imbalanced
- Cardiac output, Decreased
- Breathing pattern, Ineffective
- Infection, Risk for
- Skin integrity, Risk for impaired
- Pain, Acute
- Comfort, Impaired
- Activity intolerance
- Coping, Ineffective
- Family processes, Interrupted
- Therapeutic regimen management, Ineffective

NURSING INTERVENTIONS

1. Monitor and maintain fluid balance.
    a. Assess hydration status frequently.
    b. Monitor ascites by monitoring abdominal girth.
    c. Closely monitor edematous areas, report changes as indicated.
    d. Measure and record weight daily, report changes as indicated.
    e. Record input and output accurately.
    f. Administer diuretics as ordered and assess effectiveness.

    g. Replace fluids lost because of interstitial fluid shifts.

    h. Monitor types of fluids and administration rate to avoid fluid overload and cerebral edema while maintaining adequate circulating volume.

    i. Promote bed rest during periods of severe edema and periods of rapid weight loss during diuresis.

2. Perform measures to correct electrolyte imbalance as indicated.

3. Encourage and support nutritional intake and proper nutritional status.

    a. Continually monitor appetite and nutritional intake.

    b. Complete calorie counts and nutritional screens as indicated.

    c. Provide diet high in calories and protein.

    d. Decrease sodium intake (avoidance of high-sodium foods, diet with no added salt).

    e. Avoid extreme salt restriction or extremely high protein foods because these may be undesirable to children and/or lead to paradoxical problems.

    f. Allow child as many dietary choices as possible, provide child's favorite foods as allowed.

    g. Offer food in small quantities in attractive manner.

    h. Support family in providing calm, relaxed atmosphere during mealtimes (avoid high-pressure feeding or disruptive events).

    i. Consider intravenous, nasogastric, or nasojejunal feedings if client is unable to maintain proper nutritional status.

    j. Collaborate with clinical nutritionist as indicated.

4. Frequently reassess cardiovascular status and institute supportive measures as indicated.

5. Assess adequacy of ventilation and promptly implement airway stabilization methods as indicated; encourage client to cough and deep breathe.

6. Maintain skin integrity and prevent infection.

    a. Practice good hand-washing and aseptic technique.

    b. Provide daily bath.

    c. Gently cleanse eyes with warm saline.

    d. Keep perianal area and skin folds clean and dry.

    e. Frequently reposition and turn.

    f. Prevent pressure ulceration with pressure relief/reduction surfaces; avoid placing hard objects (tubing, cables) under child.

    g. Avoid restrictive clothing, armbands, and tape.

    h. Maintain sterility of all invasive lines and perform dressing changes and site care as needed and on schedule.

    i. Monitor for signs of infection and implement appropriate interventions as indicated.

7. Monitor for pain and provide pain relief measures as needed (see Appendix H).

    a. Assist child to find comfortable positions.

    b. Administer analgesics as needed.

    c. Use nonpharmacologic pain relief methods as appropriate.

    d. Continually reevaluate effectiveness of pain relief measures.

8. Provide emotional support to child and family (see the Supportive Care section in Appendix J).

🔺 Discharge Planning and Home Care

Provide child and parents with developmentally appropriate verbal and written instruction regarding home management of the following (see Appendix K):

1. Disease process: include expected clinical progress and signs of relapse.

2. Medications: outline dose, route, schedule, side effects, and complications.

3. Nutrition: follow high-protein, low-salt diet guidelines.

4. Prevention of infection: avoid live virus vaccination and other conditions that may lead to infection while receiving high-dose steroids or immunosuppressive therapy.

5. Skin care: assess for breakdown, prevent breakdown.

6. Pain management: institute nonpharmacologic pain measures and give analgesic agents (see Appendix H).

7. Activity: limit as needed, promote return to normal activity level as symptoms resolve.
8. Follow-up care: provide as indicated.

CLIENT OUTCOMES

1. Child will maintain fluid-electrolyte and acid-base balance within appropriate limits.
2. Child will have optimal nutrition, growth, and development.
3. Child and family will adhere to treatment regimen without occurrence of complications.
4. Child will maintain optimal comfort level and coping with illness.

REFERENCES

Hazinski MF: *Handbook of pediatric critical care,* Philadelphia, 1999, WB Saunders.

Loghman-Adham M et al: Acute renal failure in idiopathic nephrotic syndrome, *Clin Nephrol* 47(2):76, 1997

McKinney ES et al: *Maternal-child nursing,* Philadelphia, 2000, WB Saunders.

Orth SR et al: The nephrotic syndrome, *N Engl J Med* 338(17):1202, 1998.

Potts NL, Mandleco BL, editors: *Pediatric nursing: caring for children and their families,* Clifton Park, NY, 2002, Delmar.

58

◈

Neuroblastoma

◈

PATHOPHYSIOLOGY

Neuroblastomas are soft, solid tumors originating from neural crest cells that are precursors of the adrenal medulla and sympathetic nervous system. Neuroblastomas can be present wherever sympathetic nervous tissue is found. Primary tumor sites are usually in the abdomen, either in the adrenal gland or paraspinal ganglia. Less common primary sites include the paraspinal area of the thorax, the neck, and the pelvis. Usually encapsulated, neuroblastomas often impinge on adjacent tissues and organs. Bone and bone marrow involvement are common. The etiology of neuroblastoma is unknown.

INCIDENCE

1. Neuroblastoma is the most common extracranial solid tumor of childhood and the most common neoplasm of infants. It is the second most common type of childhood tumor.
2. Approximately 500 new cases are diagnosed each year in the United States.
3. The estimated incidence is 1 in 10,000 births.
4. Neuroblastoma most commonly occurs in children between birth and age 4 years.
5. The unique phenomenon of spontaneous tumor regression and maturation into benign forms may allow many cases of neuroblastoma to go undetected.
6. Prognosis is favorable if diagnosis is made before 12 months of age and if the disease is stage I, II, or IVS (see Medical and Surgical Management section in this chapter).

CLINICAL MANIFESTATIONS

(Depends on tumor location)

1. Symptoms related to retroperitoneal, adrenal gland, or paraspinal mass
   a. Firm, nontender, irregular abdominal mass that crosses midline
   b. Altered bowel and/or bladder function
   c. Vascular compression with edema of lower extremities
   d. Back pain, weakness of lower extremities
   e. Sensory loss
   f. Loss of sphincter control
2. Symptoms related to neck or thoracic mass
   a. Cervical and supraclavicular lymphadenopathy
   b. Congestion and edema of face
   c. Respiratory dysfunction/distress
   d. Headache
   e. Ecchymotic orbital proptosis
   f. Miosis
   g. Ptosis
   h. Exophthalmos
   i. Anhidrosis

COMPLICATIONS

Depending on the location of the tumor, lower extremity weakness or paralysis. Bone marrow failure may occur with bone marrow metastasis.

LABORATORY AND DIAGNOSTIC TESTS

1. Complete blood count—to detect anemia caused by many secondary factors (e.g., hemorrhage, disseminated intravascular coagulation)
2. Urinary levels of catecholamines (vanillylmandelic acid and homovanillic acid)—tumor markers that are elevated due to overproduction by tumor cells or defective storage within tumor cells
3. Neuron-specific enolase level—elevated due to correlation with amount of active neuronal tissue

4. Level of GD2 (sugar-containing lipid molecules)—present on surface of human neuroblastoma cells; detection confirms presence of neuroblastoma
5. Ferritin level—increase correlates with poorer prognosis
6. Bone marrow aspiration and biopsies—to reveal marrow involvement, confirm diagnosis, and allow staging
7. Chest radiographic study—to delineate primary thoracic neuroblastoma and vertebral and paravertebral involvement
8. Abdominal ultrasonography—to reveal location of mass and any impingement on other organs
9. Computed tomography—to determine if tumor is operable
10. Magnetic resonance imaging—to detect intraspinal involvement

MEDICAL AND SURGICAL MANAGEMENT

The International Staging System for Neuroblastoma standardizes definitions for diagnosis, staging, and treatment, and it categorizes disease according to radiographic and surgical findings, plus bone marrow status.

Localized tumors are divided into stages I, II, and III, depending on features of the primary tumor and the status of regional lymph nodes. Disseminated disease is divided into stages IV and IVS (S is for special), depending on the presence of distant cortical bone involvement, extent of bone marrow disease, and features of the primary tumor.

Children with favorable prognostic features usually require no treatment, minimal treatment, or surgical resection alone. Complete surgical resection is the only therapy required for those with stage I tumors. Surgery may also suffice for stage II tumors, but chemotherapy is widely used and sometimes supplemented with local radiotherapy. Stage IVS neuroblastoma has a high rate of spontaneous regression, and management may be limited to low-dose chemotherapy and close observation.

Stage III and IV neuroblastomas require intensive therapy, including chemotherapy, radiation therapy, surgery, autologous or allogeneic bone marrow transplant, bone marrow rescue, metaiodobenzylguanidine administration, and immunotherapy with monoclonal antibodies specific to neuroblastoma.

Medication consists of simultaneous or rotating use of multiagent chemotherapy:

1. Cyclophosphamide—inhibits DNA replication
2. Doxorubicin—interferes with nucleic acid synthesis and blocks DNA transcription
3. VP-16 (etoposide)—causes metaphase arrest and inhibits nucleic acid and protein synthesis

NURSING ASSESSMENT

1. Refer to Appendix A for system-specific assessments.
2. Be aware that physical assessment depends on tumor site and related system. Palpation of tumor site should be avoided.
3. Be aware that assessment of child with neuroblastoma should encompass all aspects of medical treatment, including chemotherapy, surgery, radiation, and bone marrow transplantation.
4. Assess child for verbal and nonverbal expressions of pain (see Appendix H).
5. Assess child's and family's coping responses.
6. Assess child's level of development (see Appendix B).

NURSING DIAGNOSES

- Infection, Risk for
- Pain
- Fluid volume, Excess
- Mobility, Impaired physical
- Therapeutic regimen management, Ineffective
- Growth and development, Delayed
- Family processes, Interrupted

NURSING INTERVENTIONS
Surgical Phase

1. Prepare child for clinical staging procedures with age-appropriate approach (see the Preparation for Procedures or Surgery section in Appendix J).
2. Monitor for signs of infection.

3. Monitor respiratory function.
4. Provide fluid support.

Chemotherapy and/or Radiation Phase

1. Assess tumor site using observation and inspection; palpation is contraindicated.
2. Minimize side effects of multiagent chemotherapy.
   a. Bone marrow suppression
   b. Nausea and vomiting
   c. Anorexia and weight loss
   d. Oral mucositis
   e. Pain
3. Observe for medication or transfusion reactions.
4. Assess skin integrity.
5. Monitor for signs of infection.
6. Monitor physical and emotional growth and development of child (see Appendix B).
7. Teach parents about medications their child is receiving.
8. Refer child and/or siblings to child life specialist.
9. Refer family to social services for support and resource utilization (see Appendixes J and L).
10. Assess for pain using age-appropriate technique (see Appendix H).
11. Provide pain management (see Appendix H).

Discharge Planning and Home Care

Instruct parents about home care management (see Appendix K).

1. Signs of infection and guidelines on when to seek medical attention
2. Wound care
3. Home care of child's central venous access device, including site care, dressing change, flushing, cap change, and emergency care
4. Medication administration (provide written information)
5. Compliance with treatment and medical appointments
6. Special nutritional needs
7. Potential behavioral changes in child and/or siblings

CLIENT OUTCOMES

1. Child and family will demonstrate ability to cope with life-threatening illness.
2. Child will be free of infection.
3. Child and family will understand home care and long-term follow-up needs.

REFERENCES

Alcoser P, Rodgers C: Treatment strategies in childhood cancer, *J Pediatr Nurs* 18(2):103, 2003.

Ball J, Bindler R, editors: *Pediatric nursing: caring for children*, East Norwalk, Conn, 1995, Appleton & Lange.

Bryant R: Managing side effects of childhood cancer treatment, *J Pediatr Nurs* 18(2):113, 2003.

Foley G et al, editors: *Nursing care of the child with cancer*, ed 2, Philadelphia, 1993, WB Saunders.

Kline N, Sevier N: Solid tumors in children, *J Pediatr Nurs* 18(2):96, 2003.

Tuffs A: Neuroblastoma screening does not reduce mortality, *BMJ* 324(7342):867, 2002.

Young G et al: Recognition of common childhood malignancies, *Am Fam Physician* 61(7):2144, 2000.

59

❖

Nonaccidental Trauma

❖

OVERVIEW OF THE PROBLEM

The lives of youth in America's major cities are being devastated by violence. Health care professionals and professional organizations (such as the American Medical Association and California Teachers Association) have acknowledged violence affecting children in the United States as a public health emergency. Examples of crimes committed by and against youth are rape, robbery, homicide, and aggravated assault. Many fights on school grounds are ending in death, and an alarming number of students are carrying guns and weapons. Since 1990 the childhood mortality rate has decreased; however, violence is increasing. The only age group in the United States for which morbidity and mortality have not improved since 1960 is adolescents. Nurses in a variety of settings must be prepared to care for affected children.

INCIDENCE

1. In 2000 the arrest rate for youths aged 10 to 17 years was 7327 per 100,000 youths.
2. In 1997 almost 1 million children were victims of abuse and neglect.
3. The juvenile violent crime rate in 2000 was lower than that in 1980.
4. Males are seven times more likely to be arrested for a violent crime than females.
5. The second leading cause of injury and death in 15- to 19-year-old teenagers in the United States is gunshot wounds. Every year 4000 children and teenagers are killed by gunfire.

6. Youths living in disadvantaged urban areas are at greater risk for becoming victims of crime and committing it.
7. Incidence is higher in African American individuals than in white individuals.
8. Approximately 6% of high school seniors in the United States carry firearms and other weapons to school.
9. The percentage of students reporting the presence of street gangs in their schools has increased from 15% to 28%.
10. Children classified as being at "high risk" for violence are younger than previously reported. Those in the 10- to 14-year-old age group are at greater risk than those in the 15- to 19-year-old age group.
11. Each year 3 million to 10 million children observe their mothers being abused, and husbands who abuse their wives are 150% more likely to abuse their children than those who do not.
12. The Centers for Disease Control and Prevention (1996) has reported that four causes account for 72% of all the mortality and much of the morbidity in the U.S. population aged 5 to 24 years:
    a. 29% of mortalities: motor vehicle accidents
    b. 20% of mortalities: homicides
    c. 12% of mortalities: suicide
    d. 11% of mortalities: other accidents such as falls, fire, drownings

CLINICAL MANIFESTATIONS

1. Injury-specific manifestations (such as trauma marks, imprint burns, immersion burns, spiral fractures, human bite marks, and head injuries)
2. Difficulty sleeping
3. Enuresis and/or encopresis
4. School problems
5. Aggression
6. Unexplained weight loss or gain
7. Loss of appetite
8. Admitted "gang" involvement
9. Involvement in high-risk behaviors (substance abuse, criminal activity)

COMPLICATIONS

1. Bleeding from wounds such as gunshot wounds and stab injuries
2. Organ damage
3. Permanent disabilities
4. Death

LABORATORY AND DIAGNOSTIC TESTS

1. Complete blood count
2. Radiographic studies
3. Various diagnostic tests, depending on site of injury

MEDICAL MANAGEMENT

Management is specific to the injuries, for example, surgery, casting, and wound care. Medications may include pain medications and antibiotics as indicated.

NURSING ASSESSMENT

1. Assess for risk factors and high-risk behaviors.
2. Assess verbal and nonverbal pain behaviors.
3. Assess for presence of injuries.
4. Assess psychosocial factors affecting youth and family.

NURSING DIAGNOSES

- Tissue integrity, Impaired
- Knowledge, Deficient
- Injury, Risk for
- Trauma, Risk for
- Infection, Risk for
- Skin integrity, Impaired
- Pain
- Self-esteem, Chronic low
- Family processes, Interrupted
- Violence, Risk for
- Self-harm, Risk for
- Social interactions, Impaired

NURSING INTERVENTIONS

1. Education of children and parents—distribute information packets, discuss preventive and interventional strategies
2. Prevention, especially of risk-taking behaviors such as violence and substance abuse; prevention is the No. 1 intervention
3. Initiation of steps to decrease gang activity and violence in schools through collaboration with school officials in developing programs
4. Pain management (see Appendix H)
5. Wound or surgical site care
6. Prevention of infection
7. Encouragement of positive social activities
8. Promotion of self-esteem through referral to community programs, peer support groups, mental health counseling
9. Promotion of use of conflict-resolution skills to deal with confrontational situations

🏠 Discharge Planning and Home Care

1. Refer family and youth to preventive and educational programs in community (Box 59-1).
2. Refer family and youth to support groups and counseling.

BOX 59-1
Resources

Brady Center to Prevent Gun Violence
1225 Eye Street NW, Suite 1100
Washington, DC 20005
Phone: 202-289-7319

Children's Safety Network
National Center for Education in Maternal and Child Health
2000 15th Street N, Suite 701
Arlington, VA 22201-2617
Phone: 703-524-7802
Fax: 703-524-9335
E-mail: rcsnceolgumedlib.dml.georgetown.edu

Continued

BOX 59-1

Resources—cont'd

Council for Safe Families
210 W 90th Street, Suite 2B
New York, NY 10024
Hotline: 212-914-5800

National SAFEKIDS Campaign
11 Michigan Avenue NW
Washington, DC 20010-2970
Phone: 202-939-4993

- American Academy of Pediatrics: http://www.aap.org—Access to publications, books, and articles
- Convention on the Rights of the Child: http://www.unicef.org/crc—Has information on children's rights, programs, publications, statistics
- National Clearinghouse on Child Abuse and Neglect Information: http://www.calib.com/nccanch—Contains publications, statistics, programs for children and families, adoption information
- Prevent Child Abuse America: http://www.preventchildabuse.org—Provides information on abuse prevention, publications, listing of offices
- United Nations Background Note on Children's Rights: http://www.un.org./rights/dpi1765e.htm—Offers information on children's rights
- U.S. Department of Health and Human Services Children's Bureau: http://www.acf.dhhs.gov/programs/cb—Provides information on laws and publications

3. Teach family/youth to perform wound or surgical site care.
4. Stress importance of follow-up care.

CLIENT OUTCOMES

1. Youth will express relief from pain.
2. Youth will demonstrate decrease or absence of risk-taking behaviors.
3. Youth and family will attend community prevention and education programs.

REFERENCES

Lemmey D et al: Intimate partner violence: mothers' perspectives of effects on their children, *MCN* 26(2):98, 2001.

Lieberman R: Early warning signs warrant attention, *California Educator* 3(5):8, 1999.

Mulryan K et al: Protecting the child, *Nursing* 30(7):39, 2000.

Muscari M: Prevention: are we really reaching today's teens? *MCN* 24(2):87, 1999.

Office of Juvenile Justice and Delinquency Prevention: *Statistical briefing book,* Jan 20, 2002, available online at http://ojjdp.ncjrs.org/ojstatbb/html/qu276.html, accessed June 8, 2003.

Posnick-Goodwin S: School: is it still a safe haven? *California Educator* 3(5):6, 1999.

Velsor-Friedrich B, Ferguson SL: Guns killing our children: a status report, *J Pediatr Nurs* 16(2):127, 2001.

60

❖

Non-Hodgkin's Lymphoma

❖

PATHOPHYSIOLOGY

Non-Hodgkin's lymphoma (NHL) is a highly malignant neoplasm of the lymphatic system and lymphoid tissue. As is the case with most childhood neoplasms, the cause of NHL has not been identified. Several factors, including viral infections, immunodeficiency, chromosomal aberration, chronic immunostimulation, and environmental exposure, have been implicated in precipitating malignant lymphomas.

Childhood NHL tends to have a rapid onset and is characterized by aggressive, widespread disease that generally shows a quick response to treatment. Common sites of involvement include the intraabdominal, mediastinal, peripheral nodal, and nasopharyngeal areas. Common extralymphoid sites include bone, skin, bone marrow, testes, and the central nervous system (CNS). With aggressive therapy, the survival rate is 90% for children with localized NHL and 60% to 70% for those with advanced disease.

Because several classification systems for NHL have been proposed, categorization remains complex. NHL can be divided into three types: (1) lymphoblastic, (2) small noncleaved cell, and (3) large cell. Favorable prognosis is indicated by the following:

1. Lymph node involvement
2. An extranodal site in the nasopharynx or oropharynx, or other isolated extranodal site, with or without lymphadenopathy
3. Gastrointestinal involvement, with or without regional lymphadenopathy, limited to the mesentery

INCIDENCE

1. NHL is the third most common malignancy in children.
2. NHL occurs from infancy through adolescence, with a peak incidence between ages 7 and 11 years.
3. Males are affected more often than females, in a 3:1 ratio.
4. Incidence of NHL is approximately 1.5 times that of Hodgkin's disease.
5. The 3-year survival rate for all children with NHL is 50% to 80%.

CLINICAL MANIFESTATIONS

Intraabdominal Involvement

1. Possible symptoms mimicking appendicitis (pain, right lower quadrant tenderness)
2. Intussusception
3. Ovarian, pelvic, retroperitoneal masses
4. Ascites
5. Vomiting
6. Diarrhea
7. Weight loss

Mediastinal Involvement

1. Pleural effusion
2. Tracheal compression
3. Superior vena cava syndrome
4. Coughing, wheezing, dyspnea, respiratory distress
5. Edema of upper extremities
6. Mental status changes

Primary Nasal, Paranasal, Oral, and Pharyngeal Involvement

1. Nasal congestion
2. Rhinorrhea
3. Epistaxis
4. Headache
5. Proptosis
6. Irritability
7. Weight loss

COMPLICATIONS

The major complication is tumor lysis syndrome (as a result of treatment).

1. Hyperuricemia
2. Hyperkalemia
3. Hyperphosphatemia
4. Hypocalcemia

LABORATORY AND DIAGNOSTIC TESTS

1. Bone marrow biopsy—to identify malignant cells with bone marrow involvement
2. Lumbar puncture—to determine presence of malignant cells in CNS
3. Complete blood count—diagnostic for bone marrow dysfunction; may show elevated white blood cell count, decreased hemoglobin level, hematocrit, and platelet count
4. Liver and kidney function tests—liver function test values may be elevated with liver involvement; kidney function test values may be elevated with kidney involvement
5. Lactate dehydrogenase level—elevated due to tumor lysis
6. Serum uric acid level— elevated due to cellular tumor load
7. Epstein-Barr virus test—positive result has been associated with NHL
8. Bone scan—diagnostic
9. Chest radiograph—diagnostic
10. Computed tomography and magnetic resonance imaging—diagnostic

MEDICAL MANAGEMENT

Current therapy for NHL is based on the stage of the disease, immunophenotype, and histopathology. Treatment for NHL is multiagent chemotherapy to eradicate the disease and to prevent further dissemination.

The following medication regimens may be used:

1. For stage I and II disease (localized lymphomas)
   a. Induction therapy
      i. Vincristine—inhibits cell division at metaphase

    ii. Prednisone—used in conjunction with
        antineoplastic agents
    iii. Doxorubicin—interferes with nucleic acid
         synthesis
    iv. Cyclophosphamide—blocks DNA, RNA, and
        protein synthesis
  b. Continuation therapy
    i. Mercaptopurine—interferes with normal cellular
       metabolism
    ii. Methotrexate—interferes with mitotic process by
        inhibiting uptake of folinic acid
2. For stage III and IV disease (advanced lymphomas)—
   COMP drug regimen
  a. Cyclophosphamide (Cytoxan)
  b. Oncovin (vincristine)
  c. Methotrexate
  d. Prednisone
3. CNS-protective medications
  a. Methotrexate
  b. Cytosine arabinoside—interferes with normal
     cellular metabolism
  c. Hydrocortisone—decreases edema caused by tumor
     necrosis

NURSING ASSESSMENT

1. Assess child's physiologic status (see Appendix A).
  a. Signs and symptoms of NHL
  b. Involvement of other body systems (e.g.,
     gastrointestinal, respiratory)
  c. Adverse effects of treatment
  d. Signs and symptoms of tumor lysis syndrome
     (hypocalcemia, hyperphosphatemia, hyperkalemia, and
     hyperuricemia)
2. Assess child and family for psychosocial needs (see the
   Supportive Care section in Appendix J).
  a. Knowledge of disease and treatment regimen
  b. Body image
  c. Family structure
  d. Family stressors

> e. Coping mechanisms
> f. Support systems
3. Assess child's level of development (see Appendix B).

NURSING DIAGNOSES

- Injury, Risk for
- Fluid volume, Excess
- Pain
- Nutrition: less than body requirements, Imbalanced
- Anxiety
- Activity intolerance, Risk for
- Therapeutic regimen management, Ineffective
- Coping, Ineffective
- Coping, Compromised family

NURSING INTERVENTIONS
Diagnosis and Staging Phase

1. Provide preprocedural education to child and family (see the Preparation for Procedures or Surgery section in Appendix J).
2. Prepare child for diagnostic procedures with age-appropriate approach (see the Preparation for Procedures or Surgery section in Appendix J).
3. Observe for signs and symptoms of systems involvement.
   a. Respiratory distress
   b. Superior vena cava syndrome
   c. CNS changes
4. Refer to child life specialist as appropriate for preprocedural preparation.
5. Assist and support child in collection of laboratory specimens.
6. Provide anticipatory guidance and family crisis intervention.

Treatment Phase

1. Monitor cardiorespiratory status.
2. Prepare for treatment-induced emergencies.
   a. Metabolic crises
   b. Hematologic crises
   c. Space-occupying tumors

3. Administer chemotherapeutic agents (see the Medical Management section in this chapter).
4. Assess for signs of extravasation.
   a. Cell lysis
   b. Tissue sloughing
5. Minimize side effects of chemotherapy.
   a. Bone marrow suppression
   b. Nausea and vomiting
   c. Anorexia and weight loss
   d. Oral mucositis
   e. Pain
6. Monitor for signs and symptoms of infection.
7. Monitor for signs and symptoms of relapse.
   a. CNS changes
   b. Infection
   c. Tumor recurrence
   d. Leukemic conversion
8. Provide ongoing emotional support to child and family (see the Preparation for Procedures or Surgery section in Appendix J).
9. Refer to child life specialist for continued coping strategies.
10. Provide ongoing education about treatment and medications.
11. Refer family to social services for support and resource utilization.
12. Monitor for tumor lysis syndrome.

🔺 Discharge Planning and Home Care

Instruct child and parents about home care management.
1. Signs of infection and when to seek medical attention
2. Care of child's central venous access device, including site care, dressing change, flushing, and emergency care
3. Medication administration (provide written information)
4. Importance of compliance with treatment and medical procedures

5. Proper nutrition for optimal weight gain and health maintenance
6. School attendance and/or activity restrictions
7. Signs and symptoms of relapse
8. Potential behavioral changes in child and/or siblings
9. Access to support services, such as parent support groups (see Supportive Care section in Appendix J and Appendixes K and L)

CLIENT OUTCOMES

1. Child and family will demonstrate ability to cope with life-threatening illness.
2. Child will be free of infection.
3. Child and family will understand home care and long-term follow-up needs.

REFERENCES

Foley G et al, editors: *Nursing care of the child with cancer,* ed 2, Philadelphia, 1993, WB Saunders.

Parker BR: Leukemia and lymphoma in childhood, *Radiol Clin North Am* 35(6):1495, 1997.

Shad A, Magrath I: Non-Hodgkin's lymphoma, *Pediatr Clin North Am* 44(4):863, 1997.

Young G et al: Recognition of common childhood malignancies, *Am Fam Physician* 61(7):2144, 2000.

61

❖

Osteogenic Sarcoma and Amputation

❖

PATHOPHYSIOLOGY

Osteogenic sarcoma is a tumor found in the diaphysis of a long bone (femur, radius, ulna, proximal humerus, or ilium). It also can affect the flat bones, which include the head, pelvis, and spine. The most common sites of occurrence are the femur and the knee, followed in order by the tibia, humerus, pelvis, jaw, fibula, and ribs. The clinical course takes the following sequence: (1) the normal bone is destroyed and is replaced by tumor cells, which results in osteoid tissue and bone; (2) growth penetrates the cortex and extends beyond it (radiating spindles of bone are characteristic of this process); and (3) the tumor extends through the bone marrow cavity. Metastasis occurs through veins and involves the lungs first.

INCIDENCE

1. Osteogenic sarcoma is the most common bone tumor in children. It is the third most common malignancy in children and accounts for approximately 5% of neoplasms in children.
2. It occurs most commonly during the adolescent growth period and in young adulthood.
3. It is uncommon before age 10 years.
4. Age range of peak incidence is 10 to 15 years.
5. More males than females are affected.
6. Sixty percent to 80% of those with nonmetastatic osteogenic sarcoma will be long-term survivors after treatment with surgery and chemotherapy.

CLINICAL MANIFESTATIONS

Symptoms are gradual in onset. The child may have symptoms for 6 to 9 months before treatment is sought. Children often present with a history of a minor injury while participating in sports. The symptoms are as follows:

1. Local pain during activity and more severe pain with passage of time (most common symptom)
2. Limping or gait variation
3. Limitation of joint motion
4. Joint tenderness
5. Local edema

COMPLICATIONS

Pathologic fractures occur with larger lesions and many times are the symptoms seen initially.

LABORATORY AND DIAGNOSTIC TESTS

1. Serum alkaline phosphatase levels—to confirm diagnosis; elevated because of osteoid production
2. Tissue biopsy—reveals presence of malignant cells
3. Anteroposterior lateral radiographic studies—to detect presence of soft tissue mass associated with destructive bone lesion, and calcification
4. Skeletal bone scan—to detect presence of metastatic bone lesions
5. Computed tomography and magnetic resonance imaging—to determine extent of disease and metastasis

MEDICAL AND SURGICAL MANAGEMENT

An important component of treatment of osteogenic sarcoma is surgery. Osteogenic sarcoma is resistant to radiation therapy; therefore, the most important prognostic factor is the ability of the physician to resect the tumor. Type of surgery is determined by the age of the child and tumor size and location. It may be either an amputation or a limb salvage. Because of the availability of new chemotherapy regimens, amputation is no longer the surgery of choice. Both procedures are performed to excise the tumor and obtain a biopsy specimen for diagnosis.

Complications of amputation are the following:

1. Reactive hyperemia—reddened skin, particularly at pressure points; subsides as keratoma layer forms
2. Contact dermatitis—most often caused by contact with prosthetic materials (e.g., polyester resins, chrome)
3. Infections—including fungal and pyogenic infections (e.g., furuncles)
4. Epidermal cysts—evident at points of friction at or near brim of socket; most often caused by ill-fitting prosthesis
5. Stump edema syndrome—consisting of worsening reactive hyperemia, which results in oozing and capillary rupture
6. Terminal bone overgrowth
7. Bony spurs—developing at corners or margins of amputation as a result of periosteal irritation
8. Neuroma
9. Phantom limb—feelings of pain and sensation in the amputated limb
10. Stump scarring—caused by inguinal weight bearing and increased shearing force at stump-socket interface

After surgery, chemotherapy is given. The chemotherapy regimens contain various combinations of the following: methotrexate, doxorubicin, bleomycin, cyclophosphamide, cisplatin, and ifosfamide. When methotrexate is given, leucovorin calcium is given to reverse the action of the methotrexate and decrease its toxicity. Leucovorin calcium is given after the infusion of methotrexate. The dosage of leucovorin calcium is equivalent to the amount of methotrexate administered. Allopurinol is also given with chemotherapy to decrease the level of uric acid, which is a by-product of chemotherapy.

When a limb salvage procedure is to be performed, chemotherapy may be given prior to surgery in an attempt to promote the success of the surgery by decreasing the tumor size preoperatively. Chemotherapy may also be given postoperatively to ensure complete tumor destruction.

NURSING ASSESSMENT

1. Assess child's and family's emotional response to upcoming surgery and need for information.
2. Postoperatively, assess for impending signs and symptoms of complications, such as signs of infection and swelling at stump or surgical site.
3. Assess for wound drainage and signs and symptoms of infection.
4. Assess child's response to chemotherapy.
5. Assess continuously child's and family's coping.
6. Assess child's and family's ability to manage home treatment regimen.
7. Assess child's and family's use of community resources.

NURSING DIAGNOSES

- Infection, Risk for
- Tissue integrity, Impaired
- Mobility, Impaired physical
- Injury, Risk for
- Pain
- Body image, Disturbed
- Fluid volume, Excess
- Therapeutic regimen management, Ineffective
- Coping, Ineffective
- Family processes, Interrupted
- Growth and development, Delayed
- Caregiver role strain, Risk for

NURSING INTERVENTIONS
Preoperative Care

1. Prepare operative site according to hospital procedure.
2. Encourage use of exercises to strengthen muscles.
3. Provide emotional support to child and parents.
   a. Provide active listening to concerns.
   b. Encourage expression of feelings of loss.
   c. Provide anticipatory information about emotional responses to surgery.

4. Provide preoperative information to decrease anxiety about unknown aspects (see the Preparation for Procedures or Surgery section in Appendix J).
5. Prepare child before laboratory and diagnostic testing.
   a. Complete blood count (CBC) (see the Preparation for Procedures or Surgery section in Appendix J)
   b. Urinalysis
   c. Bone scan
   d. Radiographic studies
   e. Type and cross-match of blood

Postoperative Care

1. Monitor for signs of complications and report immediately (see the Complications section in this chapter).
2. Observe and monitor for signs of hemorrhage every hour for 24 hours, then every 4 hours.
3. Promote patency and healing of surgical site (after amputation).
   a. Apply pressure dressing (figure eight) to stump.
   b. Institute range-of-motion exercises according to physical therapist's orders.
   c. Reinforce exercise program with physical therapist.
   d. Cleanse stump and socket every day with soap and water; dry thoroughly.
   e. Avoid use of skin lotions (can cause maculation and superficial infection).
4. Position child correctly to prevent deformities (after amputation).
   a. Trendelenburg's position
   b. Pillow beneath knee for 24 hours to decrease edema
   c. After 24 hours, no pillow beneath knee (causes flexion of knee)
   d. Prone position for several hours every day (to prevent hip flexion and contracture)
   e. No external rotation or abduction of limb to be amputated
5. Monitor for pain; administer pain medication (refer to Appendix H).

6. Promote use of and adaptation to prosthetic device (after amputation).
   a. Perform prosthetic fitting immediately after surgery because this promotes stump maturation, early ambulation, and resumption of normal activities.
   b. Encourage expression of feelings about having a disability.
   c. Explain restrictions on activities.
7. Monitor administration of chemotherapy.
   a. Provide adequate hydration (hydrate 12 hours before infusion of chemotherapy).
   b. Record intake and output hourly.
   c. Measure specific gravity to assess hydration.
   d. Monitor urine pH and Hematest results (majority of medication is excreted in urine in the first 24 hours); urine needs to be alkaline or its precipitates in kidney will cause tubular necrosis.
   e. Assist with collection of specimens for blood chemistry analysis, CBC, and platelet count.
   f. Assist with collection of urine for urinalysis.
8. Monitor for child's or adolescent's untoward and therapeutic responses to chemotherapy.
   a. Oral and gastrointestinal tract ulcerations
   b. Diarrhea
   c. Ulcerative stomatitis (hemorrhagic enteritis and death can occur)
   d. Skin reactions—urticaria, rashes
   e. Cystitis—inflammation of urinary tract
   f. Nausea and vomiting
9. Minimize negative consequences of chemotherapy.
   a. Provide good mouth care.
   b. Urge child or adolescent to stop smoking.
   c. Advise child or adolescent to stay out of sun (methotrexate can cause skin blotches).
   d. Push fluids.
   e. Administer antiemetics.
   f. Provide bland, soft diet.
   g. Elevate head of bed.
   h. Teach self-hypnosis and relaxation techniques.

10. Monitor for complications.
    a. Pneumothorax (symptoms: shortness of breath, dyspnea, chest pain)
    b. Depression of hematologic values 10 days after methotrexate administration
    c. Renal toxicity—dysuria, oliguria (monitor intake and output)
11. Provide emotional support to parents and child (see the Preparation for Procedures or Surgery section in Appendix J).

🏠 Discharge Planning and Home Care
Chemotherapy Regimen

1. Instruct parents and child/adolescent about home care management.
   a. Take leucovorin calcium on time (wake up child if necessary).
   b. Take antiemetic for nausea and vomiting.
   c. Drink increased amount of fluids (2 qt per day); milk tends to increase mucous secretions.
   d. Check urine for pH.
   e. Stay out of sun.
2. Refer to community resources for follow-up (see Appendix L).

Postoperative Care

1. Instruct child and parents about stump care or surgical site care.
2. Provide reinforcement information about physical therapy regimen.
3. Refer to school nurse and clinic and advise them about child's status (refer to the Special Education section in Appendix L).
4. Explore compliance potential by asking about following items:
   a. Means of transportation
   b. Resources for child care
   c. Finances
   d. Level of motivation

e. Understanding of need for long-term follow-up every 3 to 4 months until growth is complete

CLIENT OUTCOMES

1. Child will achieve remission.
2. Side effects of chemotherapy experienced by child will be minimized.
3. Child and family will adhere to home treatment regimen and outpatient physical therapy regimen as prescribed.

REFERENCES

Alcoser P, Rodgers C: Treatment strategies in childhood cancer, *J Pediatr Nurs* 18(2):103, 2003.

Bryant R: Managing side effects of childhood cancer treatment, *J Pediatr Nurs* 18(2):113, 2003.

Foley GV et al, editors: *Nursing care of the child with cancer,* ed 2, Philadelphia, 1993, WB Saunders.

Hudson M et al: Patient satisfaction after limb-sparing surgery and amputation for pediatric malignant bone tumors, *J Pediatr Oncol Nurs* 15(2):60, 1998.

Papagelopoulos PJ et al: Current concepts in the evaluation and treatment of osteosarcoma, *Orthopedics* 23(8):858, 2000.

Wittig JC et al: Osteosarcoma: a multidisciplinary approach to diagnosis and treatment, *Am Fam Physician* 65(6):1123, 2002.

62

❖

Osteomyelitis

❖

PATHOPHYSIOLOGY

Osteomyelitis is an infection of the bone that can occur in any bone in the body. The most common locations are the femur and the tibia. The humerus and the hip are rarely affected. The skull is a common location in infants. Usually a predisposing condition such as poor nutrition or poor hygiene exists.

Bacterial emboli reach the small arteries in the metaphysis, where circulation is sluggish. An abscess forms and replaces bone, causing increased pressure and secondary necrosis. This abscess eventually can rupture into the subperiosteal space. The infection spreads beneath the periosteum, thrombosing vessels and causing increased necrosis. The cycle of impaired circulation is thus established. A sinus can form and extend the infection to the skin. Extension to a joint results in septic arthritis. The condition can become chronic and thus quite resistant to therapy, often requiring involved surgical intervention. The epiphysis is usually spared because it has a separate circulation.

Any organism is capable of causing osteomyelitis, either by the direct *(exogenous)* route or by seeding through the blood-stream from an infection elsewhere *(hematogenous* route*)*. Exogenous sources include contamination from penetrating wounds, open fractures, or surgical wounds, or secondary extension through an abscess, burn, or wound. The hematogenous route is more common; sources include furuncles, skin abrasions, upper respiratory tract infections, otitis media, abscessed teeth, and pyelonephritis. The hematogenous form is often subacute because the preceding infection is frequently treated with antibiotics.

437

INCIDENCE

1. The highest incidence of osteomyelitis is found in 5- to 14-year-olds.
2. Osteomyelitis is twice as common in males as in females.

CLINICAL MANIFESTATIONS

1. Pain of abrupt onset—point tenderness above bone and swelling and warmth over bone
2. Fever
3. Possible dehydration
4. Unwillingness to move limb or bear weight
5. Holding of extremity in semiflexed position (muscle spasm)
6. Irritability
7. Poor appetite
8. Local signs of inflammation and infection (warmth, erythema, drainage, decreased range of motion)
9. Lethargy

COMPLICATIONS

Pathologic fractures occur as complications of osteomyelitis.

LABORATORY AND DIAGNOSTIC TESTS

1. Complete blood count—marked leukocytosis, indicates presence of infection
2. Erythrocyte sedimentation rate—elevated, indicates presence of infection
3. Blood culture and sensitivity test—positive culture in 50% of cases; common causative organisms vary with age and other factors; determine causative organism and preferred antibiotic
   a. All ages—staphylococci, primarily *Staphylococcus aureus*
   b. Young children—*Haemophilus influenzae*
   c. Neonates—coliforms *(Escherichia coli)*
   d. Sickle cell anemia—*Salmonella* organisms
   e. Foot—*Pseudomonas* organisms
4. Radiographic studies—negative first 10 to 12 days until bone destruction occurs (soft tissue swelling is evident early)

5. Computed tomography or magnetic resonance imaging— shows bone involvement
6. Bone scan—often positive early for inflammation
7. Direct needle aspiration/biopsy—confirms diagnosis and provides site specimen for culture (best method for diagnosis)

MEDICAL AND SURGICAL MANAGEMENT

Intravenous antibiotics are begun after blood has been drawn for culture. Antibiotics are administered for a minimum of 4 weeks and usually are administered for 6 weeks, depending on duration of symptoms, response to treatment, and sensitivity of the organism. Intravenous antibiotics may be administered on an outpatient basis or at home, or the child may be given oral antibiotics to complete the course at home to decrease costs. The type of antibiotic used to treat osteomyelitis depends on the results of culture and sensitivity testing. Bed rest may be prescribed, and the affected extremity is usually immobilized with a cast or splint. Surgery may be performed to drain the area and remove necrotic bone. During surgery, polyethylene tubes are placed in the bone—one for instilling an antibiotic solution (usually the upper tube) and the other for drainage. Local débridement may be performed to remove the source of infection and cleanse the area.

NURSING ASSESSMENT

1. See the Musculoskeletal Assessment section in Appendix A.
2. Assess pain—location, duration, intensity, description (refer to Appendix H).
3. Assess nutritional status—usually, poor appetite; assess adequacy of caloric intake, as well as intake of protein and fluids.

NURSING DIAGNOSES

- Infection, Risk for
- Hyperthermia
- Pain
- Tissue perfusion, Ineffective
- Therapeutic regimen management, Ineffective
- Nutrition: less than body requirements, Imbalanced

NURSING INTERVENTIONS

1. Immobilize extremity to facilitate healing and prevent complications.
   a. Apply splint, bivalved cast, or complete cast with window.
   b. Allow no weight bearing (high risk of pathologic fracture).
      i. Use gurney or wheelchair; elevate extremity slightly.
      ii. Use active range-of-motion exercises on unaffected extremity after inflammation subsides.
2. Provide pain relief measures (see Appendix H).
   a. Allow comfortable position.
   b. Support affected limb on pillows.
   c. Use care in turning and moving child.
   d. Monitor child's response to analgesia and sedation as necessary.
3. Use contact precautions if any drainage occurs.
   a. Refer to institutional procedures manual for isolation techniques.
4. Monitor child's response to antibiotic irrigation of site (up to 6 weeks).
   a. For first 3 days, expect blood, debris, and pus (have tendency to clog tubes).
      i. Reversing flow direction of tubes at intervals can prevent blockage; do so with physician consultation only.
      ii. Physician may elect to irrigate with heparin and saline solution if blockage occurs.
      iii. Use prescribed suction (usually low suction).
   b. If tubes are functioning properly, wound and dressing should remain dry.
   c. Maintain records of instillation and output (clarity, color, and volume of drainage); often up to 1000 ml/day is instilled.
   d. When tubes are removed, usually instillation tube (upper) is removed first, with drainage tube left until no further drainage occurs.
   e. Sudden pain at site of irrigation may indicate blockage of drainage tube.

5. Monitor child's response to medications.
   a. Antibiotics
   b. Antipyretics
   c. Sedatives
   d. Antihistamines
6. Provide cast care.
   a. Monitor skin temperature; casting creates concern for thermoregulation in young infants and children.
   b. Monitor color, heat, sweating, tenderness, capillary refill, and motion of digits.
   c. Keep cast clean and dry.
   d. Perform child/family teaching (place nothing inside cast).
   e. Consult physician regarding use of diphenhydramine (Benadryl) for itching.
7. Promote adequate nutritional intake.
   a. Promote high-caloric intake (juices, gelatin, Popsicles).
   b. Appetite usually returns when acute symptoms subside.
8. Monitor for signs of infection and alterations in thermoregulation.
   a. Increased temperature (institute cooling measures)
   b. Signs of inflammation
   c. Drainage or musty odor with cast
9. Provide age-appropriate diversional activities (see the relevant section in Appendix B).
10. Provide emotional support to parents (see the Supportive Care section in Appendix J).

🔺 Discharge Planning and Home Care

1. Instruct parents about elements of rehabilitation (see Appendix K).
   a. Risk of fracture
   b. Necessity for hospitalization
   c. Necessity for operations

2. Instruct parents about administration of antibiotics. Home referral may be made (e.g., percutaneous intravenous central catheter lines may be inserted).
   a. Therapeutic responses
   b. Side effects—because many antibiotics used have negative renal, audiologic, and hepatic effects, these systems must be monitored closely during therapy (intravenous medication may be prescribed if treatment is longer than 3 weeks)

CLIENT OUTCOMES

1. Child will be free of infection.
2. Child will be free of disease complications.
3. Child and family will learn to cope effectively with home treatment regimen.

REFERENCES

Branom RN: Is this wound infected? *Crit Care Nurs Q* 25(1):55, 2002.

Carek P et al: Diagnosis and management of osteomyelitis, *Am Fam Physician* 63(12):2413, 2001.

Chou KJ: Case of the month. Leg pain in a 26-day-old girl, *Emerg Off Pediatr* 10(6):188, 1997.

Morrissy RT, editor: *Lovell and Winter's pediatric orthopaedics,* ed 4, Philadelphia, 1996, JB Lippincott.

63

❖

Otitis Media

❖

PATHOPHYSIOLOGY

Otitis media is an inflammation of the middle ear. Children 6 years of age and younger are at particular risk for otitis media because their eustachian tubes are shorter and more horizontal, and lack the cartilaginous support found in older children and adults. This allows the eustachian tubes to collapse, which causes negative pressure in the middle ear. In turn, there is impaired drainage of middle ear fluid and possible reflux of pharyngeal secretions into this normally sterile area. The eustachian tubes of infants and children with cleft palate or Down syndrome are also wider, so they remain open; this allows bacteria to travel easily from the nasopharynx into the middle ear and thus further predisposes such children to infection. Otitis media is the most frequently encountered condition in office visits of children under the age of 15 years in the United States. Among childhood diseases, it is second in prevalence only to the common cold, accounting for one in three pediatric sick visits in this country. Two types of otitis media are common in clinical pediatrics: acute otitis media and otitis media with effusion.

Acute Otitis Media

Acute otitis media is characterized by fluid in the middle ear with signs and symptoms of ear infection (bulging eardrum usually accompanied by pain; or perforated eardrum, often with drainage of purulent matter). The pathogens most commonly associated with otitis media include *Streptococcus pneumoniae* (25% to 50% of cases), *Haemophilus influenzae* (15% to 30% of cases), *Moraxella catarrhalis* (3% to 20% of cases), viruses, and certain anaerobes. In the neonate, gram-negative enteric organisms or *Staphylococcus aureus* may also be the causative organisms. Group A *Streptococcus* and *S. aureus* (2% to 3% combined) were less common causes of acute otitis media in the pediatric population during the 1990s. *Chlamydia pneumoniae* infections may also be seen, most frequently in children aged 8 to 16 months.

Otitis Media with Effusion

Otitis media with effusion is characterized by fluid in the middle ear without signs and symptoms of ear infection. No definitive causative agent has been identified, although otitis media with effusion is seen more commonly in children with allergies or viral upper respiratory infections, and in those recovering from acute otitis media.

INCIDENCE

1. Otitis media occurs most often in children between 3 months and 3 years of age; age ranges of peak incidence are 5 to 24 months and 4 to 6 years.
2. Seventy percent of affected children have one episode by age 3 years, with one third having more than three episodes. The younger the child at the time of the first infection, the greater the chance of recurrent infections.
3. Boys have more ear infections than girls.
4. Children are more likely to experience repeated episodes if a parent and/or sibling also had ear infections.
5. Children with craniofacial conditions such as a cleft lip/palate and Down syndrome are also at greater risk. Fifty percent of children with cleft palate have chronic otitis media before surgical correction.
6. Children placed in large group day care settings from an early age have greater exposure to all causative bacteria and viruses from other children.
7. Exposure to an area with high pollution and/or allergens and to winter or spring weather conditions presents risk and increases the incidence of ear infections.
8. Children exposed to passive (second-hand) cigarette smoke have a significantly higher rate of otitis media.

9. Infants who are bottle-fed, especially while lying down, experience more ear infections than breast-fed infants.

CLINICAL MANIFESTATIONS
Acute Otitis Media

1. Red tympanic membrane, often bulging with no visible bony landmarks, immobile to pneumatic otoscopy (application of positive or negative pressure pulse to middle ear using bulb insufflator attachment on otoscope)
2. Complaint of ear pain (otalgia), or fussiness and ear pulling in preverbal child
3. Fever, ranging from 100° to 104° F (present in about one half of children)
4. Anorexia (common)
5. Anterior cervical lymphadenopathy
6. Transient conductive hearing loss lasting at least 2 to 4 weeks after acute infection

Otitis Media with Effusion

1. Dull yellow to gray tympanic membrane, often retracted with poor mobility on pneumatic otoscopy
2. Feeling of fullness or itch deep in ear
3. Mild to moderate conductive hearing loss for duration of effusion

COMPLICATIONS
Common

1. Tympanic membrane rupture with otorrhea
2. Short-term conductive hearing loss

Unusual

1. Long-term or permanent hearing loss
2. Meningitis
3. Labyrinthitis
4. Mastoiditis
5. Brain abscess
6. Acquired cholesteatoma (filling of sac in middle ear with epithelium or keratin)

LABORATORY AND DIAGNOSTIC TESTS

1. Pneumatic otoscopy—to visualize tympanic membrane and test tympanic membrane mobility
2. Tympanogram—to measure tympanic membrane compliance and stiffness
3. Culture and sensitivity testing—only available if tympanocentesis (needle aspiration of middle ear via tympanic membrane) is performed
4. Hearing evaluation—recommended for child who has had bilateral otitis media with effusion 3 months or longer

MEDICAL MANAGEMENT

The efficacy of therapy with steroids, decongestants, and antihistamines in the resolution of otitis media has not been proved. Their use should not be encouraged. Tonsillectomy and/or adenoidectomy are not recommended for the treatment of otitis media with effusion in the absence of specific tonsil/adenoid pathology.

The first-line antibiotic medication most often prescribed is amoxicillin/ampicillin, given in a 10-day course for children younger than 2 years of age. A shorter course may be considered for older children and those with mild disease. The second-line medication regimen (to be used when an amoxicillin-resistant organism is suspected) includes amoxicillin with clavulanate (Augmentin, a second-generation cephalosporin), cefaclor, or co-trimoxazole. In the penicillin-allergic child, azithromycin may be used.

Myringotomy is a surgical procedure in which pressure-equalizing tubes are inserted into the tympanic membrane. This allows ventilation of the middle ear, relieves the negative pressure, and permits drainage of fluid. The tubes usually fall out after 6 to 12 months. Complications that may result include atrophy of the tympanic membrane, tympanosclerosis (scarring of the tympanic membrane), chronic perforation, and cholesteatoma.

Initial Management

1. Observation *or* antibiotic therapy (optional at this time): In most cases, otitis media with effusion resolves spontaneously within 3 months.

2. Environmental risk factor control (optional): Parents should be encouraged to avoid exposing their children to passive smoking.
3. Myringotomy is *not* recommended for initial management of otitis media with effusion in an otherwise healthy child.

Management After 3 Months

If the child has *hearing in the normal range,* as indicated by a hearing threshold level of better than 20 dB in the better-hearing ear, the following are recommended:

1. Observation *or* antibiotic therapy (remains optional at this time): In most cases, otitis media with effusion resolves spontaneously.
2. Environmental risk factor control (optional): Parents should be encouraged to avoid exposing their children to passive smoking.

If the child has *bilateral hearing deficits* of 20 dB hearing threshold level or worse, the following are recommended:

1. Antibiotic therapy *or* bilateral myringotomy with tympanostomy tubes: Either one or both may be chosen to manage bilateral otitis media with effusion that has lasted a total of 3 months in an otherwise healthy child aged 1 to 3 years who has a bilateral hearing deficit.
2. Environmental risk factor control (optional): Parents should be encouraged to avoid exposing their children to passive smoking.

Management After 4 to 6 months

1. Bilateral myringotomy with tympanostomy tubes is recommended to manage bilateral otitis media with effusion that has lasted a total of 4 to 6 months in an otherwise healthy child aged 1 to 3 years who has a bilateral hearing deficit.
2. Environmental risk factor control (optional): Parents should be encouraged to avoid exposing their children to passive smoking.

NURSING ASSESSMENT

1. Assess for verbal and nonverbal pain behaviors.
2. Assess for elevated temperature (100° to 104° F).

3. Assess for enlarged lymph glands in neck area.
4. Assess nutritional status and adequacy of caloric fluid intake.
5. Assess for hearing loss.
6. Assess for speech loss/development.

NURSING DIAGNOSES

- Pain
- Comfort, Impaired
- Sensory perception, Disturbed
- Communication, Impaired verbal

NURSING INTERVENTIONS

Acute Otitis Media

1. Treat and instruct family to treat child with analgesics and/or antipyretics as needed for symptoms.
   a. Fever
   b. Ear pain
2. Offer small amounts of fluids frequently with cup or spoon if breast or bottle is refused, because sucking may cause increased ear pain in younger child.
   a. Nonnutritive (pacifier) sucking may be source of comfort to equalize pressure and/or relieve ear "popping" (chewing sugar-free gum may have same desired effect for older child).
   b. Caution parents against bottle-feeding child while child is lying down.
3. Be aware that increased fluid intake is vital to any child with fever or illness to prevent dehydration and promote healing.
4. Instruct family about safe and effective use of prescribed antibiotic.
5. Monitor and instruct family to observe for (and report) common allergic or adverse reactions to antibiotic therapy (e.g., diarrhea, nausea/vomiting, skin rash/urticaria). Serious dermatologic, hematologic, renal, hepatic, neurologic, endocrine, and/or cardiorespiratory reactions are *rare*.

6. Monitor and instruct family to observe for signs of complications with acute otitis.
   a. Ear drainage
   b. No improvement of signs and symptoms with treatment, especially after 48 hours of appropriate antibiotic therapy
   c. Stiff neck, severe fussiness and irritability (meningitis), dizziness with clumsiness or falling (labyrinthitis)

Otitis Media with Effusion

1. Educate family about course of disease and lack of definitive cause and treatment.
2. Support child and family if conductive hearing loss is present; reassure them that this is likely to resolve spontaneously.
3. If myringotomy is required, supply age-appropriate explanations of procedure to child and parents (see Appendix J).

Postoperative Care

Monitor child's response to surgical intervention (myringotomy with insertion of tympanostomy tubes).

1. Vital signs (increased temperature indicates infection)
2. Otorrhea from ears
3. Presence of bleeding
4. Pain (provide comfort measures and pain medications as needed—see Appendix H)
5. Hearing status
6. Speech development

Discharge Planning and Home Care

1. Instruct child and parents about maintaining patency of tympanostomy (e.g., when child is swimming or bathing, use ear plugs).
2. Instruct about limiting child's activities until fully recovered.
   a. Avoid rigorous activities.

    b. Provide frequent rest periods.

    c. Allow return to school after child receives medical approval.

3. Educate about importance of avoiding exposure of children to passive cigarette smoke; if household members or child care providers are unable to quit smoking, smoking should be done outdoors, away from child.

CLIENT OUTCOMES

1. Child will be free of pain as demonstrated by verbal and nonverbal behaviors.
2. Child's activity level and appetite will return to normal.
3. Child will demonstrate no hearing loss.
4. Child will demonstrate no speech delay.

REFERENCES

Asch-Goodkin J: Acute otitis media: what the evidence says, *Contemp Pediatr* 19 (suppl):4, 2002.

Takata GS et al: Evidence assessment of management of acute otitis media: I. The role of antibiotics in treatment of uncomplicated acute otitis media, *Pediatrics* 108(2):239, 2001.

US Department of Health and Human Services: Clinical practice guideline, otitis media with effusion in young children, AHCPR Pub No 94-0622, Washington, DC, 1994, US Government Printing Office.

US Department of Health and Human Services: Managing otitis media with effusion in young children, clinical practice guideline, quick reference guide for clinicians, No 12, AHCPR Pub No 94-0623, Washington, DC, 1994, US Government Printing Office.

US Department of Health and Human Services: Otitis media with effusion, middle ear fluid in children: parent guide, clinical practice guideline, No. 12, AHCPR Pub No 94-0624, consumer version, Washington, DC, 1994, US Government Printing Office.

RESOURCES

Agency for Healthcare Research and Quality (AHRQ) Publications Clearinghouse

P.O. Box 8547

Silver Spring, MD 20907-8547

Website: http://www.ahcpr.gov

Phone: 800-358-9295

Toll-free TDD service (hearing impaired only): 888-586-6340

American Academy of Pediatrics: http://www.aap.org

American Medical Association and Nemours Foundation: Childhood infections: otitis media, Kidshealth website, available at http://www.kidshealth.org, accessed June 10, 2003.

64

❖

Patent Ductus Arteriosus

❖

PATHOPHYSIOLOGY

Patent ductus arteriosus (PDA) is the persistent patency of the ductus arteriosus after birth, which results in the shunting of blood directly from the aorta (higher pressure) into the pulmonary artery (lower pressure). This left-to-right shunting causes the recirculation of increased amounts of oxygenated blood in the lungs, which raises demands on the left side of the heart. The additional effort required of the left ventricle to meet this increased demand leads to progressive dilation and left atrial hypertension. The cumulative cardiac effects cause increased pressure in the pulmonary veins and capillaries, which results in pulmonary edema. The pulmonary edema leads to decreased diffusion of oxygen and hypoxia, with progressive constriction of the arterioles in the lungs. Pulmonary hypertension and failure of the right side of the heart ensue if the condition is not corrected through medical or surgical treatment. Most PDAs are a left-to-right shunting of blood, but right-to-left ductal shunting may occur with associated pulmonary disease, left heart obstructive lesions, and coarctation of the aorta. Closure of the PDA depends primarily on the constrictor response of the ductus to the oxygen tension in the blood. Other factors affecting ductus closure include the action of prostaglandins, pulmonary and systemic vascular resistances, the size of the ductus, and the condition of the infant (premature or full term). PDA occurs more frequently in premature infants; it is also less well tolerated in these infants because their cardiac compensatory mechanisms are not as well developed and left-to-right shunts tend to be larger.

INCIDENCE

1. Precise incidence varies depending on gestational age.
2. Approximately 15% of infants with PDAs have additional cardiac defects (coarctation of the aorta, ventricular septal defect, aortic stenosis).
3. Incidence in full-term infants is 1 in 2500 to 5000 live births.
4. Overall incidence in premature infants is 20% to 75%.
5. PDA is present in 60% to 70% of infants with congenital rubella infection.
6. PDA occurs three times more often in girls than in boys.

CLINICAL MANIFESTATIONS

Manifestations of PDA in premature infants are often clouded by other problems associated with prematurity (e.g., respiratory distress syndrome). Signs of ventricular overload are not apparent for 4 to 6 hours after birth. Infants with small PDAs may be asymptomatic; infants with large PDAs may manifest signs of congestive heart failure (CHF):

1. Persistent murmur (systolic, then continuous; heard best at left upper sternal border)
2. Tachycardia (apical pulse higher than 170 beats/min)
3. Prominent to bounding pulses
4. Hyperactive precordium (result of increased left ventricular stroke volume)
5. Tachypnea (respiratory rate higher than 70 breaths/min)
6. Wide pulse pressure (higher than 25 mm Hg)
7. Increased ventricular requirement (associated with pulmonary problems)
8. Metabolic acidosis (may not be present)

COMPLICATIONS

1. Hepatomegaly (rare in premature infants)
2. Necrotizing enterocolitis
3. Concurrent pulmonary disorder (e.g., respiratory distress syndrome or bronchopulmonary dysplasia)
4. Gastrointestinal (GI) hemorrhage (decreased platelet count)
5. Hyperkalemia (decreased urinary output)

6. Arrhythmias (digitalis toxicity)
7. Failure to thrive

LABORATORY AND DIAGNOSTIC TESTS

1. Chest radiographic study—prominent or enlarged left atrium and left ventricle (cardiomegaly); increased pulmonary vascular markings
2. Echocardiography—left atrial to aortic root ratio greater than 1.3:1 in full-term infants or greater than 1.0 in preterm infants (caused by increased left atrial volume as a result of left-to-right shunt)
3. Doppler color flow mapping—used to evaluate blood flow and its direction
4. Electrocardiography (ECG)—findings vary with degree of severity: no abnormality noted with small PDA; left ventricular hypertrophy with large PDA
5. Cardiac catheterization—performed only when further evaluation of confusing echocardiographic or Doppler findings is needed or when additional defects are suspected to be present

MEDICAL MANAGEMENT

Interrupting the left-to-right flow of blood is the goal of management for the uncomplicated PDA. When the shunt is hemodynamically significant, conservative measures may be tried initially. Conservative management consists of fluid restriction and medications. Furosemide (Lasix) is used along with fluid restriction to promote diuresis and minimize the effects of cardiovascular overload. Fluid restriction alone is unlikely to cause PDA closure and in combination with diuretics may lead to electrolyte abnormalities and dehydration as well as caloric deprivation, which impairs growth.

Indomethacin (Indocin) may be used if fluid management and diuretics fail to significantly decrease the left-to-right ductal shunting. Indomethacin, a prostaglandin inhibitor, promotes closure of the ductus. It works best in newborns younger than 13 days old and is not effective after 4 to 6 weeks of life. Its side effects include transitory changes in renal function, increased incidence of occult blood loss via the GI tract, and inhibition of platelet function for 7 to 9 days. Prophylactic administration of indomethacin soon after birth in very premature infants has also been advocated to decrease the incidence of PDA, intraventricular hemorrhage, and mortality. Uncertainty exists about routine early prophylactic use of indomethacin, however, because of the possible negative effects of the drug on neonatal vasoregulation and cerebral blood flow. Contraindications for the use of indomethacin are as follows:

1. Blood urea nitrogen (BUN) levels higher than 30 mg/dl
2. Creatinine levels higher than 1.8 mg/dl
3. Urine output of less than 0.6 ml/kg/hr over the preceding 8 hours
4. Platelet count lower than 60,000/mm³, because it prolongs platelet activity
5. Stool Hematest results higher than 3+ (or moderate to large) because GI bleeding has been reported
6. Clinical or radiographic evidence of necrotizing enterocolitis
7. Evidence of enlarging central nervous system hemorrhage
8. Sepsis, proven or strongly suspected

The ductus reopens in 30% of those treated with indomethacin but may close in response to a second course of treatment.

The use of digitalis is controversial and is contraindicated in premature infants. Digitalis increases the force of contraction of the heart, increases the stroke volume and cardiac output, and decreases cardiac venous pressures. It is used to treat CHF and selected cardiac arrhythmias.

Medical management also includes prophylactic administration of antibiotics to prevent bacterial endocarditis. In older children, there are no exercise restrictions if no evidence of pulmonary hypertension is present.

Surgical management consists of PDA ligation. Two major groups of children have been identified as requiring this surgery. The first includes infants with CHF, usually premature neonates who did not respond to indomethacin therapy. Children older than 6 months of age whose ductus did not close spontaneously (and who are at risk for pulmonary hypertension and subacute endocarditis) make up the second group.

Both groups require a left thoracotomy incision. Bypass is unnecessary. Infants are usually at greater risk for complications, so the PDA is doubly ligated in a comparatively quick procedure. For older children, surgery is advised during their preschool years and is performed by dividing the ductus between clamps and suturing the ends closed. Coil closure of the PDA to plug the ductus during cardiac catheterization or video-assisted transthoracic endoscopic closure of the PDA can also be performed on infants older than 3 to 6 months of age.

The hemodynamic results of PDA ligation are truly curative, in contrast to the palliative procedures of many heart surgeries. Closure decreases the pulmonary flow while increasing the systemic flow, creating normal hemodynamics. Unfortunately, if severe pulmonary hypertension existed before surgery, closure will not reverse this process.

NURSING ASSESSMENT

1. See the Cardiovascular Assessment and Respiratory Assessment sections in Appendix A.
2. Assess hydration status.
3. Assess child's temperature.
4. Assess postoperative pain.
5. Assess child and family coping strategies.

NURSING DIAGNOSES

- Cardiac output, Decreased
- Tissue perfusion, Ineffective
- Fluid volume, Excess
- Thermoregulation, Ineffective
- Infection, Risk for
- Injury, Risk for
- Family processes, Interrupted

NURSING INTERVENTIONS

1. Monitor cardiac and respiratory status (may need to monitor as often as every hour during acute phase).
2. Observe and report signs of changes in cardiac status (color, vital signs, peripheral perfusion, level of consciousness, activity level, signs of CHF).

3. Observe and report signs of respiratory distress and changes in respiratory status.
4. Monitor and report responses to ventilator assistance.
5. Assess for and maintain optimal hydration status.
   a. Limit intake of fluids (65 to 100 ml/kg/day).
   b. Monitor urinary output.
   c. Observe for signs of fluid overload.
6. Promote and maintain optimal body temperature.
   a. Use radiant warmer.
   b. Keep child covered.
7. Monitor action and side effects of medications.
   a. Diuretics (e.g., furosemide)—decreases fluid overload, increases urinary output
   b. Indomethacin—inhibits prostaglandins, promotes closure of PDA
   c. Digitalis—increases contractility of heart (monitor serum levels)
8. Monitor response to and side effects of blood transfusions.
9. Promote process of attachment between parents and infant.
10. Provide developmentally appropriate stimulation activities (see the relevant section in Appendix B).

Preoperative Care

1. Allow parents to express feelings; despite its being relatively minor heart surgery, PDA repair is still overwhelming to parents.
2. Prepare child for surgery by obtaining assessment data.
   a. Complete blood count, urinalysis, serum glucose level, BUN level
   b. Baseline electrolyte levels
   c. Blood coagulation studies
   d. Type and cross-match of blood
   e. Chest radiographic study, ECG
3. Because older child is usually preschool age, prepare him or her accordingly; do not tell child that surgery will make him or her "feel better," because child is usually asymptomatic.

Postoperative Care

1. Monitor child's or infant's cardiac status (see the Cardiovascular Assessment section in Appendix A).
   a. Vital signs (temperature, apical pulse, respiratory rate, blood pressure)
   b. Arterial blood pressure and central venous pressure
   c. Peripheral pulses—quality and intensity
   d. Capillary refill time
   e. Presence of ascites (rare)
   f. Arrhythmias
2. Monitor for and report signs and symptoms of complications.
   a. Atelectasis
   b. Bleeding
   c. Chylothorax
   d. Hemothorax
   e. Pneumothorax
   f. Phrenic nerve damage
   g. Recurrent laryngeal nerve damage
3. Treat chylothorax if present.
   a. Provide and monitor child's intake of medium-chain-triglyceride diet.
   b. Monitor for signs of respiratory distress.
4. Provide intensive pulmonary toilet.
   a. Perform postural drainage and percussion.
   b. Change child's position every 2 hours.
   c. Encourage deep breathing and use of spirometer hourly.
   d. Encourage coughing; if child cannot cough, use suction.
5. Provide intensive pain control, because pain with thoracotomy incision is usually greater than that with median sternotomy.
6. Monitor child's response to medications.
   a. Diuretics
   b. Digitalis
7. Provide emotional support to infant or child during hospitalization.
   a. Use age-appropriate explanations before treatments.

b. Encourage, through age-appropriate means, child's expression of fears and anxieties (e.g., verbal expression, play, drawings).
c. Encourage parental expression of feelings.

🔺 Discharge Planning and Home Care

1. Instruct parents to observe for and report signs of cardiac or respiratory distress.
2. Instruct parents about administration of medications.
3. Provide parents with name of physician or nurse to contact for medical or health care follow-up.
4. Instruct parents about principles of infection control and well-child care (e.g., use of prophylactic medications before dental care).
5. Encourage and instruct parents about providing developmentally appropriate stimulation activities (see the relevant section in Appendix B).

CLIENT OUTCOMES

1. Adequate cardiac output will be achieved.
2. Respiratory compromise will be reduced.

REFERENCES

Flanagan MF et al: Cardiac disease. In Avery GB et al, editors, *Neonatology*, ed 5, Philadelphia, 1999, Lippincott Williams &Wilkins.

Fryer DC: Patent ductus arteriosus. In Fryer DC, editor: *Nadas' pediatric cardiology*, St Louis, 1992, Mosby.

Koehne PS et al: Patent ductus arteriosus in very low birth weight infants: complications of pharmacological and surgical treatment, *J Perinat Med* 29(4):327, 2001.

Lott JW: Assessment and management of cardiovascular dysfunction. In Kenner C et al, editors: *Comprehensive neonatal nursing*, Philadelphia, 1998, WB Saunders.

Montoya KD, Washington RL: Cardiovascular diseases and surgical interventions. In Merenstein GB, Gardner SL, editors, *Handbook of neonatal intensive care*, ed 5, St Louis, 2002, Mosby.

Skinner J: Diagnosis of patent ductus arteriosus, *Semin Neonatol* 6(1):49, 2001.

65

❖

Pneumonia

❖

PATHOPHYSIOLOGY

Pneumonia is an inflammation or infection of the pulmonary parenchyma. Pneumonia is attributable to one or more agents: viruses, bacteria (mycoplasmas), fungi, parasites, or aspirated foreign substances. The pattern of the illness depends on the following: (1) causative agent, (2) age of the child, (3) child's reaction, (4) extent of lesions, and (5) degree of bronchial obstruction. The clinical features of viral, mycoplasmal, and other bacterial pneumonia are listed in Box 65-1.

INCIDENCE

1. Pneumonia accounts for 10% to 15% of all respiratory infections, especially during the fall and winter months. The incidence in children younger than 5 years of age is 40 in 1000; in children 9 to 15 years of age, the incidence drops to 9 in 1000.
2. Viral pneumonia occurs more frequently than bacterial pneumonia, representing about 70% to 80% of all cases. Respiratory syncytial virus (RSV) accounts for 50% of all pneumonia cases.
3. Pneumonia is more severe and more common in infancy and early childhood.
   a. Neonatal causes: group B streptococci, *Chlamydia trachomatis*
   b. Two months to 2 years: usually viral, especially RSV (2 to 5 months)
   c. Over 2 years: usually *Streptococcus pneumoniae* and *Mycoplasma pneumoniae*

BOX 65-1
Clinical Features of Bacterial, Viral, and Mycoplasmal Pneumonia

Bacterial Pneumonia

Chlamydia trachomatis, Chlamydia pneumoniae, staphylococcal, streptococcal (90% of bacterial cases), and pneumococcal pneumonia occur most frequently.

Initial symptoms
Mild rhinitis
Anorexia
Listlessness
Progresses to abrupt onset
Acute onset of high fever
Toxic appearance
Productive cough, diminished breath sounds, rales on auscultation
Rapid and shallow respiration (50 to 80 breaths/min), dyspnea
Nasal flaring, retractions, expiratory grunt
Increased white blood cell count
Younger than 2 years of age—vomiting and mild diarrhea
Older than 5 years of age—headache and chills, often complaint of chest and abdominal pain
Chest radiographic finding of lobar pneumonia

Viral Pneumonia

Causative viruses include respiratory syncytial virus (RSV; usually in infants 2 to 5 months old), parainfluenza virus, adenovirus, and enterovirus.

Initial symptoms
Cough, usually nonproductive
Rhinitis
Progresses to insidious or abrupt onset
Range of symptoms—mild fever, slight cough, and malaise to high fever, severe cough, and prostration
Tachypnea, although infants with RSV infection may have apnea
Scattered rales, rhonchi, wheezing
Normal or slight change in white blood cell count
Chest radiographic finding of transient lobar infiltrates

Continued

BOX 65-1

Clinical Features of Bacterial, Viral, and Mycoplasmal Pneumonia—cont'd

> *Mycoplasmal Pneumonia (Most Common Type in Children Older than 5 Years of Age)*
>
> **Initial symptoms**
> Low-grade fever
> Chills
> Pharyngitis
> Headache and malaise
> Anorexia
> **Progresses to**
> Persistent, nonproductive cough, usually for 3 to 4 weeks
> Dry, hacking cough—blood-streaked sputum
> Rhinitis
> Rales, rash, and wheezing
> Chest radiographic findings vary, interstitial infiltrates
> Fatigue

4. Twenty-five percent to 75% of children with bacterial pneumonia have a concurrent viral infection.

CLINICAL MANIFESTATIONS

Major clinical signs include the following (see Box 65-1 for specific clinical manifestations):

1. Cough
2. Dyspnea
3. Tachypnea
4. Pale, dusky, or cyanotic appearance (usually late sign)
5. Decreased or absent breath sounds
6. Retractions of chest wall: intercostal, substernal, diaphragmatic, or supraclavicular
7. Nasal flaring
8. Abdominal pain (caused by irritation of diaphragm by adjacent infected lung)
9. Paroxysmal cough simulating pertussis (common in smaller children)
10. Older child does not appear ill

COMPLICATIONS

1. Chronic interstitial pneumonia
2. Chronic segmental or lobar atelectasis
3. Airway damage
4. Pleural effusion
5. Pulmonary calcification
6. Pulmonary fibrosis
7. Obliterative bronchitis and bronchiolitis
8. Persistent atelectasis

LABORATORY AND DIAGNOSTIC TESTS

1. Chest radiographic studies
2. Pulse oximetry
3. Blood gas measurement
4. Complete blood count with differential
5. Blood culture and Gram stain
6. Tuberculin skin test—rules out tuberculosis if child does not respond to treatment; use purified protein derivative but is nonreactive in 10% of children with pulmonary tuberculosis
7. Gram stain and culture of sputum, if available—usually for children older than 10 years of age; if tuberculosis is suspected, morning gastric aspirate collection may be ordered in children unable to produce sputum
8. Culture of pleural fluid—specimen of fluid from pleural space obtained to identify causative agents such as bacteria and viruses
9. Bronchoscopy—used to visualize and manipulate main branches of tracheobronchial tree; tissue obtained for diagnostic testing, therapeutically used to identify and remove foreign bodies
10. Lung biopsy—during thoracotomy, lung tissue is excised for diagnostic studies

MEDICAL MANAGEMENT

Medical treatment is primarily supportive and includes improving oxygenation with oxygen and respiratory treatments. Antibiotics are used to treat bacterial pneumonia based on culture and sensitivity testing. Hospitalization depends on the severity of the illness, the child's age, the need for supplemental oxygen, the suspected organism, and the adequacy of the home environment. If pleural effusion occurs, thoracentesis or chest tube drainage may be warranted.

NURSING ASSESSMENT

1. See the Respiratory Assessment section in Appendix A.
2. Assess patency of airway.
3. Assess for signs of respiratory distress and response to oxygen therapy. Monitor oxygen saturation levels.
4. Assess for signs of dehydration.
5. Assess child's response to medications.
6. Assess family's ability to manage home treatment regimen.

NURSING DIAGNOSES

- Breathing pattern, Ineffective
- Fluid volume, Risk for deficient
- Body temperature, Risk for imbalanced
- Activity intolerance

NURSING INTERVENTIONS

1. Monitor airway and maintain patency.
   a. Place child in semi-Fowler position, allowing child to choose position of comfort. Turn and reposition frequently to avoid pooling of secretions.
   b. Provide oxygen therapy as ordered by physician.
   c. Perform postural drainage, percussion, and vibration as needed and tolerated by child.
   d. Use play to encourage older child to cough. Encourage child to use incentive spirometer.
   e. Perform bulb or deep suction as needed.
   f. Provide for adequate rest; plan nursing care to conserve child's strength.
2. Monitor for signs of respiratory distress and response to oxygen therapy.
   a. Monitor vital signs and respiratory status, including breath sounds. Monitor oxygen saturation levels frequently.
   b. Change child's clothing and linens frequently to prevent chilling, if placed into mist tent.
   c. Observe for signs of complications (see Complications section in this chapter).

3. Monitor for and maintain optimal hydration status.
   a. Monitor administration of intravenous (IV) fluids. Encourage frequent consumption of oral fluids.
   b. Strictly record intake and output.
   c. Monitor for dehydration.
4. Monitor child's therapeutic response to and side effects from medications (if given, only for bacterial pneumonia).
5. Control fever with antipyretics.
6. Teach parents how to care for infant on IV and oxygen therapy.

🔊 Discharge Planning and Home Care

1. Instruct parents in administration of medications.
   a. Appropriate dose, route, and schedule, and need to complete entire medication course
   b. Side effects
   c. Child's response
2. Provide information to parents about measures for infection control and prevention.
   a. Avoid exposure to infectious contacts.
   b. Adhere to immunization schedule.
3. Children will have period of time when they tire easily and need additional rest periods and frequent, small feedings.

CLIENT OUTCOMES

1. Child's respiratory rate, oxygen saturation, and arterial blood gas levels will be within age-acceptable parameters without use of supplemental oxygen.
2. Child will have adequate hydration.
3. Child's temperature will remain within normal range.
4. Child will participates in self-care activities with minimal to no complaints of difficulty breathing.

REFERENCES

Correa AG: Diagnostic approach to pneumonia in children, *Semin Respir Infect* 11(3):131, 1996.

Garzon LS, Wiles L: Management of respiratory syncytial virus with lower respiratory infection in infants and children, *AACN Clin Issues* 13(3):421, 2002.

Judavji T et al: A practical guide for the diagnosis and treatment of pediatric pneumonia, *Can Med Assoc J* 156(5):S703, 1997.

66

❖

Poisoning

❖

INCIDENCE

1. Accidents (includes poisoning) are the leading cause of death in children 1 to 4 years old.
2. Most poisonings take place in the home; the most common location is the child's own residence, and the second most common is the grandparents' home.
3. Times of peak incidence are mealtimes, weekends, and holidays.
4. The peak age of incidence is between 1 and 3 years, when a child is autonomous and exploring.
5. A child who has had a poisoning episode is more likely to have a second episode than is a matched control to have a first.

CLINICAL MANIFESTATIONS

The manifestations depend on the agent that is ingested. The following are some examples:

1. Nausea
2. Tachycardia or bradycardia
3. Salivation
4. Dilated pupils
5. Diarrhea
6. Metabolic acidosis
7. Hyperthermia or hypothermia
8. Seizures
9. Lethargy
10. Dry mouth
11. Stupor
12. Delirium
13. Coma

COMPLICATIONS

1. Respiratory arrest
2. Cardiac arrest
3. Esophageal or tracheal corrosion, if caustic substance is ingested
4. Shock, acute respiratory distress syndrome
5. Congestive heart failure, renal failure, or liver failure
6. Cerebral edema, convulsions

LABORATORY AND DIAGNOSTIC TESTS

1. Blood toxicology screen
2. Urine toxicology screen
3. Blood gas analysis
4. Electrolyte levels

MEDICAL MANAGEMENT

Acute poisoning management consists of the following:
1. Elimination of the poison from the body—ipecac, gastric lavage
2. Adsorption and inactivation of the poison—activated charcoal
3. Administration of specific antidotes, if appropriate
4. Provision of supportive measures—intravenous fluids; respiratory support; treatment of shock, congestive heart failure, cerebral edema, and convulsions

NURSING ASSESSMENT

1. Take detailed history (agent ingested, dose, time of ingestion, underlying problems of child, age and weight of child, signs and symptoms produced, treatment rendered).
2. Perform complete system-by-system assessment (see Appendix A).
3. After child is stabilized or during well-child visit around 6 months of age, assess child-proofing of home.

NURSING DIAGNOSES

- Injury, Risk for
- Anxiety
- Knowledge, Deficient

NURSING INTERVENTIONS

1. Monitor child during decontamination procedures and until stable.
2. Provide emotional support to child and family (refer to the Supportive Care section in Appendix J).

🏠 Discharge Planning and Home Care

Teach parents about poison-proofing at home and poison management.

1. Make sure that all poisonous substances and medicines remain in their original containers, have child-resistant caps, and are out of reach of children.
2. Have syrup of ipecac available; parents should give only after consultation with physician or poison control center.
3. Post poison control center number on telephone.

CLIENT OUTCOMES

1. Child will have minimal injuries related to poisoning.
2. Parents will express their fears and concerns.
3. Parents will understand child's developmental level as it relates to child-proofing home and supervising child appropriately.

REFERENCES

Abbruzzi G, Stork CM: Pediatric toxicologic concerns, *Emerg Med Clin North Am* 20:223, 2002.

Kohen DE et al: Maternal reports of child injuries in Canada: trends and patterns by age and gender, *Inj Prev* 6:223, 2002.

Marchi AG et al: Severity grading of childhood poisoning: the multicentre study of poisoning in children (MSPC) score, *J Toxicol Clin Toxicol* 33(3):223, 1995.

Osterhoudt KC: The toxic toddler: drugs that can kill in small doses, *Contemp Pediatr* 17:73, 2000.

Vernon DD, Gleich MC: Poisoning and drug overdose, *Crit Care Clin* 13(3):647, 1997.

67

◆

Renal Failure: Acute

◆

PATHOPHYSIOLOGY

Acute renal failure (ARF) is the abrupt reduction or cessation of renal function secondary to a variety of disease processes (i.e., hypoxemia, shock, severe dehydration, hemorrhage, new-onset renal disease). Decreased renal functioning results in a reduction in the glomerular filtration rate. The predominant signs of renal failure are (1) oliguria or anuria, (2) electrolyte imbalances, (3) acid-base imbalances, and (4) impaired secretion of waste products (urea and creatinine).

The three types of renal failure are prerenal (hypoperfusion), intrarenal (intrinsic renal), and postrenal (obstructive). Acute prerenal failure results from decreased blood flow to the kidneys. Subsequent renal hypoxia causes cellular edema, injury, and cell death. Acute intrarenal failure results from injury to the kidney tissue. Acute postrenal failure is due to urinary outflow obstruction. The disease processes that result in renal failure are categorized according to type in Box 67-1.

INCIDENCE

1. Incidence and prognosis vary according to age, cause, associated problems, underlying condition, geographic location, and type of treatment.
2. ARF in infants and children is most frequently caused by prerenal failure (hypoperfusion).
3. ARF is common in critically ill infants and children and can significantly affect outcome (mortality and morbidity).
4. High rates of mortality related ARF (up to 78%) are associated with a combination of ARF and multisystem organ failure.

BOX 67-1

Causes of Acute Renal Failure

Prerenal (Hypoperfusion)

Severe dehydration (prolonged vomiting, diarrhea, decreased oral intake)

Shock (cardiogenic, septic, anaphylactic, hypovolemic, neurogenic)

Cardiac failure (congenital heart disease, myocardial dysfunction, cardiomyopathy, myocarditis)

Vascular fluid shifts (third-space losses, hemorrhage, burns, peritonitis)

Renal artery thrombosis

Hypoxic-ischemic events

Renal vasoconstriction or hypotension caused by medications

Intrarenal (Intrinsic)

Unresolved prerenal failure resulting in kidney cell damage

Congenital kidney abnormalities (polycystic kidney disease, renal dysplasia, bilateral agenesis, glomerular maturation arrest)

Glomerulonephritis

Interstitial nephritis

Acute tubular necrosis (prolonged ischemia)

Systemic lupus erythematosus

Hemolytic-uremic syndrome

Renal vein or artery thrombosis

Renal vasculitis

Thrombotic thrombocytopenia purpura (TTP)

Nephrotoxic agents (tumor lysis, cytotoxic therapy, hyperalimentation, antibiotics, diuretics, anesthetics, salicylates, radiographic contrast dye, heavy metals, organic solvents, pesticides)

Postrenal (Obstruction)

Renal calculi

Fungal balls

Ureterocele

Ureteral thrombosis

Structural abnormalities (ureteropelvic stenosis, urethral structure, urethral valves)

Tumors (Wilms', teratoma)

Vesicoureteral reflux

Neurogenic bladder

Injury (inflammation)

CLINICAL MANIFESTATIONS

Each type of ARF has a unique clinical manifestation. Azotemia is the cardinal sign of ARF, regardless of type. Although oliguria/anuria is frequently associated with ARF, individuals with *nonoliguric ARF* may have normal or increased urine output. Intrinsic ARF manifests in four phases: onset, oliguric, diuretic, and recovery. The onset phase begins with the precipitating event and continues until the individual develops oliguria. The oliguria/anuria (low-output) phase continues until the kidney begins to produce urine. The diuretic (high-output) phase begins with a sudden onset of diuresis and continues until urine output normalizes. The recovery phase begins with the stabilization of laboratory values and continues until normal renal function returns.

In critically ill children, the precipitating disease process frequently overshadows clinical manifestations of ARF. Although symptoms will vary with different disease processes, the most common symptoms associated with ARF are the following:

1. Azotemia (increased blood urea nitrogen [BUN] level)
2. Increased serum creatinine levels
3. Oliguria and/or anuria
4. Fluid retention and edema
5. Electrolyte imbalance
6. Acid-base imbalance
7. Hypertension, cardiac arrhythmias
8. Central nervous system (CNS) dysfunction
9. Pallor, anemia

COMPLICATIONS

1. Fluid balance complications (fluid overload, intravascular volume depletion from third-space losses, pulmonary edema, ascites causing lung compression)
2. Complications from electrolyte imbalances (arrhythmias, cardiac arrest, seizures)
3. Cardiovascular complications (congestive heart failure, hypertension, hypotension, arrhythmias, shock, cardiac arrest)
4. Respiratory complications (tachypnea, pulmonary edema, respiratory failure)

5. Neurologic complications
   a. Altered level of consciousness (lethargy, coma)
   b. Seizures (from uremia, hyponatremia, hypocalcemia, hypertension)
   c. Intracranial bleeding (neonates)
6. Bleeding (from coagulopathies)
7. Infection (from immunocompromise)
8. Skin breakdown (pruritus, poor healing, malnutrition)
9. Malnutrition (from decreased caloric intake, vomiting, diarrhea, protein loss)

LABORATORY AND DIAGNOSTIC TESTS

1. Blood tests
   a. BUN and serum creatinine levels—increased
   b. Serum sodium and calcium levels—decreased
   c. Serum potassium and phosphorus levels—increased
   d. Serum pH and bicarbonate (HCO_3) levels—decreased (metabolic acidosis)
   e. Hemoglobin level, hematocrit, platelet count—decreased (with decreased white blood cell count and platelet function)
   f. Serum albumin level—decreased
   g. Serum glucose level—decreased (particularly in infants)
   h. Serum uric acid level—increased
   i. Blood cultures—positive (with systemic infection)
2. Urine tests
   a. Urinalysis—red blood cells (RBCs) and/or casts
   b. Urine electrolyte levels, osmolality, and specific gravity—vary with disease process and stage of ARF
3. Electrocardiogram (ECG)—changes associated with electrolyte imbalance and heart failure
4. Chest and abdominal radiographic studies—fluid retention, kidney presence and size
5. Ultrasonography—kidney size, urinary tract obstruction, tumors, cysts
6. Other radiographic imaging (intravenous pyelography, radionuclide studies, renal arteriogram)—obstruction, blood flow, kidney structures, renal function

MEDICAL MANAGEMENT

1. Determine the type of ARF through evaluation of the child's history, symptoms, and laboratory results.
2. Stabilize the fluid and electrolyte balance.
   a. Enforce strict intake and output monitoring.
   b. Administer fluids as needed to maintain adequate circulation.
   c. Administer diuretics to assist in the elimination of excess fluid.
   d. Correct electrolyte imbalances.
      i. Correct hyperkalemia (Kayexalate, glucose, insulin, calcium gluconate, sodium bicarbonate, dialysis, continuous renal replacement therapy [CRRT]).
      ii. Increase serum sodium, calcium, and glucose levels with intravenous (IV) infusions.
3. Initiate peritoneal dialysis, hemodialysis or CRRT as indicated.
   a. Fluid volume overload causing congestive heart failure or pulmonary edema
   b. Intractable hyperkalemia
   c. Intractable acidosis
   d. Severe uremic symptoms
   e. Change in neurologic status
   f. Bleeding
   g. Intractable hypernatremia
   h. Severe calcium imbalances
   i. Inability to support nutritional status because of fluid overload
   j. Severely elevated BUN level
4. Support cardiovascular function.
   a. Decrease excess fluids.
   b. Control hypertension (antihypertensives).
   c. Maintain circulating volume (fluid bolus as needed).
   d. Provide inotropic support as indicated for heart failure.
5. Support respiratory function (oxygen, mechanical ventilation).
6. Control bleeding and anemia (blood product administration, minimization of needle sticks).

7. Prevent infection (antibiotics, minimization of invasive procedures).
8. Support nutrition (IV nutrition with adequate protein, nasogastric/nasojejunal continuous feeding, low-salt diet).

NURSING ASSESSMENT

1. Assess for signs and symptoms of fluid volume excess.
   a. Local edema (periorbital area, face, extremities, external genitalia; dependent edema) progressing to generalized edema
   b. Pulmonary congestion progressing to pulmonary edema
   c. Ascites with taut and shiny skin over abdomen
   d. Intake greater than output
   e. Weight gain
2. Assess for signs of electrolyte and glucose imbalance.
   a. Monitor serum electrolyte levels every 4 to 12 hours; decrease frequency when stabilized.
   b. Assess for signs of hyperkalemia.
       i. ECG: peaked T waves, wide PR interval, heart blocks, widened QRS, ventricular fibrillation
       ii. Clinical signs: muscle cramping, abdominal pain, diarrhea, muscle twitching
   c. Assess for signs of signs of hypocalcemia.
       i. CNS: tetany, anxiety, seizures
       ii. Cardiovascular: hypotension
       iii. Neuromuscular: Trousseau's sign, Chvostek's sign, muscle cramping
   d. Assess for signs of hyponatremia.
       i. CNS: apathy, weakness, dizziness, lethargy, encephalopathy, seizures
       ii. Cardiovascular: hypotension
       iii. Gastrointestinal (GI) : nausea, abdominal cramping
   e. Assess for signs of hypermagnesemia.
       i. CNS: depressed CNS, peripheral neuromuscular function, and deep tendon reflexes
       ii. Cardiovascular: hypotension, cardiac arrhythmias, depressed cardiac functioning
   f. Assess for hyperphosphatemia.
       i. Monitor serum magnesium levels.

      ii. Usually asymptomatic until levels are very high (more than 10 mEq/L).
  g. Assess for hypoglycemia.
     i. CNS: headache, slurred speech, irritability, confusion, lethargy, coma
     ii. Cardiovascular: tachycardia
     iii. Muscular: weakness, tremors, hypotonia, poor feeding
     iv. Sweating
     v. Hunger
3. Assess for signs of uremia.
  a. CNS: lethargy, confusion, seizures
  b. Cardiovascular: hypotension, hypertension
  c. GI: nausea, vomiting, anorexia
  d. Hematologic: anemia, thrombocytopenia, platelet dysfunction, increased bleeding time
4. Assess for signs of decreased cardiovascular functioning (hypotension, hypertension, shock, congestive heart failure, cardiac dysrhythmias, fluid volume deficit).
  a. Blood pressure (hypotension or hypertension)
  b. Central venous pressure (increased or decreased)
  c. Heart rate and rhythm
  d. Distal perfusion (pulses, capillary refill, temperature, color)
5. Assess for signs of ineffective breathing pattern.
  a. Respiratory rate and pattern (tachypnea, abdominal breathing, shallow breathing, apnea)
  b. Use of accessory muscles (retractions, shoulder shrugging)
  c. Nasal flaring
  d. Grunting (infants)
  e. Cyanosis
  f. Respiratory acidosis
6. Assess for signs of decreased neurologic functioning (lethargy, coma, seizures, intracranial bleeds in neonates) from shock, uremia, electrolyte imbalance, decreased cerebral perfusion, cerebral edema.
7. Assess for bleeding disorders (disseminated intravascular coagulation, GI bleeding, intracranial bleeding).

8. Assess for signs of anemia (pallor, decreased serum hemoglobin level and hematocrit, lethargy, weakness) from deficient RBC production and/or RBC destruction.
9. Assess for signs of infection (fever, increased white blood cell count, septic shock).
10. Assess for skin breakdown from pruritus, malnutrition, edema, and decreased ability to heal.
11. Assess for signs of failure to thrive and malnutrition (lethargy, weakness, poor feeding, decreased appetite, vomiting, failure to gain weight, inadequate caloric intake).
12. Assess child's comfort level.
13. Assess child's level of activity and coping response.
14. Assess family's ability to manage their child's long-term care.

NURSING DIAGNOSES

- Fluid volume, Excess
- Fluid volume, Risk for deficient
- Acid-base imbalance
- Cardiac output, Decreased
- Breathing pattern, Ineffective
- High risk for neurologic status changes
- Infection, Risk for
- Skin integrity, Risk for impaired
- Nutrition: less than body requirements, Imbalanced
- Comfort, Impaired
- Coping, Ineffective

NURSING INTERVENTIONS

1. Monitor and maintain fluid balance.
   a. Frequently assess hydration status.
   b. Accurately record input and output.
   c. Replace fluids lost as a result of interstitial fluid shifts as needed to maintain adequate vascular volume.
   d. Monitor type of fluids and administration rate to avoid fluid overload and cerebral edema while maintaining adequate circulating volume.

    e. Administer diuretics as ordered and assess effectiveness.

    f. Monitor and record weight daily.

2. Monitor serum electrolyte and glucose levels and implement corrective measures as indicated.

3. Monitor acid-base balance and implement corrective measures as indicated.

4. Frequently reassess cardiovascular status and institute supportive measures as indicated.

5. Assess breathing pattern and promptly implement airway stabilization methods as indicated; encourage coughing and deep breathing.

6. Monitor neurologic functioning and promptly report deterioration in status.

7. Assess for signs of bleeding and implement bleeding precautions (use of soft toothbrush, minimization of needle sticks, avoidance of invasive procedures).

8. Monitor for signs of anemia and implement corrective measures as indicated (blood transfusion, medication); use minimum volumes for blood draws.

9. Assess for signs of infection and implement preventive measures.

    a. Practice good hand-washing and aseptic technique.

    b. Perform care for all invasive catheters and lines.

    c. Protect child from infectious contacts.

10. Monitor for signs of skin breakdown and implement corrective measures.

    a. Administer medications for pruritus.

    b. Turn frequently; avoid placing on hard surfaces (tubing, monitor cables).

    c. Perform mouth and skin care.

    d. Use pressure relief surface as needed.

11. Assess for signs of malnutrition and provide nutritional support.

    a. Administer parenteral nutrition as indicated.

    b. Assess tolerance of enteral feeds via oral, nasogastric, or nasojejunal route.

    c. For oral feedings, offer appetizing foods while implementing dietary restrictions.

    d. Monitor caloric intake.

    e. Collaborate with nutritionist as indicated.

12. Assess child's comfort level and implement pain control measures (see Appendix H).

13. Assess coping responses and provide therapeutic environment for child and family.

    a. Encourage child and parents to express feelings of concern about child's condition.

    b. Provide developmentally appropriate information and reinforce data provided to child and parents (see the Preparation for Procedures or Surgery section in Appendix J).

14. Assess family's ability to manage their child's long-term care and provide supportive measures as indicated.

Discharge Planning and Home Care

If ARF has not resolved before discharge, provide child and parents with developmentally appropriate verbal and written instruction regarding home management of the following (see Appendix K):

1. Disease process (include expected clinical process and signs of complications)

2. Medications (dose, route, schedule, side effects, and complications)

3. Skin care

4. Nutrition

5. Prevention of infection

6. Follow-up care

CLIENT OUTCOMES

1. Child's fluid-electrolyte and acid-base status will be within normal limits.

2. Child will not demonstrate signs and symptoms of complications related to ARF.

3. Child will demonstrate normal growth and development.

4. Child and family will demonstrate sense of mastery in dealing with disease process.

REFERENCES

Bernhardt J: Renal and genitourinary disorders. In Deacon P, O'Neill P, editors: *Core curriculum for neonatal intensive care nursing,* ed 2, Philadelphia, 1999, WB Saunders.

Goldberg EA, Meyers K: Advanced practice nursing in pediatric nephrology, *Nurs Clin North Am* 32(1):125, 2001.

Goldstein S et al: Outcome in children receiving continuous venovenous hemofiltration, *Pediatrics* 107(6):1309, 2001.

Mackenzie DL: When *E. coli* turns deadly, *RN* 62(7):28, 1999.

McKinney ES et al: *Maternal-child nursing,* Philadelphia, 2000, WB Saunders.

Potts NL, Mandleco BL, editors: *Pediatric nursing: caring for children and their families,* Clifton Park, NY, 2002, Delmar.

Rainey KE et al: Successful long-term peritoneal dialysis in a very low birth weight infant with renal failure secondary to feto-fetal transfusion syndrome, *Pediatrics* 106(4):849, 2000.

68

◆

Renal Failure: Chronic

◆

PATHOPHYSIOLOGY

Chronic renal failure (CRF) is the irreversible deterioration of renal function occurring over a course of months to years. End-stage renal disease (ESRD) is the progression of CRF that results in the inability to maintain balance of body substances (buildup of fluid and waste products) using conservative treatment. ESRD occurs when less than 10% of renal function remains. Causes of CRF include a variety of congenital and acquired disorders, including (1) glomerular disease (e.g., pyelonephritis, glomerulonephritis, glomerulopathy), (2) obstructive uropathies (e.g., vesicoureteral reflux), (3) renal hypoplasia or dysplasia, (4) inherited renal disorders (e.g., polycystic kidney disease, congenital nephrotic syndrome, Alport's syndrome), (5) vascular neuropathies (e.g., hemolytic-uremic syndrome [HUS], renal thrombosis), and (6) kidney loss or damage (e.g., severe renal trauma, Wilms' tumor). Although renal disease secondary to diabetes mellitus and/or high blood pressure is a relatively common cause of ESRD in adults, these disorders are not usually seen in children.

CRF is associated with a variety of biochemical dysfunctions. Sodium and fluid imbalances result from the kidney's inability to concentrate urine. Hyperkalemia occurs due to decreased potassium secretion. Metabolic acidosis results from impaired reabsorption of bicarbonate and decreased ammonia production. Bone demineralization and impaired growth result from secretion of parathyroid hormone, elevation of plasma phosphate level (decreasing serum calcium level), acidosis (causing calcium and phosphorus release into the bloodstream), and impaired intestinal calcium absorption. Anemia results from impaired red blood cell (RBC) production, decreased RBC life span, and an increased tendency to bleed (due to impaired platelet function). Uremia occurs with a buildup of blood urea, creatinine, and waste products. Encephalopathy and neuropathy have been associated with the accumulation of uremic toxins. Malnutrition results from poor appetite, nausea, and vomiting. Altered growth and sexual maturation have been associated with altered nutrition and a variety of biochemical processes in CRF.

INCIDENCE

1. The incidence of CRF in children is estimated at 1 in 100,000. Incidence is highest in adolescents and in males. The incidence of ESRD is approximately 13 in 1 million.
2. The most frequent causes of CRF in younger children are congenital renal and urinary tract malformations (e.g., renal hypoplasia, renal dysplasia, obstructive uropathies, vesicoureteral reflux).
3. Acute renal diseases such as glomerulonephritis, HUS, and pyelonephritis most frequently cause acquired CRF in older children.

CLINICAL MANIFESTATIONS

Although the child's symptoms will vary with different disease processes, the most common symptoms associated with CRF are the following:

1. Fluid imbalance
   a. Fluid overload—edema, oliguria, hypertension, congestive heart failure
   b. Vascular volume depletion—polyuria, decreased fluid intake, dehydration
2. Electrolyte imbalance
   a. Hyperkalemia—cardiac rhythm disturbances, myocardial dysfunction
   b. Hypernatremia—thirst, stupor, tachycardia, dry membranes, increased deep tendon reflexes, decreased level of consciousness
   c. Hypercalcemia and hyperphosphatemia—irritability, depression, muscle cramps, paresthesias, psychosis, tetani, Trousseau's sign, Chvostek's sign

     d. Hypokalemia—decreased deep tendon reflexes, hypotonia, electrocardiogram (ECG) changes

3. Uremic neuropathy and encephalopathy
   a. Itching (uremic frost skin deposits)
   b. Muscle cramps and weakness
   c. Slurred speech
   d. Paresthesia of palms and/or soles
   e. Poor concentration, memory loss
   f. Drowsiness
   g. Signs of elevated intracranial pressure (ICP)
   h. Seizures
   i. Coma

4. Metabolic acidosis—tachypnea, decreased serum bicarbonate

5. Anemia and blood cell dysfunction
   a. Pallor
   b. Weakness
   c. Bleeding—stomatitis, bloody stools

6. Growth and development dysfunction
   a. Abnormal bone growth (small for age)
   b. Delayed sexual development and menstrual irregularities
   c. Malnutrition and muscle wasting
   d. Bone pain
   e. Poor appetite
   f. Activity intolerance (related to manifestations of CRF)

7. Psychosocial dysfunction
   a. Anxiety
   b. Altered self-image
   c. Depression
   d. Isolation from peers

COMPLICATIONS

1. Fluid balance complications—fluid overload or intravascular volume depletion
2. Complications from electrolyte imbalances—cardiac dysrhythmias, cardiac arrest, seizures
3. Cardiovascular complications—congestive heart failure, hypertension, left ventricular hypertrophy, arrhythmias, cardiac arrest, hypotension (with dehydration)

4. Neurologic complications—altered level of consciousness, increased ICP, seizures, coma
5. Respiratory complications—fluid overload, pulmonary edema, respiratory failure
6. Bleeding and anemia
7. Hypoglycemia
8. Infection
9. Skin breakdown—pruritus, uremic frost, decreased healing
10. Hypertensive retinopathy
11. Osseous and dental malformation (renal rickets)
12. Malnutrition and growth retardation
13. Delayed sexual development
14. Mental retardation

LABORATORY AND DIAGNOSTIC TESTS

1. Blood tests
   a. Blood urea nitrogen and serum creatinine levels—increased
   b. Serum potassium level—increased (decreased with diuretics and/or restricted intake)
   c. Serum sodium level—increased (decreased with hemodilution and/or restricted intake)
   d. Serum calcium level—decreased
   e. Serum phosphorus level—increased
   f. Serum pH and bicarbonate (HCO_3) level—decreased (metabolic acidosis)
   g. Hemoglobin level, hematocrit, platelet count—decreased (with decreased white blood cell count and platelet function)
   h. Serum glucose level—decreased (most common in infants)
   i. Serum uric acid level —elevated
   j. Blood cultures—positive results (with systemic infection)
2. Urine tests
   a. Urinalysis—RBCs and/or casts
   b. Urine electrolyte levels, osmolality, and specific gravity—vary with disease process

   c. Twenty-four-hour urine sodium collection—quantifies sodium secretion
3. Electrocardiogram—changes associated with electrolyte imbalance and/or heart failure
4. Chest and abdominal radiographic studies—changes associated with fluid retention and structural abnormalities
5. Diagnostic procedures
   a. Renal biopsy
   b. Renal scan, renal arteriogram
   c. Renal ultrasonography
   d. Magnetic resonance imaging, computerized axial tomography

MEDICAL MANAGEMENT

1. Stabilize the fluid and balance.
   a. Administer diuretics to assist in the elimination of excess fluid.
   b. Closely monitor intake and output, and weight.
   c. Administer fluids as needed to maintain adequate circulation.
2. Correct electrolyte and glucose imbalances.
   a. Correct hyperkalemia (Kayexalate, glucose, insulin, calcium gluconate, sodium bicarbonate, dialysis, continuous renal replacement therapy [CRRT], and restriction of dietary potassium).
   b. Administer calcium (by mouth or intravenous [IV] route) and encourage dietary calcium intake.
   c. Restrict dietary sodium.
   d. Administer phosphate binders.
   e. Correct hypoglycemia.
3. Support cardiovascular and respiratory function.
   a. Limit excess fluids.
   b. Control hypertension (antihypertensive medications).
   c. Maintain circulating volume.
   d. Provide cardiac medications as indicated for heart failure.
   e. Provide respiratory assistance (oxygen, mechanical ventilation) as needed.
4. Prevent infection (administer antibiotics, avoid invasive procedures or lines, prevent skin breakdown).

5. Support nutrition (adequate protein, enteral tube feedings as needed, multivitamins).
6. Control bleeding and anemia (blood products, recombinant human erythropoietin, iron).
7. Initiate dialysis (peritoneal dialysis, hemodialysis, CRRT as indicated for untreatable, severe complications of CRF: fluid volume overload [congestive heart failure or pulmonary complications], electrolyte imbalance, acidosis, central nervous system dysfunction, bone deformation and/or bone marrow depression).
8. Initiate renal transplantation as appropriate.

NURSING ASSESSMENT

1. See the Renal Assessment section in Appendix A.
2. Assess for signs of fluid volume excess and electrolyte imbalance.
   a. Local edema (periorbital area, face, external genitalia, extremities) progressing to generalized edema
   b. Pulmonary congestion progressing to pulmonary edema
   c. Ascites with taut and shiny skin over abdomen
   d. Weight gain and decreased output
   e. Signs of hyperkalemia, hypocalcemia, hyponatremia, hypermagnesemia, and hypoglycemia
3. Assess for signs of decreased cardiac output (fluid volume deficit, cardiovascular dysfunction) and respiratory compromise (fluid volume excess, pulmonary edema).
4. Assess for signs of infection (fever, increased white blood cell count, positive culture results, shock).
5. Assess for signs of uremia: neurologic (lethargy, confusion, seizures), cardiovascular (hypotension, hypertension), respiratory (respiratory compromise), gastrointestinal (nausea, vomiting, anorexia, bloody diarrhea, unpleasant breath odor), hematologic (anemia, thrombocytopenia, platelet dysfunction, increased bleeding time), and skin (uremic frost, severe itching, mouth and lip sores).
6. Assess for signs of life-threatening complications: sepsis, shock, fluid overload, severe hypertension, heart failure, respiratory failure, severe electrolyte imbalance, severe

acidosis, disseminated intravascular coagulation, coma, and seizures.

7. Assess for signs of malnutrition, growth retardation, bone deformity.
8. Assess child for growth and biopsychosocial and faith development (see Appendix B).
9. Assess child's comfort level and level of activity.
10. Assess child's coping response to long-term illness, alteration in development, treatment regimen, possibility of renal transplant and/or death.
11. Assess family's ability to cope with their child's long-term needs and provide effective care.

NURSING DIAGNOSES

- Fluid volume, Excess
- Fluid volume, Risk for deficient
- Urinary elimination, Impaired
- Cardiac output, Decreased
- Breathing pattern, Ineffective
- Gas exchange, Impaired
- Skin integrity, Risk for impaired
- Injury, Risk for
- Infection, Risk for
- Nutrition: less than body requirements, Imbalanced
- Growth and development, Delayed
- Comfort, Impaired
- Coping, Ineffective
- Family processes, Interrupted
- Therapeutic regimen management, Ineffective

NURSING INTERVENTIONS

1. Monitor fluid-electrolyte and acid-base balance.
   a. Accurately record input and output and assess hydration status frequently.
   b. Record weight frequently (daily).
   c. Maintain fluid limit.
   d. Administer diuretics and monitor response.
   e. Monitor serum electrolyte and glucose levels and implement corrective measures as indicated.

    f. Administer dialysis therapy as ordered.

    g. Monitor acid-base balance and implement corrective measures as indicated.

2. Support cardiovascular and pulmonary functioning.

    a. Monitor for fluid volume overload. Administer diuretics and dialysis as ordered.

    b. Monitor for signs of dehydration. Replace fluids as needed to maintain adequate circulating volume.

    c. Monitor for ECG changes related to electrolyte imbalance.

    d. Monitor vital signs, including blood pressure; administer antihypertensives as indicated.

    e. Administer blood products as ordered; assess for transfusion reaction. Use minimum volumes for blood draws.

    f. Assess adequacy of ventilation and promptly implement airway stabilization methods as indicated; encourage client to cough and breathe deeply.

3. Maintain skin integrity and prevent infection.

    a. Provide daily bath, frequent mouth care and skin care.

    b. Assist child with turning and prevent pressure ulceration (use pressure relief/reduction surfaces; avoid hard objects [tubing, cables] under child).

    c. Use bleeding precautions (soft toothbrush, avoidance of needle sticks).

    d. Avoid contact of child with infectious visitors.

    e. Maintain sterility of all invasive lines and perform dressing changes and site care as needed and on schedule.

    f. Monitor for signs of infection (fever, lethargy, nausea, vomiting, diarrhea, increased white blood cell count, wound infection) and begin antibiotic therapy promptly.

    g. Administer medications for pruritus.

4. Promote growth and nutrition (work with dietitian).

    a. Assist child in finding appetizing choices in low-potassium, low-sodium, low-phosphorus, high-calcium, high-protein diet.

    b. Monitor caloric intake.

   c. Monitor child's growth status by assessing growth trends.

   d. Administer enteral or IV nutrition as needed (assess tolerance of feedings).

   e. Administer vitamins, calcium supplements, and phosphate binders as indicated.

5. Assess child's comfort level and implement pain control measures (see Appendix H)

6. Assess coping responses and provide psychosocial support for child and family (see Supportive Care section in Appendix J).

🏠 Discharge Planning and Home Care

Provide child and parents with developmentally appropriate verbal and written instruction regarding home management of the following (see Appendix K):

1. Disease process (include expected clinical progress and signs of complications)
2. Medications (dose, route, schedule, side effects, and complications)
3. Prevention of infection (wound and/or line care if indicated)
4. Skin care and bleeding precautions
5. Nutrition (dietary restrictions and supplements)
6. Home dialysis therapy (if indicated)
7. Follow-up care and long-term treatment plan
8. Child's developmental needs
9. Community resources and support services (see Appendix L)

CLIENT OUTCOMES

1. Child will maintain fluid-electrolyte and acid-base balance within appropriate limits.
2. Child will be free of infection.
3. Child and family will adhere to treatment regimen without occurrence of complications.
4. Child will have optimal growth and development.

REFERENCES

Baer C: Care of the critically ill chronic renal failure patient, *Crit Care Nurs Clin North Am* 10(4):433, 1998.

Kopple JD et al: Clinical practice guidelines for nutrition in chronic renal failure: pediatric guidelines, *Am J Kidney Dis* 35(suppl 2):105, 2000.

McKinney ES et al: *Maternal-child nursing,* Philadelphia, 2000, WB Saunders.

Meleski DD: Families with chronically ill children: a literature review examines approaches to helping them cope, *Am J Nurs* 102(5):47, 2002.

Munford PR: Psychosocial adjustment and treatment of children and adolescents with ESRD. In Nissenson AR, Fine R, editors: *Dialysis therapy,* ed 3, Philadelphia, 2002, Harley & Belfus.

Potts NL, Mandleco BL, editors: *Pediatric nursing: caring for children and their families,* Clifton Park, NY, 2002, Delmar.

Rader BL, Watkins SL: Psychosocial development and adherence to medical regimens in children with chronic renal failure. In Fine R et al, editors: *CAPD/CPPD in children,* ed 2, Boston, 1998, Kluwer Academic Publishers.

Wassner SJ: Growth in children with ESRD. In Nissenson AR, Fine R, editors: *Dialysis therapy,* ed 3, Philadelphia, 2002, Harley & Belfus.

69

❖

Respiratory Distress Syndrome

❖

PATHOPHYSIOLOGY

Respiratory distress syndrome (RDS), or hyaline membrane disease, results from the absence, deficiency, or alteration of the components of pulmonary surfactant. Surfactant, a lipoprotein complex, is an ingredient of the filmlike surface of each alveolus that prevents alveolar collapse. It is secreted from type II respiratory cells in the alveoli. When surfactant is inadequate, alveolar collapse occurs and hypoxia results. Pulmonary vascular constriction and decreased pulmonary perfusion then occur, which lead to progressive respiratory failure.

INCIDENCE

1. The incidence of RDS shows an inverse relationship to gestational age: the younger the infant, the greater the risk of RDS. However, the occurrence of RDS appears to be more dependent on lung maturity than on actual gestational age.
   a. Diagnosed in 25% of infants at 34 weeks' gestation and in 80% of infants at less than 28 weeks' gestation
2. The severity of RDS is decreased in infants whose mothers received corticosteroids 24 to 48 hours before delivery. There appears to be an additive effect in improved lung function when antenatal steroid therapy is combined with postnatal surfactant administration.
3. RDS occurs twice as often in males as in females.

4. Incidence increases in full-term infants in the presence of certain factors.
   a. Diabetic mother who delivers at less than 38 weeks' gestation
   b. Perinatal hypoxia

CLINICAL MANIFESTATIONS

The following symptoms are observed in the first 2 to 8 hours of life:

1. Tachypnea (more than 60 breaths/min)
2. Intercostal and sternal retractions
3. Audible expiratory grunting
4. Nasal flaring
5. Cyanosis as hypoxemia increases
6. Decreasing lung compliance (paradoxical seesaw respirations)
7. Systemic hypotension (peripheral pallor, edema, capillary filling delayed by more than 3 to 4 seconds)
8. Decreased urinary output
9. Decreased breath sounds with rales
10. Tachycardia as acidosis and hypoxemia progress

RDS is a self-limiting disease. Improvement is typically seen 48 to 72 hours after birth when type II alveolar cell regeneration occurs and surfactant is produced. Presentation and duration of symptoms can be altered with administration of artificial surfactant.

COMPLICATIONS

1. Acid-base imbalance
2. Air leaks (pneumothorax, pneumomediastinum, pneumopericardium, pneumoperitoneum, subcutaneous emphysema, pulmonary interstitial emphysema)
3. Pulmonary hemorrhage
4. Chronic lung disease of infancy, 5% to 10%— see Chapter 14
5. Apnea
6. Systemic hypotension
7. Anemia

8. Infection (pneumonia, septicemia—transplacental or nosocomial)
9. Altered infant development and parenting behaviors

Complications Associated with Intubation

1. Endotracheal tube complications (displacement, dislodgement, occlusion, atelectasis after extubation, palatal grooves)
2. Tracheal lesions (erosion, granuloma, subglottic stenosis, necrotizing tracheobronchitis)

Complications Associated with Prematurity

1. Patent ductus arteriosus, often associated with pulmonary hypertension
2. Intraventricular hemorrhage
3. Retinopathy of prematurity
4. Neurologic impairment

LABORATORY AND DIAGNOSTIC TESTS

1. Chest radiographic studies
   a. Diffuse reticulogranular pattern in superimposed air bronchograms
   b. Central lung markings and heart border that are difficult to see; hypoinflated lungs
   c. Possible presence of cardiomegaly when other systems also involved (infants of diabetic mothers, infants with hypoxia or congestive heart failure)
   d. Large thymic silhouette
   e. Whiteout (uniform granularity) in air bronchograms, indicating severe disease if present in first few hours
2. Arterial blood gas values—hypoxemia with respiratory and/or metabolic acidosis
3. Complete blood count
4. Serum electrolytes, calcium, sodium (Na^+), potassium (K^+), glucose levels
   Lecithin/sphingomyelin ratio and phosphatidylglycerol levels are beneficial in determining timing for labor induction or elective cesarean deliveries as a means of preventing RDS.

MEDICAL MANAGEMENT

1. Improve oxygenation and maintain optimal lung volume.
   a. Maintenance of arterial partial pressure of oxygen (PaO_2) of 50 to 80 mm Hg, arterial partial pressure of carbon dioxide ($PaCO_2$) of 40 to 50, pH of at least 7.25
   b. Surfactant replacement via endotracheal tube (ET)
   c. Continuous positive airway pressure via nasal prongs to prevent volume loss during expiration or mechanical ventilation via ET for severe hypoxemia (PaO_2 lower than 50 to 60 mm Hg) and/or hypercapnia ($PaCO_2$ higher than 60 mm Hg)
   d. Transcutaneous monitoring and pulse oximetry
   e. Aerosol administration of bronchodilators
   f. Chest physiotherapy
   g. Additional cardiorespiratory measures (high-frequency ventilation, extracorporeal membrane oxygenation, nitric oxide, liquid ventilation)
2. Maintain temperature stabilization.
3. Provide appropriate fluid, electrolyte, and nutritional intake.
4. Monitor arterial blood gas levels, hemoglobin level and hematocrit, and bilirubin level.
5. Transfuse blood as needed to maintain hematocrit, for optimal oxygenation.
6. Maintain arterial line for monitoring of PaO_2 and blood sampling.
7. Administer medications as indicated.
   a. Diuretics to minimize interstitial edema
   b. Sodium bicarbonate ($NaHCO_3$) for metabolic acidosis
   c. Antibiotics for associated infection
   d. Analgesics for pain and irritability
   e. Theophylline as a respiratory stimulant
   f. Vasopressors (dopamine, dobutamine)
   g. Corticosteroids to enhance lung maturity
   h. Bronchodilators
8. See Chapter 14 for management of ongoing problems.

NURSING ASSESSMENT

1. See the Respiratory Assessment section in Appendix A.
2. Assess child's cardiorespiratory status.

3. Assess child's oxygenation.
4. Assess child's hydration status.
5. Assess child's nutritional status.
6. Assess child's developmental level (see Appendix B).
7. Assess infant-family interaction.
8. Assess family's ability to cope with home care needs (see Appendix K).

NURSING DIAGNOSES

- Gas exchange, Impaired
- Airway clearance, Ineffective
- Breathing pattern, Ineffective
- Nutrition: less than body requirements, Imbalanced
- Hypothermia
- Tissue perfusion, Ineffective
- Growth and development, Delayed
- Parenting, Impaired
- Fluid volume, Excess
- Therapeutic regimen management, Ineffective

NURSING INTERVENTIONS

1. Maintain cardiorespiratory stability.
   a. Monitor depth, symmetry, and rhythm of respirations.
   b. Monitor rate, quality, and murmurs of heart sounds.
   c. Assess responsiveness to medical interventions: mechanical ventilation, aerosol administration, and surfactant replacement therapy.
   d. Monitor Pao_2 through pulse oximetry and/or transcutaneous monitoring.
   e. Monitor arterial blood gases and laboratory data.
   f. Monitor blood pressure and fluctuations with activity and treatments.
   g. Administer medications as indicated.
2. Optimize oxygenation.
   a. Monitor correlation between environment, positioning, and transcutaneous monitoring readings.
   b. Coordinate delivery of routine care and procedures and cluster care as appropriate.
   c. Maintain ET or nasal prong position and patency.

    d. Suction as needed. Insert suction catheter only as far as end of ET tube.

    e. Administer sedatives and analgesics as needed.

    f. Maintain temperature stability.

3. Maintain appropriate fluid, nutrient, and caloric intake.

    a. Maintain intravenous access as needed.

    b. Administer feedings via most appropriate route for medical and developmental status.

    c. Record weight daily and length and head circumference weekly.

    d. Monitor and record intake and output (including blood products, urine, and stool); check pH and specific gravity.

4. Promote normal growth and development (see Appendix B).

    a. Maintain therapeutic environment with controlled handling and appropriate stimulation.

    b. Identify individual stress and interaction cues.

    c. Coordinate nursing care and procedures with tolerance level of infant.

    d. Facilitate parent-infant interaction by teaching parents infant cues and encouraging parents to hold infant, to participate in kangaroo care, and to provide some routine care for infant (e.g., feeding and bathing).

5. Incorporate other immediate family members (siblings) into infant's care as soon as appropriate.

🔺 Discharge Planning and Home Care

1. Monitor readiness for discharge (see Chapter 14)

2. Provide appropriate discharge instructions for parents (see Chapter 14).

CLIENT OUTCOMES

1. Infant will have optimal lung functioning with gas exchange and oxygenation sufficient for tissue perfusion and growth.

2. Infant will meet growth and development parameters appropriate for corrected age.

3. Parents will be competent in care of their infant.

REFERENCES

Clark RH et al: A comparison of the outcomes of neonates treated with two different natural surfactants, *J Pediatr* 139(6):828, 2001.

Cools F, Offringa M: Meta-analysis of elective high frequency ventilation in preterm infants with respiratory distress syndrome, *Arch Dis Child Fetal Neonatal Ed* 80(1):F15, 1999.

Fanaroff A, Martin R, editors: *Neonatal-perinatal medicine: diseases of the fetus and infant,* ed 7, St Louis, 2001, Mosby.

Karinski DA et al: The use of inhaled glucocorticosteroids and recovery from adrenal suppression after systemic steroid use in a VLBW premature infant with BPD: case report and literature discussion, *Neonatal Netw* 19(8):27, 2000.

Kenner C, Lott J, editors: *Comprehensive neonatal nursing: a physiologic perspective,* ed 3, Philadelphia, 2003, WB Saunders.

Merenstein G, Gardner S, editors: *Handbook of neonatal intensive care,* ed 5, St Louis, 2002, Mosby.

Morris DS et al: Extracorporeal membrane oxygenation (ECMO): a treatment for neonates in respiratory failure, *Infant Toddler Interv Transdisciplinary J* 10(4):215, 2000.

Rais-Bahrami K, Short BL: The current status of neonatal extracorporeal membrane oxygenation, *Semin Perinatol* 24(6):406, 2000.

Sweet D, Halliday H: Current perspectives on the drug treatment of neonatal respiratory distress syndrome, *Paediatr Drugs* 1(1):19, 1999.

70

❖

Respiratory Syncytial Viral Infection

❖

PATHOPHYSIOLOGY

Respiratory syncytial virus (RSV) is a highly contagious pathogen. Its primary effect is on the lower respiratory tract. RSV has an incubation period of 5 to 8 days, after which it usually causes upper respiratory tract infection symptoms. The primary mode of transmission (similar to that of other respiratory pathogens) is contact with respiratory secretions by direct handling of infected individuals or objects contaminated with the virus.

INCIDENCE

1. Annual epidemics occur during winter and early spring.
2. RSV affects any age group, but most often small children and infants younger than 2 years of age.
3. It tends to cause more severe illness in very young and debilitated children. Infants aged 6 weeks to 3 months and those with cardiac problems, pulmonary problems, or immune diseases are generally made most ill by RSV infection.

CLINICAL MANIFESTATIONS

1. Rhinorrhea and pharyngitis—usually first symptoms
2. Progression to coughing and wheezing
3. Associated otitis media
4. Lower respiratory tract symptoms: bronchiolitis, pneumonia, and apnea
5. Air hunger, retractions, increased respiratory rate, and cyanosis
6. Hypoxemia

COMPLICATIONS

1. Respiratory distress leading to respiratory failure
2. Apnea

LABORATORY AND DIAGNOSTIC TESTS

1. Complete blood count with differential
2. Chest radiographic studies
3. Nasal washing examination (enzyme immune assay)
4. Nasopharyngeal viral culture

MEDICAL MANAGEMENT

Treatment of this viral infection is supportive and based on the severity of the symptoms. In mild cases, humidified oxygen and intravenous fluids are administered. Children undergo suctioning for the mechanical removal of secretions. Children with significant respiratory distress may require endotracheal intubation and mechanical ventilation. Children identified at high risk for significant respiratory compromise, i.e., those with immune deficiency, bronchopulmonary dysplasia, or heart disease, will be evaluated for drug therapy.

Ribavirin, an antiviral drug, may be administered. RespiGam, an RSV immune globulin, provides passive immunoprophylaxis. Administration is limited and costly, and monthly consecutive intravenous infusions throughout the RSV "season" are required. Recently, palivizumab (Synagis), a humanized monoclonal antibody, was approved for intramuscular injection and is given monthly for five doses in children in high-risk groups.

NURSING ASSESSMENT

1. See the Respiratory Assessment section in Appendix A.
2. Assess ability to clear airway.
3. Assess hydration status.

NURSING DIAGNOSES

- Breathing pattern, Ineffective
- Gas exchange, Impaired
- Tissue perfusion, Ineffective
- Knowledge, Deficient

NURSING INTERVENTIONS

1. Suction as needed to clear airway.
2. Implement pulmonary toilet.
3. Position child with head of bed elevated; allow position of comfort.
4. Administer oxygen (may require use of bronchodilator).
5. Provide adequate fluid intake (intravenous and oral).
6. Strictly monitor intake and output.
7. Weigh client daily.
8. Provide small, frequent meals.
9. Institute contact precautions.
10. Encourage parental education, especially in hand-washing.

🏠 Discharge Planning and Home Care

1. Instruct parents in pulmonary toilet as indicated.
2. Provide family education regarding transmission of virus and prevention of reinfection.

CLIENT OUTCOMES

1. Child's respiratory function will return to normal.
2. Child will have effective airway clearance.

REFERENCES

American Academy of Pediatrics: Respiratory syncytial virus. In Pickering LK, editor: *2000 Red book: report of the Committee on Infectious Diseases,* ed 25, Elk Grove Village, Ill, 2000, The Academy.

Behrman R et al, editors: *Nelson textbook of pediatrics,* ed 16, Philadelphia, 2000, WB Saunders.

Cooper KE: The effectiveness of ribavirin in the treatment of RSV, *Pediatr Nurs* 27(1):95, 2001.

Hockenberry M: *Wong's nursing care of infants and children,* ed 7, St Louis, 2003, Mosby.

Malhostra A, Krilov L: Influenza and respiratory syncytial virus: update on infection, management and prevention, *Pediatr Clin North Am* 47(2):353, 2000.

71

❖

Reye's Syndrome

❖

PATHOPHYSIOLOGY

Reye's syndrome is a noninflammatory encephalopathy that is associated with fatty infiltration of the viscera and for which no other chemical or clinical explanation can be found.

Typically, symptoms are seen following a viral illness, but a definitive cause has not been identified. Viral infections most strongly associated with the onset of Reye's syndrome are influenza types A and B and varicella. In addition, the use of aspirin has been strongly linked to the onset of the syndrome, but it is not involved in every case. Although the American Academy of Pediatrics and the Centers for Disease Control and Prevention have issued warnings against the use of salicylates in children with possible varicella or influenza infection, the link between salicylates and Reye's syndrome remains a topic of intense discussion.

The widespread organ dysfunctions that accompany Reye's syndrome have led to speculation that the syndrome is the result of a universal mitochondrial insult from an unknown source. Abnormalities related to hepatic failure may occur, including enzyme elevations, coagulation disorders, and alterations in carbohydrate, amino acid, and lipid metabolism. Cerebral edema and neuronal necrosis are possible, and the usual cause of death is severe cerebral edema and brain tissue herniation. Other multisystem failures may occur, including myocardial failure, dehydration and shock, acute renal failure, peptic ulcers, pancreatitis, sepsis, and hypoglycemia.

Morbidity and mortality rates vary greatly from study to study, but overall, mortality rates have decreased dramatically in recent years. Early recognition and improved treatment are the most significant factors contributing to increased survival. The severity of the illness at the time of diagnosis correlates with the likelihood of recovery. Some children survive with profound intellectual and neurologic damage, whereas others have minimal to no sequelae. Psychiatric problems, including attention-focusing problems, anxiety disorders, and depression, are common in survivors. Vocal and speech disorders are also frequently reported disabilities.

INCIDENCE

1. Reye's syndrome is the major cause of noninfectious neurologic death following a viral illness in the pediatric age group.
2. Reye's syndrome occurs in infants and children of all age groups, with the highest incidence in children 5 to 14 years of age.
3. No gender preference is noted.
4. Reye's syndrome occurs most frequently in winter months.
5. Reye's syndrome usually appears 5 to 7 days after a viral illness has resolved.

CLINICAL MANIFESTATIONS
Phase I

1. Recovery from viral illness
2. Improvement of condition

Phase II

1. Acute deterioration about 5 to 7 days following phase I
2. Vomiting
3. Fever
4. Altered mental status that may deteriorate rapidly
5. Tachypnea
6. Hyperpnea
7. Increased intracranial pressure
8. Sluggish pupillary response
9. Seizures
10. Coma

See Table 71-1 for one of a variety of staging systems that establish criteria to assess the severity of Reye's syndrome.

TABLE 71-1
Staging of Reye's Syndrome

Criterion	Stage				
	I	II	III	IV	V
Level of consciousness	Lethargy; follows verbal commands; vomiting; sleepiness	Combativeness or stupor; verbalizes inappropriately; disorientation	Coma	Coma; seizures	Coma; no respirations; flaccid paralysis
Posture	Normal	Normal	Decorticate	Decerebrate	Flaccid
Response to pain	Purposeful	Purposeful or nonpurposeful	Decorticate	Decerebrate	None
Pupillary reaction	Brisk	Sluggish	Sluggish	Sluggish	None
Oculocephalic reflex ("doll's eyes")	Normal	Conjugate deviation	Conjugate deviation	Inconsistent or absent	None

Modified from National Institutes of Health Consensus Development Conference, March 1981; and Lovejoy FH et al: *Am J Dis Child* 128:136, 1974.

COMPLICATIONS

1. Encephalopathy
2. Cerebral herniation
3. Hepatic failure
4. Multiple organ failure
5. Gastrointestinal hemorrhage
6. Pancreatitis (severe complication with poor prognosis)

LABORATORY AND DIAGNOSTIC TESTS

1. Serum transaminase values—elevated alanine aminotransferase and aspartate aminotransferase, to at least 1.5 to 2 times normal values
2. Prothrombin and partial thromboplastin times—prolonged
3. Serum glucose level—decreased
4. Serum amylase level—elevated
5. Serum lactic dehydrogenase level—elevated
6. Serum ammonia level—hyperammonemia; elevated to at least twice normal levels
7. Serum creatinine phosphokinase level—elevated
8. Serum lipase level—elevated
9. Serum bilirubin level—usually normal
10. Liver biopsy—to define histopathologic features (usually in infants and atypical cases only)
11. Lumbar puncture—to rule out bacterial meningitis or viral encephalitis (controversial), elevated opening pressure
12. Computed tomography—to rule out other causes of encephalopathy
13. Electroencephalogram—to predict survival

MEDICAL MANAGEMENT

Medical management is supportive and is based on the child's stage of illness. Children with stage I Reye's syndrome must be hospitalized for close observation because progression of symptoms may occur rapidly. Intravenous hydration with a high-dextrose solution is needed to keep serum glucose levels normal. Children with stage II to V Reye's syndrome require aggressive therapy in a pediatric intensive care unit. Measures must be implemented to normalize intracranial pressure and provide support to failing systems. Restoration of a normal temperature and prevention of infection are priorities. The following medications may be used:

1. Anticoagulants
2. Sedatives
3. Vitamin K—for prothrombin deficiencies
4. Mannitol—osmotic diuretic for control of intracranial hypertension
5. Vecuronium—for paralysis of skeletal muscles, to enhance ventilation

NURSING ASSESSMENT

1. See the Neurologic Assessment section in Appendix A.
2. Assess respiratory pattern.
3. Assess hydration status.

NURSING DIAGNOSES

- Tissue perfusion, Ineffective
- Fluid volume, Deficient
- Hyperthermia
- Nutrition: less than body requirements, Imbalanced
- Anxiety

NURSING INTERVENTIONS

1. Maintain patency of airway.
   a. Monitor respiratory status.
   b. Check patency of endotracheal tube and airway.
   c. Check ventilator settings.
   d. Irrigate and suction as needed.
2. Monitor neurologic status with serial measures.
   a. Report any deterioration or questionable findings; intervention may be required on an emergency basis.
   b. Monitor level of consciousness.
      i. General appearance
      ii. Arousability
      iii. Orientation
      iv. Restlessness

   c. Monitor vital signs.
     i. Respiratory pattern
     ii. Blood pressure
     iii. Heart rate
     iv. Temperature
   d. Check pupils (pupils equal in size, react to light, accommodate [PERLA]).
   e. Monitor reaction to pain.
   f. Check head circumference (check fontanelles).
   g. Use Glasgow Coma Scale (see the Neurologic Assessment section in Appendix A).

3. Avoid increase in intracranial pressure.
   a. Keep head in midline.
   b. Elevate head of bed 30 to 45 degrees.
   c. Avoid knee flexion.
   d. Avoid use of restraints.
   e. Avoid letting child cry.
   f. Provide calm, quiet environment.

4. Maintain adequate nutrition and fluid balance.
   a. Monitor nasogastric tube drainage.
   b. Monitor for residuals before feedings.
   c. Monitor infusion of hypertonic glucose and electrolytes.
   d. Monitor central venous pressure and arterial pressure.
   e. Monitor intake and output.

5. Administer medications and monitor child's response.
   a. Therapeutic response
   b. Side effects

6. Monitor for complications.
   a. Atelectasis
   b. Hypoxia
   c. Respiratory disorders
   d. Coma
   e. Seizures
   f. Increased secretion of antidiuretic hormone

7. Prevent skin breakdown through frequent skin care, change of position, and use of pressure mattress or sheepskin pad.

8. Provide lubrication to eyes to prevent drying and ulceration.
9. Use cooling measures.
10. Provide environmental stimulation (e.g., auditory and tactile), because child may be able to hear and feel even though unresponsive.

🔺 Discharge Planning and Home Care

1. Instruct parents about long-term management.
   a. Administration of medications
   b. Level of exercise
   c. Infection control
2. Give anticipatory guidance related to recovery.
   a. Abnormalities present in early phase of recovery often improve or disappear completely in 6 to 12 months; most common sequelae are motor and intellectual deficits.
   b. Hearing impairments have been reported and may require individual evaluation.
   c. Voice and speech disorders such as aphonia, slurred speech, and dysfluency may occur; severely impaired voice function does not necessarily imply that child is intellectually impaired.

CLIENT OUTCOMES

1. Child's neurologic function will be maximized.
2. Family will understand rehabilitation plan.
3. Child's nutritional status will be normalized.

REFERENCES

Behrman R et al, editors: *Nelson textbook of pediatrics*, ed 16, Philadelphia, 2000, WB Saunders.

Hazinski MF: *Nursing care of the critically ill child,* ed 3, St Louis, 1996, Mosby.

Hockenberry M: *Wong's nursing care of infants and children*, ed 7, St Louis, 2003, Mosby.

Mascarella J, Hudson D: Dysimmune neurologic disorders, *AACN Clin Issues Crit Care Nurs* 2(4):675, 1991.

Orlowski JP: Whatever happened to Reye's syndrome? Did it ever really exist? *Crit Care Med* 27(8):1582, 1999.

72

❖

Rheumatic Fever: Acute

❖

PATHOPHYSIOLOGY

Acute rheumatic fever is an inflammatory disease that follows a group A beta-hemolytic *Streptococcus* infection. This disease causes pathologic lesions in the heart, blood vessels, joints, and subcutaneous tissue. The symptoms of rheumatic fever are manifested approximately 1 to 5 weeks after the infection occurs. The initial symptoms, as well as the severity of the disease, are widely varied. Arthritis, in the form of migratory polyarthritis, is the most common symptom (75%) that is initially seen. Symptoms can be classified as cardiac and noncardiac and may develop gradually. Diagnosis is based on the revised Jones criteria from the American Heart Association (Box 72-1). Meeting of two major criteria or one major and two minor criteria indicates an increased possibility of rheumatic fever. Prognosis depends on the severity of cardiac involvement.

INCIDENCE

1. One out of 2000 children between the ages of 5 and 15 years is affected.
2. Crowded living conditions increase the risk of developing acute rheumatic fever.
3. Frequency is increased in males.
4. Incidence is increased among children who have previously had rheumatic fever.
5. A 30% to 67% incidence of heart disease is seen 10 years after an individual has had rheumatic fever.
6. Incidence has increased in the United States and Europe since the late 1980s, possibly as a result of an increase in

BOX 72-1
Revised Jones Criteria

Major Criteria
- Arthritis
- Carditis
- Erythema marginatum
- Subcutaneous nodules
- Sydenham's chorea

Minor Criteria
- Previous history of rheumatic fever
- Arthralgia
- Elevated levels of acute phase reactants
- Prolonged PR interval visible on electrocardiogram
- Fever

Evidence of Streptococcal Infection
- Positive culture
- Scarlatiniform rash
- Elevated level of streptococcal antibodies

From Stollerman G et al: Jones criteria (revised) for guidance in the diagnosis of rheumatic fever, *Circulation* 32:664, 1965. By permission of the American Heart Association, Inc.

virulent strains or changes in medical management of acute pharyngitis.

CLINICAL MANIFESTATIONS

1. Arthritis—painful, warm, red, and swollen joints; migratory in nature, with knee, elbow, wrist, ankle most often affected
2. Arthralgia
3. Low-grade fever that usually spikes in late afternoon
4. Chest pain (symptom of carditis)
5. Shortness of breath (symptom of carditis)
6. Tachycardia—especially during rest or sleep
7. Bradycardia
8. Complaints of sore throat

9. Chorea
10. Subcutaneous nodules
11. Abdominal pain (symptom of carditis)
12. Cough (symptom of carditis)

COMPLICATION

Acquired heart disease is the primary complication of acute rheumatic fever.

LABORATORY AND DIAGNOSTIC TESTS

1. Echocardiography—to diagnose pericarditis
2. Pericardiocentesis—to diagnose pericarditis
3. Chest radiography—to detect cardiomegaly
4. Electrocardiography—atrioventricular block and prolonged PR segment are present in carditis
5. Antistreptolysin O (ASO) titer—increased
6. Antihyaluronidase antibody titers—increased in presence of streptococcal antibodies
7. Nicotinamide adenine dinucleotidase (NADase), anti-NADase, and antideoxyribonuclease B levels—increased in presence of streptococcal antibodies
8. Streptozyme—streptococcal antibody test; can be performed in lieu of ASO titer
9. Erythrocyte sedimentation rate—increased with inflammation
10. C-reactive protein level—increased with inflammation
11. Throat culture—to diagnose *Streptococcus* infection
12. White blood cell count—increased with infections

MEDICAL MANAGEMENT

Treatment includes the administration of antibiotics to eliminate any residual streptococci and to prevent recurrent infections. Corticosteroids are used to treat acute cases of carditis. The child is closely observed to detect progressive cardiac abnormalities (valvulitis). The remaining management is symptom-related and may include short-term bed rest to conserve energy and decrease pain, aspirin to minimize arthritic pain, and nutritional support.

NURSING ASSESSMENT

1. See the Cardiovascular Assessment and Musculoskeletal Assessment sections in Appendix A.
2. Assess for pain.
3. Assess temperature stability.
4. Assess activity level.
5. Assess nutritional status.

NURSING DIAGNOSES

- Activity intolerance
- Pain
- Hyperthermia
- Cardiac output, Decreased
- Family processes, Interrupted
- Anxiety
- Nutrition: less than body requirements, Imbalanced
- Knowledge, Deficient

NURSING INTERVENTIONS

1. Conserve child's energy during acute phase of disease.
   a. Maintain bed rest until laboratory results and clinical status improve.
   b. As condition improves, monitor gradual increase in level of activity.
2. Monitor child's response to and possible untoward effects of prescribed medications.
   a. Assess for signs of clinical improvement.
   b. Monitor for side effects of following medications: aspirin—bleeding tendencies, tinnitus; corticosteroids—cushingoid symptoms, increased weight gain, mood swings, psychotic behavior; antibiotics (penicillin)—allergic rash, anaphylaxis.
3. Provide pain relief measures (for arthralgia).
   a. Minimize handling.
   b. Use bed cradle for sheets.
   c. Maintain proper body alignment.
   d. Administer aspirin.
   e. Change child's position every 2 hours.

4. Implement age-appropriate safety precautions (for chorea and muscle weakness).
5. Use cooling measures as needed.
6. Support and maintain nutritional status (child may be anorexic during acute phase).
   a. Offer small, frequent meals (include fluids).
   b. Incorporate child's food preferences.
   c. Encourage independence in eating when possible (muscle weakness may impose limits); choose items from menu; arrange foods attractively on tray; arrange meal schedule.
   d. Offer high-quality, nutritious foods.
7. Provide emotional support to child and family.
   a. Encourage parents to express feelings.
   b. Encourage child to share feelings of helplessness, shame, and fear regarding manifestations of disease (e.g., chorea, carditis, and muscle weakness).
   c. Act as child and family advocate and liaison with members of health care team.
   d. Encourage child's contact with peers.
   e. Encourage involvement in age-appropriate recreational and diversional activities.

🔺 Discharge Planning and Home Care

Instruct parents about methods of secondary prevention.

1. Observe for signs and symptoms of recurrence.
2. Administer prophylactic antibiotics (oral formulations administered on continuous basis; intramuscular [IM] formulations administered once per month) and explain rationale for use.
3. Obtain follow-up throat culture 4 or 5 days after oral penicillin is discontinued, 3 weeks after IM penicillin G benzathine is discontinued.
4. Assist in planning activities if child is to remain in bed after hospitalization.
5. Alert dentist about child's condition before any dental care is performed.

CLIENT OUTCOMES

1. Child's musculoskeletal and cardiac function will return to normal.
2. Pain will be eliminated.
3. Child and family will understand home care instructions and importance of follow-up visits and prophylactic antibiotics.

REFERENCES

Behrman R, Kliegman R, editors: *Nelson essentials of pediatrics,* ed 4, St Louis, 2002, Mosby.

Hockenberry M: *Wong's nursing care of infants and children,* ed 7, St Louis, 2003, Mosby.

Hoekelman R et al: *Primary pediatric care,* ed 4, St Louis, 2001, Mosby.

Stollerman G: Rheumatic fever, *Lancet* 349(9056): 935, 1997.

73

◆

Scoliosis

◆

PATHOPHYSIOLOGY

Scoliosis, a frequently occurring orthopedic problem, is the lateral curvature of the spine with a Cobb angle of more than 10 degrees accompanied by vertebral rotation. It can occur anywhere along the spine. Curvatures in the thoracic area are the most common, although curvatures of the cervical and lumbar areas are the most deforming. There are two basic forms of scoliosis: functional and structural. Functional scoliosis is secondary to a preexisting problem such as poor posture or unequal leg length. This form of scoliosis can be corrected through exercises or the use of shoe lifts. Structural scoliosis results from the congenital deformity of the spinal column. This condition often occurs in children with myelomeningocele and muscular dystrophy. Scoliosis is also seen in children with cerebral palsy and osteogenesis imperfecta. The structural form of scoliosis can be classified into three basic types: (1) infantile, which occurs during the first year of life (more than 20% of affected children have spontaneous resolution); (2) juvenile, which occurs between 5 and 6 years of age (bracing is used for management); and (3) adolescent, which is not evident until 11 years of age (when skeletal maturation occurs). Management of scoliosis may include nonsurgical and/or surgical methods. Most spinal curvatures do not progress more than 20%. The curvature is flexible initially and becomes rigid with age.

INCIDENCE

1. Familial tendency is noted in one third of diagnosed cases.

2. Male-female ratio of occurrence is 1:6.
3. Adolescent scoliosis is the most common form.

CLINICAL MANIFESTATIONS

Localized lordosis, axial rotation, and lateral curvature of the spine are the major clinical manifestations of scoliosis.

1. Asymmetry of hips
2. Asymmetry of shoulders
3. Shortened trunk
4. Associated skin and soft tissue changes
5. Patches of hair in sacral area
6. Unequal leg lengths
7. Asymmetric scapulae
8. Malalignment of trunk and pelvis
9. Asymmetry of flanks
10. Asymmetry of breasts

COMPLICATIONS

1. Urinary problems (most common)
2. Neurologic problems
3. Cardiopulmonary impairment

LABORATORY AND DIAGNOSTIC TESTS

1. Forward bending test, or Adam's position—to assess inequality of flank and ribs (screening test)
2. Cobb diagnostic method—to assess angle of curvature on radiographic studies
3. Anteroposterior and lateral radiographic studies of spine—to evaluate curvature of spine
4. Three-dimensional computerized tomography
5. Magnetic resonance imaging

MEDICAL MANAGEMENT

1. Curves of less than 20 degrees require evaluation every 3 to 12 months.
2. The Milwaukee brace is used for treatment of lateral curvature of 20 to 40 degrees; the brace consists of neck ring and pelvic girdle, and it must be worn 23 hours a day until curvature is corrected.

3. The Orthoplast jacket is a molded plastic jacket that is used for the same purpose as the Milwaukee brace.
4. The Charleston bending brace is worn at night.

SURGICAL MANAGEMENT

A posterior spinal fusion is the treatment of choice for a spinal curvature greater than 40 degrees or for a curve that progressively worsens in spite of nonsurgical treatment. Spinal fusion provides a permanent method of halting the progressive worsening of the spinal curvature. Several different types of instrumentation are used to stabilize the spine internally, including the Harrington rod, Luque rod (segmental spinal instrumentation), and Dwyer cables. Use of the Luque rod instrumentation is a more recent and preferred technique in the surgical correction of scoliosis. During the surgery, bone chips from the posterior iliac crest are positioned on top of the spine. External immobilization with the use of a body cast is then not needed because greater internal immobilization is achieved with this technique.

Anterior thoracic discectomy procedures with endplate ablations and posterior spinal fusions are recommended for individuals with severe scoliosis. Video-assisted thoracoscopic surgery is used in some institutions to release the anterior spine of these individuals.

NURSING ASSESSMENT

1. See the Musculoskeletal Assessment section in Appendix A.
2. Assess for asymmetry of flank, ribs, scapulae, and hips.
3. Assess for malalignment of trunk and pelvis.

NURSING DIAGNOSES

- Knowledge, Deficient
- Injury, Risk for
- Mobility, Impaired physical
- Gas exchange, Impaired
- Fluid volume, Risk for deficient
- Pain
- Therapeutic regimen management, Ineffective
- Body image, Disturbed

NURSING INTERVENTIONS
Preoperative Care

1. Prepare child/adolescent and family before procedures for sequence of events and sensations that will be experienced.
   a. Complete blood count—to assess for anemia
   b. Blood chemistry analysis—to assess for electrolyte imbalances
   c. Coagulation studies (prothrombin)
   d. Radiography of skull
   e. Pulmonary function tests—to assess for pulmonary complications
   f. Arterial blood gas values—to assess for pulmonary complications
   g. Myelography—to rule out genitourinary and neurologic abnormalities
   h. Spinal radiography—to assess curvature of spine
2. Prepare child/adolescent for surgery (see the Preparation for Procedures or Surgery section in Appendix J).
3. Orient child/adolescent to intensive care unit and treatment procedures used postoperatively (e.g., blow gloves and spirometer).

Postoperative Care

1. Monitor for signs and symptoms of potential complications.
   a. Monitor arterial lines.
   b. Monitor temperature, respirations, blood pressure, and pulse every 1 to 2 hours until stable, then every 4 hours.
   c. Auscultate breath sounds; report changes in respiratory status (increased respirations, increased congestion, color change, chest pain, dyspnea).
   d. Monitor for spinal nerve trauma—observe lower extremities for warmth, sensation, movement, pulses, and pain.
   e. Monitor for paralytic ileus—auscultate bowel sounds.
   f. Monitor dressing for intactness and signs of complications.
      i. Note bleeding along incision.
      ii. Monitor for signs of infection.

2. Promote proper body alignment.
    a. Turn child/adolescent every 2 hours (log roll only).
    b. Monitor for reddened areas and pressure.
    c. Keep child/adolescent flat in bed until doctor orders activity (flat with log rolling only until body jacket arrives [not always ordered with Harrington rod because child is out of bed by 2 to 4 days after surgery]).
    d. Institute passive range-of-motion exercises second postoperative day.
3. Promote pulmonary ventilation.
    a. Monitor vital signs as often as every 2 hours.
    b. Have child/adolescent cough, turn, and deep breathe as often as every 2 hours.
    c. Use incentive spirometer every 2 hours.
    d. Monitor respiratory status every 2 hours until stable, then every 4 hours.
4. Monitor fluid and electrolyte balance.
    a. Monitor and record intake and output—intravenous fluids, urine, nasogastric drainage.
    b. Monitor bowel sounds.
    c. Advance diet as tolerated (clear liquid to regular diet).
    d. Monitor for signs and symptoms of dehydration and fluid overload (dehydration—decreased urinary output, increased specific gravity, doughy skin, dry mucous membranes; fluid overload—increased apical pulse, increased respiratory rate, pulmonary congestion, dyspnea, edema [initially of extremities]).
5. Provide pain relief measures as necessary (may have epidural catheter and/or patient-controlled anesthesia) (see Appendix H).
    a. Medicate routinely every 2 to 4 hours for first 72 hours.
    b. Medicate before procedures.
    c. Provide diversional activities and relaxation techniques.

🔺 Discharge Planning and Home Care
Postoperative Care

1. Instruct child/adolescent and family about various aspects of care (vary according to procedure).
   a. Physical restrictions
   b. Use of body cast or jacket (thoracic-lumbar-sacral orthotics)
   c. Equipment (e.g., firm mattress), log-rolling technique
   d. Signs of infection (increased temperature, odor from cast)
   e. Incision site care
2. Encourage child/adolescent and family to express fears and body image concerns.
3. Refer to community resources (public health nurse, home health nurses) (see Appendixes K and L).
4. Encourage adherence to follow-up care regimen (clinic visits for 6 to 12 months postoperatively).

Nonsurgical Interventions

1. Instruct child/adolescent and parents in use of Milwaukee brace or Orthoplast jacket.
   a. Application and removal of brace or jacket
   b. Cleaning of brace or jacket
   c. Skin inspection for pressure sores or skin breakdown
   d. Bathing before application
   e. Use of undergarments
2. Instruct child/adolescent and parents in use of exercises and reinforce instruction.
3. Instruct child/adolescent and parents about participation in sports and recreational activities.
4. Encourage child/adolescent to express feelings of concern and inadequacy concerning brace.
   a. Distortion of body image
   b. Feelings of rejection by peers
5. Initiate community referrals (see Appendix L).
   a. School nurse to facilitate school adaptation
   b. Financial assistance resources to cover costs incurred in treatment of condition
6. Instruct child/adolescent and family about cast care.
   a. Skin care (use alcohol only)

b. Assessment for sensation and movement
c. Exercise for unaffected extremities
d. Assessment for signs of infection (musty odor, drainage on cast)
e. Petal cast edges

CLIENT OUTCOMES

1. Child will maintain proper body alignment.
2. Child will have minimal pain during first 72 hours postoperatively.
3. Child and family will understand various aspects of postoperative home care.

REFERENCES

Bridwell KH: Surgical treatment of adolescent idiopathic scoliosis: the basics and the controversies, *Spine* 19(9):1095, 1994.

Lamontagne LL et al: Anxiety and postoperative pain in children who undergo major orthopedic surgery, *Appl Nurs Res* 14(3):119, 2001.

Lonstein JE, Winter RB: The Milwaukee brace for the treatment of adolescent idiopathic scoliosis: a review of one thousand and twenty patients, *J Bone Joint Surg Am* 76(8):1207, 1994.

Lonstein JE, Winter RB: To brace or not to brace: the true value of school screening, *Spine* 22(12):1283, 1996.

Nymberg SM, Crawford AH: Video-assisted thoracoscopic releases of scoliotic anterior spines, *AORN J* 63(3):561, 1996.

Oestreich AE et al: Scoliosis circa 2000: radiologic imaging perspective. Diagnosis and pretreatment evaluation, *Skeletal Radiol* 27(11):591, 1998.

Payne WK et al: Does scoliosis have a psychological impact and does gender make a difference? *Spine* 22(12):1380, 1997.

Pinto WC et al: Common sense in the management of adolescent idiopathic scoliosis, *Orthop Clin North Am* 25(2):215, 1994.

Puno RM et al: Surgical treatment of idiopathic thoracolumbar and lumbar scoliosis in adolescent patients, *Orthop Clin North Am* 25(2):275, 1994.

Sapontzi-Krepia DS et al: Perceptions of body image, happiness and satisfaction in adolescents wearing a Boston brace for scoliosis treatment, *J Adv Nurs* 35(5):683, 2001.

Skaggs DL, Bassett GS: Adolescent idiopathic scoliosis: an update, *Am Fam Physician* 53(7):2327, 1996.

US Preventive Services Task Force: Screening for adolescent idiopathic scoliosis: policy statement, *Nurse Pract* 19(9):39, 1994.

Winter S: Preoperative assessment of the child with neuromuscular scoliosis, *Orthop Clin North Am* 25(2):239, 1994.

74

❖

Seizure Disorders

❖

PATHOPHYSIOLOGY

Seizure is a sudden, transient alteration in brain function as a result of abnormal neuronal activity and excessive cerebral electrical discharge. This activity can be partial or focal, originating in a specific area of the cerebral cortex, or generalized, involving both hemispheres of the brain. Clinical manifestations vary, depending on the area(s) of brain involvement. The types of seizure affecting children and adolescents are listed in Box 74-1. If a small area of the brain is affected, a focal (localized) seizure may occur: however, if the electrical discharge continues, the seizure may become generalized.

The causes of seizure include perinatal factors, anoxia, congenital malformations of the brain, genetic factors, infectious disease (encephalitis, meningitis), febrile illness, metabolic disorders, trauma, neoplasms, toxins, circulatory disturbances, and degenerative diseases of the nervous system. Seizures are termed *idiopathic* when no identifiable cause can be found.

Epilepsy is a disorder characterized by recurrent unprovoked seizures that are of primary cerebral origin, which indicates underlying brain dysfunction. Epilepsy is not a disease in itself.

INCIDENCE

1. At least one seizure will occur in 3% of all children by the age of 15 years; *most* will occur with fever. An estimated 0.5% to 1% of all children will experience at least one febrile seizure.
2. Nine percent of the general population will experience seizures at some time in life.

BOX 74-1

Types of Seizure: International Classification

Partial (Focal, Local) Seizures

Simple partial seizures

- Consciousness is not impaired; may include one or a combination of the following:
  1. Motor signs—twitching of the face, hand, or one side of the body; usually the same movement with every seizure and may become generalized
  2. Autonomic signs and symptoms—vomiting, sweating, flushing, pupil dilation
  3. Somatosensory or special sensory symptoms—hearing of music, feeling of falling in space, paresthesias
  4. Psychic symptoms—déjà vu, fear, panoramic vision

Complex partial seizures

- Impairment of consciousness, although the seizure may begin as a simple partial seizure
- May include automatisms or automatic movements—lip smacking, chewing, repetitive picking, or other hand movements
- May be without automatisms—staring

Generalized Seizures (Convulsive or Nonconvulsive)

Absence seizures

- Impairment of awareness and responsiveness
- Characterized by staring usually lasting less than 15 seconds
- Abrupt onset and ending, after which the child is alert and attentive
- Usually begin between ages 4 and 14 years and often resolve by age 18 years

Myoclonic seizures

- Sudden, involuntary jerks of a muscle or muscle group
- Often observed in healthy people when falling asleep, but when pathologic involve synchronous jerks of the neck, shoulders, upper arms, and legs
- Usually last less than 5 seconds and occur in clusters
- Usually no or only brief alteration in level of consciousness

Tonic-clonic seizures (grand mal)

- Begin with loss of consciousness and a tonic portion, a generalized stiffening of muscles in the limbs, trunk, and face lasting less than a minute; often preceded by an aura
- Possible loss of bladder and bowel control

Continued

BOX 74-1

Types of Seizure: International Classification— cont'd

- Absent respirations and cyanosis
- Tonic portion followed by clonic movements of the upper and lower extremities
- Lethargy, confusion, and sleep in the postictal phase

Atonic seizures

- Sudden loss of tone that may cause the eyelids to droop, the head to nod, or the individual to fall to the ground
- Brief and occurring without warning

Status Epilepticus

- Usually, generalized tonic-clonic seizures that are repeated
- Consciousness is not regained between seizures
- Potential for respiratory depression, hypotension, and hypoxia
- Requires immediate emergency medical treatment

3. One of every 100 children will have epilepsy, or recurring seizures.
4. Infections and metabolic disorders are the most common causes of seizure in children.
5. The cause is unknown in 50% of cases, although many children will be noted to be febrile.
6. Fifty percent of seizures are indicative of acute or chronic central nervous system disorders.

CLINICAL MANIFESTATIONS

See Box 74-1 for clinical manifestations.

COMPLICATIONS

1. Aspiration pneumonia
2. Asphyxia
3. Mental retardation
4. Physical injuries, especially laceration of forehead and chin

LABORATORY AND DIAGNOSTIC TESTS

1. Electroencephalography (EEG)—used to help define type and focus of seizure
   a. Diagnosis of epilepsy does not depend solely on abnormal EEG findings.
   b. Natural sleep is preferred during EEG, although sedation with monitoring may be indicated.
2. Computed tomography (CT)—uses radiographic studies more sensitive than the ordinary to detect differences in tissue density
3. Magnetic resonance imaging—produces image using magnetic field and radio waves; particularly helpful in demonstrating brain regions (posterior fossa and sellar region) not clearly seen on CT scan
4. Positron emission tomography—for evaluation of intractable seizures to assist in localizing lesions, metabolic alterations, or blood flow in brain (involves intravenous [IV] injection of radioisotopes)
5. Evoked potentials—used to determine integrity of brain sensory pathways (absent or delayed response may be indicative of pathologic condition)
6. Laboratory tests ordered on basis of child's history and examination
   a. Lumbar puncture for cerebrospinal fluid analysis—used primarily to rule out infection
   b. Complete blood count—used to rule out infection as causative agent; in cases in which trauma is suspected, hematocrit and platelet count may be evaluated
   c. Electrolyte panel—serum electrolytes, total calcium, and magnesium often ordered for first-time seizure and in children younger than 3 months of age, in whom electrolyte and metabolic causes are more common (blood glucose test may be especially helpful in young infant or child with prolonged seizure to rule out hypoglycemia)
   d. Toxic screen of serum and urine—used to rule out ingestion of toxic substance

   e. Monitoring of levels of antiepileptic drugs—used in
      early phase of management and if compliance is in
      question (see therapeutic levels given in the Medical
      Management section of this chapter)

MEDICAL MANAGEMENT

Antiepileptic drug therapy is the mainstay of medical management. Single-drug therapy is the most desirable, with the goal of
establishing a balance between seizure control and adverse side
effects. The drug of choice is based on seizure type, epileptic
syndrome, and client variables. Drug combinations may be
needed to achieve seizure control. Complete control is achieved
in only 50% to 75% of children with epilepsy.

   The mechanisms of action of antiepileptic drugs are complex and have not been well defined. Anticonvulsants may
reduce neuronal firing, facilitate the activity of inhibitory
amino acids, or reduce slow, rhythmic firing of thalamic neurons. The following are commonly used anticonvulsants:

1. Phenobarbital—indications: myoclonic seizures, tonic-
   clonic seizures, status epilepticus; therapeutic level:
   15 to 40 μg/ml
2. Phenytoin (Dilantin)—indications: partial seizures,
   tonic-clonic seizures, status epilepticus; therapeutic
   level: 5 to 20 μg/ml
3. Carbamazepine (Tegretol)—indications: partial
   seizures, tonic-clonic seizures; therapeutic level:
   4 to 12 μg/ml
4. Valproic acid (Depakene)—indications: atypical absence
   seizures, myoclonic seizures, tonic-clonic seizures, atonic
   seizures, especially useful for mixed-seizure disorders;
   therapeutic level: 50 to 120 μg/ml
5. Primidone (Mysoline)—indications: occasionally used
   to treat tonic-clonic seizures; therapeutic level:
   4 to 12 μg/ml
6. Ethosuximide (Zarontin)—indications: absence seizures;
   therapeutic level: 40 to 100 μg/ml
7. Clonazepam (Klonopin)—indications: absence seizures,
   tonic-clonic seizures, infantile spasm; therapeutic level:
   15 to 18 μg/ml

Vagus nerve stimulation is gaining increasing popularity and credibility as a treatment option for children with intractable seizures.

NURSING ASSESSMENT

1. See the Neurologic Assessment section in Appendix A.
2. Refer to Box 74-1 for specific types of seizure disorders.

NURSING DIAGNOSES

- Injury, Risk for
- Body image, Disturbed
- Coping, Risk for compromised family
- Coping, Ineffective

NURSING INTERVENTIONS

Seizures

1. Protect child from injury.
   a. Do not attempt to restrain child or give food, liquids, or medications by mouth.
   b. If child is standing or sitting so that there is threat of falling, ease child down to prevent fall.
   c. Do not place anything in child's mouth.
   d. Loosen restrictive clothing.
   e. Prevent child from hitting anything sharp by padding any objects that might be contacted and removing any sharp objects from area. Pad bed rails.
   f. Turn child on side to facilitate clearing airway of secretions.
2. Maintain detailed observation and recording of seizure activity to assist in diagnosis or assessment of medication response.
   a. Time of onset and any precipitating events
   b. Aura (some type of warning that seizure is coming)
   c. Type of seizure or description of motor movements and level of consciousness
   d. Length of seizure
   e. Interventions during seizure (medication or safety measures)
   f. Postictal phase
   g. Vital signs

3. Provide for sleep or rest after seizure.
4. Monitor child's adverse reactions to medications.
5. Monitor drug levels.

Status Epilepticus

1. Stabilize patent airway; suction as needed.
2. Provide supplemental 100% oxygen by face mask.
3. Obtain IV access for anticonvulsant or other medication; with administration of lorazepam, diazepam, phenytoin, or phenobarbital, prepare for respiratory depression and further airway management if needed.
4. Monitor vital signs.

🔺 Discharge Planning and Home Care

1. Provide information about seizures and address any misconceptions family may have.
2. Stress importance of taking medication regularly and complying with physician follow-up to monitor growth and development, and evaluate for any subtle side effects.
3. List what steps family should take to manage seizures as they occur and when to access emergency medical care.
4. Provide anticipatory guidance regarding safety.
   a. Procurement of medic-alert bracelet
   b. Practice of water safety—swimming only with competent person (knowledgeable in life saving) in close proximity
   c. Avoidance of unprotected heights
   d. Possible restrictions on operating machinery, hot appliances, or automobiles
5. Assist in understanding process by which healthy self-concept is developed.
6. Refer to National Epilepsy Foundation for information and support.
7. Refer child and family for support and counseling as needed.

CLIENT OUTCOMES

1. Child will be free of physical injury.
2. Seizure activity will be prevented or controlled.
3. Child will have positive self-esteem and self-image that enhance wellness.
4. There will be minimal changes in family dynamics due to having child with chronic condition.

REFERENCES

Amar AP et al: Vagus nerve stimulation for control of intractable seizures of childhood, *Pediatr Neurosurg* 4(34):218, 2001.

Hay W et al: *Current pediatric diagnosis and treatment,* Stamford, Conn, 2003, McGraw-Hill/Appleton-Lange.

Huff K: Seizures and epilepsy. In Berkowitz C, editor: *Pediatrics: a primary care approach,* ed 2, Philadelphia, 2000, WB Saunders.

Mandleco BL, Potts NL: Neurological alterations. In Potts NL, Mandleco BL, editors: *Pediatric nursing: caring for children and their families,* Clifton Park, NY, 2002, Delmar.

75

❖

Serious Bacterial Infection

❖

PATHOPHYSIOLOGY

Infants and toddlers with a serious bacterial infection often present with nonspecific signs of illness. The younger the child, the more difficult it is to recognize bacterial infection. If a serious bacterial infection is suspected, urgent investigation, which is called a septic workup, and immediate intravenous antibiotic therapy are required to prevent the illness from becoming more severe and to prevent rapid spread to other sites of the body.

The risk of serious bacterial illness is generally believed to be higher in infants under 3 months of age with fever than in older infants with fever. Infants and toddlers with serious bacterial infection present with the following:

1. Septicemia—presence of microorganisms in the blood with localized or systemic disease in an ill-appearing child.
2. Occult bacteremia—bacteremia in children with a benign clinical appearance and no apparent source of serious infection (e.g., pneumonia, urinary tract infection [UTI]). Factors increasing the risk of bacteremia are young age, high fever, and high white blood cell (WBC) count.

INCIDENCE

1. In febrile infants with a rectal temperature of 100.4° F (38.0° C) or higher under 3 months of age, the prevalence of serious bacterial illness is approximately 5% to 18%.
2. The risk of occult bacteremia in children 3 to 36 months of age with fever but without localizing signs is approximately 2% to 10%.

3. *Streptococcus pneumoniae* now accounts for most infections following the initiation of routine immunizations for *Haemophilus influenzae* type B.

CLINICAL MANIFESTATIONS

1. "Not doing well"
2. Fever (hypothermia common in neonates)
3. Apnea, tachypnea
4. Duskiness, mottling, cyanosis
5. Tachycardia
6. Poor feeding, weight loss
7. Vomiting, diarrhea
8. Fussiness, irritability, lethargy
9. Hypotonicity
10. Rash, petechiae, purpura
11. Bulging fontanelle, seizure activity

COMPLICATIONS (IF NOT TREATED)

1. Meningitis
2. Septic shock
3. Death

LABORATORY AND DIAGNOSTIC TESTS

1. Complete blood count with differential
2. Erythrocyte sedimentation rate, C-reactive protein level
3. Blood culture
4. Urinalysis and urine culture of specimen obtained by catheterization or suprapubic tap (20% of children with UTI have normal urinalysis but have subsequent positive culture results)
5. Lumbar puncture, spinal fluid for culture
6. Stool smear for WBCs if gastroenteritis is suspected
7. Chest radiographic studies (if symptoms suggest pneumonia)

MEDICAL MANAGEMENT

The goals of therapy are to control the fever and treat the underlying process causing the fever. Bacterial infection should be treated with appropriate antimicrobial therapy. Febrile infants younger than 1 month of age and any toxic-appearing child younger than 36 months of age should receive intravenous antibiotics in the hospital with 48 to 72 hours of observation.

NURSING ASSESSMENT

1. Monitor vital signs closely.
2. See the Respiratory Assessment and Neurologic Assessment sections in Appendix A.
3. Assess for signs of dehydration.
4. Assess child's response to medications.

NURSING DIAGNOSES

- Infection, Risk for
- Hypothermia
- Hyperthermia
- Nutrition: less than body requirements, Imbalanced
- Anxiety
- Knowledge, Deficient

NURSING INTERVENTIONS

1. Monitor child's vital signs and neurologic status (especially anterior fontanelle) as often as every 2 hours.
2. Monitor child's hydration status.
3. Observe for rashes, petechiae, and/or purpura.
4. Institute isolation procedures; keep child in isolation for 24 hours after antibiotics are started.
5. Sponge or bathe with tepid water and unbundle child to reduce fever.
6. Administer antipyretics.
7. Administer intravenous antibiotics, monitor for side effects.
8. Provide emotional support to child during lumbar puncture and other tests; restrain child to prevent injury (refer to Appendix J).
9. Provide emotional support to family; provide and reinforce information about condition and hospitalization (refer to Appendix J).

🏠 Discharge Planning and Home Care

1. Instruct parents about administration of medications and monitoring of side effects.
2. Instruct parents to follow up with health care provider, as instructed.

CLIENT OUTCOMES

1. Child will be free of infection.
2. Child's body temperature will be maintained within normal limits.
3. Child will have consistent weight gain.
4. Family will use effective coping mechanisms in managing anxiety.
5. Family will understand home care and follow-up care.

REFERENCES

Alpern ER et al: Occult bacteremia from a pediatric emergency department: current prevalence, time to detection, and outcome, *Pediatrics* 106(3):505, 2000.

Jaskiewicz JA: Febrile infants at low risk for serious bacterial infection: an appraisal of the Rochester criteria and implications for management, *Pediatrics* 94(3):390, 1994.

Prober GG: Managing the febrile infant: no rules are golden, *Contemp Pediatr* 16(6):48, 1999.

Rosenthal M: Clues offered in diagnosing a child with fever of unknown origin, *Infect Dis Child* May 2000.

76

Short Bowel Syndrome

PATHOPHYSIOLOGY

Short bowel syndrome (SBS) is the syndrome of malabsorption and malnutrition that occurs because of a congenitally malfunctioning bowel or because of resection of small bowel necessitated by congenital or acquired conditions (Box 76-1). Symptoms of SBS include chronic diarrhea, impaired nutrient absorption, malnutrition, and poor growth and development. In addition, many affected children are dependent on parenteral nutrition (PN) over the long term, which can lead to liver dysfunction and disease.

SBS has three characteristic stages:

1. Stage I: immediate postoperative period (7 to 10 days) after enterostomy is created
   a. Intractable diarrhea with massive fluid and electrolyte losses
   b. Dependence on PN
   c. Possible bowel mucosa atrophy
2. Stage II: from 2 weeks to up to 1 year after surgery
   a. Gastric acid hypersecretion leading to quick intestinal transit time and diarrhea, impaired pancreatic enzyme function, and gastric ulcers
   b. At end of stage II, stabilization of diarrhea and progression of enteral feeding, signaling adaptive hyperplasia of intestinal mucosa, including elongation of both intestinal villi and crypts

BOX 76-1
Etiology of Short Bowel Syndrome

Congenital

- Multiple intestinal atresias
- Gastroschisis
- Omphalocele
- Cloacal exstrophy
- Malrotation and volvulus
- Long-segment Hirschsprung's disease
- Meconium ileus
- Intussusception
- Superior mesenteric artery deformities

Acquired

- Necrotizing enterocolitis
- Volvulus
- Inflammatory bowel disease
- Trauma
- Arterial or venous thrombosis
- Intussusception

  3. Stage III: up to 2 years after surgery (many children do
     not reach this stage; stomas are usually reanastomosed
     at this time)
     a. Control of diarrhea
     b. Increased tolerance of enteral nutrition (EN)
Adaptation of the bowel is dependent on the following:
  1. Intestinal length: Most surgeons agree that 25 cm of
     small bowel without an intact ileocecal valve (ICV) or
     15 cm of small bowel with an intact ICV is necessary for
     tolerance of enteral feedings.
  2. ICV: This is important but not absolutely necessary
     (depending on bowel length). The ICV slows intestinal
     transit time, which increases nutrient and fluid
     absorption. In addition, the ICV prevents
     contamination of the small bowel with colonic flora and
     therefore decreases bacterial overgrowth, translocation,
     and sepsis.

3. Region of the intestine: The adaptive response is greater in the ileum than in the jejunum. During intestinal adaptation in the ileum morphologic changes in the crypts and villi allow the ileum to take over some of the functions of the jejunum. The reverse is not true.

4. The presence of EN: Early and aggressive initiation and advancement of EN, especially human breast milk, protein hydrolysate formulas, or amino acid–containing formulas, appear to promote intestinal adaptation.

5. Age: Because intestinal length doubles between the second trimester of pregnancy and full term (a full-term infant's bowel length is 250 to 300 cm), preterm infants have a greater capacity for adaptation.

6. Individual response: Liver tolerance of chronic PN, number and virulence of infections, and development of bowel obstructions from strictures or adhesions all seem to play an important role in the overall outcome.

Survival rate is reported to be 80% to 94%, with death occurring secondary to liver disease and sepsis. Cost of treatment can range from $150,000 to $500,000 per client each year.

CLINICAL MANIFESTATIONS

1. Diarrhea, ranging from acute to chronic
2. Poor tolerance of EN
3. Poor and inconsistent growth—evidence of failure to thrive
4. Malnutrition (poor carbohydrate and fat absorption)
5. Jaundice
6. Anemia

COMPLICATIONS

Early Signs and Symptoms

1. Fluid-electrolyte imbalance—particularly in early postoperative period
2. Diarrhea
3. Sepsis
4. Gastric acid hypersecretion

5. Skin breakdown, especially on buttocks, perineum, and enterostomy site

Late Signs and Symptoms

1. Nutritional deficiencies, poor growth and development
2. Poor healing
3. Osteopenia
4. Oral aversion
5. Difficulty advancing enteral feedings
6. Vitamin and mineral deficiency
7. Need for multiple surgeries, particularly for bowel obstructions
8. Gallbladder disease
9. Hepatomegaly indicative of liver disease

LABORATORY AND DIAGNOSTIC TESTS

1. Complete blood count (CBC) with differential and platelet count—may be increased or decreased white blood cell count with sepsis, decreased platelets, and anemia secondary to liver dysfunction
2. Serum electrolyte, glucose, blood urea nitrogen, creatinine levels—to assess fluid and electrolyte imbalances, tolerance of PN
3. Liver function test—to assess liver tolerance of PN
4. Alkaline phosphatase levels—to assess liver function and monitor course of cholestasis
5. Dipstick testing or urinalysis for protein, glucose, blood, and ketones—to assess tolerance of PN
6. Gastric pH—to assess presence of gastric acid hypersecretion
7. Stool Hematest, test for reducing substances, stool Ictotest—to assess tolerance of EN, check for presence of bile in stool
8. Abdominal radiographic study—to check for dilated or obstructed loops of bowel
9. Ultrasonography of liver and gallbladder—to check for cholestasis and gallstones
10. Liver scan—uses radioactive isotope to help determine liver function
11. Liver biopsy—to diagnose liver disease

MEDICAL MANAGEMENT

The medical management of SBS focuses on the minimization of symptoms through medication and diet therapy until intestinal adaptation can occur. Surgical interventions are offered as needed.

Medications

The following medications may be used for the complications indicated.

1. Diarrhea
   a. Loperamide (Imodium)—an antidiarrheal opioid agent that slows transit time, thereby increasing absorption of water and nutrients
   b. Cholestyramine—bile-salt binder to decrease secretory diarrhea
   c. Octreotide acetate (Sandostatin)—decreases secretory diarrhea by inhibiting exocrine and endocrine, gastrointestinal, and pancreatic secretions (little is known about effects in infants; decreases insulin and growth hormone levels)
2. Gastric acid hypersecretion: ranitidine (Zantac)—H_2 blocker to increase gastric pH, slow transit time, and prevent ulcers and breakdown at anastomosis site (gastric acid hypersecretion should be temporary [up to 6 months]; medications in this class may promote bacterial overgrowth of the small intestine)
3. Liver dysfunction
   a. Phenobarbital—increases liver enzyme induction
   b. Ursodiol (Actigall)—increases bile excretion; absorbed in ileum
   c. Cholecystokinin—initiates gallbladder contractions
4. Intestinal bacterial overgrowth
   a. Trimethoprim (Bactrim)—use a half-dose for antibiotic prophylaxis to "sterilize" the intestine and to prevent bacterial overgrowth, translocation, and sepsis
   b. Metronidazole (Flagyl)—same as trimethoprim
   c. Probiotics (Lactobacillus GG)—live, human-derived microorganisms that improve intestinal microbial balance

  5. Vitamin and mineral deficiency
     a. ADEKs drops—fat-soluble vitamin supplementation
     b. Cyanocobalamin (B_{12})—injections usually needed after first few months as child is weaned off PN
     c. Mineral supplements—zinc aids in healing; selenium plays role in antioxidant system

Nutritional Interventions

1. Stage I
   a. Provide PN in a central venous catheter to supply sufficient calories, proteins, and amino acids for healing and sustained growth.
   b. Replace fluid and electrolytes lost in abnormal quantities, particularly sodium, with a replacement fluid other than PN.
   c. Once postoperative gastrointestinal motility has returned, provide minimal enteral nutrition of human breast milk or dilute formula and advance aggressively in both strength and volume as tolerated. Rates as low as 1 ml/hr may prevent mucosal atrophy and decrease intestinal adaptation time.
2. Stages II and III
   a. Begin cycling of PN. Although this remains highly debated, it appears to decrease incidence of cholestasis and allows for some time with greater freedom of movement for the child.
   b. Continue to advance enteral feedings with human breast milk or an elemental formula such as Alimentum (Ross Laboratories, Columbus, Ohio) or Pregestimil (Mead Johnson, Evansville, Indiana). If the infant is premature, change gradually to premature formula as tolerated.
   c. Provide enteral feedings through continuous infusion into the stomach, through either an orogastric or a gastrostomy tube. Continuous feedings will maximize absorption.
   d. Begin oral motor stimulation program.
   e. Increase feedings until stool volume output increases by 50% or is greater than about 40 to 50 ml/kg/day and/or significant malabsorption occurs.

   f. Provide mineral supplements such as zinc and selenium.
   g. Delete copper and manganese if liver dysfunction
      occurs.
   h. Introduce strained baby foods as tolerated when
      developmentally appropriate. Infant cereals and meats
      are most well tolerated.

SURGICAL MANAGEMENT

Surgical interventions are designed to slow transit time,
increase mucosal surface area, or increase intestinal length.

   Indications for surgical intervention include poor tolerance
of EN; numerous complications of PN, such as multiple
catheter-related infections, limiting venous access; and liver
dysfunction and disease. The following surgical options may be
used.

   1. Surgeries to slow intestinal transit time
      a. Intestinal valve—the creation of an intestinal valve to
         slow transit time (clinical experience is limited)
      b. Reversed intestinal segment—the interposition
         of a 3 to 6 cm (in pediatric clients) segment of
         bowel in which peristalsis is opposite to normal
         direction; most effective when placed in the distal
         bowel (limited to those who have longer small bowel
         length)
      c. Colon interposition—the interposition of a segment
         of colon between two segments of small bowel; this
         may slow transit time by virtue of the colon's
         inherently slow peristalsis, increasing absorption of
         fluids and electrolytes (small number of cases
         reported)
      d. Reverse electrical intestinal pacing—the application
         of electrical signals to the distal region of the small
         bowel to initiate retrograde peristalsis and thereby
         slow transit time (no successful clinical reports but
         further study is needed)
   2. Surgeries to increase mucosal surface area
      a. Tapering enteroplasty—reduces the caliber of
         dilated small bowel while preserving intestinal
         length; this should theoretically increase peristalsis

and decrease bacterial overgrowth (clinical experience is limited)

  b. Neomucosa—the transplantation or patching of intestine with new mucosa that has been grown from a cut edge of normal bowel (remains experimental; only done in animal trials to date)

3. Surgeries to increase intestinal length
  a. Bianchi intestinal lengthening procedure—the division of a segment of dilated bowel and creation of an end-to-end anastomosis, which results in a doubling of length
  b. Iowa procedure—a two-step surgery in which first a segment of bowel is secured to the undersurface of the liver or the posterior abdominal wall musculature to help bowel develop neovascularization; once this occurs (over a period of time) a second surgery is performed allowing for longitudinal division of the bowel (limited clinical use but promising early results)
  c. Small bowel transplantation—has had limited success but survival rates have improved with more effective immunosuppressive therapy (reserved for those with end-stage liver disease, complete intestinal failure, or lack of venous access)
  d. Multiorgan transplantation (liver and small bowel)—has had limited success (reserved for those with end-stage liver disease)

NURSING ASSESSMENT

1. See the Gastrointestinal Assessment section in Appendix A.
2. Assess for fluid and electrolyte imbalances.
3. Assess hydration status.
4. Assess child's tolerance of PN.
5. Assess child's readiness for and tolerance of EN.
6. Assess child for presence of pain (see Appendix H).
7. Assess for signs and symptoms of infection.
8. Assess for signs of skin breakdown.
9. Assess child's height and weight, head circumference, and pattern of growth (see Appendix I).
10. Assess child's response to medications.

11. Assess family's response to hospitalization and child's condition.
12. Assess family's readiness for discharge and ability to manage home treatment regimen.

NURSING DIAGNOSES

- Fluid volume, Deficient
- Pain
- Infection, Risk for
- Nutrition: less than body requirements, Imbalanced
- Skin integrity, Risk for impaired
- Growth and development, Delayed
- Family processes, Interrupted
- Therapeutic regimen management, Ineffective
- Caregiver role strain, Risk for

NURSING INTERVENTIONS

1. Assess for fluid and electrolyte imbalances, hydration status, and tolerance of PN.
   a. Monitor vital signs, perfusion, and mucous membranes.
   b. Monitor urine output and dipstick findings.
   c. Monitor serum and urine electrolytes and serum glucose.
   d. Monitor serum nutritional laboratory test results.
2. Monitor readiness for and tolerance of EN.
   a. Record and monitor intake, stool and enterostomy output, and emesis.
   b. Measure abdominal girth.
   c. Perform Hematest on stool.
   d. Test stool for reducing substances.
3. Monitor for verbal and nonverbal pain behaviors; implement nonpharmacologic and pharmacologic pain measures (see Appendix H).
4. Assess for any signs or symptoms of infection.
   a. Monitor serum CBC, differential, and platelets as ordered.
   b. In newborn infants, monitor for temperature, glucose instability, lethargy, and poor perfusion.
   c. In older children, monitor for poor feeding, increased temperature, and irritability.

5. Monitor for growth deficiencies.
   a. Record weight daily.
   b. Record length and head circumference weekly (see Appendix I).
   c. Plot growth parameters on growth chart (see Appendix I).
   d. Monitor serum laboratory results, assessing nutritional status.
6. Monitor for therapeutic and adverse effects of medications.
7. Monitor for appropriate growth and development (see Appendix B).
   a. Initiate developmental evaluation and treatment plan.
   b. Initiate oral stimulation program.
   c. Encourage age-appropriate use of toys and age-appropriate activities.
   d. Encourage contact with peers (older children).
8. Support family.
   a. Involve parents and family in client's care.
   b. Encourage therapeutic communication.
   c. Consider evaluation by and support from social worker.
   d. Assist family in identifying and utilizing resources and support systems.
9. Educate family on client care and discharge planning.

🔺 Discharge Planning and Home Care

1. Instruct family about home administration of nutrition.
   a. PN—how to obtain and administer
   b. EN—how to obtain, mix, and administer
2. Instruct family about medications—administration and desired and undesired effects.
3. Instruct family about care of central venous catheter.
4. Instruct family about enterostomy care (if applicable).
5. Arrange follow-up appointments with specialists and primary care physician.
6. Arrange any developmental and/or oral stimulation program follow-up (see Appendixes B and L).

7. Employ family support strategies.
   a. Assist family in identifying support systems.
   b. Encourage open communication.
   c. Encourage family to participate in child's care.

CLIENT OUTCOMES

1. Client will be able to be weaned from PN to EN.
2. Client will be free of infections.
3. Family will be able to adhere to treatment regimen.

REFERENCES

Andorsky DJ et al: Nutritional and other postoperative management of neonates with short bowel syndrome correlates with clinical outcomes, *J Pediatr* 139(1):27, 2001.

Bilodeau JA: A home parenteral nutrition program for infants, *J Obstet Gynecol Neonatal Nurs* 24(1):72, 1995.

Hwang ST, Shulman RJ: Update on management and treatment of short gut, *Clin Perinatol* 29(1):181, 2002.

Warner BW et al: What's new in the management of short gut syndrome in children, *J Am Coll Surg* 190(6):725, 2000.

Wessel J: Short bowel syndrome. In Groh-Wargo et al, editors: *Nutritional care for high risk newborns*, ed 3, Chicago, 2000, Precept Press.

77

◆

Sickle Cell Anemia

◆

PATHOPHYSIOLOGY

Sickle cell anemia, or homozygous sickle cell disease (Hb SS), is an inherited autosomal recessive disorder. The basic defect is a mutant autosomal gene that effects a substitution of valine for glutamic acid on the beta chain of hemoglobin. The result is a person with the disease or with sickle cell trait (heterozygous form Hb AS). There are other variants of sickle cell anemia, with Hb SC, Hb SB thalassemia, Hb SD, and Hb SE being the most common. Sickled red blood cells are crescent shaped, have decreased oxygen-carrying capacity, and have a greater destruction rate than do normal red blood cells. The life span of sickled cells is diminished to 10 to 30 days (normal is 120 days). Sickled cells are extremely rigid because of the gelled hemoglobin, cellular dehydration, and an inflexible membrane. The rigid cells become trapped in the circulatory system, which leads to a vicious cycle of infarction and progressive sickling.

Splenic hypofunction and, later, splenic atrophy result in reticuloendothelial failure and an incidence of infection that is 600 times higher in children with sickle cell disease than in the normal population. Children are born with fetal hemoglobin, which consists of a gamma chain; therefore, until approximately 6 months of age, when the hemoglobin begins to change to the adult type, symptoms of the disease do not usually occur (Box 77-1).

Sickle cell crises result from physiologic changes producing a decrease in oxygen available to the hemoglobin, which are typically precipitated by dehydration, infection, and hypoxia. Sickling of cells results in clumping of red blood cells in the vessels, decreased oxygen transport, and increased destruction of red blood cells. Ischemia, infarct, and tissue necrosis result from the obstruction of vessels and decreased blood flow. Three types of crisis occur: (1) vasoocclusive (painful), (2) splenic sequestration, and (3) aplastic. Sickle cell crises occur less frequently with age. Mortality in the first years of life is usually caused by infection and sequestration crisis.

INCIDENCE

1. Incidence of sickle cell trait among African Americans is estimated at 1 in 12, and incidence of sickle cell disease is estimated at 1 in 375. The disease has also been reported occasionally in those from certain areas of the Mediterranean basin, the Middle East, and India. Approximately 2000 infants are born with sickle cell disease each year in the United States.
2. Death occurs most frequently in children 1 to 3 years of age from organ failure or thrombosis of major organs, most commonly the lungs and brain.
3. With new treatments, 85% of affected individuals survive to the age of 20 years; 50% survive beyond 50 years.

CLINICAL MANIFESTATIONS

1. Vasoocclusive crisis (painful crisis) results from ischemia in tissue distal to occlusion. Crises can occur when the child has an illness that causes dehydration or a respiratory infection that lowers oxygen exchange. Other precipitating events can be exposure to cold, anesthesia, high altitudes, or extremely strenuous exercise. Fifty percent of children will have a vasoocclusive crisis by 1 year of age and close to

BOX 77-1

Early Detection: Newborn Screening Programs

- Morbidity and mortality can be significantly reduced with newborn screening and early intervention.
- Screening should include prenatal, maternal, and neonatal screening.
- Public education is critical for effective neonatal screening. Target groups include day care centers, schools, and the media.

100% will suffer from one by the age of 6 years.
Vasoocclusive crisis is characterized by the following symptoms:

a. Irritability
b. Vomiting
c. Fever
d. Anorexia
e. Pain in extremities, back, or chest
f. Dactylitis (hand-and-foot syndrome)—decreased range of motion and inflamed extremities (common in young infants)
g. Abdominal crisis
h. Cerebrovascular accidents (CVAs)
i. Ocular hemorrhages

2. Sequestration crisis (usually seen in children 5 to 36 months of age, with 76% of cases occurring before age 2 years) is due to the sequestration of sickled blood within the spleen over a period of hours, which rapidly decreases the hemoglobin level (blood pooled in the spleen is not available to the general circulation). Children are subject to fatal splenic rupture and/or splenic atrophy. Signs and symptoms of sequestration crisis are as follows:

a. Rapid and massive enlargement of spleen (splenomegaly)
b. Rapid fall in hemoglobin level, anemia
c. Tachycardia, dyspnea, pallor, syncope, and weakness (common)
d. Nausea, vomiting
e. Sudden, severe abdominal pain
f. Enlargement of liver
g. Circulatory collapse and shock

3. Aplastic crisis results from a transient suppression of red cell production while hemolysis continues at the same rate. It often occurs in association with an infection when the strong compensatory mechanism is depressed (parvovirus B19, *Salmonella*, *Streptococcus*, *Mycoplasma*, Epstein-Barr virus infections). Aplastic crisis typically occurs in children younger than 10 years. Signs and symptoms of aplastic crisis are as follows:

   a. Weakness, fatigue, dizziness
   b. Pallor
   c. Fever
   d. Dyspnea
   e. Anorexia
   f. Arthralgia
   g. Tachycardia
   h. Decreased hemoglobin level, hematocrit, and reticulocyte count
   i. Shock

COMPLICATIONS

1. Increased risk of bacterial infection primarily due to hypofunctional spleen, e.g., overwhelming sepsis, meningitis (children with sickle cell anemia have 36 times greater incidence of pneumococcal meningitis), pneumococcal pneumonia, *Salmonella* osteomyelitis
2. Delayed onset of puberty
3. Impaired fertility
4. Priapism
5. Gallstones
6. Leg ulcers
7. Chronic heart, liver, and kidney disease
8. Proliferative retinopathy
9. Depression, isolation, and low self-esteem
10. Enuresis
11. Risk for drug addiction (actual prevalence in this population is low, according to recent literature)
12. Strained parent-child relationships
13. CVAs (10%, especially between ages of 3 and 10 years)
14. Avascular necrosis
15. "Acute chest syndrome"—respiratory distress with cough and tachypnea, high fever, chest pain, and infiltrate on chest radiographic studies

LABORATORY AND DIAGNOSTIC TESTS

1. Hemoglobin electrophoresis, preferably at birth for all infants as part of newborn screening—this test can quantify percentage of hemoglobin S present. If disorder is

not identified at birth, diagnosis is rarely made before 6 to 12 months of age.

2. Tests of fetal blood or fetal cells—these tests make prenatal diagnosis possible between 9 and 11 weeks' gestation.

MEDICAL MANAGEMENT

Medical management focuses on pain control, oxygenation, hydration, and careful monitoring for complications of vasoocclusion. Administration of prophylactic penicillin to prevent septicemia should be initiated at 2 to 3 months of age and continued through 5 to 6 years of life. Immunizations are crucial to protect these children from infection. Specifically required are (1) pneumococcal conjugate vaccine (PCV7), 4 doses between 2 months and 2 years of age; (2) pneumococcal polysaccharide vaccine (PPV23) starting at 2 years of age; and (3) influenza vaccine every fall for children over 6 months of age. Meningococcal vaccine is sometimes recommended for asplenic children.

Transcranial Doppler ultrasonography is being used in some centers to identify children who are at high risk for developing a first stroke. Subsequent initiation of a long-term transfusion program for those with abnormal test results may decrease the incidence of stroke.

Hypertransfusion programs (transfusion every 3 to 4 weeks) for children who have had CVAs, progressive pulmonary disease, and possibly debilitating vasoocclusive crisis is a current treatment (90% effective). The iron overload leads to hemosiderosis (iron deposits on organs), with the following complications occurring: cardiomyopathy, cirrhosis, insulin-dependent diabetes mellitus, hypothyroidism, hypoparathyroidism, delayed growth, and delayed sexual development. Deferoxamine (Desferal) administered either subcutaneously or by intravenous transfusion at regular intervals will chelate the iron so that it can be excreted through the urine or bile to help reduce these complications.

Analgesics are used to control pain during a crisis period. Antibiotics may be used, because infection can trigger the crisis. Folic acid supplementation may be considered for children with significant hemolysis. Daily administration of oral hydroxyurea is an effective pharmacologic intervention, although use in children has not been well studied. Treatment with hydroxyurea, which increases levels of fetal hemoglobin, has been shown to reduce pain events, hospital admissions, and the need for blood transfusions. The only cure is thought to be a bone marrow transplant, which also involves risks. This may be a promising treatment modality in the near future.

NURSING ASSESSMENT

See the Cardiovascular Assessment and Respiratory Assessment sections in Appendix A and the Pain Assessment section in Appendix H.

NURSING DIAGNOSES

- Tissue perfusion, Ineffective
- Comfort, Impaired
- Infection, Risk for
- Injury, Risk for
- Growth and development, Delayed
- Coping, Compromised family
- Coping, Ineffective
- Therapeutic regimen management, Ineffective

NURSING INTERVENTIONS

1. Prevent or minimize effects of sickle cell crisis.
   a. Encourage avoidance of temperature extremes and high altitudes.
   b. Be aware that early assessment and action are keys to prevention of and intervention in crisis episode.
   c. Avoid cold and vasoconstriction during pain episode; cold promotes sickling.
   d. Provide for and promote hydration (one and one half to two times maintenance levels).
      i. Maintain strict intake and output.
      ii. Assess for signs of dehydration.
   e. Promote oxygenation of tissues; monitor for signs of hypoxia—cyanosis, hyperventilation; increased apical pulse, respiratory rate, and blood pressure; and mental confusion.

2. Provide frequent rest periods to decrease oxygen expenditure.
3. Monitor use of oxygen equipment.
4. Administer and monitor use of blood products and chelation therapy; assess for signs of transfusion reaction—fever, restlessness, cardiac dysrhythmias, chills and shaking, nausea and vomiting, chest pain, red or black urine, headache, flank pain, and signs of shock or renal failure.
5. Monitor for signs of circulatory overload—dyspnea, increased respiratory rate, cyanosis, chest pain, and dry cough.
6. Relieve or minimize pain (see Appendix H).
   a. Moist heat for first 24 hours
   b. Whirlpool or walking tank, especially if swelling has occurred
   c. Therapeutic exercises
   d. Administration of analgesics as ordered based on pain assessment. Acetaminophen with codeine may be adequate for mild to moderate pain. More severe crisis may be treated with intermittent or continuous intravenous morphine. Patient-controlled analgesia systems have been used effectively in children as young as 5 years of age.
   e. Use of nonpharmacologic methods such as guided imagery (see Appendix H).
7. Prevent infection.
   a. Assess for signs of infection—fever, malaise or irritability, and inflamed and swollen soft tissue and lymph nodes.
   b. Be aware that children are particularly susceptible to pneumococcal sepsis and pneumonia (children younger than 3 to 4 years of age) and *Salmonella* osteomyelitis.
8. Monitor for signs of complications.
   a. Infection
   b. Splenomegaly
   c. Heart, liver, kidney, joint disease
   d. Leg ulcers
   e. Stroke
   f. Decreased vision

g. Chest pain or dyspnea

h. Delay in growth and development

i. Vascular collapse and shock

9. Provide age-appropriate explanation to child about hospitalization and procedures (see Appendix J).

10. Ensure good nutrition. Metabolic rate of children with sickle cell disease has been demonstrated to be higher than that of children without the disease.

11. Provide emotional support to child and family (see the Supportive Care section in Appendix J).

    a. Encourage performance of normal activities. School absences may put child behind expected grade level (see Appendixes B and L).

    b. Encourage networking with other children and families who have sickle cell anemia.

    c. Delayed puberty occurs frequently. Adolescent often needs additional support.

12. Encourage parents to screen their family members.

    a. Newborn screening for hemoglobinopathies

    b. Screening of siblings for disease and trait

13. Identification at birth makes possible early prophylaxis against infections. Use of prophylactic penicillin is recommended beginning in newborn period (2 to 3 months of age).

🔺 Discharge Planning and Home Care

1. Provide genetic counseling.

2. Counsel child on appropriate play, leisure activities, and sports participation (to prevent hypoxia resulting from strenuous physical exertion and excessive life stress).

3. Provide parent teaching and anticipatory guidance about prevention of infection to ensure that child is seen by physician at first signs of illness; teach parents procedure for taking temperature and methods to decrease temperature.

4. Provide parents with information about routine immunization. Child should have annual vision screening.

CLIENT OUTCOMES

1. Child's respiratory rate, oxygen saturation, and arterial blood gas levels will be within normal limits, cyanosis will be absent, and urine output will be higher than 1 ml/kg/hr.
2. Child will indicate relief from pain.
3. Child and family will understand importance of medical follow-up and know when to seek medical attention.
4. Child will have minimal vasoocclusive, sequestration, and aplastic crises.
5. Child will demonstrate regular observable growth and achieve age-appropriate developmental milestones (see Appendix B).
6. Family will seek genetic counseling for other children.
7. Parents will be able to accurately describe disease process and identify special precautions necessary to prevent sickle cell crisis.

REFERENCES

American Academy of Pediatrics, Health supervision for children with sickle cell disease, policy statement, *Pediatrics* 109(3):526, 2002.

Jakubik LD, Thompson M: Care of the child with sickle cell disease: acute complications, *Pediatr Nurs* 26(4):373, 2000.

Preiss DJ: The young child with sickle cell disease, *Adv Nurse Pract* 6(6):33, 1998.

Sickle Cell Information Center, Sickle Cell Information—Clinician Summary, available at http://www.scinfo.org, accessed June 27, 2003.

78

❖

Spina Bifida

❖

PATHOPHYSIOLOGY

Two distinct types of failure of fusion of the vertebral laminae of the spinal column occur: spina bifida occulta and spina bifida cystica.

Spina bifida occulta is a defect in closure in which the meninges are not exposed on the surface of the skin. The vertebral defect is small, usually involving the lumbosacral region. External abnormalities (present in 50% of cases) may include a hair tuft, nevus, or hemangioma. A pilonidal sinus may require surgical closure if it becomes infected.

Spina bifida cystica is a defect in closure that results in protrusion of the spinal cord and/or its coverings. *Meningocele* is a protrusion that includes the meninges and a sac containing cerebrospinal fluid (CSF); it is covered by normal skin. No neurologic abnormalities are present, and the spinal cord is not involved. Hydrocephalus occurs in 20% of cases. A meningocele usually is in the lumbosacral or sacral area. Surgical correction is usually performed within days of birth.

Myelomeningocele is a protrusion of the meninges and a portion of the spinal cord, as well as a sac containing CSF. The lumbar or lumbosacral area is most often the site. The lumbosacral area is affected in 42% of cases, the thoracolumbar area in 27%, the sacral area in 21%, and the thoracic or cervical in 10%. Infants with a myelomeningocele are prone to injury during the birth process. Hydrocephalus occurs in most affected children (85% to 90%); about 60% to 70% have a normal intelligence quotient, but impairments of conceptual reasoning abilities are common. Children with both myelomeningocele and hydrocephalus have other central nervous system malformations, of which Arnold-Chiari deformity is the most common. Surgical intervention usually is performed at birth with neurosurgery for shunt placement to prevent hydrocephalus if indicated. More recently, experimental fetal surgical procedures (done about 7 weeks prior to birth) have demonstrated the potential to reduce the symptoms of spina bifida.

The specific cause of spina bifida is unknown. Multiple factors such as heredity and environment are thought to interact to produce these defects. The neural tube is normally complete 4 weeks after conception. The following have been identified as causative factors: low levels of maternal vitamins, including folic acid; the taking of clomiphene and valproic acid; and hyperthermia during pregnancy. It is estimated that nearly 75% of neural tube defects could be prevented if women took vitamins, including folic acid, before conception. Widespread public health efforts are now directed to encouraging women to take daily folic acid supplements (400 µg daily) for 1 to 3 months before becoming pregnant.

Advances in interdisciplinary care have improved the long-term outcome for affected children. Treatment improvement, with the use of medications and neurosurgery, has contributed to extending their life spans.

Diminished self-esteem is common in children and adolescents with this condition. Adolescents express concerns about sexual adequacy, social mastery, peer relationships, and physical maturity and attractiveness. The perceived severity of disability is more directly related to *self-perception* of the disability than to the actual disability of the adolescent.

INCIDENCE

1. Annually, approximately 4000 infants are born with spina bifida in the United States.
2. In the United States, the incidence is 1 in 1000 live births.
3. The risk of the disorder increases by 5% with the second child.
4. Girls are more often affected than boys.
5. Nearly 72% of children with spina bifida have latex or natural rubber allergies.

6. Between 80% and 90% of individuals with myelomeningocele have shunts.

CLINICAL MANIFESTATIONS

A varying degree of dysfunction affecting the skeleton, skin, and genitourinary tract results from spina bifida, depending on the portion of the spinal cord involved:

1. Motor, sensory, reflex, and sphincter abnormalities— may occur in varying degrees
2. Flaccid paralysis of legs; loss of sensation and reflexes
3. Hydrocephalus
4. Scoliosis
5. Bladder and bowel functions varying from normal to ineffective

COMPLICATIONS

Birth-related complications of spina bifida include the following:

1. Cerebral palsy
2. Mental retardation
3. Optic atrophy
4. Epilepsy
5. Osteoporosis
6. Fractures (caused by decreased muscle mass)
7. Painless ulcerations, injuries, decubiti

Other long-term complications include the following:

1. Shunt infections
2. Ventriculitis
3. Meningitis
4. Increased intracranial pressure due to blocked shunt
5. Blocked shunt (may be asymptomatic)
6. Tethered cord syndrome
7. Benign intracranial hypertension
8. Visual deficits
9. Latex sensitization and allergy
10. Decubitus ulcer
11. Slit ventricle syndrome
12. Obesity
13. Bowel and bladder problems
14. Mobility limitations

15. Tendonitis
16. Gastrointestinal disorders
17. Orthopedic problems (foot deformities, bowed legs, dislocated hips, spinal curvature)
18. Impaired sexual and reproductive functioning
19. Learning disabilities
20. Depression, anxiety disorders, low self-esteem, altered body image

LABORATORY AND DIAGNOSTIC TESTS

1. Diagnostic examinations: chest radiographic study, ultrasonography, computed tomography, magnetic resonance imaging, amniocentesis
2. Antenatal period testing: serum alpha fetoprotein level between 16 and 18 weeks of gestation, ultrasonography of fetus, amniocentesis if other tests are inconclusive
3. Routine preoperative testing: complete blood count, urinalysis, culture and sensitivity testing (C and S of urine), blood type and cross-match, chest radiographic study

MEDICAL AND SURGICAL MANAGEMENT

Surgical repair of myelomeningocele is performed in the neonatal period to prevent rupture. Surgical repair of the spinal lesion and shunting of CSF in infants with hydrocephalus is performed at birth. Skin grafting is necessary if the lesion is large. Children with spina bifida are at risk for latex sensitization and allergy because they are exposed to surgeries and procedures in which latex gloves come into direct contact with blood vessels and mucosa. Risk factors associated with the development of latex sensitization and allergy are atopic diathesis and number of surgeries. Children who have latex allergy have clinical symptoms, whereas those with latex sensitization have immunoglobulin E antibodies with no clinical symptoms. Whether the child has latex allergy or sensitization, avoidance of contact with latex is recommended.

Prophylactic antibiotics are administered to prevent meningitis. Nursing interventions will depend on the presence and extent of dysfunction of various body systems. In addition, children with myelomeningocele will undergo a number of surgeries depending on their clinical problems, such as tethered spinal cord, orthopedic problems, decubitus ulcers, and shunt requiring revision.

The following medications may be used depending on the child's clinical needs:

1. Antibiotics—used prophylactically to prevent urinary tract infections (selection depends on C and S)
2. Anticholinergics—used to increase bladder tone
3. Stool softeners and laxatives—used for bowel training and evacuation of stool
4. Medications to control or treat other medical and mental health problems such as epilepsy, depression.

NURSING ASSESSMENT

1. See the Musculoskeletal Assessment and Neurologic Assessment sections in Appendix A.
2. Assess parents' interactions with their infant and ability to cope with their child's condition.
3. Assess extent of motor and sensory involvement, and presence of reflexes.
4. Assess for signs and symptoms of dehydration or fluid overload.
5. Assess parents' need for preoperative and postoperative information and support (see Appendix J).
6. Assess for wound drainage and signs of infection.
7. Assess for increased intracranial pressure.
8. Assess parents' and child's ability to manage home treatment regimen (see Appendix K).
9. Assess parents' and child's needs for community services (see Appendix L).

NURSING DIAGNOSES

- Mobility, Impaired physical
- Infection, Risk for
- Injury, Risk for
- Urinary elimination, Impaired
- Bowel incontinence
- Skin integrity, Impaired

- Body image, Disturbed
- Sexuality patterns, Ineffective
- Family processes, Interrupted
- Growth and development, Delayed
- Nutrition: more than body requirements, Imbalanced
- Therapeutic regimen management, Ineffective
- Caregiver role strain, Risk for

NURSING INTERVENTIONS
Preoperative Care

1. Encourage parental expression of grief over loss of "perfect" child.
   a. Feelings related to guilt, self-blame
   b. Feelings of anger about child's condition
   c. Feelings of inadequacy for procreating infant
   d. Feelings of being overwhelmed with the situation and the unknown
2. Provide emotional support to parents (see the Supportive Care section in Appendix J).
3. Monitor infant's vital signs and neurologic status.
   a. Evaluation of temperature, apical pulse, respiratory rate, and blood pressure as often as every 2 hours
   b. Neurologic assessment (see the Neurologic Assessment section in Appendix A)
4. Promote optimal preoperative hydration and nutritional status.
   a. Monitor for dehydration or fluid overload.
   b. Monitor administration of maintenance fluids (by mouth or intravenous [IV] route).
   c. Monitor and record intake and output.
   d. Record weight daily.
5. Maintain integrity of defect; prevent further injury.
   a. Monitor for signs and symptoms of infection—fever, drainage, odor, swelling, and redness.
   b. Maintain child in prone position.
   c. Maintain sterility of dressing.
6. Prepare parents and infant for surgery (refer to institutional manual for specific guidelines) (see Appendix J).

Postoperative Care

1. Maintain nutritional and fluid intake.
   a. Assess for signs of dehydration or fluid overload.
   b. Monitor for bowel sounds.
   c. Monitor administration of IV fluids.
   d. Monitor and record intake and output.
   e. Monitor and record weight daily.
2. Monitor for signs and symptoms of infections.
   a. Fever (obtain blood C and S when infant is febrile)
   b. Drainage from surgical site
   c. Redness and inflammation
3. Promote healing of surgical site; use sterile technique when changing and reinforcing dressing.
   a. Avoid use of latex gloves and other latex-containing medical products.
4. Monitor vital signs and neurologic status.
   a. Monitor temperature, pulse, respirations, and blood pressure.
   b. Perform neurologic assessment (see the Neurologic Assessment section in Appendix A).
   c. Monitor head circumference.
5. Provide emotional support to parents (see the Supportive Care section in Appendix J).

🔺 Discharge Planning and Home Care

1. Instruct parents about long-term management of bowel and bladder training.
   a. Bladder training
      i. Prevention of bladder infections
      ii. Modification of diet for bladder control
      iii. Prevention of decubiti, increase in range of motion and mobility, and importance of skin care
      iv. Prevention of skin trauma, especially burns
      v. Preparation and information about surgical procedures: augmentation, enterocystoplasty, artificial urinary sphincter, urethral sling, abdominal stoma, urinary diversion

        vi. Preparation and information on methods for assessing renal functioning: urine cultures, measurement of serum electrolyte levels, renal scans, intravenous pyelograms, ultrasonography

    b. Bowel training—to implement regular evacuation program

        i. High-fiber diet with bulking agents

        ii. Use of stool softeners (i.e., glycerin suppositories)

        iii. Use of digital stimulation

        iv. Use of laxatives (casanthranol [Peri-Colace])

2. Provide information to parent and child about techniques to facilitate mobility and independence.

    a. Use of casting, corrective appliances (encouraged not only to provide mobility and independence but also to prevent osteoporosis and contractures)

    b. Use of wheelchairs and assistive devices

        i. Prevention of complications such as decubitus ulcers

        ii. Problem solving with malfunctions and equipment problems

        iii. Access to service providers for equipment repairs and maintenance

    c. Physical therapy regimen

        i. Reinforce importance of adherence to exercises and daily activities.

        ii. Coordinate services with physical therapist such as scheduling of appointments, integrated approach to providing services.

    d. Preparation and information on surgical procedures to treat medical needs and long-term complications

3. Instruct parents on importance of having child avoid all contact with latex or natural rubber.

    a. Notify health care professionals in all settings, such as dentists, school nurses.

    b. Review sources of latex in home and community

        i. Clothing

        ii. Art supplies

        iii. Diapers

      iv. Sneakers

      v. Toys (water toys, dolls)

4. Provide education to parents about normal growth and development and deviations from norm (see Appendix B).

   a. Call attention to special problems and needs of child with disability.

   b. Encourage positive expectations and hope for acquisition of developmental milestones with goal of living as independently and productively as possible.

   c. Act as liaison with parents, teachers, and school to establish developmentally and intellectually appropriate expectations (see Appendix L).

      i. If special education student, work with family and individualized education plan (IEP) team to ensure that health-related needs that interfere with learning are considered in developing IEP objectives (See Appendix L)

   d. Instruct adolescents and provide information about areas of concern such as recreational programs, procurement of driver's license, postsecondary programs, and peer relationships.

   e. Provide sexual and reproductive counseling (based on evaluation of genital responsiveness).

   f. Provide career/vocational counseling.

      i. Refer youth and family to secondary and postsecondary educational resources, job training youth programs in community.

   g. Provide counseling about independent living in inclusive community settings.

   h. Provide counseling on weight control measures as needed.

      i. Promote acquisition of self-advocacy and self-determination skills.

CLIENT OUTCOMES

1. Child will function at developmentally appropriate level.
2. Child will experience minimal complications associated with spina bifida.

3. Child will be well hydrated and will maintain weight within normal parameters.
4. Child will be free of infection.
5. Child and parents will demonstrate ability to maintain long-term home care and keep child free of complications, with child eventually assuming responsibility for self-care.
6. Parents will demonstrate ability to access services and supports as needed for their child's long-term management needs.
7. Child will demonstrate ability to function as independently as is developmentally possible.

REFERENCES

Behrman R et al, editors: *Nelson textbook of pediatrics*, ed 16, Philadelphia, 2000, WB Saunders.

Centers for Disease Control and Prevention: Economic burden of spina bifida—United States, 1980-1990, *MMWR* 38(15):264, 1989.

Centers for Disease Control and Prevention: Prevention program for reducing risk for neural tube defects—South Carolina, 1992-1994, *MMWR* 44(8):141, 1995.

Centers for Disease Control and Prevention: Recommendations for the use of folic acid to reduce the number of cases of spina bifida and other neural tube defects, *MMWR* 41:1, 1992.

Dise JE, Lohr ME: Examination of deficits in conceptual reasoning abilities associated with spina bifida, *Am J Phys Med Rehabil* 77(3):247, 1998.

Hoeman SP: Primary care for children with spina bifida, *Nurse Pract* 22(9):60, 1997.

Hunt G et al: Link between the CSF shunt and achievement in adults with spina bifida, *J Neurol Neurosurg Psychiatry* 67(5):591, 1999.

Kallen K: Maternal smoking, body mass index, and neural tube defects, *Am J Epidemiol* 147(12):1103, 1998.

King J et al: Bowel training in spina bifida: importance of education, patient compliance, age, and anal reflexes, *Arch Phys Med Rehabil* 75:243, 1994.

Kirpalani H et al: Quality of life in spina bifida: importance of parental hope, *Arch Dis Child* 83(4):293, 2000.

Nieto A et al: Efficacy of latex avoidance for primary prevention of latex sensitization in children with spina bifida, *J Pediatr* 140(3):370, 2002.

Rudolph A, editor: *Rudolph's pediatrics*, ed 20, East Norwalk, Conn, 1996, Appleton & Lange.

79

◆

Substance-Related Disorders

◆

PATHOPHYSIOLOGY

Substance-related disorders are a major public health problem affecting young people in the United States. They are the leading cause of preventable death in 15- to 24-year-olds. Substances used can be any of a number of drugs taken for toxic or side effects. Such substances include alcohol, amphetamines, cannabis, cocaine, hallucinogens, inhalants, nicotine, opioids, anxiolytics, and phencyclidine (PCP) (see Table 79-1). The effects of substance intoxication vary widely depending on the individual and the substance used. Generally, intoxication causes physiologic, cognitive, and psychosocial effects. A diagnosis of substance abuse is made when drug use causes adverse consequences such as physically hazardous behaviors, legal problems, and interference with school functioning.

A more serious problem is substance dependence. Prolonged heavy use of a substance results in dependence. Over time, increasing amounts of the substance are needed to achieve intoxication; this is referred to as *tolerance.* When blood concentrations of the substance diminish, unpleasant withdrawal symptoms are experienced. Once dependence develops, the individual uses the substance primarily to relieve withdrawal symptoms. Withdrawal from certain drugs such as alcohol and benzodiazepines (i.e., Valium) is potentially life threatening. Hospitalization to manage detoxification may be indicated.

Alcohol, tobacco, and marijuana are the substances most frequently abused by children and adults. Inhalant use, which is often perceived as harmless by adolescents, accounts for a large

TABLE 79-1
Common Classes of Drugs and Their Effects

Class of Drug	Psychophysiologic Effect	Common Symptoms
Stimulants (amphetamine, nicotine, caffeine, cocaine)	Increased alertness and activity, increased central nervous system activity	Restlessness, agitation, sweating, dilated pupils, dry mouth, diarrhea, increases in pulse and temperature
Depressants (barbiturates [phenobarbital, thiopental sodium, amobarbital, butabarbital, secobarbital])	Decreased central nervous system activity, anxiety reduction, sleep induction	Respiratory depression, pupil constriction and/or lateral nystagmus, lethargy, drowsiness
Nonbarbiturate sedatives (methaqualone, flurazepam, glutethimide, methyprylon)	Same as barbiturates	Dilated pupils, hypotension, fluctuating levels of consciousness
Narcotics/opiates (morphine, heroin, meperidine, methadone, others)	Pain reduction	Similar to barbiturates, evidence of injection
Minor tranquilizers (diazepam, chlordiazepoxide)	Reduction of anxiety, muscle relaxation	Drowsiness, poor muscle coordination, confusion, skin rash, nausea

Continued

TABLE 79-1
Common Classes of Drugs and Their Effects—cont'd

Class of Drug	Psychophysiologic Effect	Common Symptoms
Hallucinogens (LSD, [lysergic acid diethylamide]; mescaline; DMT [dimethyltryptamine]; STP [dimethoxy-4-methylamphetamine]; PCP [phencyclidine hydrochloride])	Alterations in sensation, emotional status, and awareness	Hallucinations, perceptual changes, psychosis
Volatile solvents (glue, cement, various sprays, gasoline, some cleaning solutions)	Central nervous system depression	Similar to barbiturates

From Haas M et al, editors: *The school nurse's source book of individualized healthcare plans*, vol 1, North Branch, Minn, 1993, Sunrise River Press, p 413.

number of deaths of teenagers. Both inhalant and heroin use are on the rise in the United States.

A number of psychosocial, developmental, cultural, attitudinal, and personality factors put the youth at risk for drug experimentation. The most significant predictor for substance use is drug use by peers. Other risk factors include poor self-image, problems with school performance, difficult temperament, hyperactivity, and genetic predisposition. Risk factors include problems associated with family dysfunction, including abuse and neglect, overly rigid or permissive parents, parental rejection, and divorce. The following are factors associated with resistance to illicit substance use: nurturing parents, positive school experience, negative attitudes toward drugs, committed religious attitudes, positive self-esteem, and social competence.

Generally, the younger the age of initial drug use, the higher the risk for serious long-term health consequences and adult abuse. Cigarette, alcohol, and marijuana use has been associated with ready access to these substances in the child's home.

Gateway phenomenon is a term denoting the pattern of using an increasing variety of substances, ultimately leading to polysubstance abuse. Evidence for this phenomena is that youth who smoke tobacco and drink alcohol are more likely to use marijuana, and those who use marijuana are more likely to use cocaine. An adolescent may initially begin using to achieve a false sense of maturity, but eventually he or she is likely to develop drug dependence. Substance abuse is associated with depression, low self-esteem, risk for school underachievement, teenage pregnancy, and delinquency. Illicit drug use creates a greater risk of contracting human immunodeficiency virus (HIV) infection and hepatitis C.

INCIDENCE

1. The prevalence rate depends on the substance.
2. Sixty-four percent of high school seniors have experimented with illicit drugs.
3. Nearly 50% of teenage suicides and accidental deaths have been associated with illegal substance use.
4. Six percent of high school seniors report using illicit drugs on a regular basis.

5. Nearly 90% of adolescents 18 years and younger report having used alcohol.
6. During the past decade, the use of inhalant drugs (glue, aerosols) has increased threefold in the 12- to 17-year age group.
7. During the past decade, marijuana and inhalants have become the two most commonly used illicit drugs by the 12- to 17-year age group.
8. Substance abuse is generally higher in males than in females.

CLINICAL MANIFESTATIONS

1. Craving for substance
2. Reddened eyes
3. Signs of trauma—from needle use, injuries due to intoxication, violent behaviors
4. Changes in level of consciousness, coordination, alertness
5. Behavioral changes
6. Isolation of self from family members and friends
7. See Table 79-1 for symptoms related to specific classes of drugs

COMPLICATIONS

1. Deterioration of health status
2. Inadequate or poor nutritional status
3. Erosion of nasal septum (from cocaine use)
4. Cardiac arrhythmias (from use of stimulants)
5. Myocardial infarction
6. Respiratory arrest (from overdose)
7. Cerebrovascular accident
8. Sudden death due to causes identified in items 4 through 7
9. HIV infection, subacute bacterial endocarditis, hepatitis, tetanus from use of contaminated needle

LABORATORY AND DIAGNOSTIC TESTS

1. Toxicologic analysis used for identification of substance, differential diagnosis

2. Blood and urine levels of substance—indicate type of substance used and time of use
3. Psychologic evaluations

MEDICAL MANAGEMENT

Treatment for substance abuse is typically done on an outpatient basis. Inpatient hospitalization is indicated if the client is suicidal or requires detoxification. Comprehensive treatment programs include individual and group psychotherapy, family therapy, recreational therapy, and social skills training. Intensive initial treatment, whether provided on an inpatient or outpatient basis, is associated with positive outcomes. It is important that the youth be connected to community resources that can support achievement of long-term outcomes. Linkages to education, training, rehabilitation, and job development programs can be of assistance.

Prevention efforts that emphasize development or enhancement of protective factors are most effective. These programs emphasize resistance to peer pressure and highlight that most children and youth do not use drugs. Interactive learning models such as role playing and small-group learning sessions are more effective than educational programs. Prevention programs should be targeted to specific audiences: universal, selective, or indicated. Universal programs address the needs of the general public, selective programs provide outreach to at-risk populations such as children of abusing parents, and indicated programs are directed to youth who use illicit substances.

NURSING ASSESSMENT

1. Obtain thorough history of illegal/illicit drugs of choice, time of last use, amount used, frequency and duration of use, and routes of administration (intravenous, oral, and inhalant forms provide more rapid effect).
2. Conduct physical assessment with emphasis on respiratory, cardiovascular, and neurologic systems (see Appendix A).
3. Note any signs of trauma or injury (e.g., needle puncture marks).
4. Assess for depression and suicide potential.

5. Assess for youth and family drug- and alcohol-related problems.
6. Obtain information about school performance.
7. Assess level, type, and frequency of social activities, after-school activities, and peer relationships.
8. Assess level and quality of family and social support.

NURSING DIAGNOSES
- Coping, Ineffective
- Coping, Compromised family
- Injury, Risk for
- Knowledge, Deficient
- Social interaction, Impaired
- Self-esteem, Chronic low

NURSING INTERVENTIONS
1. Intervene immediately if signs of depression or suicidal tendency are evident.
2. Refer for medical evaluation, because abruptly stopping drug (particularly alcohol) may cause withdrawal symptoms.
3. Refer to counseling/psychotherapy services.
4. Treatment program should target audience, emphasizing protective factors and incorporating interactive methods.
5. Encourage sharing of feelings, active listening to youth's concerns.
6. Promote use of positive coping strategies; focus on emphasizing youth's strengths.
7. Provide support for problem solving with positive use of alternative strategies.
8. Encourage linkages to community-based resources and services.

🔺 Discharge Planning and Home Care
1. Provide realistic and credible information about risks and consequences associated with drug use.
2. Provide parental anticipatory guidance on need to create clearly delineated expectations for their youth's behavior and their responsibility to serve as appropriate role models.

3. Provide parental anticipatory guidance regarding use of home drug test kits—that they have limitations and can generate false-positive results, and that their use does not substitute for open communication or parental supervision.
4. Provide information to parents about relationship between their use of tobacco and alcohol, and youth and adolescent substance use and abuse.
5. Treatment programs need to include comprehensive interdisciplinary approach that involves juvenile justice, social services, mental health services, and primary care.

CLIENT OUTCOMES

1. Adolescent will stop or decrease illicit drug use.
2. Adolescent will develop more positive coping skills.
3. Family members will learn to communicate and interact with each other more effectively.

REFERENCES

American Psychological Association: *Diagnostic and statistical manual of mental disorders*, ed 4, text revision *(DSM-IV-TR)*, Washington, DC, 2000, The Association.

Bachman J et al: Explaining recent increases in students' marijuana use: impacts of perceived risks and disapproval, 1976 through 1996, *Am J Public Health* 88(6):887, 1998.

Belcher H, Shinitzky H: Substance abuse in children: prediction, protection and prevention, *Arch Pediatr Adolesc Med* 152(10):952, 1998.

Bruner A, Fishman M: Adolescents and illicit drug use, *JAMA* 280(7):597, 1998.

Centers for Disease Control and Prevention: Morbidity and Mortality Weekly Report (MMWR) surveillance summaries—youth risk behavior surveillance—United States, 1995, Atlanta, 1995, The Centers.

Cornwall A, Blood L: Inpatient versus day treatment for substance abusing adolescents, *J Nerv Ment Dis* 186(9):580, 1998.

Kalb K: Substance abuse. In Haas M, editor: *The school nurse's source book of individualized healthcare plans*, North Branch, Minn, 1993, Sunrise River Press.

Neumark Y et al: The epidemiology of adolescent inhalant drug involvement, *Arch Pediatr Adolesc Med* 152(8):781, 1998.

80

❖

Sudden Infant Death Syndrome

❖

PATHOPHYSIOLOGY

Sudden infant death syndrome (SIDS) is defined as "the sudden death of an infant under 1 year of age which remains unexplained after a thorough case investigation, including performance of a complete autopsy, examination of the death scene, and review of the clinical history" (National Institute of Child Health and Human Development). The autopsy findings are the following: External examination reveals a body that appears well developed and nourished. A small amount of mucous or watery or bloody secretions is present at the nares. Cyanosis of the lips and nail beds is almost always present. The internal examination indicates a subacute inflammation of the upper respiratory tract and petechiae on the pleura, pericardium, and thymus (found in 80% of cases). There is pulmonary edema and congestion. The autopsy reveals symptoms of chronic hypoxemia including brainstem changes; persistence of brown fat, especially around the adrenals; and hepatic erythropoiesis. Some of these autopsy findings are demonstrated in about 80% of SIDS cases, but their absence does not exclude the diagnosis. Risk factors associated with the occurrence of SIDS are listed in Box 80-1. The pathophysiology of SIDS is unclear, but current research focuses on the following explanations:

1. Abnormalities of the central nervous system—particularly delayed myelination or gliosis (or scarring) in the respiratory control areas of the brainstem

BOX 80-1
Risk Factors

Infant

- Prematurity, particularly with birth weight of <2500 g
- Low birth weight for gestational age
- African American or Native American heritage
- Male gender (risk increased by 50%)
- Multiple births
- Low Apgar scores
- Central nervous system disturbances
- Respiratory disorders such as bronchopulmonary dysplasia
- Neonatal intensive care history

Maternal

- Low socioeconomic status
- Low educational level
- Young married mother <20 years old
- History of smoking during pregnancy
- History of drug abuse (including marijuana, methadone, cocaine, heroin, or psychedelics)
- High parity
- Short interpregnancy interval
- Anemia

2. Primary cardiac arrhythmias, particularly bradycardia secondary to a decrease in vagal nerve tone and bradycardia occurring simultaneously with central apnea and prolonged QT interval
3. Carbon dioxide rebreathing—particularly associated with the prone sleeping position and use of soft bedding
4. Airway obstruction—from pharyngeal collapse, which could be exacerbated by the prone sleeping position
5. Impaired temperature regulation and its effects on the respiratory pattern, chemoreceptor sensitivity, and cardiac control
6. Possible infectious agents—viral septicemia

INCIDENCE

1. SIDS is the most common cause of death before 1 year of age.
2. Incidence has declined significantly since 1989 due to public education efforts.
3. SIDS occurs in 1 of every 1000 live births in the general public.
4. Since 1992, the SIDS rate has decreased by more than 40% with the introduction of the supine sleeping position recommendation.
5. Age range of peak incidence is 2 to 3 months; SIDS is uncommon before 2 weeks of age or after 6 months of age.
6. SIDS has seasonal occurrence in the winter months, particularly January.
7. Occurrence of death is most frequently between midnight and 9 AM.
8. Ethnic distribution is as follows: 2.5 to 6.0 of every 1000 live births for Native Americans and African Americans; and 1.0 to 2.5 of every 1000 live births for Asians, whites, and Latinos.
9. SIDS accounts for an estimated 7000 to 10,000 infant deaths per year worldwide.

NURSING ASSESSMENT

1. Assess infant, familial, and maternal risk factors (see Box 80-1) associated with SIDS.
2. Assess family's ability to manage in-home apnea monitoring as appropriate for selected groups of infants (see Appendix K).
3. Assess family's need for support and resources during acute grieving period.

NURSING DIAGNOSES

- Family processes, Interrupted
- Grieving, Dysfunctional
- Therapeutic regimen management, Ineffective

NURSING INTERVENTIONS
Prevention

1. Complete thorough history taking and physical examination to identify presence of risk factors.
2. Perform newborn teaching with parents before discharge, stressing need for follow-up care with pediatrician and use of American Academy of Pediatrics 2000 updated guidelines recommending prone sleeping position (Box 80-2).
3. Promote compliance with American Academy of Pediatrics and "Back to Sleep" recommendations. Outreach efforts are directed to parents, health care professionals, and child care workers. "Back to Sleep" program was initiated jointly by U.S. Public Health Service, American Academy of Pediatrics, SIDS Alliance, and Association of SIDS and Infant Mortality Programs. Recommendations include the following:
   a. Put infant in supine sleeping position.
   b. Use crib conforming to Consumer Product Safety Commission and ASTM (formerly American Society for Testing and Materials) safety standards.
   c. Do not allow infant to sleep on soft surfaces.
   d. Do not use soft materials or objects as props under infant's head.
   e. Do not place soft objects in crib.
   f. Do not allow co-sleeping.
   g. Protect infant from second-hand smoking by parent/caretaker.
   h. Avoid overheating with excessive clothing or room temperature.
4. Refer mothers who use tobacco to smoking cessation programs.
5. Monitor ability of family members to participate in in-home apnea monitoring and use cardiopulmonary resuscitation when applicable (see Appendix K).
6. Refer family to appropriate community-based support group (i.e., Compassionate Friends, Candlelighters).

BOX 80-2
Modifiable Risk Factors

- Prone sleeping
- Soft sleep surfaces and loose bedding
- Overheating
- Maternal smoking during pregnancy
- Co-sleeping
- Preterm birth and low birth weight

Care After SIDS

1. Support family during acute grieving period.
2. Counsel parents and reassure them that they are not responsible for infant's death.
3. Encourage parents to express their feelings of guilt and remorse.
4. Employ therapeutic listening skills to assist parents in grieving process.
5. Allow sufficient privacy for parents to be alone with infant as needed.

BOX 80-3
Sudden Infant Death Syndrome Resources

American Sudden Infant Death Syndrome Institute
275 Carpenter Drive, Suite 100
Atlanta, GA 30328
800-232-SIDS

National Sudden Infant Death Syndrome Foundation
10500 Little Patuxent Parkway, Suite 420
Columbia, MD 21044
800-638-7437

Sudden Infant Death Syndrome Clearing House
8201 Greensboro Drive, Suite 600
McClean, VA 22102
703-821-8955

🛖 Discharge Planning and Home Care

1. During bereavement period, refer family to appropriate resources to deal with issues such as long-term grief (Box 80-3).
2. Follow up with phone call and sympathy card from staff.

CLIENT OUTCOMES

1. Family will be knowledgeable about community resources.
2. Family will demonstrate appropriate grieving behaviors.

REFERENCES

American Academy of Pediatrics, Task Force on Infant Sleep Position and Sudden Infant Death Syndrome: Changing concepts of sudden infant death syndrome: implications for infant sleeping environment and sleep position, *Pediatrics* 105(3):650, 2000.

Assessment of infant sleeping positions—selected states, *MMWR* 47(41):873, 1998.

Gaffney K: Infant exposure to environmental tobacco smoke, *J Nurs Sch* 33(4):343, 2001.

Gibson E et al: Infant sleep position following new AAP guidelines, *Pediatrics* 96(1 pt 1):69, 1995.

Gilbert-Barness E, Barness L: Sudden infant death: a reappraisal, *Contemp Pediatr* 12(4):88, 1995.

Helweg-Larsen K, Irgens L: Breast feeding and the sudden infant death syndrome in Scandinavia, 1992-95, *Arch Dis Child* 86(6):400, 2002.

Hunt CE: Sudden infant death syndrome and subsequent siblings, *Pediatrics* 95(3):430, 1995.

Moriarty H et al: Differences in bereavement reactions within couples following death of a child, *Res Nurs Health* 19(6):461, 1996.

Paris J et al: Risk factors for sudden infant death syndrome: changes associated with sleep position recommendations, *J Pediatr* 139(6):771, 2001.

Peeke K et al: Infant sleep position: nursing practice and knowledge, *MCN Am J Matern Child Nurs* 24(6):301, 1999.

Pollack HA: Sudden infant death syndrome, maternal smoking during pregnancy, and the cost-effectiveness of smoking cessation intervention, *Am J Public Health* 91(3):432, 2001.

Vance JC et al: Psychological changes in parents eight months after the loss of an infant from stillbirth, neonatal death, or sudden infant death syndrome—a longitudinal study, *Pediatrics* 96(5 pt 1):933, 1995.

81

◆

Suicide

◆

PATHOPHYSIOLOGY

Suicide, the third leading cause of death among youth in the United States, is on the rise. Risk of suicide is the most frequent reason for inpatient psychiatric hospitalizations of adolescents. Suicidal behaviors represent a continuum ranging from the completed act to suicide attempts to self-inflicted injury. Suicidal ideations are recurrent thoughts of death and of killing oneself. Suicidal ideations do not necessarily include a plan or intention to kill oneself but may be a precursor to suicidal behavior. A carefully formulated suicide plan is an indicator that the youth has serious intentions of carrying out his or her plan.

Contributing factors to youth suicide are complex and fall within the following areas: intrapersonal problems, family problems, major life changes, and demographics. Adolescents who have emotional problems or psychiatric illnesses (i.e., mood, anxiety, and personality disorders) are at risk. Family history of emotional problems, multiple family moves, problematic parent-child relationships, sexual abuse, emotional neglect, parental divorce, and family violence are risk factors for suicide. Significant recent life changes such as loss of a parent, end of a romantic relationship, and a recent move are also associated with suicidal behaviors. Demographic risk factors include being a member of a single-parent family or in a noncustodial living arrangement, being male, and being in one's late teens. Ready access to firearms in the home is positively associated with suicide attempts.

Cluster suicides have been identified among adolescents who imitate their peers in committing suicide. Females use less violent methods of suicide than do males. Suicide methods used by adolescents include poisoning, shooting (higher rate for males), hanging (higher rate for males than for females), jumping from a high place, jumping out of a car, inhaling carbon monoxide fumes, drowning, and overdose of medications.

INCIDENCE

1. Rates of mood disorders are estimated to be less than 1% among preschoolers, 2% to 5% among grammar school–aged children, and 5% to 7% among adolescents.
2. Suicide accounts for 12% of the mortality rate for those aged 5 to 24 years.
3. Suicide is the third leading cause of death in 15- to 19-year-olds and the fourth leading cause in 10- to 14-year-olds.
4. Suicide is the third leading cause of death among African Americans aged 15 to 19 years, especially among youth living in the southern United States.
5. For every suicide among high school students, there are 350 unsuccessful suicide attempts.
6. Suicide rates are highest in fall and winter.
7. Adolescent suicide risk increases sevenfold with maternal suicide attempts and fivefold with marital discord.
8. Use of firearms is the method most often employed in completed suicides among those 10 to 14 years old, followed by hanging and drug overdose.
9. Use of firearms, hanging, and drug overdose are the methods used most often by 15- to 24-year-olds who complete suicide.
10. Males are five times more likely to commit suicide than females.
11. The highest risk group for suicide is white males 15 to 19 years old, who account for 72.2% of suicides.

CLINICAL MANIFESTATIONS

1. Prolonged unhappiness, sadness, tearfulness, moodiness
2. Social withdrawal from friends, family, and usual social activities

3. Acting out and aggressive behaviors, fighting with peers and/or siblings
4. Delinquent behaviors: stealing, lying, property destruction (e.g., graffiti)
5. Sleep disorders and disturbances such as nightmares, excessive sleeping, insomnia
6. Eating disorders; changes in weight and appetite
7. Changes in school performance
8. Somatic complaints such as abdominal pain, headaches
9. Feelings of shame and guilt
10. Low self-esteem as evidenced by self-deprecating remarks, sense of worthlessness, and behavior
11. Diminished and poor school performance
12. Sense of hopelessness and despair

TREATMENT APPROACHES

The suicide risk must be assessed by a professional. Assessment *must* include inquiry into suicidal ideation, plan, intention, and available means to carry out suicide plan. If the child or youth reports suicidal ideations with a plan, and the means and the intention to carry out the plan, the individual should be continually supervised or monitored until he or she is evaluated by a mental health professional. Children and youth who attempt suicide must be referred immediately for services. A number of treatment approaches are used to treat children and youth who are suicidal. If the suicide risk is acute, then hospitalization will be necessary for stabilization, intensive monitoring, and comprehensive diagnostic evaluation followed by outpatient therapy. Outpatient follow-up is strongly recommended and may include a number of mental health interventions. The indicated treatment is individual and family psychotherapy. Psychotropic medications may be indicated for treatment of underlying depression. Drug and alcohol rehabilitation may be indicated for some youth.

NURSING ASSESSMENT

1. Do not be afraid to ask child or youth about suicidal thoughts and whether he or she has a plan and/or

intentions to carry out plan. Does he or she have history of past suicides attempts, access to drugs or medications, or weapons?

2. Assess for alcohol and drug use (when under influence of alcohol and other drugs that cause disinhibition, child or youth may act impulsively on suicidal thoughts).
3. Assess for significant changes in behavior (refer to Clinical Manifestations section in this chapter).
4. Assess level of social and family support.

NURSING DIAGNOSES

- Injury, Risk for
- Violence, Risk for self-directed
- Coping, Ineffective
- Coping, Compromised family
- Thought processes, Disturbed

NURSING INTERVENTIONS

1. Recognize warning signs of mood disorders and suicidal behaviors.
2. Identify children and youth at risk for suicide and refer for comprehensive interdisciplinary treatment services (e.g., crisis intervention team).
3. Refer child or youth to psychotherapist, school psychologist, or counselor.
4. Encourage sharing of feelings, active listening to child's or youth's concerns.
5. Promote use of positive coping strategies; focus on emphasizing child's or youth's strengths.
6. Provide support for problem solving and positive use of alternative strategies.
7. Restrict access to firearms and lethal weapons.
8. Provide access number for crisis hotline.
9. Elicit contract from child or youth not to harm self.
   a. Ask child or youth, "Are you able to verbally contract not to harm yourself and can you inform (name of specific adult) if you have thought of harming yourself?"

🏠 Discharge Planning and Home Care

1. Provide information to parents about association between ready access to guns in home and increased risk of adolescent suicide. Encourage parents to limit access to firearms or remove them from home.
2. Advocate positive parent-child relationships and positive communications; refer to family-centered therapy services, parenting skills programs, psychotherapy and psychoeducational programs.
3. Facilitate referrals for children and youth to peer support programs.
4. Coordinate prevention efforts with educational and community-based colleagues focused on self-awareness for mood disorders and suicide, and methods to enhance self-esteem.

CLIENT OUTCOMES

1. Child/youth suicide plan or attempt will be prevented.
2. Child/youth will develop new, more positive coping strategies.
3. Child/youth will identify sources of support (e.g., friends, family members).

REFERENCES

Centers for Disease Control and Prevention: Morbidity and Mortality Weekly Report (MMWR) surveillance summaries—youth risk behavior surveillance—United States, 1995, Atlanta, 1995, The Centers.

Haas M, editor: *The school nurse's source book of individualized healthcare plans,* vol 1, North Branch, Minn, 1993, Sunrise River Press.

Haas M, editor: *The school nurse's source book of individualized healthcare plans,* vol 2, North Branch, Minn, 1998, Sunrise River Press.

Lipschitz D et al: Perceived abuse and neglect as risk factors for suicidal behavior in adolescent inpatients, *J Nerv Ment Dis* 187(1):32, 1999.

Muscari M: Prevention: are we really reaching today's teens? *MCN Am J Matern Child Nurs* 24(2):87, 1999.

Pagliano LA: Adolescent depression and suicide: a review and analysis of the current literature, *Can J School Psychol* 11(2):191, 1995.

Pfeffer C et al: Suicidal children grow up: relations between family psychopathology and adolescent's lifetime suicidal behavior, *J Nerv Ment Dis* 186(5):269, 1998.

Shepherd G, Klein-Schwartz W: Accidental and suicidal adolescent poisoning deaths in the United States, 1979-1994, *Arch Pediatr Adolesc Med* 152(12):1181, 1998.

82

❖

Tetralogy of Fallot

❖

PATHOPHYSIOLOGY

Tetralogy of Fallot (TOF) is a cyanotic congenital heart disorder composed of four structural defects: (1) ventricular septal defect; (2) pulmonic stenosis, which may be infundibular, valvular, supravalvular, or a combination of these, and causes obstruction of the blood flow into the pulmonary arteries; (3) right ventricular hypertrophy; and (4) varying degrees of overriding of the aorta. The ventricular septal defect is invariably large. In children with TOF, the diameter of the aorta is larger than normal, whereas the pulmonary artery is smaller than normal. Congestive heart failure (CHF) is normally associated with defects causing a large left-to-right shunting, as is found with ventricular septal defect that results in high or low output failure. In TOF, however, CHF usually does not occur, both because the pulmonary stenosis prevents high-output failure (prevents the greater pulmonary blood flow and left-to-right shunting) and because the ventricular septal defect prevents failure of the right ventricle. Hypoxia is the primary problem. The degree of cyanosis is related to the severity of the anatomic obstruction to the blood flow from the right ventricle into the pulmonary artery, as well as to the physiologic status of the child.

Most children with TOF are candidates for complete surgical repair; however, indications for total correction versus palliative treatment depend on the philosophies of the surgeon and the institution. Total correction of TOF involves closing the ventricular septal defect and removing the obstruction to the right ventricular outflow.

The most common surgical palliation is a modified Blalock-Taussig shunt, which is placement of a Gore-Tex shunt from the subclavian artery to a branch of the pulmonary artery. The procedure is usually done before 2 years of age to enhance pulmonary blood flow. The degree of surgical risk depends on the diameter of the pulmonary arteries; risk is less than 10% if the diameter of the pulmonary arteries is at least one third of the aortic diameter.

INCIDENCE

1. TOF affects boys and girls equally.
2. Incidence is higher with older maternal age.
3. Few affected individuals survive beyond 20 years without surgery.
4. TOF accounts for 10% to 15% of all congenital defects.
5. There is a 5% mortality rate (slightly higher in infants) for individuals who undergo cardiac repair, and a 10% mortality rate for those who have shunts.
6. Unsatisfactory results are experienced by 10% of survivors.

CLINICAL MANIFESTATIONS

1. Cyanosis—appears after neonatal period, although children with mild degree of right ventricular outflow obstruction may be acyanotic
2. Hypercyanotic spells during infancy, also known as "Tet spells"
   a. Increased rate and depth of respiration
   b. Sudden onset of dyspnea
   c. Alteration in consciousness, central nervous system irritability that can progress to lethargy and syncope and ultimately result in seizures, cerebrovascular accident, and death (occurs in 35% of cases)
3. Clubbing
4. Initially normal blood pressure—can increase after several years of marked cyanosis and polycythemia
5. Classic squatting position—decreases venous return from lower extremities and increases pulmonary blood flow and systemic arterial oxygenation
6. Failure to thrive

7. Anemia (if severe hypoxia and polycythemia are present)—contributes to worsening of symptoms
8. Decreased exercise tolerance
9. Acidosis
10. Murmur (systolic ejection murmur at upper left sternal border)
11. Knee- or head-to-chest position assumed during spells or after exercise

COMPLICATIONS

The following are hemodynamic consequences of TOF:

1. Severe hypoxia
2. Sudden death from dysrhythmias

The following complications may occur after Blalock-Taussig anastomosis:

1. Bleeding—especially prominent in children with polycythemia
2. Cerebral embolism or thrombosis—risk greater with polycythemia, anemia, or sepsis
3. CHF if shunt is too large
4. Early occlusion of shunt
5. Hemothorax
6. Persistent right-to-left shunt at atrial level, especially in infants
7. Persistent cyanosis
8. Phrenic nerve damage
9. Pleural effusion

LABORATORY AND DIAGNOSTIC TESTS

1. Radiography of chest—indicates increase or decrease in pulmonary flow, size of heart and borders
2. Electrocardiogram (ECG)—indicates right ventricular hypertrophy, left ventricular hypertrophy, or both
3. Arterial blood gas values—reflect obstructive pulmonary blood flow (increased partial pressure of carbon dioxide [Pco_2], decreased partial pressure of oxygen [Po_2], and decreased pH)
4. Hematocrit or hemoglobin level—monitors viscosity of blood and detects iron deficiency anemia

5. Echocardiogram—detects septal defect, aortic position, and pulmonic stenosis
6. Cardiac catheterization—increased systemic pressures in right ventricle; decreased pulmonary artery pressures with decreased arterial hemoglobin saturation
7. Platelet count—usually decreased
8. Barium swallow test—demonstrates displacement of trachea to left of midline
9. Radiography of abdomen—detects existence of other possible congenital anomalies

MEDICAL MANAGEMENT

The following medications may be used:

1. Oxygen—used to dilate the pulmonary vasculature
2. Diuretics (e.g., furosemide [Lasix], potassium-sparing diuretics)—used to promote diuresis, decrease fluid overload; used in the treatment of edema associated with CHF
3. Digitalis—increases the force of contraction of the heart, the stroke volume, and cardiac output and decreases cardiac venous pressures; used to treat CHF and selected cardiac arrhythmias (rarely given before correction unless shunt is too large)
4. Iron—used to manage anemia
5. Propranolol (Inderal), a beta-blocker—reduces heart rate and decreases force of contraction and myocardial irritability; used to prevent or treat hypercyanotic spells
6. Morphine, an analgesic—increases pain threshold; also used to treat hypercyanotic spells by depressing the respiratory center and cough reflex
7. Sodium bicarbonate, a potent systemic alkalizer—used to treat acidosis by replacing bicarbonate ions and restoring buffering capacity of body

SURGICAL MANAGEMENT
Blalock-Taussig Anastomosis

A Blalock-Taussig subclavian pulmonary anastomosis is a palliative intervention generally recommended for children who are not candidates for corrective surgery. The subclavian artery opposite the side of the aortic arch is ligated, divided, and anastomosed to the contralateral pulmonary artery. The advantages of this shunt procedure are the ability to construct very small shunts that grow with the child and the ease of shunt removal during definitive repair. The modified Blalock-Taussig anastomosis is essentially the same but uses a prosthetic material, usually polytetrafluoroethylene. With this shunt, the size can be better controlled, and removal is easier because most complete repairs are performed at a young age.

The hemodynamic consequence of the Blalock-Taussig shunt is to allow systemic blood to enter the pulmonary circulation through the subclavian artery, which increases pulmonary blood flow under low pressure and avoids pulmonary congestion. Blood flow allows stabilization, improving cardiac and respiratory status until the child grows enough for corrective surgery to be safe. Collateral circulation will develop to ensure adequate arterial flow to the arm, although a blood pressure reading will not be obtainable in that arm.

Definitive Repair

Historically, complete repair of TOF was postponed until the preschool years. Currently it can be accomplished in 1- and 2-year-old children. Indications for surgery at a young age include severe polycythemia (hematocrit higher than 60%), hypercyanotic ("Tet") spells, hypoxia, and decreased quality of life. A median sternotomy incision is made, and cardiopulmonary bypass is established, with deep hypothermia added for some infants. If a previous shunt is in place, it is removed. Unless the repair cannot be completed through the right atrium, a right ventriculotomy is avoided because of the potential for impaired ventricular function. The right ventricular outflow obstruction is resected and widened, using Dacron with pericardial backing. Care is taken to avoid pulmonary insufficiency. The pulmonary valve is incised. The ventricular septal defect is closed with a Dacron patch to complete the operation. In cases of severe right ventricular outflow tract obstruction, a conduit may be inserted.

NURSING ASSESSMENT

1. See the Cardiovascular Assessment section in Appendix A.
2. Assess child's level of activity and acquisition of developmental milestones (preoperatively) (see Appendix B).
3. Assess for changes in cardiopulmonary status.
4. Assess for signs and symptoms of potential associated problems (complications): bleeding, CHF, arrhythmias, persistent pulmonary regurgitation, low cardiac output, pulmonary hypertension, pleural effusion, electrolyte imbalances, fluid overload, hepatomegaly, and neurologic complications.
5. Assess for postoperative pain (see Appendix H).

NURSING DIAGNOSES

- Activity intolerance
- Anxiety
- Fear
- Cardiac output, Decreased
- Tissue perfusion, Ineffective
- Fluid volume, Excess
- Fluid volume, Risk for deficient
- Infection, Risk for
- Injury, Risk for
- Family processes, Interrupted
- Coping, Ineffective
- Nutrition: less than body requirements, Imbalanced
- Growth and development, Risk for delayed
- Therapeutic regimen management, Risk for ineffective

NURSING INTERVENTIONS
Maintenance Care

1. Monitor for changes in cardiopulmonary status.
2. Monitor and maintain hydration status.
    a. Intake and output; specific gravity
    b. Signs of dehydration

3. Monitor child's response to medications (see the Medical Management section in this chapter).
   a. Iron—for iron deficiency anemia and polycythemia
   b. Antibiotics—administered before, during, and after surgery as prophylaxis against subacute bacterial endocarditis
   c. Diuretics (furosemide)—for CHF before or after surgery
   d. Digitalis—for CHF before or after surgery
   e. Morphine—to alleviate hypercyanotic spells
   f. Propranolol—to alleviate hypercyanotic spells (long-term management)
   g. Sodium bicarbonate—if documented acidosis develops
4. Provide foods high in iron (to treat iron deficiency anemia) and protein (to promote healing).
   a. Cereals, egg yolk, and meat
   b. Supplemental iron with orange juice if possible
5. Provide oxygen supplementation as needed and monitor child's response.
   a. Monitor respiratory status.
   b. Monitor color.
   c. Use and maintain respiratory equipment (oxygen mask, ventilator, or tent).
6. Protect child from potential infectious contacts and promote preventive practices (to prevent subacute bacterial endocarditis).
   a. Screen visitors for infections.
   b. Instruct child and family about good dental care.
      i. Brushing and flossing of teeth
      ii. Frequent dental checkups for detection of caries and gingival infections
      iii. Importance of antibiotic prophylaxis for dental extractions
   c. Provide close surveillance for and timely reporting of fever and abrasions for antibiotic prophylaxis.
7. Monitor for signs of complications and child's response to treatment regimen.
   a. Acidosis
   b. Anemia
   c. Brain abscess

8. Observe for phrenic nerve damage and diaphragmatic paralysis.

Preoperative Care

1. Prepare child for surgery by obtaining assessment data.
   a. Complete blood count, urinalysis, serum glucose level, and blood urea nitrogen level
   b. Baseline electrolyte level
   c. Blood coagulation studies
   d. Type and cross-match of blood
   e. Chest radiographic study and ECG
2. Use age-appropriate explanations for preparation of child (see the Preparation for Procedures or Surgery section in Appendix J).
3. Do not take blood pressure readings or make arterial punctures in potential shunt arm.

Postoperative Care

Blalock-Taussig anastomosis

1. Assess child's clinical status.
   a. Immediately after surgery, expect arm with involved subclavian artery to be cool and without blood pressure (Blalock-Taussig anastomosis).
      i. Flush blood pressure should equal mean arterial blood pressure (no blood pressure readings in shunt arm).
      ii. Note pulse pressure; wide pulse pressure indicates large shunt.
   b. Note pulses; bounding pulses indicate large shunt.
   c. Note cyanosis; hypoxemia or signs of acidosis indicate early occlusion of shunt.
   d. Assess for Horner's syndrome.
2. Monitor child for any postoperative complications.
   a. Bleeding
   b. CHF if shunt is too large or pulmonary hypertension is present
   c. Increased pulmonary blood flow and pulmonary hypertension

3. Monitor child's response to administered medications—digitalis and diuretics are administered if needed.
4. Monitor and maintain fluid and electrolyte balance.
   a. Monitor for signs of dehydration—lack of tearing, doughy skin, specific gravity higher than 1.020, and decrease in urine output or body weight.
   b. Administer fluids at 50% to 75% of maintenance volume during first 24 hours (1000 ml/m^2; then 1500 ml/m^2).
5. Promote and maintain optimal respiratory status.
   a. Perform percussion and postural drainage every 2 to 4 hours.
   b. Use suction as needed.
   c. Use spirometer, if developmentally appropriate, every 1 to 2 hours for 24 hours, then every 4 hours.
6. Monitor and alleviate child's pain (see Appendix H).
   ### *TOF corrective surgery*
1. Monitor child's clinical status, and monitor for postoperative complications.
   a. Arrhythmias
      i. Right bundle branch block caused by right ventriculotomy or ventricular septal defect repair
      ii. Complete heart block
      iii. Supraventricular arrhythmia
      iv. Ventricular tachycardia
   b. CHF caused by incision of right ventricle, which decreases pumping ability of heart (more common if pulmonary hypertension is present)
   c. Hemorrhage caused by low platelet count in children with polycythemia
   d. Low cardiac output (most common cause of death)
   e. Neurologic complications caused by thromboemboli
   f. Persistent pulmonary regurgitation
   g. Residual ventricular septal defect (affects 10% of children)
2. Monitor child's response to medications.
   a. Pressors for low cardiac output

    b. Digitalis and diuretics several weeks to months after surgery to control CHF

3. Monitor child's cardiac function hourly for 24 to 48 hours, then every 4 hours.
   a. Vital signs, including rectal temperature
   b. Color
   c. Peripheral pulses and capillary refill time
   d. Arterial blood pressure and central venous pressure
   e. Hepatomegaly
   f. Periorbital edema
   g. Pleural effusion
   h. Pulsus paradoxus
   i. Heart sounds
   j. Ascites (rare)
4. Monitor for cardiac arrhythmias.
5. Monitor for signs and symptoms of hemorrhage.
   a. Assess child's chest tube output every hour.
   b. Assess for bleeding from other sites.
   c. Maintain strict intake and output.
   d. Assess for ecchymotic lesions and petechiae.
6. Monitor and maintain child's fluid and electrolyte balance.
   a. Infuse intravenous fluids at 50% to 75% of maintenance volume for first 24 hours ($1000 \ ml/m^2$, then $1500 \ ml/m^2$).
   b. Assess for signs and symptoms of dehydration.
7. Monitor and maintain child's respiratory status.
   a. Perform chest physiotherapy.
   b. Place child in semi-Fowler position.
   c. Humidify air.
   d. Monitor for chylothorax.
   e. Provide adequate pain medications.
8. Provide for child's and family's emotional needs (see the Supportive Care section in Appendix J).
9. Monitor and alleviate child's pain (see Appendix H).
10. Provide developmentally appropriate stimulation and/or activities (see Appendix B).

🔺 **Discharge Planning and Home Care**

1. Make family aware that antibiotic prophylaxis is required for dental work and surgery.
2. Instruct family about exercise limitations, if such limitations continue.
3. Instruct parents about administration of medications and child's response to them.
4. Instruct parents about use of cardiopulmonary resuscitation.
5. Instruct parents about parenting skills.
   a. Need to maintain usual expectations for behavior and misbehavior
   b. Continuance of disciplinary measures
   c. Methods and strategies to assist child in living normally and dealing with concerns
6. Instruct parents about infection control measures.

CLIENT OUTCOMES

1. Child's vital signs will be within normal limits for age.
2. Child will participate in physical activities appropriate for age.
3. Child will be free of postoperative complications.

REFERENCES

Hockenberry M: *Wong's nursing care of infants and children,* ed 7, St Louis, 2003, Mosby.

Park M: *Pediatric cardiology for practitioners,* ed 4, St Louis, 2002, Mosby.

Spilman L, Furdon S: Recognition, understanding, and current management of cardiac lesions with decreased pulmonary blood flow, *Neonatal Netw* 17(4): 7, 1998.

83

❖

Transplantation: Bone Marrow (Hematopoietic Stem Cell Transplantation)

❖

PATHOPHYSIOLOGY

Hematopoietic stem cell transplantation (HSCT), formerly known as bone marrow transplantation, is performed for the treatment of malignancies (leukemia, lymphoma, and solid tumors), blood marrow dysfunction and failure, immunodeficiencies, and congenital metabolic disorders (Box 83-1). The bone marrow is involved in a number of functions: (1) transport of oxygen throughout the body by the erythrocytes; (2) infection protection by granulocytes, lymphocytes, and monocytes; and (3) control and prevention of bleeding by platelets. HSCT restores bone marrow, hematologic, and immune functions for conditions of bone marrow dysfunction and failure. HSCT is used to treat and prevent further progression of genetic diseases. In HSCT, donor stem cells are removed, termed *harvesting,* and then transplanted into the recipient. Once the stem cells are transplanted into the recipient, they migrate to the marrow's spaces and eventually begin to produce new cells. Additional information on the process of transplantation is provided under the Medical Management section of this chapter.

Transplantation of stem cells has been used to treat malignancies and hematologic disorders in children. Stem cells can be harvested from umbilical cord blood obtained from the placenta after birth. Umbilical cord stem cell transplants are used more in children than in adults because of the smaller amount of cells needed for children. Although there is a higher

BOX 83-1

Conditions Treated with Hematopoietic Stem Cell Transplantation

Malignancies: Leukemias, Lymphomas, and Solid Tumors

- Acute lymphocytic leukemia
- Acute myelogenous leukemia
- Acute nonlymphocytic leukemia
- Brain tumors
- Burkitt's lymphoma
- Chronic myelogenous leukemia
- Ewing's sarcoma
- Germ-cell tumor
- Hodgkin's disease
- Juvenile chronic myelogenous leukemia
- Myelodysplastic syndrome
- Neuroblastoma
- Non-Hodgkin's lymphoma
- Primitive neuroectodermal tumor
- Retinoblastoma
- Rhabdomyosarcoma
- Wilms' tumor

Bone Marrow Dysfunction/Failure

- Blackfan-Diamond anemia
- Chronic granulomatous disease
- Fanconi's anemia
- Immune dysfunction
- Infantile agranulocytosis
- Leukocyte adhesion defects
- Osteopetrosis
- Severe aplastic anemia
- Severe combined immunodeficiency syndrome
- Sickle cell disease
- Thalassemia

Immunodeficiencies

- Chédiak-Higashi syndrome
- Glanzmann's thrombasthenia
- Wiskott-Aldrich syndrome

Congenital Metabolic Disorders
- Adrenoleukodystrophy
- Hunter's syndrome
- Hurler's syndrome
- Lesch-Nyhan syndrome
- Maroteaux-Lamy syndrome
- Metachromatic leukodystrophy

incidence of delayed engraftment after cord blood transplantation, those who receive bone marrow stem cells experience a higher rate of infections and graft versus host disease (GVHD). Stem cells can also be obtained from bone marrow or peripheral blood of the individual undergoing transplantation or from a matched donor.

INCIDENCE

1. Survival rates following transplantation are 60% to 90%.
2. Ten percent of children under the age of 10 years develop GVHD between the second and tenth week after HSCT.
3. Among older children, 30% to 60% develop GVHD.
4. More than 70% of children lack a human lymphocyte antigen (HLA)–matched sibling.
5. Survival rates for persons with chronic myelogenous leukemia following transplantation are 60% to 80%.
6. Survival rates for individuals with acute leukemia following transplantation are 30% to 60%.

Epstein-Barr virus (EBV) occurs in HSCT recipients because of their depressed immune systems. Persons with normal immune systems may have EBV but have immunity to keep it under control.

CLINICAL MANIFESTATIONS

Clinical manifestations are related to occurrence of GVHD:
1. Impaired skin integrity
   a. Maculopapular rash beginning on soles, palms, and ears, and spreading throughout body

      b. Pruritus
      c. Mucositis of oral cavity
      d. Perianal redness, abscesses, fissures
  2. Respiratory infections
      a. Tachypnea
      b. Rales, rhonchi
      c. Retractions
  3. Hepatomegaly, ascites
  4. Encephalopathy
      a. Changes in vital signs
      b. Alteration in level of consciousness
  5. Renal insufficiency (increased or decreased fluid volume)
      a. Signs of fluid overload
      b. Signs of dehydration
  6. Gastrointestinal effects
      a. Diarrhea
      b. Symptoms of dehydration
      c. Weight loss
  7. Bleeding
  8. Pain

COMPLICATIONS

1. GVHD. This is the most serious complication of HSCT. GVHD occurs when transplanted T lymphocytes from the donor's bone marrow react against the host tissues. Signs and symptoms of GVHD are the following (in order of appearance): A maculopapular rash begins on the palms of the hands and soles of the feet and then spreads over the entire body. Liver dysfunction occurs, causing the child to experience left flank pain and jaundice. Elevated levels of liver enzyme are seen—serum bilirubin, alkaline phosphatase, and serum transaminases. Skin alterations include dryness, pigmentation changes, and hardening of the skin, as seen in autoimmune diseases such as scleroderma. Gastrointestinal symptoms are nausea, anorexia, abdominal pain, and diarrhea. Interstitial pneumonia can be observed during the intermediate post-HSCT period (30 days to 100 days). GVHD is

staged according to organ involvement ranging from 0 (no GVHD) to IV (extensive involvement). Chronic GVHD may occur following the acute phase up to 1 year after the transplantation. Severity of manifestations vary once vital organs are involved, and death can occur.

2. Secondary malignancies. Risk factors for the development of secondary tumors include preoperative combination chemotherapy with or without total body irradiation, viral infections, GVHD and its prophylaxis, cancer genetic predisposition, and antigenic stimulation due to lack of recipient and donor histocompatibility.
   a. Leukemia (most frequent)
   b. Lymphoma
      i. Non-Hodgkin's disease
      ii. Hodgkin's disease
   c. Nonhematologic malignancies (rare)
      i. Adenocarcinoma
      ii. Glioblastoma
      iii. Sarcoma
3. Bacterial, viral, and fungal infections (frequent cause of mortality and morbidity following transplantation). Herpes viruses are the most common agent of infection.
4. Hemorrhage
5. Hyposalivation (due to irradiation)
6. Changes in dental caries–related oral microflora (due to irradiation)
7. Relapse or recurrence of original disease

LABORATORY AND DIAGNOSTIC TESTS

1. HLA typing—to identify compatibility of potential donors
2. Mixed lymphocyte culture analyses
3. Microlymphocytotoxicity test—identifies HLAs
4. Identifications of ABO antigens
5. Complete blood count, differential, and platelet count
6. Chemistry panel, levels of electrolytes, creatinine, magnesium
7. Hepatitis screen (A, B, and C)
8. Interdisciplinary evaluations: audiology, dentistry, nutrition, ophthalmology, occupational therapy, and physical therapy

9. Chest radiographic studies and sinus studies
10. Cardiac evaluation: electrocardiogram, echocardiogram, multiple-gated acquisition
11. Pulmonary function tests
12. Viral testing: cytomegalovirus, herpes simplex virus, varicella-zoster virus, EBV, human immunodeficiency virus

MEDICAL MANAGEMENT

There are three types of hematopoietic stem cell transplants: autologous, allogenic, and syngeneic. Autologous transplantation (auto-HSCT) uses the child's own bone marrow and is performed for treatment of malignant diseases. Auto-HSCT is used as a form of consolidation therapy within the initial remission-induction therapy period or for those who have early relapse. Allogeneic transplantation (allo-HSCT), the most frequent type of HSCT, uses bone marrow from someone other than the child. The donor of choice is first a sibling, followed by a relative, parent (rarely), or closely matched unrelated donor (obtained through a national registry). Alternative donor matching options include matched unrelated donor, mismatched related donor, and unrelated cord blood donor. Syngeneic bone marrow is marrow from an identical twin. The chances of a sibling match are about 35%; parents and relatives have only a remote chance of being matches.

Critical to ensuring appropriate matching between donor and recipient is HLA typing. HLA matching is important to prevent the complication of GVHD. Rejection risk increases as the incompatibility between the donor and recipient increases. A majority of transplants are allogenic, but methods to decrease graft rejection and GVHD have improved. HLAs are protein antigens on the surface cells that are used for immune recognition. The HLA system is responsible for recognizing foreign tissues and activating an immune response. There are approximately 100 HLA antigens. The most important HLAs for matching tissue for HSCT are HLA-A, HLA-B, HLA-DR, and HLA-D antigens. The DR antigen is the most important in matching for compatibility.

Before the transplantation, a conditioning (ablative) regimen is followed. Conditioning destroys cancer cells to prevent relapse, suppresses the immune system to prevent rejection of the marrow, and enables engraftment of the infused stem cells to occur in the child's marrow. The child's bone marrow is treated with tumor antibodies to eradicate any residual disease before the donor marrow is infused into the child. The conditioning regimen involves high-dose cytotoxic drugs with or without total body irradiation. Cyclophosphamide, busulfan, cytosine arabinoside, and l-phenylalanine are used most often in the conditioning regimen. Once the conditioning is completed, the harvested marrow is infused into the child. With auto-HSCT, bone marrow is harvested from the donor's iliac crest under general anesthesia and frozen several weeks prior to the HSCT. With allo-HSCT, bone marrow is harvested and infused directly into the child. Between 10 and 21 days after the transplantation, engraftment occurs. Engraftment is demonstrated by increased white blood cell count and absolute neutrophil count (ANC).

The most serious complication of HSCT is GVHD (see the Complications section of this chapter). GVHD occurs with allo-HSCT within 30 days of the transplantation (the most critical posttransplantation period). Cyclosporine, methotrexate, antithymocyte globulin, steroids, or azathioprine (Imuran) are used to prevent or treat GVHD. Those who undergo HSCT for leukemia and experience the complications of GVHD (acute or chronic form) have less risk of experiencing relapse of their leukemia. This effect is called the graft versus leukemia effect. For 3 weeks following transplantation, the child remains immunosuppressed and receives red blood cells and platelets, because he or she is at risk for bleeding and infection. A serious complication for which to monitor during phase 2 (day 30 through day 100) is interstitial pneumonia, often caused by cytomegalovirus.

NURSING ASSESSMENT

1. Assess psychologic status before HSCT.
2. Assess for signs and symptoms of sepsis.
3. Assess for gastrointestinal complications of GVHD.
4. Assess for hepatic complications of GVHD (venoocclusive disease).

5. Assess for renal complications of GVHD.
6. Focus of assessments identified in items 2 through 5 is on monitoring for life-threatening effects.

NURSING DIAGNOSES

- Anxiety
- Tissue integrity, Impaired
- Infection, Risk for
- Fluid volume, Deficient
- Pain
- Fatigue
- Nutrition: less than body requirements, Imbalanced
- Growth and development, Delayed
- Therapeutic regimen management, Ineffective
- Body image, Disturbed
- Family processes, Interrupted

NURSING INTERVENTIONS

1. Answer parent's questions and reinforce information about research on HSCT, alternative treatments, transplant centers.
2. Answer child's questions and reinforce information using age-appropriate terminology and explanations (see Appendix J).
3. Provide orientation and reinforce information about HSCT routines, restrictions of personal items, isolation procedures and policies, average length of hospital stay.
4. Serve as service coordinator and communication liaison regarding treatment and care concerns.
5. Monitor side effects and complications of conditioning drug therapies.
6. Monitor hydration status, intake, and output.
7. Monitor for signs and symptoms of GVHD.
8. Assess pain status and administer pharmacologic and nonpharmacologic therapies (see Appendix H).
9. Monitor bone marrow infusion and assess for reactions (fever, hypertension, tachycardia, tachypnea).
10. Provide meticulous dental care, rinsing, oral therapy.

11. Provide psychosocial support as indicated by psychologic assessment and ongoing needs (see Appendix J).
12. Refer to mental health professional as needed for counseling.
13. Encourage expression of feelings using age-appropriate methods (see Appendix J).
14. Use behavioral techniques (i.e., hypnosis, muscle relaxation, visual imagery) for chemotherapy-related symptoms of anxiety, nausea, and vomiting.
15. Provide meticulous skin care.
16. Ensure adequate nutritional support.

🔺 Discharge Planning and Home Care

At selected HSCT centers, early discharge with intensive clinic follow-up and home care is being implemented. Discharge criteria under these circumstances are the following: child must be afebrile and have ANC of 500 polymorphonuclear cells/mm³ for up to 72 hours before discharge.

1. Instruct family and child about disease, long-term treatment, medication administration, symptom recognition, and complications.
2. Coordinate with school personnel. Children with autologous transplants return to school in 3 to 6 months; those with allogeneic transplants, in 9 to 12 months.
3. Instruct about long-term effects.
   a. Impaired growth
   b. Impaired fertility
   c. Restrictive lung disease and infections
   d. Cataracts
   e. Skin changes (similar to scleroderma)
   f. Musculoskeletal dysfunction
   g. Secondary cancers

CLIENT OUTCOMES

1. Child will be free of complications.
2. Child will achieve maximum potential for growth and development.

3. Parents will be competent in care of child.
4. Child will remain disease free.

REFERENCES

Alcoser P, Rodgers C: Treatment strategies in childhood cancer, *J Pediatr Nurs* 18(2):103, 2003.

Fidler P, Hibbs C: Bone marrow transplant today—home tomorrow: ambulatory care issues in pediatric marrow transplantation, *J Pediatr Oncol Nurs* 14(4):228, 1997.

Forte K: Alternative donor sources in pediatric bone marrow transplantation, *J Pediatr Oncol Nurs* 14(4):213, 1997.

Frederick B, Hanigan M: Bone marrow transplantation. In Foley G et al, editors: *Nursing care of the child with cancer,* ed 2, Philadelphia, 1993, WB Saunders.

Lennard AL, Jackson GH: Stem cell transplantation, *West J Med* 175(1):42, 2001.

Norville R et al: Virus specific cytotoxic T lymphocytes as prophylaxis for Epstein-Barr virus lymphoproliferative disease in pediatric bone marrow transplant recipients, *J Pediatr Oncol Nurs* 14(4):194, 1997.

Senior K: Umbilical cord blood transplants as good as bone marrow? *Lancet* 357(9273):2031, 2001.

84

◆

Transplantation: Organ

◆

PATHOPHYSIOLOGY

Tremendous strides have been made in pediatric transplantation in the last decade. Organ transplantation is an acceptable form of treatment for end-stage organ failure. Advances in immunosuppression, improvements in surgical techniques, and experience in postoperative management have contributed to the improved results. Kidney, liver, and heart transplantations have become routine, and lung and small bowel transplantations are increasing in numbers. Primary diseases that can lead to the need for renal transplantation include acquired diseases such as chronic glomerulonephritis, lupus erythematosus, pyelonephritis, hemolytic-uremic syndrome, and bilateral Wilms' tumor. It is also the treatment for congenital conditions such as polycystic disease, obstructive uropathy, cystinosis, and Alport's syndrome. The major problem associated with transplantation is rejection. Rejection can result from any of a variety of causes: cellular and/or humoral immune response, infection, and noncompliance with treatment regimen. Other causes of graft failure include technical failure and medication toxicity.

The major indications for liver transplantation include biliary atresia, α_1-antitrypsin deficiency, tyrosinemia, and posthepatic cirrhosis. Indications for cardiac transplantation include cardiomyopathy, hypoplastic left heart syndrome, and other lethal complex congenital heart anomalies.

The survival rates have improved significantly in recent years and range from 85% to 95% at 1 year after transplantation. Factors restricting transplantation currently are the limited availability of organs and the need for life long immunosuppression.

Growth may be delayed, but pubertal development proceeds normally after successful transplantation.

INCIDENCE

1. Occurrence of organ transplantation is 15 to 20 per 1 million population.
2. One-year graft survival rate for kidney transplants is 90%.
3. One-year graft survival rate for heart transplants is 85% to 90%.
4. One-year graft survival rate for liver transplants is 85%.
5. Survival rates are decreased with subsequent grafts.

CLINICAL MANIFESTATIONS

Refer to chapters dealing with disorders of specific organ.

COMPLICATIONS (POSTTRANSPLANTATION)

1. Hyperacute, acute, or chronic rejection
2. Poor organ function
3. Hypertension
4. Bleeding at transplant site
5. Infection (*Candida*, cytomegalovirus, other viruses)
6. Medication toxicity
7. Surgical complications
8. Increased risk of cancer

LABORATORY AND DIAGNOSTIC TESTS
Preoperative Evaluation

1. Extensive serologic studies, including chemistry panel, complete blood count (CBC) with differential, platelet count, viral screening, blood cultures
2. Meticulous search for infection, including dental examinations, sinus radiography
3. Electrocardiogram, chest radiographic study, echocardiogram, possible cardiac biopsy
4. Urinalysis, urine culture and sensitivity testing
5. Histocompatibility testing
   a. ABO blood type
   b. Antibody screening
   c. Human leukocyte antigen typing (A, B, C, D, DR)

Postoperative Evaluation

1. Metabolic panel, liver panel, CBC
2. Cyclosporine or tacrolimus levels
3. Biopsy of the transplanted organ (diagnostic for rejection)

MEDICAL MANAGEMENT

Immunosuppression regimens vary by center, but most include a combination of cyclosporine, azathioprine, tacrolimus, mycophenolate mofetil, sirolimus, and corticosteroids to prevent rejection. Rejection is treated with high-dose steroids or polyclonal or monoclonal antibodies. Other medications include nystatin as a prophylactic for *Candida* infection, antihypertensives and diuretics for hypertension and edema, antibiotics, and antacids. The average length of hospital stay following transplantation is 2 weeks. Medications must be taken for life, and close medical follow-up is required.

NURSING ASSESSMENT

1. See the Renal Assessment and Cardiovascular Assessment sections in Appendix A.
2. Assess hydration status.
3. Assess for signs and symptoms of infection.
4. Assess for signs and symptoms of rejection.

NURSING DIAGNOSES

- Infection, Risk for
- Fluid volume, Excess
- Body image, Disturbed
- Fear
- Coping, Ineffective

NURSING INTERVENTIONS
Preoperative Care

Prepare recipient and family for transplantation.

1. Provide information about presurgical routine.
2. Reinforce information given about surgery.
3. Provide age-appropriate preprocedural or preoperative preparation.

Postoperative Care

1. Monitor for and report signs of rejection.
2. Monitor vital signs and report significant changes, because they may be indicators of rejection, bleeding, infection, or hypovolemic shock.
   a. Check vital signs every hour for 24 hours; if stable, then check vital signs every 4 hours.
3. Monitor urinary output; report any significant changes.
4. Observe for drainage on dressing.
   a. Circle extent of drainage.
   b. Notify physician if drainage increases significantly.
5. Observe for child's therapeutic response to and untoward effects of medications.
6. Observe for and report signs and symptoms of possible complications.

Discharge Planning and Home Care

1. Instruct child and family about therapeutic responses and untoward reactions to medications.
2. Reinforce necessity of complying with medical regimen.
3. Reinforce information provided about nutritional needs.
4. Instruct about proper dental care (brushing and flossing).
5. Refer to appropriate community resources, clinics, agencies, or personnel for psychosocial needs.

CLIENT OUTCOMES

1. Child will have normal graft function.
2. Child will remain free of infection.
3. Child and family will understand and remain compliant with medication and follow-up regimens.

REFERENCES

Boucek MM et al: The Registry of the International Society of Heart and Lung Transplantation: first official report—1997, *J Heart Lung Transplant* 16(12): 1189, 1997.

Doelling NR et al: Medium term results of pediatric patients undergoing orthotopic heart transplantation, *J Heart Lung Transplant* 16(12):1225, 1997.

Neuman M: Evaluation of the pediatric renal transplant recipient, *ANNA J* 24(5):515, 1997.

Saunders R et al: Rapamycin in transplantation: a review of the evidence, *Kidney Int* 59:3, 2001.

85

◆

Traumatic Brain Injury

◆

PATHOPHYSIOLOGY

Traumatic brain injury (TBI) is a common injury in children and the most common cause of traumatic death. TBI is often caused by a primary injury, followed by a secondary injury. The primary injury is the actual trauma itself because it occurs after the impact on the central nervous system and may cause damage and/or death of the brain cells. A hypoxic insult may also cause a primary injury. The secondary injury is caused by the brain's response to the trauma and evolves over a period of hours to days after the injury. The secondary injury can result in the loss of cerebral autoregulation, development of cerebral edema, and breakdown of the blood-brain barrier. The secondary injury is magnified by systemic hypotension or hypertension, hypoxia, or hypercapnia.

INCIDENCE

1. Boys are affected more often than girls.
2. Concussions are the most frequent type of TBI.
3. Six hundred thousand children are treated for TBI in the emergency department each year.
4. TBI is the leading cause of acquired disability in childhood.
5. Every year, 25,000 children die from a TBI.
6. Causes of TBI vary with age:
   a. Ages 1 to 2 years—frequently results from child abuse
   b. Ages 2 to 5 years—frequently results from motor vehicle collisions in which the child was an unrestrained passenger

    c. Ages 5 to 12 years—frequently results from pedestrian injuries and falls from bikes, roller blades, all-terrain vehicles, skateboards, and so on

    d. Ages 12 to 18 years—frequently results from motor vehicle collision and violent assaults

7. Skull fractures are present in 25% of children with TBI.
8. Posttraumatic seizures develop in 10% of children with cerebral contusions.
9. Laws requiring the use of seat belts or car seats for children of all ages have been effective in reducing the frequency and severity of TBI.
10. The effectiveness of bicycle helmets for injury prevention has been clearly demonstrated, and helmets should be worn during participation in other sports and recreational activities.

CLINICAL MANIFESTATIONS

1. Bump or bruise on head
2. Headache
3. Bleeding from laceration, nose, or ears
4. Seizures
5. Vomiting
6. Irritability and agitation
7. Loss of consciousness
8. Decorticate or decerebrate posturing
9. Battle's sign—bruising over temporal area
10. Raccoon sign—bruising around eyes

COMPLICATIONS

Depending on the type, severity, and location of the head injury, deficits may be multiple and include motor, communicative, cognitive, sensory, behavioral, and emotional problems or delay in reaching developmental milestones not yet achieved. A variety of complications involving the nervous system and other organ systems may be seen. These complications can occur from either the primary or secondary injury to the brain.

Primary Brain Injury

Primary injuries include the following:

1. *Scalp lacerations* are common in infants and young children and are usually harmless unless a large amount of blood is lost so that hypovolemic shock occurs.

2. *Concussion* results from shearing and stretching forces in the brain that produce no structural damage. This is the least serious type of injury that requires close monitoring for complications. With a concussion, the child usually has a momentary loss of consciousness. Recovery generally takes place within 24 hours with a return to the preinjury level of activity and orientation.

3. *Cerebral contusion* is localized brain injury that consists of bruising, tearing, bleeding, and swelling of the brain with temporary or permanent structural damage. This may occur directly under the area of impact or on the opposite side of the brain as it hits the skull. A contusion causes a disruption of cerebral tissue to varying degrees. Signs and symptoms reflect the extent of injury and blood loss and may include loss of consciousness, mild motor and sensory deficits, changes in visual awareness, seizures, or coma.

4. *Skull fractures* may take the form of a *linear skull fracture* in which the dura mater is not penetrated; a *depressed skull fracture,* in which bone fragments are indented into the brain tissue and produce a hematoma or contusion; or a *compound skull fracture,* in which a laceration and depressed fracture are present. The skull fragment often lacerates the dura as it is displaced into the brain tissue. A *basilar skull fracture* is a break in the posterior portion of the skull that often results in a dural laceration, which leads to the leakage of cerebrospinal fluid.

5. *Hematoma* is the accumulation of blood under the skull. An *epidural hematoma* occurs when the blood collects between the skull and the dura mater. This is most common in older children and usually results from a tear of the meningeal artery. Clinically, loss of consciousness may occur, and hematoma should be suspected if there is a basal or temporal skull fracture. Children with this type of hematoma should be assessed for decreased level of consciousness, development of

headache, dilation of the pupil on the affected side, and fever. Symptoms may be delayed for hours or days if the source of bleeding is venous. A *subdural hematoma* occurs when the blood collects below the dura mater and the brain and is often associated with a contusion. This type of hematoma can become life threatening if it compresses vital centers of the brain or causes cerebral edema. Children with this type of hematoma should be assessed for loss of consciousness, unilateral pupil dilation, focal seizures, and/or hemiparesis. Treatment for symptomatic hematomas, no matter where they are located, is surgical evacuation of the hematoma by a craniotomy procedure. The prognosis for the child with a subdural hematoma is less favorable than that for a child with an epidural hematoma, even after surgical evacuation, due to the associated damage to the underlying brain tissue.

6. *Subarachnoid hemorrhage* results from a tear of the subarachnoid vessels due to the large shearing forces produced during a severe TBI. This type of hemorrhage is frequently seen in the abused child. Children should be assessed for nuchal rigidity, headache, and decreasing levels of consciousness.

7. *Diffuse axonal injury* is frequently seen in children with severe head trauma, such as those with shaken baby syndrome, and is caused by a strain on the actual nerve fibers. This results in a generalized block along the nerve pathways. This type of injury may result in widespread cerebral edema, neuronal dysfunction, and prolonged coma. The prognosis for this type of injury ranges from severe disability to death.

Secondary Brain Injury

Secondary brain injury results from the severity of the primary brain injury and may include the following:

1. *Cerebral edema* either is caused by the primary injury or is a result of hypoxia, hypercapnia, or cerebral ischemia. Edema usually peaks in 24 to 72 hours and often results in a deterioration of neurologic status. Cerebral edema

may result in increased intracranial pressure (ICP); this then may lead to decreased cerebral perfusion, which may result in irreversible brain dysfunction, herniation, and death if not treated.

2. *Meningitis* may result from an infection of the cerebrospinal fluid. Clinically, the child will develop fever, nuchal rigidity, and irritability.

LABORATORY AND DIAGNOSTIC TESTS

1. Radiographic study of skull
2. Computed tomographic scan of brain
3. Magnetic resonance imaging of brain
4. Test for presence of glucose in drainage from ears or nose

MEDICAL MANAGEMENT

Management goals are to prevent and minimize secondary injury to the brain. As with any severe injury, the first step of treatment is management of the airway, breathing, and circulation. Treatment is then based on the neurologic assessment, which includes use of the pediatric Glasgow Coma Scale (GCS). The GCS rates the child's performance in three major areas: eye opening, motor response, and verbal response. The highest score that can be achieved is 15 (least injured); the lowest is 3 (poorest outcome). Scores of 8 or lower indicate a severe brain injury; scores of 9 to 12 indicate a moderate injury; and scores of 13 to 15 indicate a minor injury.

Minor injury (GCS score of 13 through 15) with normal radiologic studies and vital signs: child may be discharged to a reliable, knowledgeable parent. Appropriate discharge instructions include the following:

1. Wake the child every 2 hours to look for changes in mental status.
2. Return to the emergency department if any of the following occur:
   a. Vomiting
   b. Sleepiness or weakness
   c. Headaches
   d. Confusion
   e. Restlessness

f. Personality changes
g. Inconsolable irritability
h. Seizures
i. Drainage or blood from nose or ears

Moderate injury (GCS score of 9 through 12): child should be admitted for observation even if radiologic studies are normal.

Severe injury (GCS score of 3 through 8): child should be admitted or transferred to a pediatric intensive care unit. May require surgical evacuation of subdural or epidural hematoma along with supportive management. ICP monitoring may be indicated to identify and manage cerebral edema.

In all cases of TBI, the goal of therapy is a return of function. In some cases, function is lost or limited, which results in disability. Factors most predictive of disability(s) in a severe injury include the GCS motor score 3 days after injury, level of oxygenation in the emergency department, presence of intracranial hematoma, length of elevation of ICP, and presence and severity of extracranial injuries. Children with a severe injury will require an intensive rehabilitation program designed to promote a return to an optimal level of function. This is best managed in a pediatric inpatient rehabilitation unit, followed by outpatient therapy. In addition to rehabilitation to address lost physical function, such as impaired motor skills of the upper and lower extremities, motor skills for language, and swallowing abilities, cognitive rehabilitation is also critical to minimize the severity of disability. For children, a return to school is a major goal. For those with a severe TBI, a special individualized education plan will need to be developed to continue with the cognitive rehabilitation. Children may also be provided with school-based physical, occupational, and speech-language therapies; services for the hearing and visually impaired; behavior management; and counseling.

NURSING ASSESSMENT

1. Assess airway, breathing, and circulation.
2. See the Neurologic Assessment section in Appendix A.
3. Assess level of consciousness.
4. Assess for signs of increased ICP.

5. Assess for skin bruising or swelling, rhinorrhea, or ear drainage.
6. Assess cause of injury and identify potential child abuse.

NURSING DIAGNOSES

- Gas exchange, Impaired (if severe)
- Tissue perfusion, Ineffective (if severe)
- Injury, Risk for
- Pain
- Knowledge, Deficient
- Family processes, Impaired
- Caregiver role strain, Risk for

NURSING INTERVENTIONS

1. Ensure that patent airway, breathing, and circulation are present. Maintain oxygen and suction at bedside.
2. Monitor for, prevent, and intervene in case of increased ICP.
   a. Elevate head of bed 30 degrees to promote venous return and decrease cerebral vasocongestion.
   b. Monitor for signs of increased ICP.
      i. Increased respiratory rate, decreased heart rate, elevated blood pressure
      ii. Decreased level of consciousness
      iii. Seizure activity
      iv. Vomiting
      v. Alteration in pupil size and reactivity
3. Ensure safe environment, restrain child if agitated.
4. Decrease external stimuli.
5. Assess for signs and symptoms of disability.
6. Apply ice to bumps and bruises.
7. Administer skin care under cervical collar, if used.
8. Educate child and parents about causes and prevention of TBI.

🔺 Discharge Planning and Home Care
Preventive Care

Instruct children and family about importance of prevention. Examples include use of helmets in sports in which injury to head is possible following a fall, prevention of pedestrian–motor vehicle or bicycle–motor vehicle accidents, and avoidance of high-risk behaviors in older children. Offer both oral and written instructions, because families can be overwhelmed at discharge.

Long-Term Care

1. Instruct in need for and administration of medications, particularly antiseizure medications.
2. Identify need for outpatient physical and occupational therapy, cognitive retraining, expressive and receptive language retraining, oral motor retraining, behavior management, and counseling.
3. Support child and family with the school reentry process.
   a. Development of individualized education plan
   b. Neuropsychologic testing
   c. Appropriate stimulation; too many competing external stimuli can increase agitation

CLIENT OUTCOMES

1. Child will return to optimal level of neurologic functioning.
2. Child will maintain adequate cerebral perfusion, and vital signs will be within normal parameters.
3. Family will demonstrate positive coping strategies in situations in which disability results from TBI.

REFERENCES

Brain Injury Association: Pediatric brain injury fact sheet, Washington, DC, 1996, The Association.

Christianson J, Phelps J: Assessment and treatment of the pediatric traumatic brain injury patient, *Nurs Spect* 8(24):12, 1998.

Curley M et al: *Critical care nursing of infants and children,* Philadelphia, 1996, WB Saunders.

Michaud LJ: Brain injury rehabilitation, 5. Acute brain injury in children, *Arch Phys Med Rehabil* 79(3):S26, 1998.

Ponsford J et al: Impact of early intervention on outcomes after mild traumatic brain injury in children, *Pediatrics* 108(6):1297, 2001.

Sander AM et al: Relationship of family functioning to progress in a post acute rehabilitation program following traumatic brain injury, *Brain Inj* 16(8):649, 2002.

Strauss DJ et al: Long-term survival of children and adolescents after traumatic brain injury, *Arch Phys Med Rehabil* 79(9):1095, 1998.

86

◆

Urinary Tract Infections

◆

PATHOPHYSIOLOGY

Urinary tract infection (UTI) is the bacterial colonization of any segment of the urinary tract. The number of organisms in the urine is higher than can be accounted for by the method of collection. The most common diagnostic criterion for UTI is the presence of at least 100,000 bacterial colonies in 1 ml of a clean midstream urine catch obtained on two consecutive specimen collections. The presence of urine and stool around the urinary meatus allows the bacteria to proliferate and ascend upward to the urethra. Children at risk are those with underlying defects of the urinary system, chronic disease, and neurologic disorders. UTI is second in frequency of occurrence to upper respiratory tract infections.

INCIDENCE

1. The female/male ratio is 9:1.
2. Age range of peak incidence in girls is 7 to 11 years.
3. Age range of peak incidence in boys is 2 to 6 years.
4. In 90% of cases the infecting organism is *Escherichia coli.*
5. Fifty-seven percent of males and 37% of females with UTIs have an underlying abnormality.
6. Incidence of symptomatic UTI is lower than that of asymptomatic UTI.
7. Of people with UTIs, 30% to 80% experience reinfection within 1 year.
8. UTI rarely leads to permanent damage, end-stage renal disease, or chronic pyelonephritis.

9. Uncircumcised boys typically experience two or three UTIs in childhood.

CLINICAL MANIFESTATIONS
Infants (Initially Seen with Vague Symptoms)

1. Colic
2. Jaundice
3. Poor eating
4. Vomiting
5. Fever
6. Lethargy
7. Irritability
8. Increased number of wet diapers
9. Growth retardation

Preschool Children

1. Fever (most common)
2. Weak urinary stream or dribbling
3. Foul-smelling urine
4. Hematuria
5. Enuresis
6. Abdominal pain
7. Frequency
8. Urgency
9. Dysuria

School-Aged Children

1. Diarrhea
2. Strong urine
3. Hematuria
4. Dysuria
5. Frequency
6. Urgency
7. Personality changes

Children of All Ages

1. Abdominal distention
2. Dehydration
3. Flank pain

4. Costovertebral angle tenderness
5. Chills and fever
6. Constipation

COMPLICATIONS

1. Reinfection
2. Chronic pyelonephritis

LABORATORY AND DIAGNOSTIC TESTS

1. Urine culture—to determine presence and amount of microorganisms (obtain sample from midstream urine or urethral catheterization)
2. Suprapubic aspiration—to obtain sterile urine
3. Intravenous pyelogram—to visualize kidney and bladder
4. Voiding cystourethrogram—to establish presence of vesicoureteral reflux and abnormalities
5. Cystoscopy—to visualize interior of bladder and urethra (not routinely performed)
6. Retrograde pyelography—to visualize contour and size of ureters and kidneys
7. Cystometry—to assess filling capacity of bladder and effectiveness of detrusor reflux

MEDICAL MANAGEMENT

Before treatment is initiated, a diagnosis needs to be made based on the child's symptoms and results of the culture and sensitivity testing identifying the organism. Most of the commonly acquired UTIs can be effectively treated with 7 to 14 days of antibiotic therapy. The most commonly used antibiotics are trimethoprim/sulfamethoxazole, nitrofurantoin, amoxicillin, sulfisoxazole, cefaclor, and ampicillin.

NURSING ASSESSMENT

1. See Renal Assessment section of Appendix A.
2. Assess urine output for frequency, urgency, presence of odor, and dysuria.
3. Assess for elevated temperature.
4. Assess for pain (see Appendix H).
5. Assess for behavioral changes.

NURSING DIAGNOSES

- Urinary elimination, Impaired
- Hyperthermia
- Pain
- Therapeutic regimen management, Ineffective
- Injury, Risk for

NURSING INTERVENTIONS

1. Monitor child's therapeutic response to and untoward effects of medication.
   a. Obtain urinalysis including culture and sensitivity test before administration of drugs.
   b. Repeat urinalysis 48 to 72 hours after antibiotics are initiated and 1 week after therapy has ended.
2. Encourage intake of fluids according to norms.
   a. First 10 kg—100 ml/kg/24 hr
   b. Second 10 kg—150 ml/kg/24 hr
   c. Above 20 kg—170 ml/kg/24 hr

🔺 Discharge Planning and Home Care

Prime concern is to prevent reinfection.

1. Instruct family and child about importance of completing 7- to 14-day course of antibiotic treatment.
2. Instruct child to void frequently (retention of urine serves to maintain infection).
3. Instruct about proper perineal cleaning (e.g., anterior-to-posterior wiping).
4. Instruct about avoidance of bubble baths.

CLIENT OUTCOMES

1. Child will be free of signs and symptoms of UTI.
2. Child will not experience recurrent UTIs.
3. Child and family will adhere to treatment regimen.

REFERENCES

Eckler JAL: Combating UTI—urinary tract infection, *Nursing 2000* 30(6):1, 2000.

Marchiondo K: A new look at urinary tract infections, *Am J Nurs* 98(3):34, 1998.

Miller K: Urinary tract infections: children are not little adults, *Pediatr Nurs* 22(6):473, 1996.

Ross JH, Kay R: Pediatric urinary tract infection and reflux, *Am Fam Physician* 59(6):1472, 1999.

Rushton HG: Urinary tract infections in children: epidemiology, evaluation, and management, *Pediatr Clin North Am* 44(5):1133, 1997.

87

◆

Ventricular Septal Defect and Repair

◆

PATHOPHYSIOLOGY

Ventricular septal defect is characterized by a septal communication that allows direct blood flow between the ventricles, usually from left to right. Such defects may vary from 0.5 to 3.0 cm in diameter. Approximately 20% of the ventricular septal defects seen in children are simple (i.e., small). Many of them close spontaneously. Approximately 50% to 60% of affected children have a moderate-size defect and show symptoms in late childhood. The defect is frequently associated with other cardiac defects. The altered physiology can be described as follows:

1. Pressure is higher in the left ventricle and promotes the flow of oxygenated blood through the defect to the right ventricle.
2. Increased blood volume is pumped into the lungs, which eventually may become congested with blood; this may lead to increased pulmonary vascular resistance.
3. If the pulmonary resistance is high, right ventricular pressure may increase, causing a reversal of the shunt; the unoxygenated blood then flows from the right ventricle to the left, which produces cyanosis (Eisenmenger's syndrome).

In a child with a simple ventricular septal defect, the clinical picture may include the presence of a murmur, mild exercise intolerance, fatigue, dyspnea during exertion, and recurrent severe respiratory tract infections. The seriousness of the condition depends on the size of the shunt and the degree of pulmonary hypertension. If the child is asymptomatic, no treatment is required; however, if congestive heart failure (CHF) develops or the child risks pulmonary vascular change or demonstrates extreme shunting, surgical closure of the defect is indicated. The ideal age range for surgery is 3 to 5 years.

With a larger defect, the child will show the same symptoms, but they will be more severe and may appear within the first month of life.

INCIDENCE

1. The male/female ratio with the defect is 1:1.
2. An increase in ventricular septal defects is seen in children with Down syndrome.
3. The surgical risk of mortality is from 10% to 25%, depending on the types of complications involved, the defect size, the age of the individual, and the degree of pulmonary vascular resistance.

CLINICAL MANIFESTATIONS

1. Characteristic sign is loud, harsh, pansystolic murmur generally heard best at left lower sternal border (large defects may not be as loud as small ones).
2. Severe overloading of right ventricle causes hypertrophy and obvious cardiac enlargement.
3. With increased pulmonary vascular resistance, dyspnea and frequent respiratory infections are common.
4. Signs of cyanosis are possible, including assumption of squatting position and decreased venous return.

COMPLICATIONS

1. CHF
2. Infective endocarditis
3. Development of aortic insufficiency or pulmonary stenosis
4. Progressive pulmonary vascular disease
5. Damage to ventricular conduction system

LABORATORY AND DIAGNOSTIC TESTS

1. Cardiac catheterization—demonstrates abnormal communication between ventricles and demonstrates degree of pulmonary vascular resistance
2. Electrocardiogram (ECG) and radiographic study—reveal left ventricular hypertrophy
3. Complete blood count (CBC)—part of routine preoperative testing
4. Routine prothrombin time (PT) and partial thromboplastin time (PTT)—preoperative testing, may reveal bleeding tendencies (usually normal)

MEDICAL MANAGEMENT

Vasopressors or vasodilators are the medications used for children with a ventricular septal defect and severe CHF in critical care settings.

1. Dopamine (Intropin)—has a positive inotropic effect on the myocardium, resulting in increased cardiac output and increased systolic and pulse pressures; has minimal or no effect on diastolic pressure; used to treat hemodynamic imbalance caused by open heart surgery (dosage regulated to maintain blood pressure and renal perfusion).
2. Isoproterenol (Isuprel)—has a positive inotropic effect on myocardium, resulting in increased cardiac output and work; decreases both diastolic and mean pressures while increasing systolic pressure.

SURGICAL MANAGEMENT: VENTRICULAR SEPTAL DEFECT REPAIR

Early repair is preferable if the defect is large. Infants with CHF may require complete or palliative surgery in the form of pulmonary artery banding if the condition cannot be stabilized medically. Because of the irreversible damage secondary to pulmonary vascular disease, surgery should not be postponed past the preschool years or if progressive pulmonary vascular resistance is present.

A median sternotomy is made and cardiopulmonary bypass is established. Hypothermia is used for some infants. For a membranous defect high in the septum, a right atrial incision allows the surgeon to repair the defect by working through the tricuspid valve. Otherwise, a right or left ventriculotomy is necessary. Generally, a Dacron or pericardial patch is placed over the lesion, although direct suturing may be used if the defect is minimal. Previous banding is removed, and any deformities caused by it are repaired.

Surgery should produce a hemodynamically normal heart, although any damage caused by pulmonary hypertension is irreversible. Complications include the following:

1. Potential aortic insufficiency (particularly if present preoperatively)
2. Arrhythmias
   a. Right bundle branch block (right ventriculotomy)
   b. Heart block
3. CHF, especially in children with pulmonary hypertension and left ventriculotomy
4. Hemorrhage
5. Left ventricular dysfunction
6. Low cardiac output
7. Myocardial damage
8. Pulmonary edema
9. Residual intraventricular septal defects if repair not complete because of presence of multiple ventricular septal defects

NURSING ASSESSMENT

1. See the Cardiovascular Assessment section in Appendix A.
2. Assess for complications.
   a. Diastolic murmur—indicates aortic insufficiency
   b. Widening pulse pressure—indicates aortic insufficiency
   c. Arrhythmias
   d. CHF
   e. Bleeding
   f. Low cardiac output, especially during first 24 hours after surgery

NURSING DIAGNOSES

- Anxiety
- Activity intolerance

- Cardiac output, Decreased
- Tissue perfusion, Ineffective
- Fluid volume, Excess
- Infection, Risk for
- Injury, Risk for
- Family processes, Interrupted
- Growth and development, Delayed
- Therapeutic regimen management, Ineffective

NURSING INTERVENTIONS
Preoperative Care

1. Prepare child with age-appropriate explanations before surgery (see the Preparation for Procedures or Surgery section in Appendix J).
2. Monitor child's baseline status.
   a. Vital signs
   b. Color of mucous membranes
   c. Quality and intensity of peripheral pulses
   d. Capillary refill time
   e. Temperature of extremities
3. Assist and support child during preoperative laboratory and diagnostic tests.
   a. CBC, urinalysis, serum glucose level, and blood urea nitrogen level
   b. Serum electrolyte levels—sodium, potassium, and chloride
   c. PT, PTT, and platelet count
   d. Type and cross-match of blood
   e. Chest radiographic study
   f. ECG

Postoperative Care

1. Monitor child's postoperative status as often as every 15 minutes for first 24 to 48 hours.
   a. Vital signs
   b. Color of mucous membranes
   c. Quality and intensity of peripheral pulses
   d. Capillary refill time
   e. Periorbital edema

    f. Pleural effusion

    g. Pulsus paradoxus or decreased pulse pressure

    h. Arterial pressures

    i. Cardiac rhythms

2. Monitor for hemorrhage.

    a. Measure chest tube output hourly.

    b. Assess for clot formation in chest tube.

    c. Assess for ecchymotic lesions and petechiae.

    d. Assess for bleeding from other sites.

    e. Record blood output for diagnostic studies.

    f. Monitor strict intake and output.

    g. Administer fluids at 50% to 75% of maintenance volume during first 24 hours.

    h. Administer blood products as indicated.

3. Monitor child's hydration status.

    a. Skin turgor

    b. Moistness of mucous membranes

    c. Specific gravity

    d. Daily weights

    e. Urine output

4. Monitor for signs and symptoms of CHF.

5. Maintain skin temperature at 36.0° to 36.5° C and rectal temperature at 37° C.

6. Monitor and maintain child's respiratory status.

    a. Have child turn, cough, and deep breathe.

    b. Perform chest physiotherapy.

    c. Humidify air.

    d. Monitor for chylothorax.

    e. Provide pain medications as needed (see Appendix H).

7. Monitor for complications (see the Complications section in this chapter).

8. Observe for skin breakdown (e.g., back of head).

9. Monitor and alleviate child's pain (see Appendix H).

10. Provide opportunities for child to express feelings through age-appropriate means (see the relevant section in Appendix B).

11. Provide emotional support to parents (see the Supportive Care section in Appendix J).

🔺 Discharge Planning and Home Care

Provide instruction to parents about the following (see Appendix K):

1. Medications
2. Time intervals for follow-up care
3. Indications for contacting physician

CLIENT OUTCOMES

1. Child's vital signs will be within normal limits for age.
2. Child will participate in physical activities appropriate for age.
3. Child will be free of postoperative complications.

REFERENCES

Devine S et al: A basic guide to cyanotic congenital heart disease, *Contemp Pediatr* 15(10):133, 1998.

Hockenberry M: *Wong's nursing care of infants and children,* ed 7, St Louis, 2003, Mosby.

Park M: *Pediatric cardiology for practitioners,* ed 4, St Louis, 2002, Mosby.

Suddaby EC, Grenier MA: The embryology of congenital heart defects, *Pediatr Nurs* 25(5):499, 1999.

Witt C: Cyanotic heart lesions with increased pulmonary blood flow, *Neonatal Netw* 17(7):7, 1998.

88

◆

Wilms' Tumor

◆

PATHOPHYSIOLOGY

Wilms' tumor is usually a single tumor that arises from the renal parenchyma. It is separated from the kidney by a membranous capsule. The tumor originates from renoblast cells located in the kidney's parenchyma. A larger tumor will extend across the midline. The tumor may extend to surrounding structures, causing obstruction of the inferior vena cava (from ascites or edema) and/or obstruction of the intestines or constipation. It is associated with congenital anomalies such as hypospadias, cryptorchidism, pseudohermaphroditism, and aniridia, as well as with hemihypertrophy, cardiac malformations, Beckwith-Wiedemann syndrome, and neurofibromatosis.

This tumor grows rapidly. Tissue type varies from "favorable" to "unfavorable" pathologic characteristics. Favorable histologic categories include multiocular cysts, nephroblastomatosis, and congenital mesoblastic nephromas. Unfavorable histologic categories includes clear-cell sarcoma, anaplasia, and rhabdoid tumor. Metastasis occurs through the bloodstream to the lungs and liver. The tumor may spread through the lymphatics to the retroperitoneal lymph nodes. The most common site for metastasis is the lungs, followed by the liver, contralateral kidney, and bone (rare). The tumor should not be palpated because this can cause seeding of the tumor elsewhere or can lead to pulmonary embolization.

INCIDENCE

1. Wilms' tumor accounts for 6% of childhood cancers and 7% of all solid tumors in children. It is the most common renal malignancy in children.

2. Age range of peak incidence is 3 to 4 years; it is rarely seen after age 7.
3. Prognosis varies according to the stage of the disease at the time of diagnosis and tumor cell histologic characteristics.
4. Overall survival rate of children with tumors having favorable histologic characteristics and with nonmetastatic disease is 90%.

CLINICAL MANIFESTATIONS

The first three symptoms are the predominant clinical manifestations.

1. Flank mass
2. Pain
3. Hematuria
4. Hypertension
5. Fever
6. Malaise
7. Weight loss, anorexia

COMPLICATIONS

1. Metastasis to lungs, bone marrow (anemia), contralateral kidney, and liver
2. Adverse reactions to chemotherapy and/or radiation therapy

LABORATORY AND DIAGNOSTIC TESTS

1. Intravenous pyelogram and abdominal radiography, computed tomography (CT), ultrasonography, and/or magnetic resonance imaging—to detect mass, tumor thrombus in renal veins, enlarged lymph nodes, and tumor relationship to adjoining structures
2. Serum glutamic-oxaloacetic transaminase, serum glutamic-pyruvic transaminase, and lactic dehydrogenase levels—elevated with liver involvement
3. Complete blood count—to assess for anemia and potential bleeding problems
4. Urinalysis—to assess for hematuria
5. Urinary catecholamine levels—tumor markers; to rule out neuroblastoma

6. Blood urea nitrogen, creatinine, and electrolyte levels—to assess renal function
7. Chest CT scan—to assess for metastasis
8. Erythropoietin levels in urine and serum—increased in presence of metastatic disease
9. Bone marrow aspiration and biopsy—to assess for bone marrow involvement (rare)

SURGICAL AND MEDICAL MANAGEMENT

Surgery is very important in the treatment of Wilms' tumor. A nephrectomy, or removal of the affected kidney, is performed. In addition to removing the tumor, the surgery also serves to provide tissue for diagnosis, histologic examination, and staging, and it provides an opportunity to explore lymph nodes and abdominal organs for involvement. Staging is the exact determination of the extent of the disease at the time of diagnosis. The National Wilms' Tumor Study Group staging system consists of five stages that reflect the extent of disease. Postoperatively, radiation therapy and/or chemotherapy are initiated.

Wilms' tumor is radiosensitive. The decision to use radiation therapy is based on the histology and stage of the tumor. The chemotherapy drugs and dosage chosen are highly individualized. The following drugs may be given: vincristine, actinomycin D, doxorubicin, cyclophosphamide, cisplatin, etoposide, and ifosfamide.

NURSING ASSESSMENT

1. See Renal Assessment section in Appendix A.
2. Assess preoperatively for enlarged abdomen in flank areas (do not palpate tumor).
3. Assess for bowel sounds and abdominal distention postoperatively.
4. Assess for preoperative and postoperative pain (see Appendix H).
5. Assess wound for drainage and signs of infection.
6. Assess child's and family's response to illness and surgery.
7. Assess child's developmental level (see Appendix B).

NURSING DIAGNOSES

- Tissue integrity, Impaired
- Injury, Risk for
- Gas exchange, Impaired
- Infection, Risk for
- Anxiety
- Pain
- Coping, Ineffective
- Family processes, Interrupted
- Therapeutic regimen management, Ineffective
- Growth and development, Delayed

NURSING INTERVENTIONS

Preoperative Care

1. Avoid palpation of abdomen to prevent seeding of tumor.
2. Monitor child's clinical status; observe for signs and symptoms of complications.
   a. Vital signs
   b. Signs and symptoms of vena caval obstruction (facial plethora and venous engorgement)
   c. Signs and symptoms of renal failure
   d. Bone pain
   e. Anemia and bleeding tendencies
   f. Hypertension
3. Provide age-appropriate preprocedural and presurgical explanations to child to alleviate anxiety (see Preparation for Procedures or Surgery section in Appendix J).
4. Encourage child and parents to express concerns and fears about diagnosis (see the Supportive Care section in Appendix J).

Postoperative Care

1. Monitor child's clinical status.
   a. Vital signs (monitor as often as every 2 hours after surgery)
   b. Intake and output
   c. Hypertension (caused by removal of kidney)
2. Monitor child's abdominal functioning.
   a. Patency of nasogastric (NG) tube
   b. Bowel sounds

    c. Signs and symptoms of obstruction from vincristine-induced ileus

    d. Postoperative adhesion formation

3. Promote fluid and electrolyte balance.
   a. Monitor infusion of intravenous solutions.
   b. Monitor for electrolyte imbalances.
   c. Monitor for metabolic alkalosis (results from NG drainage).

4. Maintain and support respiratory status.
   a. Perform pulmonary toilet.
   b. Have child turn, cough, and deep breathe.
   c. Use suction as needed.
   d. Change child's position every 2 hours.

5. Monitor incisional site for intactness and healing.
   a. Observe for signs and symptoms of drainage.
   b. Monitor for intactness.
   c. Monitor for signs and symptoms of infection (redness, warmth, inflammation).
   d. Change dressing as needed.

6. Provide for child's hygienic needs.
   a. Oral and rectal care (especially important because child is immunosuppressed)
   b. Skin care—dry between folds of skin and lubricate

7. Protect child from infection resulting from immunosuppression.
   a. Maintain reverse isolation and/or meticulous hand-washing if white blood count decreases (refer to institutional policy). No fresh flowers or plants; wash fresh fruits and vegetables well.
   b. Limit contacts with public.
   c. Dress child appropriately for weather changes.

8. Monitor side effects of radiotherapy; tumor is remarkably sensitive to radiation.

9. Monitor side effects of chemotherapy.
   a. Actinomycin D
   b. Vincristine
   c. Doxorubicin
   d. Cyclophosphamide
   e. Cisplatin

    f. Etoposide

    g. Ifosfamide

10. Monitor and alleviate child's pain (see Appendix H).
11. Provide developmentally appropriate stimulation and/or activities for child (see Appendix B).

🔺 Discharge Planning and Home Care

1. Instruct parents about various aspects of medical management.
   a. Therapeutic response to medications
   b. Untoward reactions to medications
   c. Attendance at scheduled clinic visits
   d. Monitoring of axillary and oral temperature
   e. Need to call physician if any signs or symptoms of infection are noted
2. Provide information to parents about available resources.
   a. Community (i.e., school) resources (see Appendix L)
   b. Financial resources
3. Provide emotional support and referral to support groups for parents, siblings, and affected child (see the Supportive Care section in Appendix J).

CLIENT OUTCOMES

1. Child will be free of complications.
2. Child's level of anxiety prior to procedures and surgery will be minimized.
3. Child and family will adhere to long-term treatment regimen.

REFERENCES

Foley GV et al: *Nursing care of the child with cancer,* Philadelphia, 1993, WB Saunders.

Stegbauer CC: Diagnosis and referral of Wilms' tumor, *Nurse Pract* 24(5):121, 1999.

Young G et al: Recognition of common childhood malignancies, *Am Fam Physician* 61(7):2144, 2000.

Pediatric Diagnostic Tests and Procedures

General Nursing Action

These nursing actions are applicable to all the procedures discussed in this section.

NURSING ASSESSMENT

Assess the following:
1. Developmental level of cognitive capacity as it relates to ability to understand procedure
2. Previous experience with procedure
3. Acuity level
4. Coping abilities
5. Available parental support
6. Parental understanding of procedure
7. Allergies
8. Reaction to medications taken previously

NURSING INTERVENTIONS
Preprocedural Care (See Appendix J)

1. Explain procedure, including sensory information, in age-appropriate language; younger child may want to practice selected aspects of procedure (e.g., lying on abdomen).
2. Prepare child for preparatory procedural assessment (e.g., complete blood count or urinalysis).
3. Obtain information about usual reaction and sensitivity.
4. Reinforce information given to parents about child's or infant's condition; explain purpose and anticipated outcome of procedure.

Postprocedural Care

1. Provide opportunities for child to discuss procedure and for clarification of misconceptions.
2. Monitor child's clinical status.
   a. Vital signs
   b. Level of consciousness
3. Provide foods and fluids when tolerated.
   a. Discontinue intravenous fluids when child is awake.
   b. Initially offer small amounts of clear fluids; assess tolerance before progressing to full liquids and solids.

89

◆

Cardiac Catheterization

◆

Cardiac catheterization is an invasive procedure used to measure the intracardiac pressure of the heart chambers and great vessels, as well as oxygen saturation. In addition, angiography is performed when contrast dye is injected to outline the anatomic details of any cardiac malformation. A radiopaque catheter is inserted percutaneously through a large-bore needle into the right femoral artery. Measurements of chamber pressures, oxygen saturation, cardiac output, and shunt flow, as well as pulmonary vascular resistance, are obtained and recorded (Box 89-1). In children cardiac catheterization is used primarily to accurately diagnose complex cardiac defects. Neonates and infants with congestive heart failure who appear pale, cyanotic, tachypneic, diaphoretic, fretful, or fatigued will be studied earlier than a stable child for whom the timing of further repair of a defect remains in question.

Cardiac catheterization is also performed in an interventional manner, using balloon catheters or coiled stents for such purposes as dilating stenotic valves or vessels, and using coils or umbrella catheters for closing defects. This can delay or negate the need for surgery. Cardiac catheterization is also performed for electrophysiologic studies, for studies of the heart's electrical system, and in those infants and children with dysrhythmias refractory to medication.

NURSING ASSESSMENT

1. Assess cardiopulmonary status.
   a. Respiratory rate and quality of lung sounds
   b. Color
   c. Heart rate and cardiac sounds

BOX 89-1

Normal Heart Chamber and Great Vessel Pressures and Oxygen Saturations

The pressures in the systemic circuit, or on the left side of the heart, are normally higher than those in the pulmonary circuit, or on the right side of the heart.

- Superior vena cava mean pressure: 3 to 5 mm Hg
- Right atrium mean pressure: 3 to 5 mm Hg
- Right ventricle systolic/diastolic pressure: 25/3 mm Hg
- Pulmonary artery systolic/diastolic pressure: 25/10 mm Hg
- Left atrium mean pressure: 8 mm Hg
- Left ventricle systolic/diastolic pressure: 100/6 mm Hg
- Aorta systolic/diastolic pressure: 100/60 mm Hg

It is normal for oxygen in the blood to be extracted by the tissues so that blood returns to the right side of the heart with an oxygen level about 30% lower than the level when it entered the left atrium from the lungs. Blood entering the left atrium is less than 97% to 100% saturated because there is mixing with blood passing through pulmonary arteriovenous and other small shunts.

- Right atrium saturation: 65% to 75%
- Right ventricle saturation: 65% to 75%
- Left atrium saturation: 95%
- Left ventricle saturation: 95%

    d. Dorsalis pedis (pedal) pulse quality

    e. Skin temperature and color

    f. Complete blood count (to obtain values necessary for hemodynamic calculations in the catheterization laboratory), bleeding time, and type and cross-match

2. Assess whether nothing-by-mouth orders were carried out.
3. Assess child's and parents' knowledge of procedure and level of anxiety.

NURSING INTERVENTIONS
Preprocedural Care

1. Prepare child and parents for procedure and describe cardiac catheterization room.
2. Administer sedative and monitor child's response according to institutional guidelines.
3. Mark dorsalis pedis pulse and posterior tibial pulse.

4. Record baseline oxygen saturation in infant with cyanotic heart defect.
5. Ensure safe transport to catheterization laboratory.
   a. Monitor heart rate and oxygen saturation.
   b. Provide equipment for airway management, including oxygen, suction, ventilation bag, and mask; additional airway equipment (for intubation) is needed for unstable infant or child.

Postprocedural Care

1. Assess physiologic status.
   a. Monitor vital signs every 15 minutes during first hour; every 30 minutes during second hour; then every hour for 4 hours; then every 4 hours.
   b. Assess pulses below catheterization site for quality and symmetry.
   c. Assess color and temperature of affected extremity.
2. Assess insertion site.
   a. Intactness of dressing
   b. Signs of bleeding
   c. Formation of hematoma
3. Maintain bed rest for 6 to 12 hours after catheterization if arterial catheterization was performed and for 4 to 6 hours if venous catheterization was performed (or per order of physician).
4. Begin administration of clear liquids and advance diet as tolerated.
5. Assess for other complications or adverse effects such as pain, cold stress (infants), dysrhythmias, dye reactions, or nausea and vomiting.
6. Provide opportunities for distraction, relaxation, and play.

REFERENCES

Hockenberry M: *Wong's nursing care of infants and children*, ed 7, St Louis, 2003, Mosby.

Lock JE et al: *Diagnostic and interventional catheterization in congenital heart disease*, Boston, 1987, Martinus Nijhoff.

Tremko LA: Understanding diagnostic cardiac catheterization, *Am J Nurs* 97(2):16, 1997.

Uzark K: Therapeutic cardiac catheterization for congenital heart disease—a new era in pediatric care, *J Pediatr Nurs* 16(5):300, 2001.

90

◆

Computed Tomography

◆

Computed tomography is an invasive (with use of contrast dye) or noninvasive radiographic procedure that is performed to detect differences in tissue radiodensity. It is used for the entire body; for example, it provides a 360-degree view of the brain in 1-degree increments, giving an image of the intracranial structures and showing precise location of abnormalities. It is a diagnostic tool used in the assessment of various pathologic conditions. Serial evaluations can be performed because the amount of radiation is minimal.

NURSING ASSESSMENT

1. Assess infant's or child's ability to remain still for 5 to 45 minutes.
2. Assess for allergies if contrast dye is to be administered.
3. Assess child's previous experience with and reaction to similar procedures and need for sedation.

NURSING INTERVENTIONS

1. Provide age-appropriate explanation of procedure as it is performed (include anticipation of sensations).
2. Monitor infant's or child's reaction to sedation.
   a. Record pulse, respiration, and pulse oximetry readings (and blood pressure, if special equipment is available) every 5 minutes.
   b. Monitor untoward allergic reactions.
   c. Secure infant or child safely on scanning table.
3. Monitor infant's or child's pretest reaction to contrast medium; report any signs or symptoms of allergic reaction.

4. If procedure is performed on outpatient basis, instruct parents about monitoring sedated child after procedure.
   a. Child should rest or sleep until sedation has worn off.
   b. Ensure that parents understand importance of maintaining open airway when child is sleeping from sedation (especially in car seat).

REFERENCES

Behrman R et al, editors: *Nelson textbook of pediatrics,* ed 16, Philadelphia, 2000, WB Saunders.

Hockenberry M: *Wong's nursing care of infants and children,* ed 7, St Louis, 2003, Mosby.

91

❖

Electrocardiography

❖

Electrocardiography is a noninvasive procedure that measures the electrical activity of the heart and records it on graph paper. It provides a written account of each myocardial contraction and the electrical activity generated by it. Electrocardiograms (ECGs or EKGs) can be used diagnostically to demonstrate myocardial infarction and ischemia, hypertrophy of the heart chambers, electrolyte and acid-base imbalances, and effects of various drugs. The ECG is used to detect cardiac arrhythmias and conduction defects, and it can reveal a cardiac rhythm that is typically diagnostic of a specific cardiac disorder or congenital heart defect. The ECG sinus pattern changes with age. The greatest change occurs during the first year of life, which reflects the alterations in circulation.

NURSING ASSESSMENT

1. Assess child's previous experience with procedures.
2. Assess developmental and cognitive level.
3. Assess child's and parents' understanding of procedure.

NURSING INTERVENTIONS

1. Explain procedure to child before it is performed.
2. Encourage child to ask questions.
3. Reassure child and encourage him or her to lie quietly during procedure.
4. Assist in gently holding infant or child (to limit motion during procedure).
5. Remove conduction gel after procedure is completed.

REFERENCE

Hockenberry M: *Wong's nursing care of infants and children,* ed 7, St Louis, 2003, Mosby.

92

❖

Endoscopy

❖

Fiberoptic endoscopy of the upper and lower intestines is used for the diagnosis and treatment of a variety of intestinal diseases. Endoscopy provides visualization of the mucosa of the gastrointestinal tract, allows tissue samples to be obtained, and permits performance of therapeutic procedures. Upper intestinal tract endoscopy allows direct visualization of the esophagus, stomach, and duodenum. Indications for an upper intestinal tract endoscopy include bleeding, vomiting, failure to thrive, recurrent abdominal pain, ingestion of foreign body or caustic substance, and stricture. Lower intestinal tract endoscopy allows the physician direct visualization of the mucosa of the colon. Indications for colonoscopy include bleeding, chronic inflammatory bowel disease, and chronic diarrhea. There are few contraindications to endoscopy, and it is most often performed in an outpatient setting. Conscious sedation is used not only to sedate but also to minimize discomfort during the procedure.

NURSING ASSESSMENT

1. Assess child's compliance with preprocedural preparation such as ingestion of nothing by mouth and bowel preparation as ordered.
2. Assess child's and parents' understanding of procedure.

NURSING INTERVENTIONS

1. Explain procedure to child and caregivers before it is performed.
2. Monitor vital signs including oxygen saturation during and after procedure.

3. Ensure proper positioning of child.
4. Assist with airway maintenance.
5. Observe for evidence of bleeding or excessive abdominal pain and/or distension.

REFERENCES

Gilger M: Gastroenterologic endoscopy in children: past, present and future. *Curr Opin Pediatr* 13(5):429, 2001.

Hockenberry M: *Wong's nursing care of infants and children,* ed 7, St Louis, 2003, Mosby.

93

◆

Intracranial Pressure Monitoring

◆

Intracranial pressure (ICP) monitoring detects intracranial hypertension. It is indicated for the following conditions: intracranial hypertension, tumors, hemorrhage, contusions, edema, and brain injury. It is used in children when there is a diagnosis of Reye's syndrome, lead poisoning, hydrocephalus, metabolic disorders, and/or head trauma after neurosurgery. It is an invasive procedure that requires the drilling of burr holes into the subarachnoid space for the placement of the pressure monitor into the epidural space. One of several techniques may be used. These include ventriculostomy, ventricular tap, shunt, subdural recording, intraparenchymal recording, and subarachnoid bolt. Deep sedation is induced for monitoring the child.

NURSING ASSESSMENT

Assess child's neurologic status.

NURSING INTERVENTIONS

1. Maintain functioning of ICP monitoring equipment.
   a. Report readings higher than norm.
      i. ICP higher than 15 mm Hg
      ii. Cerebral perfusion pressure (CPP) higher than 50 mm Hg (CPP equals mean arterial pressure minus ICP)
   b. Note association between elevations and sleeping and feeding respiratory rate and apical pulse.
2. Monitor for signs and symptoms of complications.
   a. Hemorrhage

    b. Infection

    c. Leakage of cerebrospinal fluid

3. Provide explanations to parents about monitoring procedures to alleviate anxiety.

4. Monitor child's response to barbiturate coma.

    a. Monitor apical pulse, respiratory rate, blood pressure, and arterial pressure every 15 minutes during acute phase, then hourly during maintenance phase.

    b. Monitor urinary output hourly during acute phase, then every 2 to 4 hours during maintenance phase.

    c. Monitor serum level of sedative.

REFERENCES

Fischer D: Neurological monitoring, *Adv Nurses Fla* 2(9):18, 2001.

Hockenberry M: *Wong's nursing care of infants and children,* ed 7, St Louis, 2003, Mosby.

March K: Intracranial pressure monitoring and assessing intracranial compliance in brain injury, *Crit Care Clin North Am* 12(4):429, 2000.

94

❖

Intravenous Pyelogram

❖

The intravenous pyelogram (IVP) makes it possible to identify the presence or absence of the kidneys and determine the size, configuration, and function of the kidneys, renal pelvis, ureters, and bladder. Distortions, strictures, scarring, and distention from obstruction can be detected using IVP. Masses may be identified by their displacement of the kidneys, ureters, or bladder. Renal function is assessed by timing the clearance of the contrast medium through the kidneys. IVP may be used to detect renal calculi or tumors, identify urinary or kidney abnormalities (e.g., hydronephrosis, vesicoureteral reflux, polycystic kidney disease, renovascular hypertension), and evaluate the renal and/or urinary system after trauma.

The procedure is performed by injecting intravenous (IV) radiopaque contrast material and assessing its passage through the kidneys, ureters, and bladder. The dye is filtered by the kidneys and passes through renal tubules. Visualization is achieved by taking a sequence of radiographs at set intervals over 30 to 45 minutes. Congenital abnormalities such as absent or displaced kidneys or horseshoe kidneys, and abnormalities of the ureter are detected by assessing size and position of the structures compared to normal. Retroperitoneal tumors are detected by assessing kidney displacement and/or compression of renal structures. Extrinsic or intrinsic tumors, cysts, stones, and scar tissue can be detected by assessing the flow of dye through the renal pelvis, ureter, and bladder. IVP after trauma to the urinary system may reveal urinary leakage outside the urinary system. Renal hematomas are detected by assessing kidney contours.

If the renal arterial blood flow is interrupted (e.g., renal artery blood clots, arterial laceration), the contrast medium may not be visualized or the clearance time may be significantly increased. If glomerular disease is present (e.g., glomerulonephritis), the delay in clearance time will reflect the decreased glomerular filtration rate.

Some individuals may experience flushing and a warm sensation after the dye is injected. Because the dyes contain iodine, there is the potential for mild to severe allergic reactions. Antihistamine, epinephrine, vasopressors, steroids, oxygen, isotonic IV fluids, and resuscitation equipment must be available in case they are needed for treating an anaphylactic response.

NURSING ASSESSMENT

1. Obtain careful history, assessing for contraindications for IVP and conditions that are more likely to lead to complications. These include allergy or sensitivity to iodine (shellfish allergy), current treatment for asthma or other severe allergies, combined renal and hepatic disease, cardiac failure, oliguria (severe renal failure), severely elevated blood urea nitrogen (BUN) level, multiple myeloma, inability to tolerate dehydration procedures, and shock. Nephrotoxic dye can negatively affect renal function in children with dehydration, increased BUN levels, and multiple myeloma.
2. Assess child's developmental level to plan preparation (see the Preparation for Procedures or Surgery section in Appendix J).
3. Assess child's previous experience with and reaction to similar procedures.

NURSING INTERVENTIONS
Preprocedural Care

1. Observe for sensitivity to iodine or shellfish. Inform radiology staff if allergy is suspected. Premedicate with steroids and diphenhydramine (Benadryl) if ordered for prophylaxis in children with suspected sensitivity to contrast material.
2. Administer cathartic, laxative, and/or enema evening before and morning of procedure as ordered. Infants and young children are generally excluded from this step. Fecal

material, barium, and gas in bowel can impair visualization of renal structures.

3. Maintain food and fluid restrictions. Frequently, solid foods are restricted 8 to 12 hours before procedure. Clear fluids may or may not be permitted according to institutional policies. For individuals with high IV infusion rates, rate may need to be decreased during hours before IVP is performed. Although slight dehydration is required to concentrate contrast medium in urinary tract, adequate hydration before and after procedure is necessary to prevent renal failure from dye.

4. Assess fluid, electrolyte, and renal status (serum BUN and creatinine levels). Report any laboratory values that indicate renal failure and/or dehydration, because dye may worsen renal function.

Postprocedural Care

1. Observe for reactions to dye. Many individuals experience transient warmth, facial flushing, and/or salty taste. Mild reactions may include nausea, vomiting, and occasionally appearance of wheals. Serious reactions are related to anaphylactic allergic reaction to dye. Promptly notify physician if any reaction occurs. Be prepared to administer antihistamines if symptoms persist. If anaphylaxis occurs (rare), be prepared to resuscitate using oxygen, positive pressure ventilation, diphenhydramine, steroids, epinephrine, and vasopressors as indicated.

2. Ensure adequate oral or IV hydration to replenish fluids and avoid dehydration. Assess for adequacy of urine output. Instruct parents that decreased urine output following procedure may indicate renal impairment.

3. Observe for signs of extravasation at IV insertion site (elevate extremity and perform warm soaks as needed).

REFERENCES

Kee JL: *Handbook of laboratory and diagnostic tests*, ed 4, Upper Saddle River, NJ, 2001, Prentice Hall.

Kee JL: *Laboratory and diagnostic tests with nursing implications*, ed 6, Upper Saddle River, NJ, 2002, Prentice Hall.

Pagana K, Pagana T: *Mosby's manual of diagnostic and laboratory tests*, St Louis, 1998, Mosby.

95

◆

Magnetic Resonance Imaging

◆

Magnetic resonance imaging (MRI) is an imaging method that provides a clear anatomic display of the body. This display provides excellent tissue discrimination, and the study may be done in any plane without the use of radiation. The MRI scan is found to be superior to the computed tomographic scan because MRI uses no radiation and it depicts subtle contrasts between body tissues. Magnetic resonance images are created by sending radio waves to the child, who is lying in an external magnetic field. The image is created from interaction of the body tissue with the radio waves in the magnetic field. To prevent artifacts caused by movement, children are frequently sedated with either chloral hydrate or pentobarbital (Nembutal).

Client and environmental safety issues are paramount in the MRI room because the magnet is always on. The resulting magnetic field will attract any ferrous object (e.g., beepers, watches, infusion pumps, and oxygen tanks) into the scanner. Individuals are screened before entry for internal and external objects that may retain heat from the radio waves and cause burns.

NURSING ASSESSMENT

1. Screen child for pregnancy or implanted metal devices before scanning (metal devices may include, but are not limited to, metal pins or screws in bones, joints, or soft tissues; Harrington rod; pacemaker; and artificial heart valve).

2. Assess for adequate oxygenation during procedure if sedated.
3. Assess child's and parents' understanding of procedure.

NURSING INTERVENTIONS

1. Do not allow anyone to enter scan room with prohibited items.
   a. Hearing aid
   b. Cochlear or lens implant
   c. Jewelry, watch, tie pin, or tie tac
   d. Cardiac pacemaker
   e. Coins, magnetic-strip credit cards, or money clips
   f. Keys, safety pins, bobby pins or hairpins, or barrettes
   g. Beeper or metal stethoscope
2. Explain procedure to parents and child before entering scan room.
3. Monitor child's reaction to sedation.
   a. Record pulse oximetry value every 5 minutes until awake.
   b. Monitor untoward allergic reactions.

REFERENCE

Hockenberry M: *Wong's nursing care of infants and children,* ed 7, St Louis, 2003, Mosby.

96

❖

Peritoneal Dialysis

❖

Peritoneal dialysis (PD) removes solutes and fluids from the blood through the peritoneum (a semipermeable membrane) by means of osmosis and diffusion. Osmosis is the movement of a solute from an area of higher concentration to an area of lower concentration. Diffusion is the random movement of particles to form a uniform concentration. The purpose of PD is to remove toxic substances, body wastes, and excess fluids using the peritoneum as an exchange surface.

The PD catheter is placed through a small abdominal incision or through a trocar-induced puncture hole into the peritoneal cavity. This catheter is connected to a system of fluid bags and tubing. Dialysis can be done manually or via a continuous dialysis-cycling machine. When the dialysis fluid remains in the abdomen (dwell time), equilibration between plasma and dialysis fluid leads to removal of solutes and excess fluid. This occurs through diffusion and convection.

Many children with chronic renal failure receive continuous dialysis at night. This allows them to be disconnected from dialysis during the day. When manual dialysis is used, the dialysis solution is introduced into the abdominal cavity via gravity flow by raising the fluid bag above the level of the child. At the completion of the dwell time, the dialysate is removed by placing the fluid bag below the level of the child and allowing the solution to drain out by gravity. Accurate record keeping of the exact amount of fluid instilled and drained is required for appropriate fluid management.

PD is most frequently used in pediatric clients for the following reasons:

1. Congenital or acquired renal disease and resulting chronic renal failure.
2. Complications of acute renal failure not controlled with medical management.
3. Severe hypervolemia with deteriorating clinical condition refractory to diuretics and medical management. Signs of deterioration may include hypertension, volume overload, worsening neurologic status, congestive heart failure, pulmonary edema, and/or hypertensive encephalopathy.
4. Ingestion of toxins (these may include salicylates, phenytoin, heavy metals, barbiturates, or other substances).
5. Severely abnormal laboratory values not responsive to medical management. These conditions may include severe hyperkalemia, severe azotemia, intractable acidosis, severe uremia, or other electrolyte imbalance (hyponatremia, hypocalcemia, hyperphosphatemia).

NURSING ASSESSMENT

1. Assess child's underlying condition, including medical diagnosis, fluid and electrolyte status, hemodynamic stability, and other related factors.
2. Assess child's ability to tolerate procedure and therapy.
3. Assess child's response to therapy and resolution of symptoms or improvement in underlying condition.
4. Assess for complications related to PD.

NURSING INTERVENTIONS

1. Prepare child for catheter placement.
   a. Assess for special risks (bleeding disorders, ventriculoperitoneal shunt, hypotension, necrotizing enterocolitis). If PD is deemed best option, proceed with caution.
   b. Perform preprocedural teaching. Obtain informed consent (see Appendix J).
   c. Monitor child's reaction to sedation and pain medication (see Appendix H).

    d. Maintain sterile technique when assisting with catheter placement (e.g., use mask and sterile gloves).

    e. Monitor child's condition and intervene as needed.

2. Monitor response to therapy.

    a. Assess laboratory test results for blood urea nitrogen level, creatinine level, and blood chemistry analysis.

    b. Assess fluid status.

    c. Assess for bowel sounds and abdominal complications.

    d. Assess nutritional status. Promote adequate nutritional intake and protein replacement.

    e. Assess comfort level and ability to resume activities of daily living. Implement interventions that increase comfort level.

    f. Monitor for sleep pattern disturbance. Promote comfort and adequate rest periods.

3. Monitor for PD-related complications.

    a. Assess for retroperitoneal bleeding from perforation (decreased hematocrit, abdominal discoloration, signs of hypovolemia).

    b. Assess for signs of dehydration (tachycardia, hypotension, sunken eyeballs, decreased peripheral perfusion, and change in level of consciousness). Hypotension may result if fluid is withdrawn too rapidly and circulatory volume is depleted.

    c. Monitor temperature because infants and young children may become hypothermic if dialysate is not warmed prior to instillation.

    d. Monitor for signs of respiratory distress (from abdominal distention, fluid overload, and hydrothorax).

    e. Assess for hyperglycemia when using dialysis solutions with glucose.

    f. Maintain patency of dialysis catheter. Assess for leakage at insertion site.

        i. Assess for catheter occlusion by monitoring ease of flow by gravity.

        ii. Reposition child as needed to improve flow (e.g., turn side to side, raise or lower head of bed, etc.).

        iii. Position catheter and tubing without kinks with fluid bags at appropriate level. Secure catheter and tubing with sterile dressing and tape or tubing immobilization device.

    iv. Keep clamps in appropriate position.

    v. Administer anticoagulants as ordered.

    vi. Irrigate dialysis catheter as ordered.

g. Monitor for infection at catheter insertion site and/or peritoneal cavity.

    i. Maintain intact system while avoiding entering line. When entering line or changing drainage bags, use sterile technique.

    ii. Maintain sterile dressing over catheter insertion site. Clean site with nonirritating solution and redress per routine and as needed when dressing is wet or soiled.

    iii. Assess for signs of infection (fever, chills, increased abdominal tenderness, redness or swelling at catheter insertion site, increased serum white blood cell count, cloudy dialysate drainage solution).

    iv. Culture dialysate fluid as ordered.

    v. Administer antibiotics as ordered intravenously or via PD catheter.

h. Control pain (back pain, cramping, and incision site pain) using analgesic agents and nonpharmacologic techniques as indicated (see Appendix H).

    i. Monitor for protein loss.

4. Prepare child and family for home PD (as appropriate) by teaching and arranging home care support and equipment (see Appendix K).

REFERENCES

Chada V, Warady BA: Adequacy of peritoneal dialysis in pediatric patients. In Nissenson AR, Fine RN, editors: *Dialysis therapy*, ed 3, Philadelphia, 2002, Harley & Belfus.

Holoway MS: Peritoneal dialysis orders in children. In Nissenson AR, Fine RN, editors: *Dialysis therapy*, ed 3, Philadelphia, 2002, Harley & Belfus.

Locking-Cusolito H et al: Sleep pattern disturbance in hemodialysis and peritoneal dialysis patients, *Nephrol Nurs J* 28(1):40, 2001.

Neu AM: Infant and neonatal peritoneal dialysis. In Nissenson AR, Fine RN, editors: *Dialysis therapy*, ed 3, Philadelphia, 2002, Harley & Belfus.

Rainey KE et al: Successful long-term peritoneal dialysis in a very low birth weight infant with renal failure secondary to feto-fetal transfusion syndrome, *Pediatrics* 106(4):849, 2000.

Warady BA et al: Peritoneal dialysis in children. In Gokal R et al, editors: *Textbook of peritoneal dialysis*, Boston, 2000, Kluwer Academic Publishers.

97

◆

pH Probe Monitoring

◆

The presence of acid reflux in the distal esophagus is detected by pH probe monitoring. A thin, flexible probe is inserted transnasally and advanced to the distal esophagus 1 to 4 cm above the lower esophageal sphincter. It is attached to a portable recording device that permits monitoring of infants and children in a physiologic setting with normal dietary intake.

Continuous pH probe monitoring is indicated for diagnosis of gastroesophageal reflux. Reflux is considered to be a decrease in pH in the esophagus to less than 4.0. Exposure of the esophagus to gastric acid is assessed by (1) cumulative time the pH is lower than 4.0, (2) frequency of reflux episodes, and (3) duration of episodes.

NURSING ASSESSMENT

1. Assess child's previous experience with procedures.
2. Assess child's and parents' understanding of procedure.

NURSING INTERVENTIONS

1. Explain procedure to child and parents before it is performed.
2. Probe should be securely taped to infant's or child's face to maintain placement. Reinforce as needed to prevent dislodgement or removal by infant or child.
3. Instruct parents to document starting and ending time of feedings, position changes, vomiting, apnea, and so on. Careful documentation is necessary to ensure accurate results.
4. Instruct family/parents to avoid placing tension on probe or electrode wire.

5. Normal pH is 5.5 to 7.0; pH readings on meter that are higher than 8 or that are negative number indicate machine malfunction.

REFERENCES

Fonkalsrud E, Ament M: Gastroesophageal reflux in childhood, *Curr Probl Surg* 33(1):3, 1996.

Hillemeier A: Gastroesophageal reflux: diagnostic and therapeutic approaches, *Pediatr Clin North Am* 43(1):197, 1996.

Hockenberry M: *Wong's nursing care of infants and children,* ed 7, St Louis, 2003, Mosby.

98

◆

Pneumogram Sleep Studies

◆

Sleep studies and polysomnography refer to the continuous and simultaneous monitoring and recording of various physiologic parameters of sleep. Polysomnography is distinguished from a sleep study by the inclusion of sleep staging. Measured parameters include electrocardiographic data, airflow, respiratory effort, oxygen saturation, end-tidal analysis, blood pressure, and the individual's activity. The recording is reviewed and interpreted by a practitioner specially trained in sleep study and polysomnography interpretation.

A sleep study or polysomnography is indicated for individuals with sleep-related breathing disorders, neuromuscular disease, or sleep-related symptoms.

NURSING ASSESSMENT

1. Assess child's previous experience with procedures.
2. Assess child's and parents' understanding of procedure.
3. Assess child's routine daily activities and sleep patterns.

NURSING INTERVENTIONS

1. Explain procedure to child and parents before it is performed.
2. Provide supportive environment with favorite toy, pillow, or music to facilitate child's sleep.

REFERENCES

American Sleep Disorders Association and Sleep Research Society: Practice parameters for the indications for polysomnography and related procedures, *Sleep* 20:406, 1997.

Bobin S et al: Childhood obstructive sleep apnea: diagnostic methods, *Pediatr Pulmonol* 16(suppl):289, 1997.

Appendixes

A

◆

Nursing Assessments

◆

MEASUREMENTS

1. Temperature
2. Pulse
3. Respirations
4. Blood pressure
5. Height
6. Weight
7. Head circumference (under 2 years of age)

CARDIOVASCULAR ASSESSMENT

1. Pulses
   a. Apical pulse—rate, rhythm, and quality
   b. Peripheral pulses—presence or absence; if present, rate, rhythm, quality, and symmetry; major differences between extremities
   c. Blood pressure—all extremities
2. Chest examination and auscultation
   a. Chest circumference
   b. Presence of chest deformity
   c. Heart sounds—murmur
   d. Point of maximum impulse
3. General appearance
   a. Activity level
   b. Height, weight
   c. Behavior—apprehensive or agitated
   d. Clubbing of fingers and/or toes

4. Skin
   a. Pallor
   b. Cyanosis—mucous membranes, extremities, nail beds
   c. Diaphoresis
   d. Abnormal temperature
5. Edema
   a. Periorbital
   b. Of extremities

RESPIRATORY ASSESSMENT

1. Breathing
   a. Respiratory rate, depth, and symmetry
   b. Pattern of breathing—apnea, tachypnea
   c. Retractions—suprasternal, intercostal, subcostal, and supraclavicular
   d. Nasal flaring
   e. Position of comfort
2. Chest auscultation
   a. Equal breath sounds
   b. Abnormal chest sounds—rales, rhonchi, wheezing
   c. Prolonged inspiratory and expiratory phases
   d. Hoarseness, cough, stridor
3. Chest examination
   a. Chest circumference
   b. Shape of chest
4. General appearance
   a. Color—pinkness, pallor, cyanosis, acrocyanosis
   b. Activity level
   c. Behavior—apathetic, inactive, restless, and/or apprehensive
   d. Height and weight

NEUROLOGIC ASSESSMENT

1. Vital signs
   a. Temperature
   b. Respirations
   c. Heart rate
   d. Blood pressure
   e. Pulse pressure

2. Head examination
   a. Fontanelles—bulging, flat, sunken
   b. Head circumference (under 2 years of age)
   c. General shape
3. Pupillary reaction
   a. Size
   b. Reaction to light
   c. Equality of responses
4. Level of consciousness (see Glasgow Coma Scale in Table A-1)
   a. Alertness—response to name and command
   b. Irritability
   c. Lethargy and drowsiness
   d. Orientation to self, others, and environment

TABLE A-1
Glasgow Coma Scale

Symptom	Score
Eyes Open	
Spontaneously	4
To speech	3
To pain	2
Not at all	1
Best Verbal Response	
Oriented to time, place, and person	5
Verbal response indicating confusion and disorientation	4
Inappropriate words making little sense	3
Incomprehensible sounds	2
None	1
Best Motor Response	
Compliance with command to move body part	5
Purposeful attempt to stop painful stimuli	4
Decorticate pain response (arm flexion)	3
Decerebrate pain response (arm extension and internal rotation)	2
None	1

5. Affect
   a. Mood
   b. Lability
6. Seizure activity
   a. Type
   b. Length
7. Sensory function
   a. Reaction to pain
   b. Reaction to temperature
8. Reflexes
   a. Superficial and deep tendon reflexes (see Table B-1 in Appendix B for infant reflexes)
   b. Presence of pathologic reflexes (e.g., Babinski's)
9. Intellectual abilities (depend on developmental level)
   a. Ability to write or draw
   b. Ability to read

GASTROINTESTINAL ASSESSMENT

1. Hydration
   a. Skin turgor
   b. Mucous membranes
   c. Intake and output
2. Abdomen
   a. Pain
   b. Rigidity
   c. Bowel sounds
   d. Vomiting—amount, frequency, and characteristics
   e. Stooling—amount, frequency, and characteristics
   f. Cramping
   g. Tenesmus

RENAL ASSESSMENT

1. Vital signs
   a. Pulse
   b. Respirations
   c. Blood pressure
2. Kidney function
   a. Flank or suprapubic tenderness
   b. Dysuria

    c. Voiding pattern—steady or dribbling

    d. Frequency or incontinence

    e. Urgency

    f. Ascites

    g. Edema—scrotal, periorbital, of lower extremities

3. Character of urine and urination

    a. Appearance—clear or cloudy

    b. Color—amber, pink, red, reddish brown

    c. Odor—ammonia, acetone, maple syrup

    d. Specific gravity

    e. Crying upon urination

4. Hydration

5. Genitalia

    a. Irritation

    b. Discharge

MUSCULOSKELETAL ASSESSMENT

1. Gross motor function

    a. Muscle size—presence of atrophy or hypertrophy of muscles; symmetry in muscle mass

    b. Muscle tone—spasticity, flaccidity, limited range of motion

    c. Strength

    d. Abnormal movements—tremors, dystonia, athetosis

2. Fine motor function

    a. Manipulation of toys

    b. Drawing

3. Gait—arm and leg swing, heel-to-toe gait

4. Posture control

    a. Maintenance of upright position

    b. Ataxia

    c. Swaying

5. Joints

    a. Range of motion

    b. Contractures

    c. Redness, edema, pain

    d. Abnormal prominences

6. Spine

    a. Spinal curvature—scoliosis, kyphosis

    b. Pilonidal dimple

7. Hips
   a. Abduction
   b. Adduction

HEMATOLOGIC ASSESSMENT

1. Vital signs
   a. Pulse
   b. Respirations
2. General appearance
   a. Signs of congestive heart failure
   b. Restlessness
3. Skin
   a. Abnormal color—pallor, jaundice
   b. Petechiae
   c. Bruises
   d. Bleeding from mucous membranes or from injection or venipuncture sites
   e. Hematomas
4. Abdomen
   a. Enlarged liver
   b. Enlarged spleen

ENDOCRINE ASSESSMENT

1. Vital signs
   a. Pulse
   b. Respirations—Kussmaul's respiration
   c. Blood pressure
2. Hydration status
   a. Polyuria
   b. Polyphagia
   c. Dry skin
   d. Excessive thirst
3. General appearance
   a. Height and weight
   b. Mood
   c. Irritability
   d. Hunger
   e. Headache
   f. Shakiness

B

◆

Growth and Development

◆

INFANT (0 TO 1 YEAR)
Physical Characteristics
Age 0 to 6 months
1. Weight
    a. Birth weight doubles by 6 months.
    b. Infant gains approximately 1½ lb/mo.
2. Height
    a. Average height at 6 months is 26 inches.
    b. Height increases at rate of 1 in/mo.
3. Head circumference
    a. Head circumference reaches 17 inches at 6 months.
    b. Circumference increases by ½ in/mo.
Age 6 to 12 months
1. Weight
    a. Birth weight triples by end of 1 year.
    b. Approximate weight at 1 year is 22 lb.
    c. Infant gains 1 lb/mo.
2. Height
    a. Most extensive growth occurs in trunk.
    b. Infant grows ½ in/mo.
    c. Total height increases by 50% by 1 year.
3. Head circumference
    a. Head circumference increases by ¼ in/mo.
    b. Circumference at 1 year is 20 inches.

Gross Motor Development
Age 1 to 4 months
1. Raises head when prone

2. Can sit for short periods with firm support
3. Can sit with head erect
4. Bounces on lap when held in standing position
5. Attains complete head control
6. Lifts head while lying in supine position
7. Rolls from back to side
8. Arms and legs assume less flexed posture
9. Makes precrawling attempts

Age 4 to 8 months

1. Holds head erect continuously
2. Bounces forward and backward
3. Rolls from back to abdomen
4. Can sit with support for short intervals

Age 8 to 12 months

1. Sits from standing position without help
2. Can stand erect with support
3. Cruises
4. Stands erect alone momentarily
5. Pulls self to crawling position
6. Crawls
7. Walks with help

Fine Motor Development

Age 1 to 4 months

1. Makes purposeful attempts to grab objects
2. Follows objects from side to side
3. Attempts to grasp objects but misses
4. Brings objects to mouth
5. Watches hands and feet
6. Grasps objects with both hands
7. Holds objects momentarily in hands

Age 4 to 8 months

1. Uses thumb and fingers for grasping
2. Explores grasped objects
3. Uses shoulder and hand as single unit
4. Picks up objects with cupped hands
5. Is able to hold objects in both hands simultaneously
6. Transfers objects from hand to hand

Age 8 to 12 months
1. Releases objects with uncurled fingers
2. Uses pincer grasp
3. Waves with wrist
4. Can locate hands for play
5. Can put objects in containers
6. Feeds crackers to self
7. Drinks from cup with help
8. Uses spoon with help
9. Eats with fingers
10. Holds crayons and makes marks on paper

Sensory Development
Age 0 to 1 month
1. Distinguishes sweet and sour taste
2. Withdraws from painful stimuli
3. Distinguishes odors—able to detect mother's scent
4. Turns head away from aversive odors
5. Discriminates sounds of different pitch, frequency, and duration
6. Responds to changes in brightness
7. Begins to track objects but easily loses location
8. Prefers human face to other objects in visual field
9. Has visual acuity of 20/400—able to focus on objects up to 8 inches away
10. Quiets at sound of voices

Age 1 to 4 months
1. Discriminates mother's face and voice from those of female stranger
2. Evidences accurate visual tracking
3. Discriminates between visual patterns
4. Distinguishes familiar and unfamiliar faces

Age 4 to 8 months
1. Responds to changes in color
2. Follows object from midline to side
3. Follows objects in any direction
4. Tries to locate sounds
5. Attempts hand-eye coordination

6. Has highly developed sense of smell
7. Reaches adult limits of visual acuity
8. Responds to unseen voice
9. Demonstrates taste preference
Age 8 to 12 months
1. Has increased depth perception
2. Knows own name

Cognitive Development (Sensorimotor Stage—Birth to 2 Years)

Child learns through physical activities and sensory modalities (Table B-1).
Age 0 to 1 month
1. Involuntary behavior
2. Primarily reflexive
3. Autistic orientation
4. No concept of self or others
Age 1 to 4 months
1. Reflexive behavior gradually replaced by voluntary movement
2. Activity centered around body
3. Makes initial attempts to repeat and duplicate actions
4. Engages in much trial-and-error behavior
5. Attempts to modify behavior in response to varied stimuli (e.g., sucking breast versus bottle)
6. Demonstrates symbiotic orientation
7. Is unable to differentiate self from others
8. Engages in activity because it is pleasurable
Age 4 to 8 months
1. Demonstrates purposeful repetition of actions
2. Demonstrates emergence of goal-directed behavior
3. Discriminates differences in intensity (sounds and sights)
4. Imitates simple actions
5. Demonstrates beginnings of object permanence
6. Anticipates future events (e.g., feedings)
7. Demonstrates awareness that self is separate from others
Age 8 to 12 months
1. Anticipates event as pleasant or unpleasant
2. Demonstrates emergence of intentional behavior
3. Demonstrates goal-directed behavior

TABLE B-1
Infant's Reflexes

Reflex	Description	Appearance	Disappearance
Babinski	Fanning of toes with upward extension when sole of foot is stroked	Birth	9 months
Galant	Arching of trunk toward stimulated side when infant is stroked along spine	Birth	Neonatal period
Moro (startle)	Sudden outward extension of arms with midline return when infant is startled by loud noise or rapid change in position	Birth	4 months
Palmar (grasp)	Grasping of object with fingers when palm is touched	Birth	4 months
Parachute	Extension forward of arms and legs in protective manner when infant is held in horizontal prone and downward-moving position	8 months	Indefinite
Placing	Attempt to raise and place foot on edge of surface when foot is touched on top	Birth	12 months
Plantar	Inward flexion of toes when balls of feet are stroked	Birth	12 months
Righting	Attempt to maintain head in upright position	Birth	24 months

Continued

TABLE B-1
Infant's Reflexes—Cont'd

Reflex	Description	Appearance	Disappearance
Rooting	Turning of head toward stimulated side of cheek when touched	Birth	6 months
Sucking	Initiation of sucking when object is placed in mouth	Birth	Indefinite
Swimming	Mimicking of swimming movement when held horizontally in water	Birth	4 months
Walking	Initiation of stepping movements when held upright with feet touching a surface	First weeks; reappears at 4-5 months	12 months

4. Evidences object permanence
5. Looks for lost objects
6. Can imitate larger number of actions
7. Understands meaning of simple words and commands
8. Associates gestures and behaviors with symbols
9. Becomes more independent of mothering figure

Language Development
Age 1 month
1. Coos
2. Makes vowel-like sounds
3. Makes whimpering sounds when upset
4. Makes gurgling sounds when content
5. Smiles in response to adult speech
Age 1 to 4 months
1. Makes sounds and smiles
2. Can make vowel sounds
3. Vocalizes
4. Babbles
Age 4 to 8 months
1. Uses increasing number of vocalizations
2. Uses two-syllable words ("boo-boo")
3. Is able to form two vowel sounds together ("baba")
Age 8 to 12 months
1. Speaks first word
2. Uses sounds to identify objects, persons, and activities
3. Imitates wide range of word sounds
4. Can say series of syllables
5. Understands meaning of prohibitions such as "no"
6. Responds to own name and those of immediate family members
7. Evidences discernible inflection of words
8. Uses three-word vocabulary
9. Uses one-word sentences

Psychosexual Development (Oral Stage)
1. Body focus—mouth
2. Developmental task—gratification of basic needs (food, warmth, and comfort) as supplied by primary caretakers

3. Developmental crisis—weaning; infant is forced to give up pleasures derived from breast or bottle feedings
4. Common coping skills—sucking, crying, cooing, babbling, thrashing, and other forms of behavior in response to irritants
5. Sexual needs—pleasurable body sensations are generalized, although focused on oral needs; infant derives physical pleasure from being held, cuddling, rocking, and sucking
6. Play—tactile stimulation provided through caretaking activities

Psychosocial Development (Trust Versus Mistrust)

1. Developmental task—development of sense of trust with primary caretaker
2. Developmental crisis—weaning from breast or bottle
3. Play—interactions with caretakers form the basis for development of relationships later in life
4. Role of parents—infant formulates basic attitudes toward life based on experiences with parents; parents can be perceived as reliable, consistent, available, and caring (sense of trust) or as the negative counterpart (sense of mistrust)
5. Plan—to provide consistent, predictable support and love that foster child's attachment to primary caretakers and sense of trust about the environment

Socialization Behavior
Age 0 to 1 month
Smiles indiscriminately
Age 1 to 4 months
1. Smiles at human face
2. Is awake greater portion of day
3. Establishes sleep-awake cycle
4. Crying becomes differentiated
5. Distinguishes familiar and unfamiliar faces
6. Prefers gazing at familiar face
7. "Freezes" in presence of strangers

Age 4 to 8 months
1. Is constrained in presence of strangers
2. Begins to play with toys
3. Fear of strangers emerges
4. Is easily frustrated
5. Flails arms and legs when upset

Age 8 to 12 months
1. Plays simple games (peekaboo)
2. Cries when scolded
3. Makes simple requests with gestures
4. Demonstrates intense anxiety with separation from primary caregiver
5. Prefers caretaker figures to other adults
6. Recognizes family members

Moral Development

Moral development does not begin until the toddler years, when initial cognition is evident.

Faith Development (Undifferentiated Stage)

Feelings of trust and interactions with caretakers form the basis for subsequent faith development.

TODDLER (1 TO 3 YEARS)
Physical Characteristics
1. Weight
   a. Toddler gains approximately 5 lb/yr.
   b. Weight gain decelerates considerably.
2. Height
   a. Height increases by approximately 3 in/yr.
   b. Body proportions change; arms and legs grow at faster rate than head and trunk.
   c. Lumbar lordosis of spine is less evidenced.
   d. Toddler is achieving less pudgy appearance.
   e. Legs have "bowing" appearance (tibial torsion).
3. Head circumference
   a. Anterior fontanelle closes by 15 months.
   b. Head circumference increases by 1 in/yr.
4. Teeth—first and second molars and canines erupt.

Gross Motor Development

Age 15 months

1. Walks alone with wide-base gait
2. Creeps up stairs
3. Can throw objects

Age 18 months

1. Begins to run; seldom falls
2. Climbs up and down stairs
3. Climbs onto furniture
4. Plays with pull toys
5. Can push light furniture around room
6. Seats self on chair

Age 24 months

1. Walks with steady gait
2. Runs in more controlled manner
3. Walks up and down stairs using both feet on each step
4. Jumps crudely
5. Assists in undressing self
6. Kicks ball without losing balance

Age 30 months

1. Can balance momentarily on one foot
2. Uses both feet for jumping
3. Jumps down from furniture
4. Pedals tricycle

Fine Motor Development

Age 15 months

1. Builds tower of two blocks
2. Opens boxes
3. Pokes fingers in holes
4. Uses spoon but spills contents
5. Turns pages of book

Age 18 months

1. Builds tower of three blocks
2. Scribbles in random fashion
3. Drinks from cup

Age 24 months

1. Drinks from cup held in one hand
2. Uses spoon without spilling

3. Builds tower of four blocks
4. Empties contents of jar
5. Draws vertical line and circular shape
   Age 30 months
1. Holds crayons with fingers
2. Draws cross figure crudely
3. Builds tower of six blocks

Psychosexual Development (Anal Stage)

1. Body focus—anal area
2. Developmental task—learning to regulate elimination of bowel and bladder
3. Developmental crisis—toilet training
4. Common coping skills—temper tantrums, negativism, playing with stool and urine, regressive behaviors such as thumb sucking, curling hair into knot, crying, showing irritability, and pouting
5. Sexual needs—sensations of pleasure are associated with excretory functions; child actively explores body
6. Play—child enjoys playing with excreta as evidenced by fecal smearing
7. Role of parents—to help child achieve continence without overly strict control or overpermissiveness

Psychosocial Development (Autonomy Versus Shame and Doubt)

1. Developmental task—learning to assert self in expression of needs, desires, and wants
2. Developmental crisis—toilet training; child experiences, for the first time, social constraints on behavior by parents
3. Common coping skills—temper tantrums, crying, physical activity, negativism, breath holding, affection seeking, play, and regression
4. Play—child initiates and seeks play opportunities and activities; seeks attention from caretakers; explores body; enjoys sensations from gross and fine motor movements; plays actively with objects; learns to interact in socially approved ways

5. Role of parents—to serve as socializing agents for basic rules of conduct; to impose restrictions for first time on child's behavior; to direct focus from primary and immediate gratification of child's needs
6. Plan—to provide consistency in setting limits on child's behavior yet encourage child's exploration with environment and learning new skills

Moral Development (Preconventional Stage)

1. Toddler's concept of right and wrong is limited.
2. Parents have significant influence on toddler's conscious development.

Faith Development (Intuitive-Projective Stage)

1. Faith beliefs are learned from parents.
2. Child imitates family's religious practices and gestures.

PRESCHOOLER (3 TO 6 YEARS)
Physical Characteristics

1. Weight
   a. Preschooler gains less than 2 kg (5 lb)/yr.
   b. Mean weight is 18 kg (40 lb).
2. Height
   a. Preschooler grows 5 to 7 cm (2 to 2½ in)/yr.
   b. Mean height is 108 cm (42 inches).
3. Posture—lordosis is no longer present.
4. Teeth—preschooler is losing temporary teeth.

Gross Motor Development
Age 36 months

1. Dresses and undresses self
2. Walks backward
3. Walks up and down stairs alternating feet
4. Balances momentarily on one foot
Age 4 years
1. Hops on one foot
2. Climbs and jumps
3. Throws ball overhand with increased proficiency

Age 5 years

1. Jumps rope
2. Runs with no difficulty
3. Skips well
4. Plays catch

Age 6 years

1. Runs skillfully
2. Runs and plays games simultaneously
3. Begins to ride bicycle
4. Draws a person with body, arms, and legs
5. Includes features such as mouth, eyes, nose, and hair in drawing

Fine Motor Development

Age 36 months

1. Strings large beads
2. Copies cross and circle
3. Unbuttons front and side buttons
4. Builds and balances 10-block tower

Age 4 years

1. Uses scissors
2. Cuts out simple pictures
3. Copies square

Age 5 years

1. Hits nail on head with hammer
2. Ties laces on shoes
3. Can copy some letters of alphabet
4. Can print name

Age 6 years

1. Is able to use a fork
2. Begins to use a knife with suspension

Sensory Development

Age 4 years

1. Has very limited space perception
2. Can identify names of one or two colors

Age 5 years

1. Can identify at least four colors
2. Can make distinctions between objects according to weight
3. Imitates parents and other adult role models

Cognitive Development (Preoperational Stage—2 to 7 Years)

Child progresses from sensorimotor behavior as a means of learning and interacting with the environment to the formation of symbolic thought.

1. Develops ability to form mental representations for objects and persons
2. Develops concept of time
3. Has egocentric perspective; supplies own meaning for reality

The following are characteristics of thoughts:

1. Animism: belief that objects have feelings, consciousness, and thoughts as humans do
2. Artificialism: belief that a powerful agent (natural or supernatural) causes the occurrence of events
3. Centration: ability to focus on only one aspect of a situation
4. Participation: belief that events occur to meet the needs and desires of the child
5. Syncretism: use of a specific explanation for an event as an answer to describe situations that are different in nature from the original one
6. Juxtaposition: rudimentary form of association and reasoning; connects two events but does not imply causal relationship
7. Transduction: rudimentary form of association and reasoning; associates nonsignificant facts in a causal relationship
8. Irreversibility: inability to reverse the process of thinking; inability to backtrack through the content of thoughts from conclusion to beginning

Language Development
Age 2 years
1. Uses two- and three-word sentences
2. Uses holophrases
3. More than half of speech is understandable
Age 3 years
1. Constantly asks questions
2. Talks whether audience present or not

3. Uses telegraphic speech (without prepositions, adjectives, adverbs, and so on)
4. Enunciates the following consonants: *d, b, t, k,* and *y*
5. Omits *w* from speech
6. Has vocabulary of 900 words
7. Uses three-word sentences (subject-verb-object)
8. States own name
9. Makes specific sound errors *(s, sh, ch, z, th, r,* and *l)*
10. Pluralizes words
11. Repeats phrases and words aimlessly

Age 4 years

1. Has vocabulary of 1500 words
2. Counts to three
3. Narrates lengthy story
4. Understands simple questions
5. Understands basic cause-effect relationships of feelings
6. Conversation is egocentric
7. Makes specific sound errors *(s, sh, ch, z, th, r,* and *l)*
8. Uses four-word sentences

Age 5 years

1. Has 2100-word vocabulary
2. Uses five-word sentences
3. Uses prepositions and conjunctions
4. Uses complete sentences
5. Understands questions related to time and quantity (how much and when)
6. Continues specific sound errors
7. Learns to participate in social conversations
8. Can name days of week

Age 6 years

1. Speech sound errors disappear
2. Understands cause-effect relationships of physical events
3. Uses language as medium of verbal exchange
4. Speech resembles adult form in terms of structure
5. Expands vocabulary according to environmental stimulation

Psychosexual Development (Phallic Stage)

1. Body focus—genitals
2. Developmental task—increased awareness of sex organs and interest in sexuality
3. Developmental crisis—Oedipal or Electra complex; castration fears; fear of intrusion to body; development of prerequisites for masculine or feminine identity; identification with parent of same sex (in families with only one parent, resolution of crisis during this stage may be more difficult)
4. Common coping skills—reaction formation; transition of negative feelings toward parent of opposite sex to positive feelings; masturbation during periods of stress and isolation
5. Temperament—amount of jealousy and behaviors vary according to child's past experiences and family environment
6. Play—dramatic play in which child enacts parental roles and same-sex roles

The following are age-specific characteristics:

1. Age 5 years—decreased sex play; child is modest and evidences less exposure; interested in where babies come from; aware of adult sex organs
2. Age 6 years—mild sex play, with increased exhibitionism; mutual investigation of sexes

Psychosocial Development (Initiative Versus Guilt)

1. Developmental task—development of conscience; increased awareness of self and ability to function in the world
2. Developmental crisis—modeling appropriate sex roles; learning right and wrong
3. Common coping skills
   a. Beginning problem-solving skills
   b. Denial
   c. Reaction formation
   d. Somatization (usually in gastrointestinal system)
   e. Regression
   f. Displacement
   g. Projection
   h. Fantasy

4. Play—child has active fantasy life; evidences experimentation with new skills in play; increases play activities in which child has control and uses self
5. Role of parents—supervision and direction are accepted by 5-year-olds; 6-year-olds respond more slowly and negatively to parental requests and directions; parents are role models for the preschooler, and their attitudes have a great influence on the child's behavior and attitudes
6. Plan—to provide appropriate play activities and self-care opportunities

Socialization Behavior

1. Sees parents as most important figures
2. Is possessive; wants things own way
3. Is able to share with peers and adults
4. Imitates parents and other adult role models

Moral Development (Preconventional Stage)

1. Preschooler sees rules as rigid and inflexible.
2. Negative consequences are viewed as punishment for misdeeds.
3. Parents are seen as the ultimate authorities for determining right and wrong.
4. Child begins process of internalizing sense of right and wrong.

Faith Development (Intuitive-Projective Stage)

1. Religious practices, trinkets, and symbols begin to have practical meaning for the preschooler.
2. God is viewed in human terms.
3. God is understood as being part of nature, such as in the trees, flowers, and rivers.
4. Evil can be imagined in frightening terms such as monsters or the devil.

SCHOOL-AGED CHILD (7 TO 12 YEARS)
Physical Characteristics

A growth spurt begins. Great variation may be normal. Developmental charts are for reference only. Girls may begin to develop secondary sex characteristics and begin menstruation during this stage. Age of onset of menstruation has decreased in the past decade.

1. Weight—child gains 2 to 4 kg (4 to 7 lb)/yr.
2. Height—at 8 years of age arms grow longer in proportion to body; height increases at age 9.
3. Teeth—child continues to lose baby teeth; has 10 to 11 permanent teeth by 8 years of age and approximately 26 permanent teeth by age 12.

Gross Motor Development

1. Age 7 to 10 years—gross motor activities under control of both cognitive skills and consciousness; gradual increase in rhythm, smoothness, and gracefulness of muscular movements; increased interest in perfection of physical skills; strength and endurance also increase
2. Age 10 to 12 years—high energy level and increased direction and control of physical abilities

Fine Motor Development

1. Shows increased improvement in fine motor skills because of increased myelinization of central nervous system
2. Demonstrates improved balance and eye-hand coordination
3. Is able to write rather than print words by age 8
4. Demonstrates increased ability to express individuality and special interests such as sewing, building models, and playing musical instruments
5. Exhibits fine motor skills equal to those of adults by 10 to 12 years of age

Cognitive Development (Concrete Operational Stage—Age 7 to 11 Years)

1. Child's thinking becomes increasingly abstract and symbolic in character; ability to form mental representations is aided by reliance on perceptual senses
2. Weighs a variety of alternatives in finding best solutions
3. Can reverse operations; can trace the sequence of events backward to beginning
4. Understands concepts of past, present, and future

5. Can tell time
6. Can classify objects according to classes and subclasses
7. Understands concepts of height, weight, and volume
8. Is able to focus on more than one aspect of a situation

Language Development

1. Uses language as medium for verbal exchange
2. Words may be recognized before their meaning is understood
3. Is less egocentric in orientation; able to consider another perspective
4. Understands most abstract vocabulary
5. Uses all parts of speech, including adjectives, adverbs, conjunctions, and prepositions
6. Incorporates use of compound and complex sentences
7. Vocabulary reaches 50,000 words at end of this period

Psychosexual Development (Latency Stage)

1. Body focus—sexual concerns become less conscious
2. Developmental task—gradual integration of previous sexual experiences and reactions (in recent years there has been increased documentation that latency is not a neutral period in the development of sexuality)
3. Developmental crisis—increased reference to preadolescent sexual concerns, beginning at approximately 10 years of age
4. Common coping skills—nail biting, dependence, increased problem-solving skills, denial, humor, fantasy, and identification
5. Role of parents—major role in educating child about rules and norms governing sexual behavior and sexuality and in influencing gender-specific behavior

The following are age-specific characteristics:

1. Age 7 years—decreased interest in sex and less exploration; increased interest in opposite sex, with beginning of girl-boy "love" feelings
2. Age 8 years—high sexual interest; increase in activities such as peeping, telling dirty jokes, and wanting more sexual information about birth and sexual lovemaking; girls—increased interest in menstruation

3. Age 9 years—increased discussion with peers about sexual topics; division of sexes in play activities; relating of self to process of reproduction; self-consciousness about sexual exposure; interest in dating and relationships with opposite sex in some children

4. Age 10 years—increasing interest in own body and appearance; many children begin to "date" and relate to opposite sex in group and couple activities

5. Age 11 to 13 years—concerns about appearance; social pressures to look thin and attractive are source of stress; misconceptions about intercourse and pregnancy are evident in many children

Psychosocial Development (Industry Versus Inferiority)

1. Developmental task—learning to develop a sense of adequacy about abilities and competencies as opportunities for social interactions and learning increase; child strives to achieve in school

2. Developmental crisis—child is in danger of developing a sense of inferiority if he or she does not feel competent in the achievement of tasks

3. Play—child enjoys engaging in loosely structured activities with peers (e.g., baseball or foursquare); play tends to be sex segregated; rough-and-tumble play is characteristic of outdoor unstructured play; personal interests, activities, and hobbies develop at this age

4. Role of family and parents—parents are becoming less significant figures as agents for socialization; association with peers tends to diminish the predominant effect parents have had previously; parents are still perceived and responded to as the primary adult authorities; expectations of teachers, coaches, and religious figures have significant impact on child's behavior

5. Plan—promote involvement in age-appropriate school-related activities (e.g., clubs and sports), after-school groups (e.g., 4-H and Boy and Girl Scouts), and social and

community groups (e.g., volunteering) to develop a sense of accomplishment and pride

Moral Development (Conventional Stage)

1. Child's sense of morality is determined by external rules and regulations.
2. Child's social relationships and contact with authority figures influence his or her sense of right and wrong.
3. Child's sense of right and wrong is strict and rigid.

Faith Development (Mythical-Literal Stage)

1. Child's beliefs are heavily influenced by authority figures.
2. Child is learning to distinguish what is natural versus what is supernatural.
3. Child begins to develop personal sense of God.

ADOLESCENT (13 TO 19 YEARS)
Physical Characteristics

Adolescence is characterized by rapid growth and initial awkwardness in gross motor activity and by heightened emotionality because of hormonal changes.

1. Somatic changes—girls mature an average of 2 years earlier than boys because of rapid maturation of central nervous system
2. Height and weight—higher averages occur in boys because of greater velocity of growth spurt and 2-year delay in puberty
3. Teeth
   a. Dentition is completed during late adolescence.
   b. Eighty percent of adolescents need to have one or more wisdom teeth removed.
4. Puberty
   a. Average age of onset is 12½ years in females and 15½ years in males (Table B-2).
   b. Nocturnal emissions are commonly reported at 14½ years (age range is 11½ to 17½ years).
   c. Menarche is identification criterion for pubertal status in girls; average age is 12½ to 13 years.

TABLE B-2
Changes During Puberty

Male	Female	Both Sexes
Thickening and strengthening of pelvic bone structure	Increase in diameter of internal pelvis	Increased broadening of body frame
Increase in size of scrotum and testicles	Enlargement of breasts, ovaries, and uterus	Darkening and coarsening of pubic hair
Increase in sensitivity of genital area	Increase in growth of labia	Increase in axillary hair
Increase in size of penis	Increase in size of vagina	Changes in vocal pitch

Gross Motor Development and Fine Motor Development

Gradual increases in gross motor and fine motor control are evidenced throughout this period. Both neurologic development and increased practice of skills account for the changes.

Common difficulties associated with physical changes during adolescence are as follows:

1. Skin problems and/or disorders
   a. Eczema
   b. Acne vulgaris
2. Poor posture
   a. Lordosis
   b. Scoliosis
3. Dentition problems
   a. Removal of wisdom teeth
   b. Malocclusion
4. Headaches
5. Weight problems and/or disorders
   a. Juvenile obesity
   b. Anorexia nervosa
   c. Bulimia

Cognitive Development (Formal Operational Stage—11 Years and Up)

The ability to think approaches a level comparable with adult competencies. The adolescent acquires the capacity to reason symbolically about more global and altruistic issues and uses a more systematic approach to problem solving. Characteristics of thinking include the following:

1. Takes another perspective into account when processing information
2. Thinking is not limited by actual circumstances; can apply theoretic concepts to hypothesized or imagined situations
3. Develops an altruistic orientation (fairness and justice)
4. Develops own value system
5. Can form deductive and inductive conclusions

Language Development

1. Uses language as medium to convey ideas, opinions, and values
2. Incorporates complex structural and grammatical forms
3. Makes evident use of slang and peer-accepted terminology

Psychosexual Development (Genital Stage)

1. Body focus—genital region
2. Developmental task—integration of developmental tasks learned in previous stages. The extent to which developmental tasks have been previously achieved and resolved will influence the extent to which the individual functions at this stage. This stage is characterized by a renewed sexual interest and sexual attraction to others (of the same or opposite sex).
3. Developmental crisis—resolving and integrating the conflicts of previous stages to function and perform as an integrated adult. This adult behavior is evidenced by the ability to engage in pleasurable intimate sexual relationships with a partner, become a responsible and caring parent, work productively, and be a contributing community member.
4. Common coping skills—increased problem-solving skills, healthy lifestyle (exercise, proper eating, and sufficient sleep), prosocial behaviors, humor, fantasy, anger, denial, use of illicit substances, aggressive and criminal behaviors, "acting out" depression, and eating disorders.
5. Role of parents—primary role of parents is to educate youth about appropriate sexual behavior and sexuality and rules of conduct in all social situations such as intimate relationships, social relationships, and work and community settings. Additionally, parents and/or adult authority figures provide reproductive counseling and discuss prevention of sexually transmitted disease.

The following are age-specific characteristics:

1. Age 14 to 16 years—concerns about appearances; social pressures to look thin and attractive are source of stress; pressure to conform to norms of peer group; social comparisons to social concepts of "popularity" influence social interactions; social relationships directed to include

opposite sex. Pairing of youths within larger social group activities becomes apparent. "Steady" or monogamous dating patterns emerge. Sexual activity is evident within this age group. Teenage pregnancy is a risk.

2. Age 17 to 19 years—concerns about appearances continue; social pressures to look thin and attractive continue to be a source of stress; pressure to conform to norms of peer group continues; social comparisons to social concepts of "popularity" continue to influence social interactions; social relationships remain directed to include opposite sex. Pairing of youths within larger social group activities continues to be apparent. "Steady" or monogamous dating patterns continue to emerge. Risks include teen age marriage, pregnancies, and sexually transmitted diseases.

Psychosocial Development (Identity Versus Role Confusion)

1. Developmental task—development of a sure sense of one's own unique individuality, based on the needs, desires, preferences, values, and belief system that have evolved continuously throughout childhood

2. Developmental crisis—adolescent feels a sense of role confusion; cannot identify accurately what factors are necessary for optimal self-growth; is heavily influenced by opinions and judgments of peers

3. Play—strenuous and structured physical activities (e.g., football and soccer) tend to be sex segregated. Heterosexual relationships evolve, laying the foundation for intimate long-term relationships. Strong, intimate friendships develop. Cliques appear, providing strong social and emotional support for teenagers. Adolescents begin to engage in adult activities (e.g., voting, drinking, and working). They use fantasy to imagine sexual encounters and relationships, and enhance sexuality by focusing on male and female stereotypic activities such as driving fast cars, wearing "sexy" clothing, and lifting weights. Romance novels become popular with adolescent girls. Activities such as shopping and spending time in clothing and department stores increase.

4. Coping skills—problem solving; use of defenses (e.g., reaction formation, displacement, identification, suppression, rationalization, intellectualization, denial, conversion reaction); use of humor; increased socialization
5. Role of parents and family—conflicts with parents may arise, primarily out of adolescent's need to be independent; parents are influential, subconsciously and unconsciously, in the adaptation and use of values and beliefs in making decisions
6. Plan—to facilitate and support social development

Moral Development (Postconventional Stage)

1. Postconventional stage is not universally attained by adolescents.
2. Adolescent may apply ideals to moral predicaments (justice, charity).

Faith Development (Individuating-Reflexive Stage)

1. Adolescent may become very religious or reject religious beliefs entirely.
2. Adolescent may regress to earlier stages to obtain comfort.
3. Acceptance and rejection of beliefs may be influenced by peer group.

C

❖

Immunizations

❖

Two major roles played by the nurse caring for infants and children are educating parents about immunizations and reviewing the immunization status of each child. The following are some risk factors for failure of children to be immunized: low educational level and/or low socioeconomic status of the parent(s), nonwhite race, young parental age, large family size, single parent, lack of prenatal care, lack of parental knowledge regarding immunizations, misconceptions regarding immunizations, and late start with immunizations. Nurses should be aware of these risk factors and target those populations for education. Ongoing active immunization efforts are necessary to ensure that infectious disease continues to be a rare occurrence in the United States. All 50 states have immunization requirements that must be met for a child to enroll in school. This has resulted in immunization rates of close to 100% for school-aged children in the United States.

Some terms must be understood. *Immunity* is the resistance to or protection against a specific disease or infectious agent. There are basically three types of immunity: active, artificial, and passive. *Active immunity* is a long-lasting immunity that results when the body is stimulated to produce its own antibodies. *Artificial immunity* is a type of active immunity in which antibody production is caused by the introduction of antigens in the form of toxoids and vaccines rather than by a specific disease entity. A *toxoid* is a bacterial toxin that has been chemically treated or heat treated to reduce its virulence without destroying its ability to stimulate the production of antibodies (e.g., the diphtheria and tetanus toxoids). A suspension of the actual microorganisms in weakened or killed form is a *vaccine*. Typhoid, pertussis, measles, mumps, and rubella are examples of diseases for which there are vaccines. Finally, *passive immunity* is a form of immediate but transient protection against infectious disease. This type of immunity can be obtained through the administration of preparations of convalescent serum or adult blood products that contain antibodies previously formed against an infectious agent. Passive immunity provides only limited protection against infectious disease.

Box C-1 gives a recommended schedule for the immunization of normal or well children. Because there are frequent

BOX C-1
ACIP, AAP, and AAFP Immunization Recommendations

HBV
- Birth to 2 months
- 1 to 4 months
- 6 to 18 months

DTP
- 2 months
- 4 months
- 6 months
- 12 to 18 months
- 4 to 6 years

HAV (Recommended in High-Risk Areas)
- 2 years
- 2 years + 6-18 months

Hib
- 2 months
- 4 months
- 6 months
- 12 to 15 months

PCV7
- 2 months
- 4 months
- 6 months
- 12-15 months

Continued

BOX C-1
ACIP, AAP, and AAFP Immunization Recommendations—cont'd

Polio (Inactivated Poliovirus)
- 2 months
- 4 months
- 6 to 18 months
- 4 to 6 years

MMR
- 12-15 months
- 4-6 years

Td
- 11-12 years

Varicella
- 12 to 18 months

Recommended Ages for Immunizations and Screenings
- 2 months: DTP, OPV, HBC, HBV
- 4 months: DTP, OPV, HBC, HBV
- 6 months: DTP, HBC, HBV
- 12 months: tuberculin test (depending on the risk of exposure, it may be administered yearly or every other year after this age), varicella vaccine (12 to 18 months)
- 15 months: MMR, HBC
- 12 to 18 months: DTP, OPV, HBC
- 15 to 18 months: DTaP, HBC
- 4 to 6 years: DTP, OPV
- 10 to 14 years: MMR
- 14 to 16 years: adult tetanus toxoid (repeated every 10 years for lifetime)

AAFP, American Academy of Family Physicians; *AAP,* American Academy of Pediatrics; *ACIP,* Advisory Committee on Immunization Practices; *DTaP,* diphtheria and tetanus toxoids and acellular pertussis vaccine; *DTP,* diphtheria and tetanus toxoids with pertussis vaccine; *HAV,* hepatitis A vaccine; *HBC, Haemophilus influenzae* type B conjugate vaccine; *HBV,* hepatitis B vaccine; *Hib, Haemophilus influenzae* type B^3 conjugate vaccine *MMR,* live measles, mumps, and rubella viruses combined in a vaccine; *PCV7,* 7-valent, pneumococcal polysaccharide-protein conjugate vaccine; *Td,* tetanus and diphtheria vaccine.

changes to the immunization schedule, the reader should double-check information with the American Academy of Pediatrics Committee on Infectious Diseases.

VARIOUS VACCINES AND TOXOIDS
Diphtheria, Tetanus, and Pertussis

A mixture of three antigens (diphtheria and tetanus toxoids and acellular pertussis vaccine) and a mineral substance that prolongs and enhances the antigenic properties by delaying absorption make up the diphtheria, tetanus, and acellular pertussis (DTaP) vaccine. Although the diphtheria toxoid does not produce absolute immunity, when it is given on the recommended schedule, protective levels of antitoxin continue for 10 years or more. There are three forms of the tetanus immunizing agent: tetanus toxoid, tetanus immune globulin (human), and tetanus antitoxin (usually horse serum). The recommended dose and route are 0.5 ml intramuscularly (IM). At age 11 or 12 a booster of tetanus and diphtheria (Td) vaccine should be given (0.5 ml IM).

Poliomyelitis

The Sabin vaccine, or oral (trivalent) poliovirus vaccine (OPV), and inactivated poliovirus vaccine (IPV) are used in providing immunity to all three types of poliovirus that cause paralytic poliomyelitis. The IPV vaccine is the preferred form. The recommended dose and route are 0.5 ml subcutaneously (SQ) or IM.

Measles, Mumps, and Rubella

Live viruses for measles, mumps, and rubella (MMR) are usually combined into one vaccine. That one vaccine may provide lifelong immunity to each disease. The rubella portion is extremely important in controlling congenital rubella syndrome. The recommended dose and route are 0.5 ml SQ.

Haemophilus Influenzae Type B

The *Haemophilus influenzae* type B vaccine is a polysaccharide inactive vaccine. Three types of this vaccine are currently available, all of which appear to be equally effective: HBOC, PRP-OMP, and PRP-D (refer to American Academy of Pediatrics guidelines for recommendations for vaccine regimen). This vaccine provides protection against the *H. influenzae* bacteria, which can cause meningitis, epiglottitis, septic arthritis, sepsis, and bacterial pneumonia. The recommended dose and route are 0.5 ml IM.

Hepatitis B

Hepatitis B is a potentially fatal viral infection that can cause cirrhosis or liver cancer. The hepatitis B virus (HBV) vaccine can be administered at different sites simultaneously with the diphtheria-tetanus-pertussis (DTP), MMR, and *H. influenzae* B conjugate (HBC) vaccines. Pain and soreness at the injection site are the most common side effects. Hepatitis B vaccine is considered appropriate for all children, for adolescents who are sexually active with multiple partners, for persons with developmental disabilities, and for health professionals. Protection is estimated to last a lifetime. The recommended dose and route are 0.5 ml IM.

Varicella

Children targeted for vaccination against varicella are infants between 12 and 18 months of age and older school-aged children who have not had varicella and who have not been previously immunized. Adolescents over the age of 13 should receive two doses of the vaccine, 4 to 8 weeks apart. This vaccine can be given with diphtheria, tetanus, DTP, polio, hepatitis B, and *H. influenzae* type B vaccines. Duration of immunity is not known. The recommended dose and route are 0.5 ml SQ.

Pneumococcal Infection

Infection with *Streptococcus pneumoniae* may cause meningitis and pneumonia. Pneumococcal infection is the leading cause of bacterial meningitis in the United States. The recommended dose and route are 0.5 ml IM.

Hepatitis A

Hepatitis A is transmitted via the oral-fecal route. Poor handwashing is a known contributor to its transmission. The recommended dose and route for the vaccine are 0.5 ml IM.

POSSIBLE REACTIONS

Slight reactions to the DTP vaccine are not unusual. Local reactions (redness and edema) at the injection site are common. Mild to moderate temperature elevations and irritability may occur, but they usually resolve within a few hours. Seizures or neurologic damage on rare occasions occur after the administration of the DTP vaccine. If severe reactions occur (such as hypotonia or seizure), the pertussis portion of the vaccine may be eliminated in future vaccinations. Very rarely, vaccine-induced disease results; however, this event usually occurs in immunosuppressed children. Fever and rash have occurred after the administration of the MMR vaccine. Side effects of the varicella vaccine include a maculopapular rash with up to five lesions at the injection site or elsewhere and pain or redness at the injection site. Possible pneumococcal vaccine side effects are soreness, redness, or swelling at the injection site or low-grade fever. Most children who receive hepatitis type A vaccine are asymptomatic; however some may have nonspecific symptoms such as fever and nausea.

CONTRAINDICATIONS

Any time an acute febrile illness is present, immunizations should be postponed. Administration of live-virus vaccines is contraindicated in individuals with leukemia, lymphoma, malignancies, or immunodeficiency diseases; children with marked sensitivity to eggs, chicken, or neomycin; children on immunosuppressive therapy; children who have recently received immune serum globulin plasma or blood products; and pregnant females. A physician's consent must be obtained before administering other immunizations to such individuals. The pertussis vaccine is contraindicated in those children with a history of previous reaction to the DTP vaccine. Anaphylactic reaction to any vaccine contraindicates future administration of that vaccine.

REFERENCES

Advisory Committee on Immunization Practices, American Academy of Pediatrics, and American Academy of Family Physicians: Recommended childhood immunization schedule—United States, 2003, available online at http://www.cispimmunize.org/pro/2002_main.html, accessed June 18, 2003.

Evers DB: Teaching mothers about childhood immunizations, *MCN* 26(5):253, 2001.

Paulson PR, Hammer AL: Pediatric immunization update 2002, *Pediatr Nurs* 28(2):173, 2002.

RESOURCES

American Academy of Pediatrics: http://www.aap.org

Children's Vaccine Program: http://www.childrensvaccine.org

ImmunoFacts: http://www.immunofacts.com

National Immunization Program of the Centers for Disease Control and Prevention: http://www.cdc.gov/nip

D

❖

Standardized Method for Taking Blood Pressure in Children

❖

1. Cuff size corresponds to the size of the child's upper right arm.
2. Essential equipment for taking blood pressures (BPs) in children and adolescents are three pediatric cuffs of differing sizes, standard adult cuff, oversized adult cuff, and thigh cuff (for taking leg BP).
3. Oversized adult cuff and thigh cuff are used for obese adolescents.
4. Guidelines for selecting appropriate BP cuff:
   a. Cuff bladder width is 40% of the arm circumference halfway between the olecranon and the acromion (Figure D-1).
   b. Cuff bladder covers 80% to 100% of the arm's circumference (Figure D-2).
   c. Obtain BP with the cubital fossa at the heart level while supporting the arm (Figure D-3).
   d. Place a stethoscope over the right arm brachial artery pulse, proximal and medial to the cubital fossa and below the bottom edge of the cuff (i.e., about 2 cm above the cubital fossa) (Figure D-3).
5. Take BP after the child or adolescent has been seated 3 to 5 minutes.
6. Average the two systolic and diastolic BP measurements to obtain an estimate of the child's BP level.

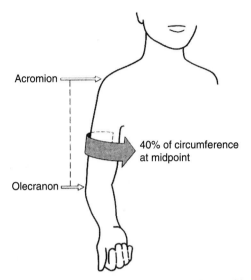

Figure D-1   Selecting the proper cuff size: cuff bladder width. (From American Academy of Pediatrics: Update on the 1987 Task Force Report on High Blood Pressure in Children and Adolescents: A Working Group Report from the National High Blood Pressure Education Program, *Pediatrics* 98(4):649, 1996.)

7. The diastolic measurement in children and adolescents is the fifth Korotkoff sound (K5), which is the last faint sound heard when taking the BP.
8. BP norms can be found in Tables D-1 and D-2. BP norms are based on the child's height percentile, age, and sex. The child's height percentile is determined by his or her placement on standardized growth charts (Appendix I).
9. The child's BP is considered within normal limits if it falls below the 90th percentile. The child's BP is considered in the high-normal range if it falls between the 90th and 95th percentiles, thereby warranting additional monitoring. BPs above the 95th percentile are hypertensive.

BPs may be taken using automated equipment. Oscillometric devices are used extensively in pediatric intensive care units.

Text continued on p. 713.

TABLE D-1
Blood Pressure Norms for Girls 1 to 17 Years of Age

Age, y	Blood Pressure Percentile*	Systolic Blood Pressure by Percentile of Height, mm Hg†							Diastolic Blood Pressure by Percentile of Height, mm Hg†						
		5%	10%	25%	50%	75%	90%	95%	5%	10%	25%	50%	75%	90%	95%
1	90th	97	98	99	100	102	103	104	53	53	53	54	55	56	56
	95th	101	102	103	104	105	107	107	57	57	57	58	59	60	60
2	90th	99	99	100	102	103	104	105	57	57	58	58	59	60	61
	95th	102	103	104	105	107	108	109	61	61	62	62	63	64	65
3	90th	100	100	102	103	104	105	106	61	61	61	62	63	63	64
	95th	104	104	105	107	108	109	110	65	65	65	66	67	67	68
4	90th	101	102	103	104	106	107	108	63	63	64	65	65	66	67
	95th	105	106	107	108	109	111	111	67	67	68	69	69	70	71
5	90th	103	103	104	106	107	108	109	65	66	66	67	68	68	69
	95th	107	107	108	110	111	112	113	69	70	70	71	72	72	73
6	90th	104	105	106	107	109	110	111	67	67	68	69	69	70	71
	95th	108	109	110	111	112	114	114	71	71	72	73	73	74	75
7	90th	106	107	108	109	110	112	112	69	69	69	70	71	72	72
	95th	110	110	112	113	114	115	116	73	73	73	74	75	76	76
8	90th	108	109	110	111	112	113	114	70	70	71	71	72	73	74
	95th	112	112	113	115	116	117	118	74	74	75	75	76	77	78

Age (Year)	Blood Pressure Percentile														
9	90th	110	110	112	113	114	115	116	71	72	72	73	74	74	75
	95th	114	114	115	117	118	119	120	75	76	76	77	78	78	79
10	90th	112	112	114	115	116	117	118	73	73	73	74	75	76	76
	95th	116	116	117	119	120	121	122	77	77	77	78	79	80	80
11	90th	114	114	116	117	118	119	120	74	74	75	75	76	77	77
	95th	118	118	119	121	122	123	124	78	78	79	79	80	81	81
12	90th	116	116	118	119	120	121	122	75	75	76	76	77	78	78
	95th	120	120	121	123	124	125	126	79	79	80	80	81	82	82
13	90th	118	118	119	121	122	123	124	76	76	77	78	78	79	80
	95th	121	122	123	125	126	127	128	80	80	81	82	82	83	84
14	90th	119	120	121	122	124	125	126	77	77	78	79	79	80	81
	95th	123	124	125	126	128	129	130	81	81	82	83	83	84	85
15	90th	121	121	122	124	125	126	127	78	78	79	80	80	81	82
	95th	124	125	126	128	129	130	131	82	82	83	84	84	85	86
16	90th	122	122	123	125	126	127	128	79	79	79	80	81	82	82
	95th	125	126	127	128	130	131	132	83	83	83	84	85	86	86
17	90th	122	123	124	125	126	127	128	79	79	79	80	81	82	82
	95th	126	126	127	129	130	131	132	83	83	83	84	85	86	86

From American Academy of Pediatrics: Update on the 1987 Task Force Report on High Blood Pressure in Children and Adolescents: A Working Group Report from the National High Blood Pressure Education Program, *Pediatrics* 98(4):649, 1996.

*Blood pressure percentile was determined by a single reading.
†Height percentile was determined by standard growth curves.

TABLE D-2
Blood Pressure Norms for Boys 1 to 17 Years of Age

Age, y	Blood Pressure Percentile*	Systolic Blood Pressure by Percentile of Height, mm Hg†							Diastolic Blood Pressure by Percentile of Height, mm Hg†						
		5%	10%	25%	50%	75%	90%	95%	5%	10%	25%	50%	75%	90%	95%
1	90th	94	95	97	98	100	102	102	50	51	52	53	54	54	55
	95th	98	99	101	102	104	106	106	55	55	56	57	58	59	59
2	90th	98	99	100	102	104	105	106	55	55	56	57	58	59	59
	95th	101	102	104	106	108	109	110	59	59	60	61	62	63	63
3	90th	100	101	103	105	107	108	109	59	59	60	61	62	63	63
	95th	104	105	107	109	111	112	113	63	63	64	65	66	67	67
4	90th	102	103	105	107	109	110	111	62	62	63	64	65	66	66
	95th	106	107	109	111	113	114	115	66	67	67	68	69	70	71
5	90th	104	105	106	108	110	112	112	65	65	66	67	68	69	69
	95th	108	109	110	112	114	115	116	69	70	70	71	72	73	74
6	90th	105	106	108	110	111	113	114	67	68	69	70	70	71	72
	95th	109	110	112	114	115	117	117	72	72	73	74	75	76	76
7	90th	106	107	109	111	113	114	115	69	70	71	72	72	73	74
	95th	110	111	113	115	116	118	119	74	74	75	76	77	78	78
8	90th	107	108	110	112	114	115	116	71	71	72	73	74	75	75
	95th	111	112	114	116	118	119	120	75	76	76	77	78	79	80

Age	BP percentile	Systolic BP by height percentile							Diastolic BP by height percentile						
9	90th	109	110	112	113	115	117	117	72	73	73	74	75	76	77
	95th	113	114	116	117	119	121	121	76	77	78	79	80	80	81
10	90th	110	112	113	115	117	118	119	73	74	74	75	76	77	78
	95th	114	115	117	119	121	122	123	77	78	78	80	80	81	82
11	90th	112	113	115	117	119	120	121	74	74	75	76	77	78	78
	95th	116	117	119	121	123	124	125	78	79	79	80	81	82	83
12	90th	115	116	117	119	121	123	123	75	75	76	77	78	78	79
	95th	119	120	121	123	125	126	127	79	79	80	81	82	83	83
13	90th	117	118	120	122	124	125	126	75	75	76	77	78	79	80
	95th	121	122	124	126	128	129	130	79	79	80	81	82	83	84
14	90th	120	121	123	125	126	128	128	76	76	77	78	79	80	80
	95th	124	125	127	128	130	132	132	80	81	81	82	83	84	85
15	90th	123	124	125	127	129	131	131	77	77	78	79	80	81	81
	95th	127	128	129	131	133	134	135	81	81	82	83	84	85	86
16	90th	125	126	128	130	132	133	134	79	79	80	81	82	82	83
	95th	129	130	132	134	136	137	138	83	83	84	85	86	87	87
17	90th	128	129	131	133	134	136	136	81	81	82	83	84	85	85
	95th	132	133	135	136	138	140	140	85	85	86	87	88	89	89

From American Academy of Pediatrics: Update on the 1987 Task Force Report on High Blood Pressure in Children and Adolescents: A Working Group Report from the National High Blood Pressure Education Program, *Pediatrics* 98(4):649, 1996.

*Blood pressure percentile was determined by a single reading.

†Height percentile was determined by standard growth curves.

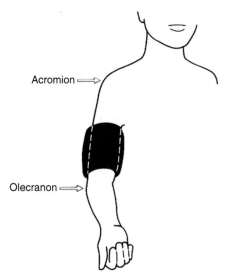

Figure D-2   Cuff bladder and arm circumference. (From American Academy of Pediatrics: Update on the 1987 Task Force Report on High Blood Pressure in Children and Adolescents: A Working Group Report from the National High Blood Pressure Education Program, *Pediatrics* 98(4):649, 1996.)

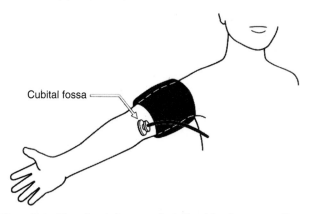

Figure D-3   Use of a stethoscope in taking blood pressure. (From American Academy of Pediatrics: Update on the 1987 Task Force Report on High Blood Pressure in Children and Adolescents: A Working Group Report from the National High Blood Pressure Education Program, *Pediatrics* 98(4):649, 1996.)

Oscillometry provides accurate systolic and diastolic pressures and mean arterial pressures and pulses. Their use is less reliable in standard clinical settings because frequent calibration is needed to ensure the accuracy of readings. Under these circumstances, the auscultation method is preferred.

REFERENCES

American Academy of Pediatrics: Update on the 1987 Task Force Report on High Blood Pressure in Children and Adolescents: A Working Group Report from the National High Blood Pressure Education Program, *Pediatrics* 98(4):649, 1996.

Perloff D et al: Human blood pressure determination by sphygmomanometry, *Circulation* 88:2460, 1993.

E

◆

Laboratory Values

◆

The following are normal laboratory values unless otherwise stated.

1. Acetone, ketone bodies (serum)
    a. Newborn to age 1 week: slightly higher than values for ages over 1 week
    b. Ages over 1 week
        i. Acetone: 0.3 to 2.0 mg/dl (51.6 to 344.0 μmol/L) (International System [SI] units)
        ii. Ketones: 2 to 4 mg/dl
2. Albumin (serum)
    a. Newborn: 2.9 to 5.4 g/dl
    b. Infant: 4.4 to 5.4 g/dl
    c. Child: 4.0 to 5.8 g/dl
3. Albumin in meconium: negative
4. Ammonia (serum)
    a. Newborn: 64 to 107 μg/dl
    b. Child: 29 to 70 μg/dl (29 to 70 μmol/L) (SI units)
5. Amylase dehydrogenase (serum)—child: 45 to 200 dye U/dl
6. Arterial blood gases
    a. Partial pressure of oxygen (Po_2): 75 to 100 mm Hg
    b. Partial pressure of carbon dioxide (Pco_2)
        i. Infant: 27 to 40 mm Hg
        ii. All other ages: 35 to 45 mm Hg
    c. pH
        i. Premature infant (cord): 7.15 to 7.35
        ii. Premature infant (age 48 hours): 7.35 to 7.5
        iii. Newborn: 7.27 to 7.47

        iv. Infant: 7.35 to 7.45
        v. Child: 7.35 to 7.45
7. Bilirubin
  a. Total
     i. Newborn: 2.0 to 6.0 mg/dl
     ii. Age 48 hours: 6.0 to 7.0 mg/dl
     iii. Age 5 days: 4.0 to 12.0 mg/dl
     iv. Age 1 month to adult: 0.3 to 1.2 mg/dl
  b. Indirect (unconjugated)—age 1 month to adult: 0.3 to 1.1 mg/dl
  c. Direct (conjugated)—age 1 month to adult: 0.1 to 0.4 mg/dl
8. Bleeding time
  a. Normal time: 2 to 7 minutes
  b. Borderline time: 7 to 11 minutes
9. Blood urea nitrogen (BUN) (serum)
  a. Newborn: 8 to 18 mg/dl
  b. Infant or child: 5 to 18 mg/dl
  c. Adolescent: 8 to 17 mg/dl
10. Calcium (serum)
  a. Premature infant: 6 to 10 mg/dl
  b. Full-term infant: 7.5 to 11 mg/dl
  c. Child: 8.8 to 10.8 mg/dl
  d. Adolescent: 8.4 to 10.2 mg/dl
11. Carotene (serum)—child: 40 to 130 µg/dl
12. Catecholamines
  a. Values for child lower than those for adult
  b. Total
     i. Random urine: 0 to 14 µg/dl
     ii. Twenty-four-hour urine: less than 100 g/24 hr
  c. Epinephrine: less than 10 ng/24 hr
  d. Norepinephrine: less than 100 ng/24 hr
  e. Metanephrines: less than 100 ng/24 hr
13. Cerebrospinal fluid (CSF)
  a. Specific gravity: 1.007 to 1.009
  b. Glucose
     i. Infant or child: 60 to 80 mg/dl
     ii. All other ages: 40 to 80 mg/dl

    c. Protein
       i. Newborn: 45 to 100 mg/dl
       ii. Child: 10 to 20 mg/dl
       iii. Adolescent: 15 to 40 mg/dl
    d. pH: 7.33 to 7.42
    e. Cell count
       i. Neonate: 0.5 polymorphonuclear cells; 0 to 5 mononuclear cells; 0 to 5 red blood cells (RBCs)/mm^3
       ii. All other ages: 0 polymorphonuclear cells; 0 to 5 mononuclear cells; 0 to 5 RBCs/mm^3

14. Cholesterol (serum)
    a. Age 1 to 4 years: less than or equal to 210 mg/dl
    b. Age 5 to 14 years: less than or equal to 220 mg/dl
    c. Age 15 to 20 years: less than or equal to 235 mg/dl

15. Copper (Cu) (serum)
    a. Newborn: 20 to 70 μg/dl
    b. Child: 30 to 190 μg/dl
    c. Adolescent: 90 to 240 μg/dl

16. C-reactive protein (CRP) (serum)—child: negative

17. Creatine phosphokinase (CPK)
    a. Infant: 20 to 31 U/L
    b. Infant to adolescent: 15 to 50 U/L

18. Creatinine (serum)
    a. Cord: 0.6 to 1.2 mg/dl
    b. Newborn: 0.3 to 1.0 mg/dl
    c. Infant: 0.2 to 0.4 mg/dl
    d. Child: 0.3 to 0.7 mg/dl
    e. Adolescent: 0.5 to 1.0 mg/dl

19. Cortisol (plasma) — child
    a. At 8 AM: 15 to 25 μg/dl
    b. At 4 PM: 5 to 10 μg/dl

20. Culture results—blood, throat, sputum, wound, skin, stool, urine: negative or no growth of pathogen

21. Electrolytes (serum)
    a. Sodium (Na$^+$)
       i. Premature infant: 132 to 140 mmol/L
       ii. Infant: 139 to 146 mmol/L
       iii. Child: 138 to 145 mmol/L
       iv. Adolescent: 136 to 146 mmol/L

b. Potassium (K^+)
   i. Infant: 4.1 to 5.3 mmol/L
   ii. Child: 3.4 to 4.7 mmol/L
   iii. Adolescent: 3.5 to 5.1 mmol/L
c. Chlorine (Cl^-): 98 to 106 mmol/L
d. Carbon dioxide (CO_2)
   i. Infant: 27 to 41 mm Hg
   ii. Child (male): 35 to 48 mm Hg
   iii. Child (female): 32 to 45 mm Hg

22. Erythrocyte sedimentation rate (ESR, sed rate)
    a. Newborn: 0 to 2 mm/hr
    b. Age 4 to 14 years: 0 to 10 mm/hr
23. Fasting blood glucose
    a. Newborn: 30 to 80 mg/dl
    b. Child: 60 to 100 mg/dl
24. Ferritin concentration (serum)—abnormal: less than 10 to 12 µg/L
25. Ferritin determination (serum)
    a. Newborn: 20 to 200 ng/ml
    b. 1 month: 200 to 500 ng/ml
    c. 2 to 12 months: 30 to 200 ng/ml
    d. 1 to 16 years: 8 to 140 ng/ml
26. Fibrin degradation products (FDP) (serum)
    a. Adult: 2 to 10 µg/ml
    b. Child: test not usually performed
27. Fibrinogen level (plasma)
    a. Newborn: 150 to 300 mg/dl
    b. Child: 200 to 400 mg/dl
28. Glucose (serum): 40 to 100 mg/dl
29. Glucose tolerance test (GTT) results (oral)—child 6 years or older:

Time (hr)	Whole Blood (mg/dl)	Serum (mg/dl)
½	<150	<160
1	<160	<170
2	<115	<125
3	60-100	70-110

30. Hematocrit (Hct)
    a. Newborn: 44% to 75%
    b. Infant: 28% to 42%
    c. Age 6 to 12 years: 35% to 45%
    d. Age 12 to 18 years (male): 37% to 49%
    e. Age 12 to 18 years (female): 36% to 46%
31. Hemoglobin (Hb)
    a. Age 1 to 3 days: 14.5 to 22.5 g/dl
    b. Age 2 months: 9.0 to 14.0 g/dl
    c. Age 6 to 12 years: 11.5 to 15.5 g/dl
    d. Age 12 to 18 years (male): 13.0 to 16.0 g/dl
    e. Age 12 to 18 years (female): 12.0 to 16.0 g/dl
32. Hemoglobin electrophoresis (hemoglobin F [Hb F])
    a. Newborn: Hb F, 50% to 80% of total Hb
    b. Infant: Hb F, 8% of total Hb
    c. Child: Hb F, 1% to 2% of total Hb after 6 months
33. Human immunodeficiency virus type 1 (HIV-1)
    (serum)—child: seronegative
34. Immunoglobulin (Ig) values (serum):

	% Total	Newborn	3 mo	6 mo	1-3 yr	4-6 yr	6-16 yr
IgG	80	650-1250	275-750	200-1100	300-1400	550-1500	700-1650
IgA	15	0-12	5-55	10-90	20-150	50-175	50-225
IgM	4	5-30	15-70	10-80	20-230	20-100	22-260
IgD	0.2	—	—	—	—	—	—
IgE	0.0002	—	—	—	<10	<25	<62

35. Iron (serum): 50 to 120 µg/dl
36. Iron concentration (serum): 30 to 70 µg/g
37. Lactic dehydrogenase (LDH) (serum)
    a. Newborn: 300 to 1500 IU/L
    b. Child: 50 to 150 IU/L; 100 to 295 U/L
38. Lead (serum)—child: normal range, 10 to 20 µg/dl
39. Lipase (serum)
    a. Infant: 9 to 105 U/L
    b. All other ages: 20 to 180 U/L
40. Magnesium (serum)
    a. Newborn: 1.4 to 2.9 mEq/L
    b. Child: 1.6 to 2.6 mEq/L

41. Osmolality (serum)—child: 270 to 290 mOsm/kg
42. Osmolality (urine)
    a. Newborn: 100 to 600 mOsm/L
    b. Child: 50 to 1200 mOsm/L; usual range, 300 to 900 mOsm/L
43. Ova and parasites (O and P) (feces)
    a. Child: negative
    b. Parasites most often found in stool: roundworms, ameba, hookworms, protozoa, tapeworms
44. Partial thromboplastin time (PTT) and activated partial thromboplastin time (APTT)
    a. Newborn to age 3 months: higher than adult times
    b. Child: higher than adult times
    c. Adult: PTT, 30 to 45 seconds; APTT, 35 to 45 seconds
45. Phosphorus (serum)
    a. Premature infant: 4.6 to 8.0 mg/dl
    b. Newborn: 5.0 to 7.8 mg/dl
46. Plasminogen (plasma)—adult: 2.5 to 5.2 U/ml; 20 mg/dl
47. Platelet count
    a. Newborn: 84,000 to 478,000/μl
    b. All other ages: 150,000 to 400,000/μl
48. Protein (serum)
    a. Premature infant: 4.2 to 7.6 g/dl
    b. Newborn: 4.6 to 7.4 g/dl
    c. Infant: 6.0 to 6.7 g/dl
    d. Child: 6.2 to 8.0 g/dl
49. Protein (urine)
    a. Values higher in children
    b. Random urine specimen: negative, 0 to 5 mg/dl; positive, 6 to 2000 mg/dl
    c. Twenty-four-hour urine specimen: 25 to 150 mg/24 hr
50. Prothrombin time (PT, pro time)
    a. Newborn: 12 to 21 seconds
    b. All other ages: 11 to 15 seconds
51. Red blood cells (RBCs)
    a. Infant (1 to 18 months): 2.7×10^6 to 5.4×10^6/mm^3

     b. Preschooler: $4.27 \times 10^6/mm^3$
     c. School-age: $4.31 \times 10^6/mm^3$
     d. Adolescent: $4.60 \times 10^6/mm^3$

52. Reticulocyte count
     a. Birth to 6 months: 3% to 7%
     b. Six months to 2 years: 0.3% to 2.2%
     c. All other ages: 0.5% to 1.5%

53. Serum glutamic-pyruvic transaminase (SGPT)
     a. Age 6 to 12 months: 16 to 36 IU/L
     b. Age 2 to 17 years: 622 IU/L

54. Serum glutamic-oxaloacetic transaminase (SGOT)
     a. Age 6 to 12 months: less than or equal to 40 IU/L
     b. Age 2 to 17 years: 10 to 30 IU/L

55. Sweat test results: negative

56. Thyroid-stimulating hormone (TSH) (serum)—newborn: less than 25 uIU/ml by the third day

57. Toxoplasmosis, rubella, cytomegalovirus, and herpes simplex (TORCH) titer—infant under 2 months: negative

58. Transferrin (serum): 200 to 400 mg/dl

59. Triglycerides (serum)
     a. Infant: 5 to 40 mg/dl
     b. Child (5 to 11 years): 10 to 135 mg/dl
     c. Adolescent or young adult (12 to 29 years): 10 to 140 mg/dl

60. Uric acid (serum)
     a. Female: 2.0 to 6.0 mg/dl
     b. Male: 3.0 to 7.0 mg/dl

61. Urinalysis
     a. Specific gravity: 1.003 to 1.035
     b. pH
          i. Infant: 5.0 to 7.0
          ii. All other ages: 4.8 to 7.8
     c. Protein: negative
     d. Blood: negative
     e. Glucose: negative
     f. Ketones: negative

62. White blood cell count (WBC)
    a. Infant: 6000 to 17,500/mm^3
    b. Preschooler: 5500 to 15,500/mm^3
    c. School-aged child: 4500 to 13,500/mm^3
    d. Adolescent: 4500 to 11,000/mm^3
63. White blood cell differential:

Cell Type	Percentage of Total	Values ($\mu l/mm^3$)
Neutrophils		
Total	61 (newborn)	—
	32 (1 yr)	—
	50-70 (>1 yr)	2500-7000
Segmented	50-65 (>1 yr)	2500-6500
Band	0-5 (>1 yr)	0-500
Eosinophils	1-3	100-300
Basophils	0.4-1.0	40-100
Monocytes	4-9 (1-12 yr)	—
	4-6 (>12 yr)	200-600
Lymphocytes	34 (newborn)	—
	60 (1 yr)	—
	42 (6 yr)	—
	38 (12 yr)	—
	25-35 (>12 yr)	1700-3500

REFERENCES

Kee JL: *Laboratory and diagnostic tests with nursing implications,* ed 4, East Norwalk, Conn, 1995, Appleton & Lange.

National Institutes of Health, NIH Clinical Center: *Pediatric laboratory values,* Feb 3, 2003, available online at http://www.cc.nih.gov/ccc/pedweb/pedsstaff/pedlab.html, accessed June 19, 2003.

Watson J, Jaffe M: *Nurse's manual of laboratory and diagnostic tests,* Philadelphia, 1995, FA Davis.

F

◆

Abbreviations

◆

<	Less than
>	Greater than
AAMR	American Association of Mental Retardation
AAP	American Academy of Pediatrics
ABS	Adaptive behavior scales
ABVD	Adriamycin, bleomycin, vinblastine, and dacarbazine
ADA	American Diabetic Association
ADHD	Attention-deficit/hyperactivity disorder
AIDS	Acquired immunodeficiency syndrome
ALL	Acute lymphoid, or lymphocytic, leukemia
ALT	Alanine aminotransferase
ALTE	Apparent life-threatening event
ANC	Absolute neutrophil count
ANLL	Acute nonlymphoid leukemia
ARF	Acute renal failure
ASO	Antistreptolysin O
AST	Aspartate aminotransferase
AT	Antithrombin
AZT	Zidovudine
BiPAP	Inspiratory and expiratory positive airway pressure
BMT	Bone marrow transplantation
BPD	Bronchopulmonary dysplasia
BUN	Blood urea nitrogen
C and S	Culture and sensitivity
CBC	Complete blood count
CDC	Centers for Disease Control and Prevention
CF	Cystic fibrosis
CHF	Congestive heart failure

CLD	Chronic lung disease
cm	Centimeter
CMV	Cytomegalovirus
CNS	Central nervous system
CO_2	Carbon dioxide
COMP	Cyclophosphamide, Oncovin, methotrexate, prednisone
CORN	Council of Regional Networks for Genetic Services
CP	Cerebral palsy
CPAP	Continuous positive airway pressure
CPP	Cerebral perfusion pressure
CPR	Cardiopulmonary resuscitation
CRF	Chronic renal failure
CSF	Cerebrospinal fluid
CT	Computed tomography
CVA	Cerebrovascular accident
DDC	Zalcitabine
DDH	Developmental dysplasia of the hip
DDI	Didanosine
DIC	Disseminated intravascular coagulation
dl	Deciliter (100 ml)
DNA	Deoxyribonucleic acid
DSM-IV	*Diagnostic and Statistical Manual of Mental Disorders,* 4th edition, text revision
DTaP	Diphtheria, tetanus, and acellular pertussis (vaccine)
DTP	Diphtheria, tetanus, and pertussis (vaccine)
ECG	Electrocardiogram
ECMO	Extracorporeal membrane oxygenation
EEG	Electroencephalogram
EI	Early intervention
EIP	Early intervention program
EN	Enteral nutrition
ESR	Erythrocyte sedimentation rate
ESRD	End-stage renal disease
ET	Endotracheal tube
FAS	Fetal alcohol syndrome
FDP	Fibrin degradation product
g	Gram

GCS	Glasgow Coma Scale
GER	Gastroesophageal reflux
GI	Gastrointestinal
GM-CSF	Granulocyte-macrophage colony-stimulating factor
GVHD	Graft versus host disease
HAV	Hepatitis A virus
Hb	Hemoglobin
HBC	*Haemophilus influenzae* type B conjugate (vaccine)
HBIG	Hepatitis B immunoglobulin
HBV	Hepatitis B virus
HCO_3	Bicarbonate
HCV	Hepatitis C virus
HDV	Hepatitis D virus
HEV	Hepatitis E virus
HFV	High-frequency ventilation
HGV	Hepatitis G virus
HIV	Human immunodeficiency virus
HLA	Human lymphocyte antigen
H_2O	Water
hr	Hour
HUS	Hemolytic-uremic syndrome
ICP	Intracranial pressure
ICV	Ileocecal valve
IDDM	Insulin-dependent diabetes mellitus
IEP	Individualized education plan
IFSP	Individualized family service plan
Ig	Immunoglobulin
IgG	Immunoglobulin G
IgM	Immunoglobulin M
IHP	Individualized health care plan
IM	Intramuscular
in	Inch
IPV	Inactivated poliovirus (vaccine)
IQ	Intelligence quotient
ITP	Idiopathic thrombocytopenic purpura; individualized transition plan
IU	International unit
IV	Intravenous
IVGG	Intravenous gamma globulin

IVIG	Intravenous immune globulin
IVP	Intravenous pyelogram
JRA	Juvenile rheumatoid arthritis
K^+	Potassium
kcal	Kilocalorie
kg	Kilogram
L	Liter
lb	Pound
LES	Lower-esophageal sphincter
LOC	Level of consciousness
m	Meter
m^2	Square meter
MAS	Meconium aspiration syndrome
mEq	Milliequivalent
mg	Milligram
μg	Microgram
min	Minute
ml	Milliliter
mm	Millimeter
mm^3	Cubic millimeter
MMR	Measles, mumps, and rubella (vaccine)
MOPP	Mechlorethamine, Oncovin, procarbazine, and prednisone
mOsm	Milliosmole
MRI	Magnetic resonance imaging
Na^+	Sodium
NADase	Nicotinamide adenine dinucleotidase
$NaHCO_3$	Sodium bicarbonate
NEC	Necrotizing enterocolitis
ng	Nanogram
NG	Nasogastric
NHL	Non-Hodgkin's lymphoma
NO	Nitric oxide
NPH	Neutral protamine Hagedorn (insulin)
NPO	Nothing by mouth
NSAID	Nonsteroidal antiinflammatory drug
OPV	Oral poliovirus (vaccine)
oz	Ounce
$Paco_2$	Partial pressure of carbon dioxide, arterial

Pao_2	Partial pressure of oxygen, arterial
PCA	Patient-controlled analgesia
Pco_2	Partial pressure of carbon dioxide
PCP	Phencyclidine; *Pneumocystis carinii* pneumonia
PCR	Polymerase chain reaction
PCV7	7-Valent, pneumococcal polysaccharide-protein conjugate vaccine
PD	Peritoneal dialysis
PDA	Patent ductus arteriosus
PERLA	Pupils equal, react to light, accommodate
pH	Hydrogen ion concentration (indicates acidity-alkalinity)
PN	Parenteral nutrition
PO	Oral; by mouth
Po_2	Partial pressure of oxygen
PPV23	Pneumococcal polysaccharide vaccine
PT	Prothrombin time
PTT	Partial thromboplastin time
RBC	Red blood cell; red blood cell count
RDS	Respiratory distress syndrome
RNA	Ribonucleic acid
ROM	Range of motion
RSV	Respiratory syncytial virus
SBS	Short bowel syndrome
SGOT	Serum glutamic-oxaloacetic transaminase
SGPT	Serum glutamic-pyruvic transaminase
SI	International System of Units (Système Internationale)
SIDS	Sudden infant death syndrome
SQ	Subcutaneous
TBI	Traumatic brain injury
Td	Tetanus and diphtheria (vaccine)
3TC	Lamivudine
TOF	Tetralogy of Fallot
TORCH	Toxoplasmosis, rubella, cytomegalovirus, and herpes simplex
TPN	Total parenteral nutrition
TT	Thrombin time
U	Unit

UTI	Urinary tract infection
VLBW	Very low birth weight
VP	Ventricular-peritoneal
WBC	White blood cell; white blood cell count
ZDV	Zidovudine

G

◆

West Nomogram

◆

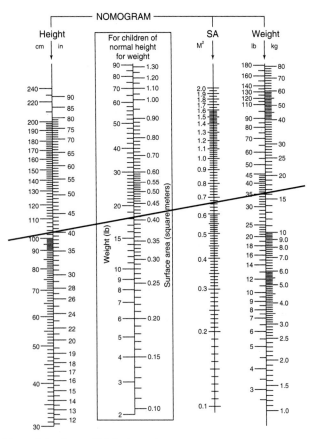

Figure G-1 See p. 729 for legend.

Figure G-1, cont'd For estimation of surface area: surface area is given by the point at which a straight line connecting height and weight intersects surface area (SA) column, or, if child is roughly of normal proportion, is given by weight alone (boxed values). Line shows SA determination (0.68 m^2) for child 41 inches tall who weighs 35 lb. (Nomogram modified from data of E. Boyd by CD West. From Behrman RE et al, editors: *Nelson textbook of pediatrics*, ed 17, Philadelphia, 2003, WB Saunders.)

H

◆

Pain in Children

◆

DEFINITIONS

The International Association for the Study of Pain (1979) defines pain as "an unpleasant sensory and emotional experience associated with actual or potential tissue damage, or described in terms of such damage." McCaffrey and Beebe (1994) state that "pain is whatever the person experiencing it says it is, existing whenever the experiencing person says it does." This definition does not necessarily imply that the child must verbalize pain. Pain may also be expressed through crying, vocalizations, or other behavioral manifestations.

PHYSIOLOGY

Pain is a complex physiologic process that can be divided into three neurochemical events: transduction, transmission, and modulation.

Transduction occurs at the site of initiation of pain. Pain receptors (nociceptors) in the periphery are stimulated by a mechanical, thermal, or chemical event. This stimulus results in the release of pain-producing substances.

Transmission of the impulse continues as it travels into the dorsal horn of the spinal cord via large, thinly myelinated A-delta fibers and small, unmyelinated C fibers. From here the impulse is carried via the anterolateral pathway on to the thalamus and then to the cortex. It is in the cortex that the impulse is perceived as pain. Many factors, including culture, past experience, the meaning of the pain, and emotional state, all contribute to the individual's perception of pain. Both transduction and transmission occur in afferent pathways.

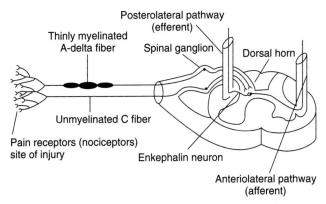

Figure H-1   Transduction, transmission, and modulation of pain.

Modulation of pain occurs in the brain at the level of the periaqueductal gray matter and medulla oblongata, as well as in the dorsal horn of the spinal cord, as endogenous opioids (enkephalins) are released in the posterolateral pathway, an efferent pathway.

Figure H-1 shows transduction, transmission, and modulation of pain in the dorsal horn.

NATURE OF PAIN

Table H-1 provides a brief overview of the types of pain with descriptions and examples of each.

PAIN ASSESSMENT

Self-report is the most accurate means of obtaining information regarding the location and intensity of the child's pain. Input from the family is very important and may be necessary if the child is unwilling or unable to report for himself or herself. Obtaining a pain history is helpful in developing a plan of care for the child. Ask questions regarding the child's previous experience with painful events, including how the child responds to pain and what methods of pain management have been successful in the past. Also learn what word the child uses to describe pain (e.g., *boo-boo, owie*). The pain assessment should be tailored to the child's developmental level.

TABLE H-1
Nature of Pain

Type	Description	Examples
Acute	Brief; associated with tissue damage or inflammation; intensity steadily diminishes over days to weeks	Surgical pain, burns, fractures
Chronic persistent	Persistent or near-persistent pain over a period of 3 months or longer	Arthritis, sickle cell crisis
Recurrent	Repetitive painful episode alternating with pain-free intervals	Headache; abdominal, chest, or limb pain
Neuropathic	Persistent pain related to persistent or abnormal excitability in the peripheral or central nervous system with no ongoing tissue injury; often described as "burning," "strange," or "pins and needles"	Amputation pain syndromes, plexus injuries, reflex sympathetic dystrophy
Psychogenic	Persistent pain that is a manifestation of a psychiatric disease	Somatization disorder, somatoform pain disorder, conversion disorder

Physiologic signs are neither specific nor sensitive indicators of pain but may be used as an adjunct to behavioral assessment and self-report in all age groups. Assess behavioral manifestations with caution, because many children will play, watch television, or sleep as a means of coping with pain. If the child is receiving sedatives in addition to analgesics, behavioral response to pain may be blunted.

Neonates and Infants (Birth to 1 Year)

Use of behavioral indexes is the best method of assessing pain in neonates. Facial grimaces, alterations in tone and activity, and crying are the most often used indicators of pain in this age group. Premature and critically ill neonates may not respond as vigorously to pain as healthy, full-term neonates. This lack of response does not indicate a lack of perception.

Behavioral indexes are also the most useful indicators of pain for infants beyond the neonatal period. In addition to facial grimaces, alterations in tone and activity, and crying, these infants demonstrate deliberate withdrawal from the painful stimulus and a wide variety of vocalizations.

Toddlers (1 to 3 Years)

Behavioral responses also continue to be the standard for pain assessment in toddlers. However, their behavioral repertoire is expanded to include rubbing the site of pain and aggressive behavior (biting, hitting, and kicking). Some toddlers are capable of verbalizing where something hurts, but they cannot describe the intensity of the pain.

Preschoolers (3 to 5 Years)

By age 3 to 4 years, most children can begin to use self-report tools such as the Oucher Scale (Figure H-2). These tools provide the most accurate measure of a child's pain. Preschoolers are better able to describe the intensity of their pain. This age group may also display aggressive behavior in response to pain.

School-Aged Children (5 to 13 Years)

The Oucher Scale is also useful for school-aged children. Children in this age group may use either the faces shown on

OUCHER

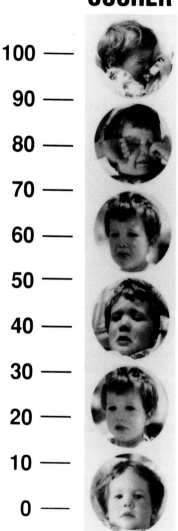

100 —

90 —

80 —

70 —

60 —

50 —

40 —

30 —

20 —

10 —

0 —

Figure H-2 The Caucasian Oucher Scale, developed and copyrighted by Judith E. Beyer, RN, PhD, 1983. This tool is also available in Hispanic and African American versions.

the scale or the numeric values. By age 7 or 8 many children can use a numeric scale. These children should have an understanding of the concept of order and number. Children in this age group can describe the intensity and location of their pain in greater detail. They may tend to act brave, demonstrating less overt behavior patterns, such as clenching their fists and teeth or remaining very still or rigid.

Adolescents (13 to 19 Years)

Any of the tools described here are useful for adolescents. They can also respond to being asked, "On a scale of 0 to 10, with 0 being no pain and 10 being the worst pain you have ever had, what is your pain now?" Adolescents are capable of describing the intensity, location, and duration of their pain. They also display a variety of behavioral responses including mood swings and regression to an earlier developmental stage. Adolescents tend to dismiss their pain and refuse intervention in the presence of their peers.

PAIN MANAGEMENT

Pain management, ideally, is a multidisciplinary effort. The pain management "team" may include any or all of the following professionals: nurse, physician, child life specialist, respiratory therapist, occupational therapist, physical therapist, and chaplain, along with the child and the family. Strategies for pain management should include both pharmacologic and nonpharmacologic approaches. The following sections describe both types of management strategies.

Pharmacologic Management

Acute pain is managed with opioid and nonopioid analgesics. Table H-2 provides a list of selected medications used for the management of acute pain in the pediatric population. Patient-controlled analgesia and epidural analgesia are described in the following sections.

Because intramuscular injections are painful and frightening for children, this route of administration should be reserved for exceptional circumstances.

TABLE H-2
Selected Medications Used to Manage Acute Pain in the Pediatric Population

Drug	Dose (mg/kg)*	Route	Frequency	Comments
Opioids				
Morphine	0.3	PO	Every 3-4 hr	The standard for opioid therapy, most commonly used opioid in neonates.
	0.1	IV	Every 3-4 hr	
Codeine	1	PO	Every 3-4 hr	Not recommended for parenteral use; decreased incremental analgesic effect with doses higher than 65 mg.
Hydromorphone	0.06	PO	Every 3-4 hr	—
	0.015	IV	Every 3-4 hr	
Hydrocodone	0.2	PO	Every 3-4 hr	Doses of aspirin and acetaminophen in combination products must be adjusted as appropriate for body weight.
Meperidine (Demerol)	0.75	IV	Every 3-4 hr	Reserved for very brief courses of opioid use in clients who have demonstrated allergy to morphine or hydromorphone; accumulation of the metabolite normeperidine may result in seizures.

Drug	Dose	Route	Interval	Comments
Methadone	0.2	PO	Every 6-8 hr	—
	0.1	IV	Every 6-8 hr	
Oxycodone	0.2	PO	Every 3-4 hr	Doses of aspirin and acetaminophen in combination products must be adjusted as appropriate for body weight.
Nonopioids				
Acetaminophen	10-15	PO or PR	Every 4 hr	No antiinflammatory activity.
Nonsteroidal antiinflammatory drugs (NSAIDs)				
Aspirin	10-15	PO	Every 4 hr	Inhibits platelet aggregation; may cause postoperative bleeding; do not administer salicylate to children with suspected or confirmed viral infection (e.g., chickenpox).
Choline magnesium salicylate	25	PO	Twice a day	May have minimal antiplatelet activity; oral liquid available; do not administer salicylate to children with suspected or confirmed viral infection (e.g., chickenpox).

Continued

TABLE H-2
Selected Medications Used to Manage Acute Pain in the Pediatric Population—cont'd

Drug	Dose (mg/kg)*	Route	Frequency	Comments
Ibuprofen	10	PO	Every 6-8 hr	Oral suspension available.
Naproxen	5	PO	Every 12 hr	Oral liquid available.
Ketoralac	0.5	IV	Every 6-8 hr	The only parenteral NSAID; has not been approved for use in the pediatric population; there are presently ongoing clinical trials regarding the use of the IM preparation as an IV preparation in the pediatric and adult populations.

IM, Intramuscular; *IV,* intravenous; *PO,* by mouth; *PR,* by rectum.
*Recommended dose for children weighing less than 50 kg.

Patient-controlled analgesia

Patient-controlled analgesia (PCA) is a method of intravenous administration of small boluses of opiates used in the treatment of postoperative pain. The child uses a hand-operated device to signal the PCA pump to deliver a bolus dose of the medication. The pump will deliver the medication directly into the child's intravenous line provided that a set period of time ("lockout interval") has passed since the previous dose. In addition to the boluses, many PCA pumps have the capability to deliver a background or continuous infusion of the opiate. Delivery of a continuous infusion helps maintain a steady therapeutic drug level even when the child is sleeping.

The child must have the cognitive ability to understand the principles of PCA. By the age of 7 most children can use PCA without difficulty. Each individual child's developmental level must be assessed prior to initiation of this method of drug administration. Teaching the child about PCA preoperatively is helpful.

Benefits of PCA include elimination of delay in analgesic administration, high levels of client satisfaction, usefulness for all types of acute pain, potential reduction in total medication requirement, and reduction in nursing staff workload.

Complications are the same as those for other methods of opiate administration—respiratory depression, urinary retention, pruritus, nausea, and vomiting.

Epidural analgesia

Epidural analgesia may be used in children who have undergone any of a variety of surgeries, including thoracic, abdominal, and genitourinary tract procedures. The epidural catheter is placed by an anesthesiologist and provides access for continuous opiate infusion or delivery of boluses of opiates and/or local anesthetics.

Compared with traditional intravenous or PCA administration of opiates, smaller doses of opiate given via an epidural catheter provide adequate pain control with less sedation. Because of the increased comfort level, the child is better able to participate in postoperative care. Additional benefits include earlier ambulation and increased ability to deep breathe. Potential side effects of epidural analgesia include respiratory depression, urinary retention, pruritus, infection, spinal headache, nausea, and vomiting.

Nonpharmacologic Management

Behavioral and other nonpharmacologic techniques may be used in conjunction with pharmacologic management of acute pain. Table H-3 lists selected nonpharmacologic pain management strategies. These techniques often allow for a reduction in the amount of analgesic required. It is important to assess the child's individual response to any strategy. Involving families in these strategies often enhances their success.

TABLE H-3
Nonpharmacologic Pain Management Techniques

Age Group	Techniques
Neonates	▪ Pacifiers ▪ Music (fetal heart sounds) ▪ Swaddling, blanket nests, or boundaries ▪ Speaking in quiet tones ▪ Minimization of noxious stimuli: frequent handling, noise, bright lights (premature neonates may be overwhelmed by increased sensory stimuli)
Infants	▪ Visual stimuli ▪ Speaking in quiet tones ▪ Pacifiers ▪ Rocking ▪ Swaddling (for younger infants) ▪ Music ▪ Cutaneous stimulation: transcutaneous electric nerve stimulation, heat, cold, massage
Toddlers	▪ Magic wands ▪ Kaleidoscopes ▪ Pop-up books ▪ Music

Continued

TABLE H-3
*Nonpharmacologic Pain Management
Techniques—cont'd*

Age Group	Techniques
Preschoolers	- Controlled breathing—blowing bubbles - Cutaneous stimulation - Magic wands - Kaleidoscopes - Pop-up books - Finding hidden picture *(Where's Waldo?)* - Listening to music or a story through a headset - Video watching - Emotive imagery—using a child's favorite superhero to "fight" the pain - Controlled breathing - Behavior rehearsal—becoming familiar with a procedure through play - Cutaneous stimulation
School-aged children	- Imagery - Listening to music or a story through a headset - Video watching - Controlled breathing - Behavior rehearsal - Cutaneous stimulation - Modeling—observing another child during a procedure; the child models or demonstrates behavior that assists in mastering the procedure (can be live or on videotape)
Adolescents	- Imagery - Music - Controlled breathing - Video watching - Cutaneous stimulation - Modeling

PROCEDURAL PAIN

Invasive procedures are essential in diagnosis and treatment for many hospitalized children. These procedures include venipuncture, intravenous catheter insertion, circumcision, cardiac catheterization, chest tube insertion, central line insertion, bone marrow aspiration, and biopsy. Some dressing changes may also cause significant pain and stress in children.

The child and the family should be adequately prepared for the procedure. The type of preparation should be based on the child's developmental level. Be aware of the environment in which the procedure is to be performed. Minimize noise, provide adequate lighting, and ensure privacy. The child's room and bed are considered safe places. Procedures should not be performed in the room or the bed unless absolutely necessary.

Allow a family member (ideally, mother and/or father, if present) to be with the child before, during, and after the procedure. The family member should be prepared for his or her role, which usually involves assisting in nonpharmacologic pain relief measures.

If anxiolytics are used to reduce anxiety associated with procedures, it is important to remember that these medications will blunt the child's response to pain but will not provide pain relief.

A key principle in the management of procedural pain is the provision of maximal treatment for the pain and anxiety of a first procedure, particularly if the child must undergo repeated procedures. This helps to reduce the development of anticipatory anxiety prior to subsequent procedures.

REFERENCES

International Association for the Study of Pain, Subcommittee on Taxonomy: Pain terms: a list with definitions and notes usage, *Pain* 6:249, 1979.

James SR et al: *Nursing care of children: principles & practice,* Philadelphia, 2002, WB Saunders.

McCaffrey M, Bebee A: *Pain: clinical manual for nursing practice,* St Louis, 1994, Mosby.

Oakes LL: Assessment and management of pain in the critically ill pediatric patient, *Crit Care Nurs Clin North Am* 13(2):281, 2001.

Rodriguez E, Jordan R: Contemporary trend in pediatric sedation and analgesia, *Emerg Med Clin North Am* 20(2):199, 2002.

I

❖

Height and Weight Growth Curves

❖

See Figure I-1 on p. 744.

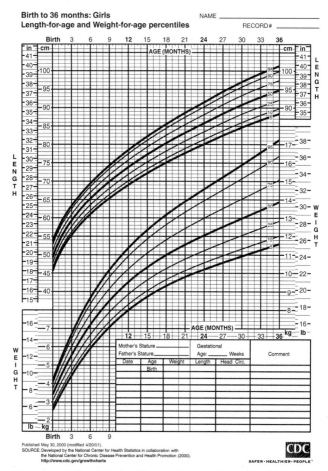

Figure I-1 Girls: birth to 36 months. Length and weight. These charts were developed by the National Center for Health Statistics in collaboration with the National Center for Chronic Disease Prevention and Health Promotion, 2000. The data on these charts are considered representative of the general United States population.

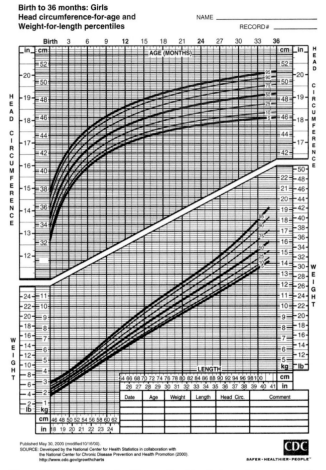

Figure I-2 Girls: birth to 36 months. Head circumference, length, and weight.

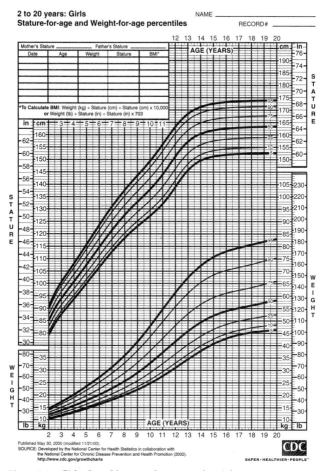

Figure I-3 Girls: 2 to 20 years. Stature and weight.

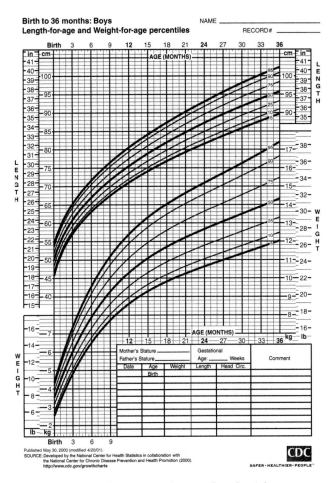

Birth to 36 months: Boys
Length-for-age and Weight-for-age percentiles

NAME _____

RECORD# _____

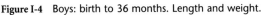

Published May 30, 2000 (modified 4/20/01).
SOURCE: Developed by the National Center for Health Statistics in collaboration with
the National Center for Chronic Disease Prevention and Health Promotion (2000).
http://www.cdc.gov/growthcharts

Figure I-4   Boys: birth to 36 months. Length and weight.

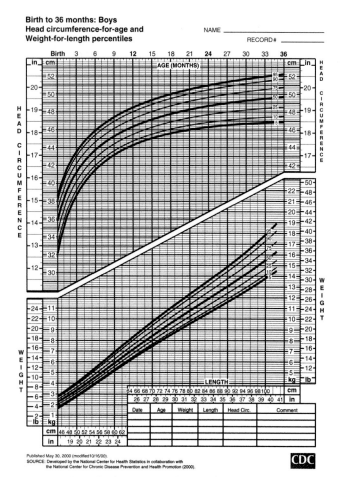

Figure I-5 Boys: birth to 36 months. Head circumference, length, and weight.

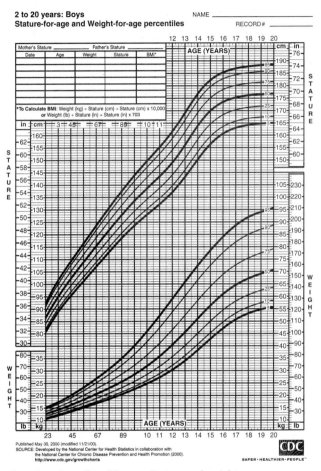

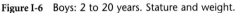

Figure I-6   Boys: 2 to 20 years. Stature and weight.

J

❖

Psychosocial Interventions

❖

PREPARATION FOR PROCEDURES OR SURGERY

1. Prepare child and parents for procedure or surgery.
   a. Provide age-appropriate explanations.
      i. For younger children, use of sensory materials such as graphics (e.g., pictures) or props (e.g., bandages, surgical mask) enhances child's comprehension.
      ii. For older children, use of illustrations such as film or pictures (e.g., anatomic figures) is helpful to supplement explanation.
   b. Explain procedure or surgery and preoperative routine in terms of sequence of events to occur, including sensory information (e.g., mouth will feel dry, child will feel sleepy).
   c. For younger children, encourage preprocedural play such as using medical equipment, doll, or stuffed animal as means of explaining procedure or surgery.
   d. Use age-appropriate means for explaining body changes following procedure or surgery and for eliciting concerns from child.
   e. Provide and reinforce information for parents about child's condition and treatment to help them answer their child's questions or relieve their own anxiety.
   f. Assure child that procedure is not being done because child is "bad."
2. Prepare child and parents emotionally for surgery.
   a. Provide understandable explanations in lay terms.
   b. Use active listening to elicit concerns.

c. Encourage expression of feelings (e.g., guilt, anger, anxiety, feeling of being overwhelmed).

d. Encourage expression of fears concerning child's well-being.

e. Provide anticipatory information about emotional responses to surgery.

f. Encourage parents to room in and participate in child's care as means of promoting security and decreasing anxiety.

g. Encourage parental participation during selected procedures; some procedures can be very traumatic for parent and convey erroneous message to younger child that parent cannot "protect" child from harm.

h. Encourage parental participation during induction of anesthesia and during recovery (if applicable).

i. Provide for parents' physical comforts (e.g., sleeping and hygiene).

j. Encourage use of preexisting support systems such as family members, close friends, and clergy.

k. Encourage incorporation of some home habits—such as use of child's blanket, praying, and storytelling—into hospital routine.

l. Assist parents in providing support and information to siblings while child is hospitalized.

m. If needed, provide information to parents about addressing sibling needs such as by disclosing information about child's clinical status, maintaining household routines, arranging for family members or friends to supplement parent caretaking activities, and communicating with school personnel.

3. Assist and support child during preoperative laboratory and diagnostic tests.

a. Prepare or provide information about upcoming procedures (e.g., complete blood count, urinalysis, laboratory and diagnostic tests).

b. Assist in collection of preoperative laboratory and diagnostic data.

    c. Prepare child for surgery by obtaining nursing assessment data such as evaluation of body systems and nursing history.

    d. Monitor child's reactions to presurgical or preprocedural preparations.

4. Monitor child's baseline status prior to surgery or procedure.

    a. Vital signs

    b. System assessment

SUPPORTIVE CARE

1. Alleviate anxiety caused by various aspects of hospital experience, including invasive procedures for diagnostic tests, pain, threatening and confusing hospital environment, unfamiliar hospital personnel, knowledge deficit pertaining to hospital routines and treatments, and age-related fears.

    a. Provide therapeutic play during all phases of illness and for each new procedure based on child's developmental level (see the previous section, Preparation for Procedures or Surgery, for additional information).

    b. Explain each procedure or hospital routine at child's and parents' cognitive levels; allow enough time for child and parents to ask questions and express anxieties.

    c. Suggest ways for parents to support their child during hospitalization and procedures (e.g., holding child after procedure).

    d. Consult parents and child about preferences among "quiet" toys and activities during acute phase of illness; encourage parents and volunteers to play with child, allowing for rest periods and then passive participation (see Appendix B).

    e. Encourage and promote socialization with peers as means to cope adaptively with effects of disease.

2. Provide emotional and other support to parents.

    a. Provide and reinforce explanations about hospital experience.

    b. Encourage use of preexisting support systems (e.g., relatives, friends, clergy).

    c. Encourage expression of feelings through active listening techniques.

    d. Provide for physical comforts (e.g., arrangements for sleeping, bathing).

    e. Refer to social services if appropriate.

    f. Refer to in-hospital parent support group; encourage parents to network with other parents in hospital for support.

3. Provide comfort measures to ease child's anxiety and discomfort of during hospitalization.

    a. Teach parents how to hold and comfort child who has intravenous support and other medical equipment.

    b. Encourage parents to participate in aspects of child's care such as bathing and feeding; however, if parents are uncomfortable or otherwise unable to provide care, they should not feel pressured to do so.

    c. Keep stimulation to a minimum; arrange procedures or treatments so as to minimize interruptions, especially at night.

    d. Teach parents nonpharmacologic pain relief measures to use with child (see Appendix H).

4. Provide developmentally appropriate visual, auditory, and tactile stimulation (see Appendix B).

5. Provide consistent nursing care to promote trust and to alleviate anxiety.

6. Encourage use of recreational and diversional activities (see Appendix B).

K

◆

Home Care

◆

1. Instruct parents verbally and with detailed written information about the following aspects of medical management to enhance adherence:
   a. Disease process—signs, symptoms, complications, and treatment regimen
   b. Administration of medications—therapeutic response to medications, untoward reactions to medications
   c. Treatment procedures—steps of procedures and schedule
   d. Activity restrictions—level of activities, schedule and types of restrictions, restriction/activity accommodations
   e. Equipment needs—care and maintenance of equipment, phone number of vendor, insurance coverage
   f. Name and phone number of appropriate follow-up contact (e.g., private medical doctor, clinic, health maintenance organization, clinical nurse specialist, nurse practitioner, case manager)
2. Instruct parents about identifying symptoms that indicate worsening of condition and need to report to physician.
3. Provide child and family with information about community support systems for long-term adaptation (member of rehabilitation team such as speech and language therapist, occupational and physical therapist).
   a. School referral
      i. School reintegration program—refer to appropriate school personnel such as school nurse, teacher, or specialist

ii. Referral for 504 plan—educational accommodations made by school to respond to child with special health care need who is a general education student for additional educational supports (placement of desk in front of classroom, uninhibited access to bathroom facilities as needed, on-site medication protocol)

b. Parent groups for ongoing support, information, and advocacy

c. Children's groups for ongoing support

d. Siblings groups for ongoing support

e. Financial resources and information about third-party providers

f. Community specialists and programs for ongoing therapy and/or services

g. Community organizations for ongoing support and information (e.g., American Cancer Society, United Cerebral Palsy)

4. Instruct parents about parenting issues.

a. Need to maintain usual expectations for behavior and misbehavior

b. Continuance with disciplinary measures, e.g., use of "time out" discipline (note that parents may need additional training for this)

c. Strategies to assist child in living normally and dealing with concerns

d. Use of child-rearing practices that avoid labeling child's behavior as deviant, because such labeling may have self-fulfilling result

e. Use of strategies that encourage interactions with peers

5. Facilitate adherence to long-term management during follow-up visits by reinforcing information pertaining to procedures and community resources to prevent complications; ask questions that explore adherence potential.

a. Means of transportation

b. Resources for child care

c. Finances

d. Level of motivation

e. Understanding of need for long-term follow-up

6. Monitor family adaptation and functioning.
   a. Ensure that all interventions take into account family's cultural, religious, educational, and socioeconomic background.
   b. Involve siblings as much as possible because they have many concerns and feelings about changes in child and in family's functioning.
   c. Consider possibility that siblings feel self-blame and guilt.
   d. Encourage parents to express feelings of insecurity and concerns about caring for child at home, as well as about long-term management and prognosis.
   e. Refer parents to support groups and/or counseling, because parental relationships may be strained as a result of intense pressures and care expectations of ill child.

❖

Community Services

❖

SPECIAL EDUCATION

Special education refers to the educational services and supports provided to children and youth with disabilities. As described later, service systems in education, developmental disabilities, rehabilitation, and job development have been developed to promote better educational and adult outcomes for infants, children, and youth with disabilities. Until recently, the emphasis of special education programs was on provision of services in segregated settings focused on limited objectives with a deficit-oriented approach. Best practice approaches foster the provision of services and supports within inclusive general education settings. That is, students who need special education services are educated in general education classrooms rather than only with other students in special education.

In educational settings, the mechanism for developing an educational plan to ensure that students in special education achieve their educational, vocational, and community life goals is described as well. The individualized education plan and the individualized transition plan describe the processes used by educators to assist students with disabilities to achieve their educational goals. Early intervention as explained in the next section refers to the system of services available to infants and toddlers who are at risk for or have disabilities.

EARLY INTERVENTION

The early intervention (EI) system was initially authorized in 1986 in the Education of the Handicapped Act amendments (Public Law [PL] 99-457) and was reauthorized with subsequent amendments, most recently in the Individuals with Disabilities Education Act (IDEA) (PL 105-17) in 1997. PL 99-457 specified the following important concepts and elements to be integrated into EI services:

1. Family-centered services
2. Culturally competent services
3. Supports and interventions that are comprehensive (biopsychosocial perspective), systematic, and functional (assessment of what the infant/toddler can do and what interventions are needed)
4. Focus on the strengths of the child and family rather than deficits
5. Incorporation of an interagency approach

EI services are provided to infants and toddlers from birth to 3 years of age. Infants who qualify for EI services are those born with Down syndrome or other genetic disorders, mental retardation, or low birth weight, or born prematurely; infants exposed in utero to illicit substances and alcohol; and those born small or large for gestational age. The goals of EI are to promote the infant's optimal growth and development and to provide services and support to families as a means of promoting their involvement in assisting their child to reach his or her optimal function. EI has been demonstrated to enhance neurodevelopmental outcomes for infants and toddlers.

Several types of EI programs are available. An EI program may be center based or home based or a combination of both. Center-based programs are situated in locations in the community where services are rendered. EI services may be provided in the family's home.

Infants and toddlers who are at risk for disabilities or who are diagnosed with disabilities are referred to EI services. Eligibility is assessed by an interdisciplinary team of professionals that includes but is not limited to a pediatrician, psychologist, nurse, occupational and physical therapists, speech and language specialist, audiologist, and family advocate. Once eligibility has been determined, an individualized family service plan (IFSP) is developed that is family centered and based on family priorities. The IFSP specifies the services and supports needed that will assist the child and family in meeting their goals. Services should be provided in the most inclusive settings possible. Infants and toddlers are referred to EI services for the following services based on the IFSP:

1. Case management/service coordination
2. Assistive technology
3. Speech therapy
4. Audiology
5. Physical therapy
6. Occupational therapy
7. Psychologic evaluation and therapy
8. Family support services
9. Health and medical services

The services provided to the infant or toddler as specified in the IFSP will take into account the following:

1. The findings of the interdisciplinary assessments/evaluations that identify the child's level of development and comprehensive needs for services.
2. The strengths and service needs of the child's family.
3. Identification of IFSP goals and objectives.
4. Proposed outcomes expected as a basis for services.
5. Identification of where and what type of services are to be offered, and who will provide them.
6. Identification of the case manager/service coordinator who is responsible for coordination of services and liaison with the family.

INDIVIDUALIZED EDUCATION PLAN

1. The individualized education plan (IEP) is the written plan for a child with a disability, as determined by an interdisciplinary process involving educational personnel with expertise in special education and related services. IEPs are written for students who receive special education services. The IEP contains the following information:
   a. Statement of the child's present level of educational performance
   b. Indication of the extent to which the child's disability affects his or her educational progress and participation in school activities
   c. Statement of annual goals and short-term objectives to achieve the goals

    d. Statement of special education and related services, supplementary aids and services, and program modifications and/or supports that will be provided in as inclusive a setting as possible for the child to meet IEP goals

    e. Extent to which the child's educational program is conducted in segregated educational settings

    f. Identification of the methods used to measure the child's progress in achieving IEP goals

    g. Identification of the methods used to inform the parents of the child's progress in meeting IEP goals

    h. Indication of whether the child will take district, state-wide achievement tests

        i. If yes, then how the student will be tested, and what, if any, accommodations will be made.

        ii. If the student will not be tested, then provision of an explanation.

2. Other considerations that are addressed in formulating the child's IEP are the following:

    a. Identification of the child's strengths

    b. Identification of parental concerns

    c. Findings of recent evaluations

    d. "Special factors"

        i. Identification of positive behavioral interventions, strategies, and supports for the child with behavioral challenges

        ii. Language needs of the child with limited English proficiency

        iii. Provision of instruction in braille for the child who is blind or visually impaired

        iv. Communication needs for the child who is deaf or hard of hearing

        v. The child's needs for assistive technology

3. According to the provisions of IDEA, the child's IEP team consists of the following individuals:

    a. The child's parents

    b. At least one regular teacher (provided the child is in general education)

c. At least one special education teacher
d. Educational representative from the school (i.e., school administrator) who has supervisory authority to ensure that IEP services will be provided
e. Educational personnel who can provide the findings and interpretation of evaluations conducted (i.e., school counselor, psychologist)
f. Other experts, such as related services personnel
g. The child as appropriate

INDIVIDUALIZED TRANSITION PLAN

The purpose of the individualized transition plan (ITP) is to plan and implement a well-thought-out direction for the ensuing years of secondary education for the student with a disability that will enable him or her to transition successfully to postsecondary settings. Each transition plan is individualized according to the student's interests, preferences, and needs— one student may desire employment while another student may choose to pursue additional education at the local community college or at a university after he or she leaves the high school setting. Transition planning is a component of the IEP.

1. Beginning at age 14 years, with an annual update thereafter, the IEP must contain a statement of the transition services the youth will need, such as academic courses and work-based learning experiences. The IEP must contain goals and benchmarks that focus on the student's transition needs in his or her course of study.

2. Beginning at age 16 years (or younger if determined as appropriate by the IEP team), the IEP must contain the following:
   a. Identification of a coordinated set of activities that are outcome oriented and are reviewed annually, promoting the movement of the student from school to postschool activities
   b. Statement of transition services, including services and linkages to interagency bodies such as the department of rehabilitation to implement the transition plan

    c. Specification of transition services in one or more of the following six areas:
      i. Instruction
      ii. Community experiences
      iii. Development of employment objectives
      iv. Postschool adult and living objectives; and, if appropriate,
      v. Daily living skills
      vi. Functional vocational evaluation
    d. Delineation of activities and services based on the student's interests, preferences, and needs
3. Related services are to be included in the IEP as needed by students.
4. If the agency does not provide a transition service specified in the IEP, then another IEP meeting is convened to develop other plans to meet transition objectives specified in the IEP.
5. One year before the student reaches the age of majority (varies according to state), the family and student are informed that IDEA rights are transferred to the youth.

STATE CHILDREN'S HEALTH INSURANCE PROGRAM

In 1997, with the passage of the Balanced Budget Act, Congress expanded the Medicaid program for children. This new legislation, establishing the State Children's Health Insurance Program (SCHIP), made it possible for states to provide health insurance coverage to uninsured children whose family income was above the financial eligibility requirements for Medicaid (up to 200% of the federal poverty level). Under this new program, the federal government annually provides states $4 billion to help with the costs of health insurance for eligible children. Each state has the flexibility to determine eligibility criteria within the following broad guidelines: (1) the individual is not currently eligible for Medicaid insurance; (2) the individual is under 19 years of age; and (3) family income is at or below 200% of the federal poverty level. SCHIP can be an expansion of the state's current Medicaid program offering the same benefits or a new program that incorporates the following standards:

1. Insurance coverage must be equivalent to that of the usual commercial health insurance plans, such as the federal employee health benefits plan.
2. States can require affordable payments and fees for insurance coverage.
3. States can institute copayments on a sliding scale for families whose incomes are above 150% of the federal poverty level.
4. States cannot require copayments for immunizations and preventive care.

For information on specific state programs, see the following website: http://www.statelocalgov.net/index.cfm.

EARLY AND PERIODIC SCREENING, DIAGNOSIS, AND TREATMENT PROGRAM

The Early and Periodic Screening, Diagnosis, and Treatment Program (EPSDTP) is a federally funded program (Medicaid) administered by each state that enables eligible poor children to receive an array of preventive health care, diagnostic, and treatment services. The goal of the program is to ensure that eligible children receive the necessary pediatric health care services to prevent childhood illnesses and disabilities. Each state is responsible for administering its own EPSDTP but must offer the assortment of services specified by federal regulations. The state EPSDTP does not provide direct services but is responsible for reimbursement and for ensuring that an adequate number of providers are available to supply services that are timely, accessible, and comprehensive. This program is for children from birth through 18 years of age. Eligible children include those whose family incomes are up to 200% of the federal poverty level. These services include the following:

1. Comprehensive medical and developmental history taking
2. Physical examination (unclothed)
3. Nutrition assessment
4. Immunizations
5. Vision and hearing screening

6. Dental screening
7. Selected laboratory tests: hematocrit, hemoglobin levels, tuberculosis screening, sickle cell anemia testing, urinalysis, serum lead levels, and Pap smear
8. Health education related to developmental level
9. Sports and camp physical examinations
10. For adolescents: smoking cessation counseling, family planning, treatment for sexually transmitted diseases
11. For children with special health care needs: additional physical examinations as needed
12. Medical problems found during routine physical examinations must be treated with program funds

Other ancillary services provided include the following:

1. Assistance with transportation needs
2. Referrals to other service programs such as Special Supplemental Nutrition Program for Women, Infants, and Children, mental health programs, Title V programs for children with special health care needs

TITLE V PROGRAM FOR CHILDREN WITH SPECIAL HEALTH CARE NEEDS

The Title V Program for Children with Special Health Care Needs is a publicly funded health care program for eligible children with special health care needs. This program was originally enacted in 1935 as Title V of the Social Security Act. Funded by federal, state, and local governments, the program provides health care, related services, and case management services to children with special health care needs whose condition meets medical eligibility requirements and whose family income meets the financial eligibility requirements. Age range of eligibility is from birth through 21 years of age. State programs are responsible for ensuring the availability of adequate numbers of professionals who meet the service standards set by program guidelines. Services received by children with special health care needs include the following:

1. Long-term specialty care services provided by an interdisciplinary team of professionals (physicians, registered nurses, social workers, nutritionists)

2. Community- and/or school-based physical therapy and occupational therapy services
3. Case management
4. Transition services
5. Necessary medical equipment and supplies such as wheelchairs, suction machines
6. Assistive technology
7. Social services
8. Nutritional consultations
9. Surgeries
10. Hospitalizations
11. Medications
12. Orthodontics (must be related to chronic condition)

SPECIAL SUPPLEMENTAL NUTRITION PROGRAM FOR WOMEN, INFANTS, AND CHILDREN

The Special Supplemental Nutrition Program for Women, Infants, and Children (WIC) designed to provide nutritious foods, nutritional education, and referrals for eligible individuals was first begun in 1972. This nonentitlement program is administered by the U.S. Department of Agriculture, so that the annual funds budgeted for the program are not sufficient to cover services for all eligible populations. This program serves children under 5 years of age who are at nutritional risk, as well as pregnant, breast-feeding, and postpartum women in low-income families (family income of no more than 185% of the federal poverty level). Services provided by WIC include the following:

1. Coupon vouchers for nutritious foods such as milk, juice, eggs, and cheese that can be redeemed at local grocery stores
2. Classes on healthy eating and health behaviors
3. Breast-feeding classes
4. Referrals to other community-based programs for health and social services

HEAD START AND EARLY HEAD START PROGRAMS

The Head Start preschool program is a federally funded developmental and family support program for low-income individuals (family income of less than $15,000/yr) serving preschool children aged 3 to 5 years and their families. More than 20 million children have participated in the Head Start program since its inception in 1965 as an initiative of President Johnson's War on Poverty. The goal of Head Start is to better prepare low-income preschool children for elementary school by providing them with enriched learning and social opportunities and health care. An additional program goal is to enable parents to learn child care skills permitting them to obtain employment in Head Start. Currently, nearly 1 million ethnically and racially diverse children (black: 33.8%; white: 29.9%; Hispanic: 29.7%; American Indian: 3.6%; Asian: 2%; Pacific Islander: 1%) are enrolled in Head Start. Thirteen percent of children enrolled in Head Start have disabilities. Most children (59%) receive medical and dental services through the EPSDTP program. The Head Start program provides a range of services to preschool children that includes child-centered early childhood development and education services based on the child's learning and development needs. These programs involve indoor and outdoor play activities such as painting, dancing, game playing, storytelling, and participating in learning projects. There are many educational and support programs for parents. Head Start staff make home visits to provide additional instruction and support. Parents play an active role in Head Start programs as volunteers to enable them to gain work experience for employment. The Early Head Start program, similar in purpose to the Head Start program, was begun in 1995 and serves infants and toddlers 3 years of age and younger, and pregnant women.

The Head Start program is administered by the Head Start Bureau of the U.S. Department of Health and Human Services. Federal funding for local programs is awarded to local public agencies, schools, and nonprofit and for-profit organizations. Eighty percent of funding comes from the federal government; the remaining funds are provided by local communities. Services provided by Head Start include the following:

1. Preschool program
2. Health care that includes medical, dental, mental health, and nutritional services
3. Referral to community-based social service agencies

SUPPLEMENTAL SECURITY INCOME PROGRAM

The Social Security Administration (SSA) administers the Supplemental Security Income (SSI) program. Eligible children with disabilities are provided SSI monthly payments. Eligibility criteria include the following: (1) family income below a designated level; (2) U.S. residency, U.S. citizenship, or, for noncitizens, connection with military service or status as designated refugee or individual granted asylum; (3) presence of blindness; (4) presence of "marked and severe functional limitation" due to physical or mental condition or combination of conditions; (5) persistence of the condition for longer than 1 year or expectation that the condition will cause the child's death; (6) family income of less than $500/mo for child; (7) resources of less than $2000 for child.

Eligibility is determined by state Disability Determination Services (DDSs) contracted by the SSA. The DDS evaluation team reviews the assessment data from doctors, teachers, counselors, therapists, and social workers on the extent to which the child's disability affects the child's level of functioning. All eligibility determinations are based on the written report and medical records for the child. No in-person interviews or evaluations are conducted. The disability evaluation specialist determines whether the child's disability corresponds to one of the 100 SSA listings of physical or mental impairments or "medically equal" or "functionally equal" impairment.

Many programs are targeted specifically at adolescents and young adults who want to work or continue their education and still receive their SSI benefits. The Plan for Achieving Self-Support (PASS) allows the individual to earn money and still receive SSI income. The PASS allows the individual to save money for education, training, or startup of a business. Individuals who earn enough money that they no longer need the SSI check may be able to continue to receive Medicaid benefits according to Section 1619(a) and 1619(b) plans.

The Impairment Related Work Expenses (IRWE) program allows individuals with disability needs to deduct from their earnings the money spent for equipment and services required to enable them to work. Deductible expenses include costs of durable medical equipment, medical supplies, job coaches, attendant care, architectural modifications to the home, and transportation services.

Students enrolled in college or a training program who are under 22 years of age can exclude earned income of up to $1620 each year from their SSI benefits. For additional information, see the following website: http://www.ssa.gov (SSA).

An SSA representative can be contacted directly at 800-772-1213 between 7 AM and 7 PM. The TTY number is 800-325-0778. The SSA recommends making phone calls after the beginning of the week and the beginning of each month.

REFERENCES

American Academy of Pediatrics, State insurance program (SCHIP), Medicaid provisions of the Balanced Budget Act of 1997 (PL 105-33), 2002, available at http://www.aap.org/advocacy/schippro.htm, accessed November 12, 2002.

Association of Maternal and Child Health Programs, Issue brief: The impact of the state's child health insurance program (SCHIP) on Title V children with special health care needs programs, updated edition, 2000, available at http://www.amchp1.org/news/Impact%20_SCHIP_CSHCN.pdf, accessed November 1, 2002.

Education of the Handicapped Act Amendments of 1986 (PL 99-457), US Code, vol 20, secs 1400 *et seq* (1986).

Individuals with Disabilities Education Act (IDEA) of 1990 (PL 101-476), US Code, vol 20, secs 1401 *et seq* (1990).

Individuals with Disabilities Education Act (IDEA) of 1991 (PL 102-119), US Code, vol 20, secs 1400 *et seq* (1991).

Individuals with Disabilities Education Act (IDEA) (PL 105-17), June 4, 1997.

Porter S et al, editors: *Children and youth assisted by medical technology in educational settings: guidelines for care*, Baltimore, 1997, Paul H. Brookes.

Los Angeles Medical Home Project, Systems of care for children with special health care needs, 2000, available at http://www.medicalhomela.org/LA%20Medical%20Home.htm, accessed October 15, 2002.

US Department of Agriculture, WIC at a glance, 2002, available at http://www.fns.usda.gov/wic/ProgramInfo/WICataglance.htm, accessed November 1, 2002.

US Department of Health and Human Services, Administration on Children, Youth and Families, Head Start facts, 2001, available at http://www.acf.hhs.gov/programs/opa/facts/headst.htm, accessed October 31, 2002.

M

◆

Breast-Feeding

◆

NORMAL PARAMETERS

1. Eight to 12 feedings/day, for 20 to 60 minutes (total for both breasts) is common in the first several weeks.
2. Allow the infant to finish the first breast before offering the second breast. Offer both breasts during each feeding. Limiting the duration of feedings can interfere with adequate milk transfer.
3. Giving additional liquid to breast-feeding infants is not necessary and should be discouraged. Some mothers will try to give a bottle after nursing to determine if the infant is getting enough. All infants will suck on a bottle even when full.

COMMON PROBLEMS

1. Sore nipples
   a. Assess for appropriate positioning; position the infant on the areola (not the nipple), ensure that the infant is held "stomach to stomach."
   b. Have the mother break suction with a finger before removing the infant from the breast.
   c. Express breast milk and let dry on the nipple, allow nipples to air dry after feeding.
   d. Begin the feeding on the less sore breast.
   e. Assess for candidiasis/thrush.
2. Engorgement
   a. Engorgement is excessive fullness to the point that the infant can breast-feed only with difficulty. If breasts are

warm and firm or hard, the mother may have a low-grade fever.

b. Ensure frequent breast-feedings. Utilize rousing techniques if the infant is sleepy.

c. Express some milk by hand or pump if the areola/nipple area is too hard for the infant to grasp.

d. Use warm, moist compresses 10 to 20 minutes before nursing.

e. Use a mild analgesic if needed.

f. Cold compresses applied to the breasts may be comforting after feeding.

g. Restricting fluids has not been shown to be an effective treatment for engorgement.

3. Refusal of baby to nurse; usually due to the following:

a. Incorrect positioning

b. Flat or inverted nipples

c. Engorgement

d. Inability of the baby to breathe; nose may be blocked by the breast or nasal congestion

4. Insufficient milk supply

a. Inability to make sufficient milk for the infant is very rare and is usually due to previous breast surgery or a hormone imbalance.

b. Infant signs:

i. Infant is restless and/or irritable during or between feedings.

ii. Infant acts "hungry all the time," sucks fists or blanket, moves head rapidly from side to side at the breast.

iii. Infant comes off the areola/nipple frequently.

iv. Infant cries or is fussy constantly, is difficult to console, is fussy immediately after a feeding.

v. Infant falls asleep at the breast.

vi. Urine output and bowel movements are inadequate.

c. Maternal signs:

i. Breasts feel soft before each feeding.

ii. Breasts did not enlarge or become tender during pregnancy.

       iii. Breasts did not become full or engorged postpartum.

       iv. Mother reports previous breast surgery.

  d. Interventions

     i. If infant is receiving sufficient breast milk for growth, reassure mother.

     ii. If infant is not growing appropriately, refer to lactation consultant.

5. Maternal medications

  a. Although the placenta permits a ready crossover of drugs to the fetus in utero, the breast serves as a formidable barrier that protects the infant. Most drugs pass through to the mother's milk but they do so in minute amounts, usually less than 1% of the maternal dose. Most are not harmful to the infant; many cannot be found when infant serum is checked.

  b. Always use a reference book specifically for breast-feeding situations. Many drug books base their recommendations on information provided by the drug manufacturer and will not suggest use in breast-feeding mothers due to inadequate research.

6. Candidiasis/thrush—common in mother and infant after antibiotic treatment.

  a. Symptoms:

     i. Nipples may be itchy or burning, may appear red or pink, shiny, or flaky.

     ii. Nipples may be cracked.

    iii. Acute pain is felt during and after nursing, which may be described as "shooting" pain.

    iv. If infection is severe, blisters that weep may appear.

     v. Mother may have a vaginal yeast infection.

    vi. Infant may have oral thrush and/or monilial diaper rash.

  b. Interventions:

     i. Treat both the mother and infant to control cross-contamination. This is one situation in which the application of breast milk to the nipple after the feeding is not recommended.

ii. Boil pacifiers, breast pump parts that touch the milk or infected area, bottle nipples, toys, etc.

iii. Expressed milk should not be frozen for later use; freezing deactivates but does not kill yeast. Milk frozen during a *Candida* outbreak may reinfect the infant when given after treatment.

7. Jaundice
   a. Effective breast-feeding does not alter the levels of bilirubin or incidence of jaundice in the first 5 days of life, but infrequent nursing and delayed onset may do so.
   b. Colostrum/breast milk has a laxative effect, stimulating the passage of meconium and lowering the bilirubin levels.
   c. If temporary supplements are needed, calorie-dense, milk-based fluids, not water or glucose water, should be used.

SEPARATION OF MOTHER AND INFANT

1. The normal frequency of feeding must be replicated when mother and infant are separated; have the mother breast-feed whenever possible and/or manually express or utilize a breast pump on the same schedule as at home.
2. Remember that nursing at the breast is less strenuous for the infant than bottle feeding.

REFERENCES

American Academy of Pediatrics Committee on Drugs, The transfer of drugs and other chemicals into human milk, policy statement, *Pediatrics* 108(3):776, 2001.

Briggs GG et al: *Drugs in pregnancy and lactation*, ed 6, Baltimore, 2001, Lippincott Williams & Wilkins.

Hale R: *Medications and mothers' milk*, ed 8, Amarillo, Tex, 1999, Pharmasoft Medical Publishing.

Lawrence RA, Lawrence RM: *Breastfeeding: a guide for the medical profession*, ed 5, St Louis, 1999, Mosby.

Riordan J, Auerbach KG: *Pocket guide to breastfeeding and human lactation*, Boston, 2001, Jones and Bartlett.

Index

Page references followed by *b, f, n,* or *t* indicate boxes, figures, notes, or tables, respectively.

A

AAMR. *See* American Association on Mental Retardation
Abbreviations, 722-727
Abdomen, 670
Abdominal radiography
  in acute renal failure, 472
  flat-plate study, 327
  in short bowel syndrome, 535
  in tetralogy of Fallot, 585
  in Wilms' tumor, 629
Abdominal ultrasonography, in neuroblastoma, 412
Abdominal-perineal pull-through procedure, 265-266
Abduction brace, 126-127
ABS. *See* Adaptive Behavior Scales
Absence seizures, 521*b*
Abuse
  child abuse and neglect, 68-76
  emotional, 68
  physical, 68
  sexual, 68, 72*b*
  substance, 567
  types of, 68
ABVD drug regimen, 222
Acetabular dysplasia, 123
Acetaminophen, 62, 196, 737*t*
Acetone, ketone bodies, 714

Acidemias. organic, 272*b*, 275, 276, 277
Acidosis, metabolic, 131*b*
ACPA/CPF (American Cleft Palate–Craniofacial Association), 88
Acquired immunodeficiency syndrome (AIDS), 226-237
  categorization of, 232*t*, 233*t*
  preventive measures, 234*b*
Actigall (ursodiol), 536
Adaptive Behavior Assessment System, 373
Adaptive Behavior Scales (ABS) (AAMR), 373
Adaptive behaviors, 373
Adderall (amphetamine), 40
ADEK drops, 537
ADHD. *See* Attention-deficit/hyperactivity disorder
Adolescents (13 to 19 years)
  cognitive development, 695
  faith development, 698
  fine motor development, 695
  formal operational stage, 695
  genital stage, 696-697
  gross motor development, 695
  growth and development, 693-698

Adolescents *(Continued)*
  HIV infection and AIDS in, 227,
      230
  individuating-reflexive stage, 698
  language development, 696
  mental retardation in, 382
  moral development, 698
  pain assessment in, 735
  pain management techniques
      for, nonpharmacologic,
      741*t*
  physical changes in, 695
  physical characteristics, 693
  postconventional stage, 698
  psychosexual development,
      696-697
  psychosocial development,
      697-698
  stature-for-age and weight-
      for-age percentiles, 746*f*,
      749*f*
Adrenal hyperplasia, congenital,
      273
Adriamycin (doxorubicin), 222
Advisory Committee on
      Immunization Practices
      (ACIP), 700*b*-701*b*
Advocacy activities, 381*b*
Aerosol generators, 113
African Americans, 70
Aganglionic megacolon,
      congenital, 212
Agency for Health Care Policy and
      Research (AHCPR)
      Publications Clearinghouse,
      450
Aggressive behavior, 373
AHCPR. *See* Agency for Health
      Care Policy and Research
AIDS, 226-237
  categorization of, 232*t*, 233*t*
  preventive measures, 234*b*
Airway clearance
  emergency measures for, 158
  maintenance of, 56

Albumin, serum
  in hemolytic-uremic syndrome,
      188
  in Kawasaki disease, 319
  in nephrotic syndrome, 402
  normal values, 714
Albuterol, 113
Alkaline phosphatase, 220, 430, 535
Alkylating agents, 405
ALL. *See* Leukemia, acute
      lymphoid or lymphocytic
Allopurinol (Zyloprim), 347
Alopecia, 353*t*
ALTEs. *See* Apparent life-
      threatening events
Amenorrhea, 7
American Academy of Family
      Physicians (AAFP), 700*b*-701*b*
American Academy of Pediatrics
      (AAP), 75*b*, 420*b*, 451
  "Back to Sleep"
      recommendations, 573
  immunization
      recommendations,
      700*b*-701*b*
American Association on Mental
      Retardation (AAMR), 373
American Cleft Palate–Craniofacial
      Association (ACPA/CPF), 88
American Diabetic Association
      (ADA), 136*b*
American Heart Association, 508*b*
American Indians, 70, 766
American Medical Association
      (AMA), 416, 451
American Sudden Infant Death
      Syndrome Institute, 574*b*
Amethopterin (methotrexate),
      345-346
Amino acid, branched-chain, 272*b*
Amino acid metabolism, disorders
      of, 271*b*
  clinical manifestations, 274, 275,
      276, 277
  of transsulfuration, 272*b*

Amino acid transport disorders, 272*b*

δ-Aminolevulinic acid, urine, 327

Ammonia, serum, 503, 714

Amobarbital, 563*t*

Amoxicillin, 446

Amoxicillin with clavulanate (Augmentin), 446

Amphetamines (Dexedrine, Dextrostat, and Adderall), 40, 563*t*

Ampicillin, 446

Amputation
    complications of, 431
    discharge planning and home care, 435
    limb salvage, 431
    positioning after, 433
    postoperative care, 433-435
    preoperative care, 432-433
    prosthetic devices after, 433-434

Amylase dehydrogenase, serum, 503, 714

Anal stage, 683

Analgesia
    epidural, 739-740
    narcotic, 196
    patient-controlled, 739

Anaphylactic shock, 355*t*

Anemia, 182
    aplastic, 10-15
    in chronic renal failure, 482
    iron deficiency, 300-305
    nursing interventions related to child undergoing chemotherapy and radiotherapy, 355*t*
    sickle cell, 543-551
    signs and symptoms, 476
    in tetralogy of Fallot, 584

Animism, 686

ANLL. *See* Leukemia, acute nonlymphoid

Ann Arbor staging system for Hodgkin's disease, 221*b*

Anoplasty, perineal, 265-266

Anorectal agenesis, 263

Anorexia nervosa, 3-9
    diagnostic criteria for, 4*b*
    nursing interventions, 8-9, 351*t*
    purging type, 4*b*
    restricting type, 4*b*

Antibiotics
    for cellulitis, 62
    for croup, 107
    for cystic fibrosis, 113
    for foreign body aspiration, 158
    for gastroenteritis, 173-174
    for nephrotic syndrome, 403
    for otitis media, 446, 447
    side effects, 442
    for spina bifida, 556

Anticholinergics, 33, 556

Anticonvulsants, 524

Antideoxyribonuclease B, 509

Antidepressants, 7

Antihyaluronidase antibody, 509

Antihypertensives, 96, 251

Antinuclear antibody test, 260, 309

Antirheumatic drugs, 312

Antistreptolysin A, 509

Anus, imperforate, 263-269

Aorta, coarctation of the, 93-99

Aplastic anemia, 10-15

Aplastic crisis, 545-546

Apnea, 16-19

Apparent life-threatening events, 20-24

Appendectomy, 26-27
    postoperative care, 28-29
    preoperative care, 27-28

Appendicitis, 25-30

ARF. *See* Renal failure, acute

Arnold-Chiari deformity, 553

Arterial blood gases
    in drowning, 146
    in hemolytic-uremic syndrome, 188
    in meconium aspiration syndrome, 359

Arterial blood gases *(Continued)*
normal values, 714-715
in respiratory distress syndrome, 492
in tetralogy of Fallot, 584
Arterial partial pressure of carbon dioxide (PaCo$_2$), 493
Arterial partial pressure of oxygen (Pao$_2$), 493
Arteriograms, 250
Arthralgia, 510
Arthritis, juvenile rheumatoid, 306-316
Artificialism, 686
Asians and Pacific Islanders, 70, 766
Asparaginase, 344-345
Aspiration, suprapubic, 618
Aspirin therapy, 320, 737*t*
Asthma, 31-35
Athetosis, 65
Attention-Deficit Disorders Evaluation Scale, 39
Attention-deficit/hyperactivity disorder, 36-42
coding, 38*b*
diagnostic criteria for, 37*b*-38*b*
Augmentin (amoxicillin with clavulanate), 446
Auscultation, chest, 668
Autonomy, 683-684
Axonal injury, diffuse, 611
Azathioprine, 312
Azithromycin, 446
AZT (zidovudine), 233
Azulfidine (sulfasalazine), 312

B

Babinski reflex, 677*t*
"Back to Sleep" recommendations (AAP), 573
Bacteremia, occult, 528
Bacterial infection
intestinal overgrowth, 536
pneumonia, 461*b*
serious, 528-531

Bactrim (trimethoprim sulfamethoxazole), 233, 536
Ballismus, 65
Bananas, rice, applesauce, and toast (BRAT) diet, 173
Barbiturates, 563*t*
Barium enema, 291
Barium swallow test, 585
Barlow's maneuver, 125*b*
Bayley Scales of Infant Development, 373
Beck Depression Inventory, 49
Becker's muscular dystrophy, 385, 386
Beckwith-Wiedemann syndrome, 628
Behavior
adaptive, 373
aggressive, 373
delinquent, 578
infant socialization, 680-681
self-injurious, 373
Behavioral activities, 380*b*
Bender Visual Motor Gestalt Test, 337
β-agonists, 33, 113
Bianchi intestinal lengthening procedure, 539
Bilirubin
in hepatitis, 203
in hyperbilirubinemia, 244
normal values, 715
in Reye's syndrome, 503
Binge eating, 4*b*, 47, 48
Biopsy
bone marrow, 630
direct needle aspiration, 439
excisional lymph node, 221
in inflammatory bowel disease, 291
liver, 194, 535
lung, 463
muscle, 387
renal, 183, 188, 260
tissue, 260, 430

Biotin, 279
Blacks, 766
Bladder training, 558-559
Blalock-Taussig anastomosis, 585-586
    complications, 584
    postoperative care, 589-590
Bleeding episodes, 193
Bleeding time, normal, 715
Bleomycin, 222, 431
Blood cell dysfunction, 482
Blood coagulation tests, 194
Blood culture and sensitivity, 146,
        365, 438
Blood pressure
    guidelines for, 249*t*
    guidelines for selecting appropriate
        cuff, 706, 707*f*, 708*f*
    high; *See* Hypertension
    norms for boys, 711*t*-712*t*
    norms for girls, 709*t*-710*t*
    standardized method for taking,
        706-713, 707*f*, 708*f*
Blood products, 12, 142, 190
Blood tests. *See also specific tests*
    in acute renal failure, 472
    in chronic renal failure, 483
    fetal, 547
    in glomerulonephritis, 183
    in nephrotic syndrome, 402-403
Blood urea nitrogen
    in drowning, 146
    in hypertension, 250
    in lead poisoning, 327
    normal values, 715
    in Wilms' tumor, 630
BMT. *See* Bone marrow
        transplantation
Bodygrams, 73*n*
Bone marrow, 593
Bone marrow aspiration
    in idiopathic thrombocytopenic
        purpura, 260
    in leukemia, 343
    in neuroblastoma, 412
    in Wilms' tumor, 630

Bone marrow dysfunction/failure,
        594*b*
Bone marrow transplantation,
        593-602
    conditions treated with, 594*b*-595*b*
Bone scans, 343, 430, 439
Bottle-nipple combinations, 89
Bowel perforation, 215
Bowel training, 559
Boys
    blood pressure norms, 711*t*-712*t*
    head circumference-for-age and
            weight-for-length
            percentiles, 748*f*
    length-for-age and weight-
            for-age percentiles, 747*f*
    stature-for-age and weight-
            for-age percentiles, 749*f*
BPD. *See* Bronchopulmonary
        dysplasia
Braces, abduction, 126-127
Brady Center to Prevent Gun
        Violence, 419*b*
Brain damage, 326
Brain infection, 375*t*
Brain injury
    primary, 609-611
    secondary, 611-612
    traumatic, 608-615
Branched-chain amino acids, 272*b*
    disorders of, 276, 277
BRAT diet (bananas, rice,
        applesauce, and toast), 173
Breast-feeding, 769-772
Breathing, 668
    ineffective, 405, 475
British Diabetic Association
        (ADA), 136*b*
Bronchiolitis, 43-46
Bronchodilators
    for chronic lung disease of
            infancy, 80
    for croup, 106, 107
    for cystic fibrosis, 113
    for foreign body aspiration, 158

Bronchopulmonary dysplasia, 77, 80
Bronchoscopy, 157, 463
Bulimia nervosa, 47-51
   diagnostic criteria for, 48*b*
   nonpurging type, 48*b*
   purging type, 48*b*
Burkholderia cepacia, 110
Burns, 52-59
   chemical, 56
   classification according to depth,
      53*b*
   deliberate or unexplained, 71*b*
   distribution of, 54*f*
   electrical, 56
   first degree (superficial), 53*b*
   flame, 56
   scald, 56
   second degree (partial
      thickness), 53*b*
   third degree (full thickness), 53*b*
Butabarbital, 563*t*

C

Caffeine, 563*t*
Calcium, serum, 220, 715
California Teachers Association,
   416
Caloric intake, 81
Calorie(s), 87*n*
   infant requirements, 87
   newborn requirements, 87
Campylobacter, 167
Campylobacter jejuni, 170*t*
Candida albicans, 150
Candidiasis/thrush, 771-772
CANDIS (Child Abuse and Neglect
   Database Instrument
   System), 75*b*
Captopril (Capoten), 96
Carbamazepine (Tegretol), 373,
   524
Carbohydrate malabsorption, 271*b*,
   276, 277
Carbohydrate metabolism,
   disorders of, 277

Carbon dioxide (CO_2)
   arterial partial pressure of
      ($Paco_2$), 493
   normal values, 717
   partial pressure of (Pco_2), 714
Cardiac catheterization, 639-641
   in patent ductus arteriosus, 454
   in tetralogy of Fallot, 585
Cardiac output, decreased, 102, 485
Cardiac status, 97-98
Cardiopulmonary assessment,
   639-640
Cardiorespiratory stability, 81
Cardiotoxicity, 353*t*
Cardiovascular assessment,
   667-668
Cardiovascular function,
   decreased, 405, 475
Caregiving, 82
Carotene, serum, 715
Cast care, 441, 518-519
Catecholamines, 411, 629, 715
CD4 counts, 233*t*
Cefaclor, 446
Celecoxib (Celebrex), 310
Cell lysis, 350
Cellulitis, 60-63
   orbital, 61*b*
   periorbital, 61*b*
Cement, 564*t*
Centers for Disease Control and
   Prevention (CDC),
   327-328, 417
Central nervous system toxicity,
   326
Centration, 686
Cerebral contusion, 610
Cerebral dysgenesis, 374*t*
Cerebral edema, 611-612
Cerebral palsy, 64-67
Cerebrospinal fluid, 715-716
CF. *See* Cystic fibrosis
Chelation therapy, 328-329, 330*t*-
   331*t*
Chemical burns, 56

Chemotherapy
for amputation, 434
complications, 434-435
discharge planning and home
care, 435
for Hodgkin's disease, 222
negative effects of, 434
for neuroblastoma, 413, 414
for non-Hodgkin's lymphoma,
424-425
nursing interventions, 223-224,
351*t*-355*t*
for osteogenic sarcoma, 431
side effects of, 224, 414
Chest auscultation, 668
Chest computed tomography, 630
Chest examination, 667, 668
Chest radiography
in acute renal failure, 472
in acute rheumatic fever, 509
in congestive heart failure, 101
in cystic fibrosis, 112
in drowning, 146
in foreign body aspiration, 157
in Hodgkin's disease, 221
in hypertension, 250
in idiopathic thrombocytopenic
purpura, 260
in leukemia, 343
in meconium aspiration
syndrome, 359
in neuroblastoma, 412
in patent ductus arteriosus, 454
in respiratory distress syndrome,
492
in tetralogy of Fallot, 584
CHF. *See* Congestive heart failure
Child abuse and neglect, 68-76
clinical manifestations of, 71*b*-72*b*
resources, 75*b*
Child Abuse and Neglect Database
Instrument System
(CANDIS), 75*b*
Child Abuse Prevention and
Treatment Act, 68

Child Behavior Checklist, 40
Child maltreatment. *See* Child
abuse and neglect
Child neglect, 68
Children's Depression Inventory, 8
Children's Safety Network, 419*b*
Chills and fever, 352*t*
Chlamydia pneumoniae, 444
Chlamydia trachomatis, 460
Chlorambucil, 403
Chlordiazepoxide, 563*t*
Chlorine (Cl⁻), 717
Cholecystokinin, 536
Cholestasis, 276
Cholesterol, serum, 250, 402, 716
Cholesterolemia, familial, 273*b*
Cholestyramine, 536
Choline magnesium salicylate, 737*t*
Chorea, 65
Christmas disease, 192
Chromosomal damage, 355*t*
Chromosomal disorders, 374*t*
Chronic lung disease of infancy,
77-84
survival rates, 78*t*
Chylothorax, 458
Circulatory overload, 549
Cisplatin, 431
Clavulanate, amoxicillin with
(Augmentin), 446
CLD. *See* Chronic lung disease
Cleaning solutions, 564*t*
Cleft lip and cleft palate, 85-92
Cleft lip and cleft palate repair, 86
postoperative care, 90-91
preoperative care, 88-90
preoperative home care, 90
Clonazepam (Klonopin), 524
Clotting factor VIII deficiency, 192
Clotting factor IX deficiency, 192
CMV infection. *See*
Cytomegaloviral infection
CNS-protective medications, 425
Coagulation screening tests, 194
Coarctation of the aorta, 93-99

Coarctectomy, 94-96
    postoperative care, 97-98
    preoperative care, 96-97
Cocaine, 563*t*
Codeine, 736*t*
Cognitive Assessment System, 372
Cognitive development
    adolescent (formal operational
        stage), 695
    infant (sensorimotor stage),
        676-679
    preschooler (preoperational
        stage), 686
    school-aged child (concrete
        operational stage),
        690-691
Cognitive disability, 369
Colitis, ulcerative, 288-289
Colon interposition, 538
Colonoscopy, 291
Colostomy
    complications, 293
    for imperforate anus, 265-266
    for inflammatory bowel disease,
        292
    temporary, 213
Colostomy care, 217
Comfort measures, 753
    in congestive heart failure, 103
    in hepatitis, 206
    in Kawasaki disease, 322
Community living activities,
    379*b*-380*b*
Community referrals, 518
Community services, 757-768
Community support systems,
    754-755
COMP drug regimen, 425
Complement levels, 309, 320
Complete blood count
    in drowning, 146
    in hemolytic-uremic syndrome,
        188
    in Hodgkin's disease, 220
    in hypertension, 250

Complete blood count *(Continued)*
    in idiopathic thrombocytopenic
        purpura, 260
    in inflammatory bowel disease,
        291
    in JRA, 309
    in Kawasaki disease, 319
    in lead poisoning, 327
    in leukemia, 342-343
    in neuroblastoma, 411
    in osteomyelitis, 438
    in seizure disorders, 523
    in short bowel syndrome, 535
    in Wilms' tumor, 629
Computed tomography, 642-643
    in cytomegaloviral infection, 120
    in Hodgkin's disease, 221
    for inborn errors of metabolism,
        278
    in neuroblastoma, 412
    nursing assessment, 642
    nursing interventions, 642-643
    in osteogenic sarcoma, 430
    in osteomyelitis, 439
    in Reye's syndrome, 503
    in seizure disorders, 523
    in Wilms' tumor, 629, 630
Concrete operational stage,
    690-691
Concussion, 610
Congenital adrenal hyperplasia, 273
Congenital aganglionic megacolon,
    212
Congenital hip dysplasia, 123-128
Congenital hydrocephalus, 238
Congenital hypothyroidism, 273
Congenital metabolic disorders,
    595*b*
Congestive heart failure, 100-104
    signs of, 101, 453
Consciousness, level of, 669
Contact precautions, 440
Continuous Performance Test, 40
Continuous positive airway
    pressure, 493

Contusion, cerebral, 610
Convention on the Rights of the Child, 420*b*
Conventional stage, 693
Copeland Symptom Checklist for Attention-Deficit Disorders, 39
Copper (Cu), serum, 220, 716
Coproporphyrin, urine, 327
Corticosteroids
  for asthma, 33
  for chronic lung disease of infancy, 80
  for croup, 106-107, 107
  for foreign body aspiration, 158
  for nephrotic syndrome, 403
Cortisol, 130*b,* 716
Co-trimoxazole, 446
Coumadin (warfarin), 320
Council for Safe Families, 420*b*
Counterregulatory hormones, 130*b*
CP. *See* Cerebral palsy
C-reactive protein, 319, 509, 716
Creatine phosphokinase, 387, 503, 716
Creatinine, 250, 630, 716
Creatinine clearance, 146
CRF. *See* Renal failure, chronic
Crohn's and Colitis Foundation of America, 298
Crohn's disease
  clinical manifestations, 290
  complications, 290
  incidence, 289
  medical management, 292
  pathophysiology, 288, 289
Cromolyn sodium and nedocromil, 33
Croup, 105-109
Cryoprecipitate, 195
Cryptosporidium, 167
Culture
  blood, 146, 365, 438
  HIV, 230
  nasopharyngeal, 365

Culture *(Continued)*
  normal values, 716
  pleural fluid, 463
  sputum, 463
  stool, 172, 291
  throat, 509
  urine, 250, 365, 618
  viral, 119
Cuprimine (penicillamine), 312
Cyanocobalamin (B_{12}), 537
Cyanosis, 583
Cyclooxygenase-2 inhibitors, 310
Cyclophosphamide (Cytoxan)
  hemorrhagic cystitis due to, 353*t*
  for ITP, 260
  for JRA, 312
  for leukemia, 347-348
  for nephrotic syndrome, 403
  for neuroblastoma, 413
  for non-Hodgkin's lymphoma, 425
  for osteogenic sarcoma, 431
  side effects, 348
Cyclosporin, 312, 403
Cystathione β-synthase deficiency, 275, 276, 278
Cystic fibrosis, 110-116
Cystitis, hemorrhagic, 353*t*
Cystometry, 618
Cystoscopy, 618
Cytarabine (cytosine arabinoside, Cytosar), 346-347
Cytomegaloviral infection, 117-122
Cytosine arabinoside (cytarabine), 346-347, 425
Cytoxan (cyclophosphamide), 347-348, 425

D

Dacarbazine, 222
Dactylitis, 545
Daunorubicin (Daunomycin), 348, 353*t*
DDAVP (desmopressin), 195
DDC (zalcitabine), 233

DDH. *See* Developmental dysplasia of the hip

DDI (didanosine), 233

DDSs. *See* Disability Determination Services

Deferoxamine (Desferal), 547

Degenerative disorders, 375t

Dehydration, 658

Delayed physical and sexual development, 355t

Demerol (meperidine), 736t

Demyelinating disorders, 375t

Dental care, 588

Depakene (valproic acid), 524

Depressants, 563t

Depression, 373

Desferal (deferoxamine), 547

Desmopressin (DDAVP), 195

Development, 673-698
  adolescent (13 to 19 years), 693-698
  delayed, 355t
  infant (0 to 1 year), 673-681
  preschooler (3 to 6 years), 684-689
  school-aged child (7 to 12 years), 689-693
  toddler (1 to 3 years), 681-684

Developmental activities, 82

Developmental dysfunction, 482

Developmental dysplasia of the hip, 123-128
  assessment criteria, 125b

Developmental needs, 58, 81

Dexedrine (amphetamine), 40

Dextrostat (amphetamine), 40

Diabetes mellitus
  energy requirements in, 136b
  insulin-dependent, 129-137
  nutritional requirements in, 136b

Diabetic ketoacidosis
  laboratory and diagnostic tests, 133
  nursing interventions, 134-135
  signs of, 131b

Diagnostic and Statistical Manual of Mental Disorders, fourth edition *(DSM-IV),* 335b

Diagnostic tests and procedures, 635-663. *See also specific conditions*

Dialysis
  hemodialysis, 190-191, 473
  peritoneal, 190-191, 473, 656-660

Diarrhea
  medications for, 536
  nursing interventions, 351t

Diazepam, 563t

DIC. *See* Disseminated intravascular coagulation

Diclofenac sodium (Voltaren), 310

Didanosine (DDI), 233

Dietary management
  BRAT (bananas, rice, applesauce, and toast) diet, 173
  of Hirschsprung's disease, 217
  plans, 136b

Diffuse axonal injury, 611

Digitalis
  for CHF, 102
  for patent ductus arteriosus, 455
  side effects, 457
  for tetralogy of Fallot, 585

Dihydrolipoyl dehydrogenase disorders, 277

Dilantin (phenytoin), 524

Dilaudid (hydromorphone), 736t

Dimercaprol, 332

Dimethoxy-4-methylamphetamine (STP), 564t

Dimethyltryptamine (DMT), 564t

Diphtheria, tetanus, and acellular pertussis vaccine, 701b

Diphtheria, tetanus, and pertussis vaccine, 702, 704
  immunization recommendations, 700b
  recommended ages for, 701b

Diplegia, 64

Disability
  cognitive, 369
  intellectual, 369
  learning, 334-339, 369
  self-perception of, 553
Disability Determination Services
    (DDSs), 767
Dislocations
  hip, 123
  unexplained, 72*b*
Disorder of written expression,
    335*b*
Disseminated intravascular
    coagulation, 137-143
Diuretics
  for chronic lung disease of
      infancy, 80
  for nephrotic syndrome, 403
  side effects, 405, 457
  for tetralogy of Fallot, 585
DMT (dimethyltryptamine), 564*t*
DNA hybridization testing, 119
Dopamine (Intropin), 623
Doppler color flow mapping, 454
Dornase alfa, 113
Down syndrome, 205, 371, 622
Doxorubicin (Adriamycin)
  cardiotoxicity, 353*t*
  for Hodgkin's disease, 222
  for neuroblastoma, 413
  for non-Hodgkin's lymphoma,
      425
  for osteogenic sarcoma, 431
Drowning, 144-149
Drug classes and effects, 563*t*-564*t*
*DSM-IV. See Diagnostic and
    Statistical Manual of Mental
    Disorders,* fourth edition
DTaP vaccine. *See* Diphtheria,
    tetanus, and acellular
    pertussis vaccine
DTP vaccine. *See* Diphtheria,
    tetanus, and pertussis
Duchenne's muscular dystrophy,
    385

Dwyer cables, 515
D-Xylulose absorption blood and
    urine test, 291
Dyskinetic cerebral palsy, 65
Dysmorphic features, 280
Dysplasia
  acetabular, 123
  bronchopulmonary, 77
  congenital hip, 123-128
  developmental, of hip, 123-128
Dystonia, 65

E

Early and Periodic Screening,
    Diagnosis, and Treatment
    Program (EPSDTP),
    763-764, 766
Early intervention programs
    (EIPs), 66
Early intervention services,
    757-759
Eating Attitudes Test, 8, 49
Eating Disorder Examination, 49
Eating Disorder Inventory, 49
Echocardiography
  in acute rheumatic fever, 509
  in Kawasaki disease, 319
  in patent ductus arteriosus,
      454
  in tetralogy of Fallot, 585
Edema, 668
  cerebral, 611-612
  reduction of, 403
Edetate disodium calcium, 332
Edetate disodium calcium
    mobilization test, 327
Education of the Handicapped Act
    amendments (PL 99-457),
    757, 758
Educational activities, 379*b*
Educational inadequacy, 376*t*
EIPs. *See* Early intervention
    programs
Eisenmenger's syndrome, 621
Electrical burns, 56

Electrocardiography, 644-645
in acute renal failure, 472
in acute rheumatic fever, 509
in chronic lung disease of
infancy, 79
in congestive heart failure, 101
in hypertension, 250
in Kawasaki disease, 319
nursing assessment, 644
nursing interventions, 644-645
in patent ductus arteriosus, 454
serial, 79
in tetralogy of Fallot, 584
Electroencephalography
in drowning, 146
for inborn errors of metabolism,
278
in Reye's syndrome, 503
in seizure disorders, 522-523
Electrolyte imbalances, 59*b*
in chronic renal failure, 481-482,
482
signs and symptoms of, 474, 485
Electrolytes, serum
in chronic lung disease of
infancy, 79
in drowning, 146
in hemolytic-uremic syndrome,
189
in hypertension, 250
in inflammatory bowel disease,
291
in meningitis, 365
in nephrotic syndrome, 403
normal values, 716-717
in seizure disorders, 523
in Wilms' tumor, 630
Electromyography, 279, 387
Emergency care
for burns, 56
for foreign body aspiration, 158
Emotional abuse, 68
Emotional support, 752-753
in acute rheumatic fever, 511
in burns, 58

Emotional support *(Continued)*
postoperative, 458-459
preoperative, 432
in sickle cell anemia, 550
Employment activities, 380*b*
Enbrel (etanercept), 312
Encephalopathy
in chronic renal failure, 482
hypertensive, 182
medical management, 328-329
Endangerment Standard, 69
Endocrine nursing assessment, 672
Endoscopy, 646-647
End-stage renal disease, 480, 481
Enema, barium, 291
Energy requirements, 136*b*
Engerix-B (hepatitis B vaccine),
205
Engorgement, 769-770
Enteric adenovirus, 168*t*
Enteroplasty, tapering, 538-539
Environmental disadvantage, 376*t*
Environmental risk factor control,
447
Enzyme-linked immunosorbent
assay, 230
Epidural analgesia, 739-740
Epidural hematoma, 610-611
Epiglottitis, 150-154
Epinephrine
for croup, 106, 107
functions of, 130*b*
Epispadias, 264*t*
EPSDTP. *See* Early and Periodic
Screening, Diagnosis, and
Treatment Program
Erythrocyte protoporphyrin
concentration, 302
Erythrocyte sedimentation rate
in acute rheumatic fever, 509
in Hodgkin's disease, 220
in inflammatory bowel disease,
291
in JRA, 309
in Kawasaki disease, 319

Erythrocyte sedimentation rate
  (Continued)
  normal values, 717
  in osteomyelitis, 438
Erythromycin, 253
Erythropoietin, 630
Escherichia coli, 167, 173
  enteroinvasive, 170*t*
  enteropathogenic, 171*t*
  enterotoxigenic, 170*t*
  in hemolytic-uremic syndrome,
      186
  in meningitis, 362
Esophageal atresia, 264*t*
Estrogen replacement, 7
Etanercept (Enbrel), 312
Ethosuximide (Zarontine), 524
Etoposide (VP-16), 413
Evoked potentials, 523
Excisional lymph node biopsy,
      221
Excretory venogram, 250
External-beam radiation therapy,
      222
Extravasation, 224, 427

F

Facial injuries, 71*b*
Factor IX, 195
Factor IX deficiency, 192
Factor VIII, 195
Factor VIII deficiency, 192
Faith development
  adolescent (individuating-
      reflexive stage), 698
  infant (undifferentiated stage),
      681
  preschooler (intuitive-projective
      stage), 689
  school-aged child (mythical-
      literal stage), 693
  toddler (intuitive-projective
      stage), 684
Falls, 71*b*
Familial cholesterolemia, 273*b*

Familial hyperlipoproteinemia,
      273*b*
Familial lipoprotein lipase
      deficiency, 273*b*
Family support, 756
  for burns, 58
  for home management, 115-116
  integration, 82
Fasting blood glucose, 717
Fatigue, 355*t*
Fatty acid oxidation defects, 276,
      277
Fatty acid oxidation disorder, 276
Feeding
  for cleft lip and cleft palate,
      89-90
  newborn, 87
Feelings, verbalization of, 58
Ferritin, serum, 302, 717
Ferritin, urinary, 412
Fetal blood tests, 547
Fever
  chills and, 352*t*
  in Kawasaki disease, 318
  measures to lower, 321
Fibrin degradation products, 717
Fibrinogen, plasma, 717
Fine motor development
  adolescent, 695
  infant, 674-675
  preschooler, 685
  school-aged child, 690
  toddler, 682-683
First aid for burns, 56
Flagyl (metronidazole), 536
Flame burns, 56
Fluid balance
  in anemia, 476-477
  in chronic renal failure, 481, 482
  in congestive heart failure, 103
  in nephrotic syndrome, 406-407
Fluid overload, 81, 481
Fluid retention, 352*t*
Fluid volume excess, 474, 485
Fluoroscopy, 157

Fluoxetine (Prozac), 373
Flurazepam, 563*t*
Follow-up appointments, 236, 315
Food(s) high in iron, 588
Foreign body aspiration, 155-159
Formal operational stage, 695
Fractures, 160-166
    increased risk of, 355*t*
    Salter-Harris classification, 160,
        161*b*
    skull, 610
    unexplained, 72*b*
Fresh frozen plasma, 142
Fresh whole blood, 142
Frozen plasma, 195
Fructose metabolism, disorders of,
    271*b*, 275, 276, 277
Furosemide (Lasix), 147, 454, 585

G

Galactose metabolism, disorders
    of, 271*b*, 275, 276, 277
Galactosemia, 273
Galant reflex, 677*t*
Galeazzi's sign, 125*b*
Gamma globulin, IV, 320
Ganciclovir, 120
Gangliosidosis
    G$_{M1}$, 273*b*
    G$_{M2}$, 273*b*
Gasoline, 564*t*
Gastric acid hypersecretion, 536
Gastroenteritis, 167-176
    acute, 168*t*-171*t*
Gastroesophageal reflux, 177-180
Gastrointestinal assessment, 670
Gateway phenomenon, 565
GCS. *See* Glasgow Coma Scale
GD2, urinary, 412
General nursing action, 637-638
Genetic blood testing, 112
Genital stage, 696-697
Genitourinary anomalies, 264*t*
GER. *See* Gastroesophageal reflux
Giardia lamblia, 167, 174

Gingiva tissue biopsy, 260
Girls
    blood pressure norms, 709*t*-710*t*
    head circumference-for-age and
        weight-for-length
        percentiles, 745*f*
    length-for-age and weight-
        for-age percentiles, 744*f*
    stature-for-age and weight-
        for-age percentiles, 746*f*
Glasgow Coma Scale (GCS), 612,
    669*t*
Glomerulonephritis, 181-185
Glucagon, 130*b*
Glucocorticosteroids, 312
Gluconeogenesis defects, 276, 277
Glucose
    fasting, 717
    in meningitis, 365
    normal values, 717
    in Reye's syndrome, 503
Glucose imbalance, 474
Glucose tolerance test, 717
Glucose-6-phosphatase deficiency,
    272*b*
Glucose-6-phosphate
    dehydrogenase deficiency,
    276
Glue, 564*t*
Glutaricaciduria type II, 277, 278
Glutethimide, 563*t*
Glycogen storage disorders, 271*b*,
    276, 277
Glycosylation, congenital disorders
    of, 277-278
Goodenough-Harris Drawing Test,
    337
Graft-*versus*-host disease
    after bone marrow
        transplantation, 596-597
    clinical manifestations, 595-596
Gram stain, 365
Grand mal (tonic-clonic) seizures,
    521*b*-522*b*
Granulocytes, 12

Grasp reflex, 677*t*

Gray Oral Reading Test—Revised, 337

Great vessel pressure, normal, 640*b*

Gross motor development
  adolescent, 695
  infant, 673-674
  preschooler, 684-685
  school-aged child, 690
  toddler, 682

Group A streptococci, 60, 444, 507

Group B *Streptococcus*, 362, 460

Growth and development, 673-698
  adolescent (13 to 19 years), 693-698
  height and weight growth curves, 744*f*-749*f*
  infant (0 to 1 year), 673-681
  preschooler (3 to 6 years), 684-689
  school-aged child (7 to 12 years), 689-693
  toddler (1 to 3 years), 681-684

Growth dysfunction, 482

Growth hormones, 130*b*

Growth promotion, 81

Guilt, 688-689

GVHD. *See* Graft-*versus*-host disease

H

Haemophilus influenzae, 443

Haemophilus influenzae type B
  in cellulitis, 60
  in epiglottitis, 150
  in meningitis, 362

Haemophilus influenzae type b
    vaccine, 702-703
  immunization
      recommendations, 700*b*
  recommended ages for, 701*b*

Hair loss, traumatic, 71*b*

Hallucinogens, 564*t*

Haloperidol (Haldol), 373

Hand-and-foot syndrome, 545

Harm Standard, 69

Harrington rod, 515

Harvesting, bone marrow, 593

HAV. *See* Hepatitis A virus

HB$_c$Ag. *See* Hepatitis B core antigen

HBIG. *See* Hepatitis B immunoglobulin

HB$_s$Ag. *See* Hepatitis B surface antigen

HBV. *See* Hepatitis B virus

HCV. *See* Hepatitis C virus

HDV. *See* Hepatitis D virus

Head circumference-for-age and weight-for-length percentiles
  for boys, 748*f*
  for girls, 745*f*

Head examination, 669

Head injury
  evaluation strategies, 375*t*
  external, 71*b*

Head Start, 765-766

Head-to-chest position, 584

Health and safety activities, 380*b*

Health insurance, 762-763

Health Resources and Services Administration (HRSA), 273-274

Hearing deficits, bilateral, 447

Heart chamber, normal, 640*b*

Heart failure, congestive, 100-104

Heart murmur, 584

Heart transplantation, 603

Heart-lung transplantation, 113-114

Height
  growth curves, 744*f*-749*f*
  West nomogram, 728*f*-729*f*

Height-for-age and weight-for-age percentiles
  for boys, 749*f*
  for girls, 746*f*

Hematest, 172, 291, 535

Hematocrit
  in drowning, 146
  in inflammatory bowel disease, 291
  in iron deficiency anemia, 302
  in nephrotic syndrome, 403
  normal values, 718
  in tetralogy of Fallot, 584
Hematologic assessment, 672
Hematoma, 610-611
Hemiparesis, 64
Hemochromatosis, neonatal, 276
Hemodialysis, 190-191, 473
Hemoglobin
  in drowning, 146
  in iron deficiency anemia, 302
  in nephrotic syndrome, 403
  normal values, 718
  in tetralogy of Fallot, 584
Hemoglobin electrophoresis, 546-547, 718
Hemolytic-uremic syndrome, 185-191
  mild, 187*b*
  recurrent, 187*b*
  severe, 187*b*
Hemophilia, 192-199
Hemophilia A, 192
Hemophilia B, 192
Hemorrhage
  signs and symptoms of, 57, 97, 141, 179-180, 349-350
  subarachnoid, 611
Hemorrhagic cystitis, 353*t*
Hepatic glycogen storage diseases, 277
Hepatitis, 200-207
Hepatitis A
  clinical manifestations, 202
  complications, 203
  pathophysiology, 200-201
Hepatitis A vaccine, 703
  immunization recommendations, 700*b*
Hepatitis A virus, 200

Hepatitis A virus antibody, 204
Hepatitis B
  clinical manifestations, 202-203
  complications, 203
  pathophysiology, 201
Hepatitis B core antigen (HB$_c$Ag), 204
Hepatitis B immunoglobulin, 205
Hepatitis B surface antigen (HB$_s$Ag), 204
Hepatitis B vaccine, 703
  immunization recommendations, 700*b*
  recommended ages for, 701*b*
Hepatitis B vaccine (Recombivax HB or Engerix-B), 205
Hepatitis B virus, 200
Hepatitis C
  clinical manifestations, 202-203
  complications, 203
  pathophysiology, 201
Hepatitis C virus, 200
Hepatitis C virus antibody, 204
Hepatitis D
  clinical manifestations, 202-203
  complications, 203
  laboratory and diagnostic tests, 204
  pathophysiology, 201
Hepatitis D virus, 200
Hepatitis E
  clinical manifestations, 202-203
  pathophysiology, 201
Hepatitis E virus, 200
Hepatitis G
  clinical manifestations, 202-203
  pathophysiology, 202
Hepatitis G virus, 200
Hepatosplenomegaly, 276
Hernia (inguinal), 208-211
Hernia repair, 209
  postoperative care, 210-211
  preoperative care, 210
Heroin, 563*t*
HEV. *See* Hepatitis E virus

HGV. *See* Hepatitis G virus
Hib vaccine. *See Haemophilus influenzae* type b vaccine
Hip
  developmental dysplasia of, 123-128
  dislocation of, 123
  subluxation of, 123
Hip dysplasia, congenital, 123-128
Hirschsprung's disease, 212-218
Hispanics, 70, 766
Histidine metabolism, disorders of, 271*b*-272*b*, 274, 275, 276, 278
HIV infection. *See* Human immunodeficiency virus (HIV) infection
Hodgkin's disease, 219-225
  Ann Arbor staging system for, 221*b*
Home care, 754-756. *See also specific conditions*
  of chronic renal failure, 488
  of croup, 108
  of cystic fibrosis, 115-116
  family compliance with, 115-116
  of Hodgkin's disease, 224
  of non-Hodgkin's lymphoma, 427-428
  preoperative, 90
Home living activities, 379*b*
Homovanillic acid, 411
Hormones, counterregulatory, 130*b*
Hospital care for burns, 56-58
Human development activities, 379*b*
Human immunodeficiency virus (HIV), 226
  antigen test, 231
  culture, 230
  DNA polymerase chain reaction test, 231
  perinatal exposure, 231
  type 1, 718

Human immunodeficiency virus (HIV) infection, 226-237
  clinical categories for children under 13, 228*b*-229*b*
  determination of immune category based on age and CD4 count, 233*t*
  mildly symptomatic, 228*b*
  moderately symptomatic, 228*b*-229*b*
  not symptomatic, 228*b*
  severely symptomatic, 229*b*
Human lymphocyte antigen typing, 597
Humidifiers, 46
Hunter's syndrome, 277
Hurler's syndrome, 277
Hydration, 97-98, 397, 670
Hydrocephalus, 238-243
Hydrocodone, 736*t*
Hydrocortisone, 425
Hydromorphone (Dilaudid), 736*t*
Hydroxychloroquine (Plaquenil), 312
Hygiene, 175
Hyperactivity-impulsivity attention-deficit/hyperactivity disorder, 36-42
  symptoms of, 37*b*-38*b*
Hyperbilirubinemia, 244-247
Hypercalcemia, 481
Hyperglycemia, 131*b*
Hyperkalemia, 59*b*
  in chronic renal failure, 481
  signs and symptoms of, 190, 474
Hyperlipoproteinemia, familial, 273*b*
Hypermagnesemia, 474
Hypernatremia, 404, 481
Hyperphosphatemia, 474-475, 481
Hyperplasia, congenital adrenal, 273
Hypersensitivity, 355*t*
Hypertension, 248-252
Hypertensive encephalopathy, 182

Hypertransfusion programs, 547
Hypertrophic pyloric stenosis, 253-258
Hyperuremia, 352*t*
Hypocalcemia, 59*b*, 190, 474
Hypoglycemia, 190, 475
Hypokalemia, 404, 482
Hyponatremia, 59*b*, 190, 404, 474
Hypospadias, 264*t*
Hypothyroidism, congenital, 273
Hypovolemic shock, 57

I

Ibuprofen, 310, 738*t*
IDDM. *See* Insulin-dependent diabetes mellitus
Identity *versus* role confusion, 697-698
Idiopathic thrombocytopenic purpura, 258-262
  acute, 259*b*
  chronic, 259*b*
  recurrent, 259*b*
IEPs. *See* Individualized education plans
Ifosfamide, 431
IFSPs. *See* Individualized family service plans
IHPs. *See* Individualized health plans
Ileostomy, 292
Immunity, 699
  active, 699
  artificial, 699
  passive, 700
Immunizations, 699-705
  for HIV infection, 233
  recommendations, 700*b*-701*b*
  recommended ages, 701*b*
  for sickle cell anemia, 547
Immunodeficiency. *See also* Acquired immunodeficiency syndrome (AIDS)
  bone marrow transplantation for, 594*b*

Immunoglobulin (Ig)
  CMV, 120
  hepatitis B, 205
  intravenous (IVIG), 260, 312
  juvenile rheumatoid arthritis, 309
  normal values, 718
Immunoglobulin A (IgA), 718
Immunoglobulin D (IgD), 718
Immunoglobulin E (IgE), 320, 718
Immunoglobulin G (IgG)
  antibody tests, 119, 204
  normal values, 718
Immunoglobulin M (IgM)
  antibody tests, 119, 204
  in Kawasaki disease, 320
  normal values, 718
Immunosuppressive therapy, 403, 605
Imodium (loperamide), 536
Impairment Related Work Expenses (IRWE), 767-768
Imperforate anus, 263-269
  associated anomalies, 264*t*
Impulsivity, 38*b*
Inactivated poliovirus vaccine, 702
Inattention, 37*b*
Inborn errors of metabolism, 270-287, 271*b*-273*b*
  evaluation strategies, 374*t*
Independence, 559
Inderal (propranolol), 96, 585
Individualized education plans (IEPs), 337, 338, 377, 759-761
  transition planning, 761-762
Individualized family service plans (IFSPs), 338, 377, 758-759
Individualized health plans (IHPs), 338
Individualized transition plans (ITPs), 761-762
Individuals with Disabilities Education Act (IDEA) (PL 105-17), 758

Individuating-reflexive stage, 698
Indomethacin (Indocin)
  contraindications to, 455
  for JRA, 310
  for patent ductus arteriosus,
      454-455
  side effects, 457
Industry *versus* inferiority, 692-693
Infants (0 to 1 year)
  "Back to Sleep"
      recommendations, 573
  calorie requirements, 87
  chronic lung disease in, 77-84
  coarctation of the aorta in, 93
  cognitive development, 676-679
  developmental dysplasia of the
      hip in, 124
  early intervention services for,
      759
  faith development, 681
  fine motor development, 674-675
  gross motor development,
      673-674
  growth and development,
      673-681
  head circumference-for-age and
      weight-for-length
      percentiles, 745*f,* 748*f*
  hemophilia in, 193
  Hirschsprung's disease in, 213
  HIV infection and AIDS in,
      227-230, 231
  hydrocephalus in, 238-239
  language development, 679
  length-for-age and weight-
      for-age percentiles, 744*f,*
      747*f*
  meningitis in, 363-364
  mental retardation in, 377-378
  moral development, 681
  near-miss sudden infant death
      syndrome, 20
  nonpharmacologic pain
      management techniques
      for, 740*t*

Infants *(Continued)*
  oral stage, 679-680
  pain assessment in, 733
  physical characteristics, 673
  psychosexual development,
      679-680
  psychosocial development, 680
  reflexes, 677*t*-678*t*
  risk factors for SIDS, 571*b*
  sensorimotor stage, 676-679
  sensory development, 675-676
  serious bacterial infection in,
      528
  shaken baby syndrome, 72*b*
  socialization behavior, 680-681
  Special Supplemental Nutrition
      Program for Women,
      Infants, and Children
      (WIC), 765
  sudden infant death syndrome,
      570-575
  urinary tract infections in, 617
Infections
  bacterial, serious, 528-531
  brain, 375*t*
  cytomegaloviral, 117-122
  HIV, 226-237
  in leukemia, 349
  protection against infectious
      contact, 234*b,* 235
  secondary, 205-206
  urinary tract, 616-620
Inferiority, 692-693
Inflammatory bowel disease,
      288-299
Infliximab (Remicade), 312
Inguinal hernia, 208-211
Initiative *versus* guilt, 688-689
Injury
  brain, 609-611
  diffuse axonal, 611
  external head, facial, and oral,
      71*b*
  head, 375*t*
  secondary brain, 611-612

Injury (*Continued*)
  skin, 71*b*
  thermal, 71*b*
  traumatic brain, 608-615
Insulin, 129, 131*b*
Insulin-dependent diabetes
    mellitus, 129-137
Intellectual disability, 369
Intelligence testing, 336
Intelligence tests, 372
International Association for the
    Study of Pain, 730
Intestinal atresia, 264*t*
Intestinal bacterial overgrowth, 536
Intestinal brush border, 271*b*
Intestinal malrotation, 264*t*
Intestinal obstruction, 28
Intestinal pacing, reverse, 538
Intestinal segment, reversed, 538
Intestinal valve, 538
Intraabdominal non-Hodgkin's
    lymphoma, 423
Intracranial pressure, increased,
    241
Intracranial pressure monitoring,
    648-649
Intravenous gamma globulin, 320
Intravenous immunoglobulin, 260,
    312
Intravenous infusion, infiltration
    of, 355*t*
Intravenous pyelography, 650-653
  in urinary tract infections, 618
  in Wilms' tumor, 629
Intropin (dopamine), 623
Intuitive-projective stage, 684, 689
Iowa procedure, 539
IPV. *See* Inactivated poliovirus
    vaccine
Iron
  foods high in, 588
  in Hodgkin's disease, 220
  in lead poisoning, 327
  normal values, 718
  for tetralogy of Fallot, 585

Iron deficiency anemia, 300-305
Iron supplements, 302-303
Irradiation, total nodal, 222
Irreversibility, 686
IRWE. *See* Impairment Related
    Work Expenses
Ischemia, 141
Isoproterenol (Isuprel), 623
ITP. *See* Idiopathic
    thrombocytopenic purpura
ITPs. *See* Individualized transition
    plans
IVGG. *See* Intravenous gamma
    globulin
IVP. *See* Intravenous pyelography

J

Jaundice
  and breast-feeding, 772
  clinical manifestations, 276
  with hypertrophic pyloric
    stenosis, 254
Joint function, maximal, 58
JRA. *See* Juvenile rheumatoid
    arthritis
Juvenile rheumatoid arthritis,
    306-316
  pauciarticular, 308, 311*t*
  polyarticular, 307-308, 311*t*
  systemic, 307, 311*t*
Juxtaposition, 686

K

K-ABC. *See* Kaufman Assessment
    Battery for Children
Kaufman Assessment Battery for
    Children (K-ABC), 373
Kawasaki disease, 317-324
Keto acid disorders, 272*b*, 276, 277
Ketoacidosis, diabetic, 131*b*
Ketonuria, 131*b*
Ketorolac, 738*t*
Key Math—Revised, 337
Kidney function, 670-671
Kidney transplantation, 603

Kids Eating Disorder Survey, 8, 49
Klonopin (clonazepam), 524
Knee or head-to-chest position, 584
Kussmaul respirations, 131*b*

L

Laboratory values, 714-721
Lacerations, scalp, 610
Lactated Ringer's solution, 173
Lactic dehydrogenase
   in Kawasaki disease, 319
   normal values, 718
   in Reye's syndrome, 503
   in Wilms' tumor, 629
Lactobacillus GG, 536
Lamivudine (3TC), 233
Language development
   adolescent, 696
   infant, 679
   preschooler, 686-687
   school-aged child, 691
Language tests, 337
Laparoscopy, 255
Laparotomy, surgical staging, 221
Laryngoscopy, 157
Lasix (furosemide), 147, 454, 585
Latex allergy, 559-560
Lead, blood, 327
Lead, serum, 718
Lead poisoning, 325-333
   intervention guidelines, 330*t*-331*t*
   screening guidelines, 327-328, 330*t*-331*t*
Learning disabilities, 334-339, 369
   DSM-IV criteria, 335*b*
   not otherwise specified, 335*b*
Lecithin/sphingomyelin ratio, 492
Leiter International Performance Scale—Revised (Leiter-R), 373
Length-for-age and weight-for-age percentiles
   for boys, 747*f*
   for girls, 744*f*

Lesch-Nyhan syndrome, 275, 276, 278
Leukemia, 340-356
   acute lymphoid or lymphocytic (ALL), 340-341, 341-342
   acute nonlymphoid (ANLL), 340, 341, 342
   bone marrow transplantation for, 594*b*
Leukopenia, 354*t*, 394
Leukotriene modifiers, 33
Life-threatening events, apparent, 20-24
Limb salvage, 431
Lip, cleft, 85-92
Lipase, serum, 503, 718
Lipid metabolism, disorders of, 273*b*, 275, 276, 277
Lipoprotein electrophoresis, 250
Lipoprotein lipase deficiency, familial, 273*b*
Listeria monocytogenes, 362
Liver and small bowel transplantation, 539
Liver biopsy, 194, 503, 535
Liver dysfunction, 536
Liver function tests, 194, 220, 535
Liver scan, 343, 535
Liver transplantation, 603
Long-term care
   adherence to, 755
   for Reye's syndrome, 506
   for traumatic brain injury, 615
Loperamide (Imodium), 536
LSD (lysergic acid diethylamide), 564*t*
Lumbar puncture, 343, 503
Lung biopsy, 463
Lung disease, chronic, of infancy, 77-84
Lung transplantation, 113-114
Luque rod, 515
Lymph node biopsy, excisional, 221
Lymphangiography, 221

Lymphoid or lymphocytic leukemia, acute (ALL), 340
Lymphoma
  advanced, 425
  bone marrow transplantation for, 594*b*
  localized, 424-425
  non-Hodgkin's, 422-428
Lysergic acid diethylamide (LSD), 564*t*
Lysosomal enzymes, disorders of, 273*b*, 274, 275
Lysosomal storage disorders, 276, 277

M

Magnesium, serum, 718
Magnetic resonance imaging, 654-655
  for inborn errors of metabolism, 278
  in neuroblastoma, 412
  in osteogenic sarcoma, 430
  in osteomyelitis, 439
  in seizure disorders, 523
  in Wilms' tumor, 629
Malignancy
  after bone marrow transplantation, 597
  bone marrow transplantation for, 594*b*
Malnutrition, 376*t*
Managing Your Child's Crohn's Disease and Ulcerative Colitis, 298
Mannitol (Mannitor), 147
Maple syrup urine disease
  clinical manifestations, 274, 275, 277
  screening for, 273
MAS. *See* Meconium aspiration syndrome
Matching Familiar Figures Test, 40
Math tests, standardized, 337
Mathematics disorder, 335*b*

Matulane (procarbazine), 222
McBurney's point, 25
Mead Johnson cleft lip/palate nurser, 89
Mean corpuscular volume, 302
Mean hemoglobin concentration, 302
Measles, mumps, and rubella vaccine, 702, 704
  immunization recommendations, 701*b*
  recommended ages for, 701*b*
Measurements, 667
Mechlorethamine (nitrogen mustard), 222
Meconium aspiration syndrome, 357-361
Mediastinal non-Hodgkin's lymphoma, 423
Medicaid, 767
Medications. *See also specific medications by name*
  for acute pain, 736*t*-738*t*
  for ADHD, 40
  for anorexia nervosa, 7
  antihypertensive, 96
  CNS-protective, 425
  drug classes and effects, 563*t*-564*t*
  maternal, 771
  for neuroblastoma, 413
  for non-Hodgkin's lymphoma, 424-425
  for respiratory distress syndrome, 493
  for Reye's syndrome, 504
  for short bowel syndrome, 536-537
  for spina bifida, 556
  for tetralogy of Fallot, 585
Megacolon, congenital aganglionic, 212
Mellaril (thioridazine), 373
Memory function tests, 337
Meningitis, 362-368, 612
Meningocele, 552

Menkes' syndrome, 275
Mental retardation, 369-384
    diagnostic criteria for, 370*b*
    etiologic risk factors, 374*t*-376*t*
    operational definition of, 371*b*
    perinatal onset, 375*t*
    postnatal onset, 375*t*-376*t*
    prenatal onset, 374*t*-375*t*
    support areas and representative
        support activities for,
        379*b*-381*b*
Meperidine (Demerol), 563*t*, 736*t*
Mercaptopurine (Purinethol), 346,
        425
Mescaline, 564*t*
Metabolic acidosis, 131*b*, 482
Metabolic disorders
    congenital, 595*b*
    types, 270-273
Metabolism, inborn errors of,
        270-287
    evaluation strategies, 374*t*
Methadone, 563*t*, 737*t*
Methaqualone, 563*t*
Methotrexate (Amethopterin)
    complications, 435
    for JRA, 312
    for leukemia, 345-346
    for non-Hodgkin's lymphoma,
        425
    for osteogenic sarcoma, 431
    side effects, 345-346
Methylmalonate metabolism,
        disorders of, 272*b*
Methylphenidate (Ritalin), 40, 373
Methylxanthines, 33
Methyprylon, 563*t*
Metronidazole (Flagyl), 536
Microphage activation syndrome,
        309
Microscopy, 119
Middle ear infection, 443-451
Milk supply, insufficient, 770-771
Millard repair, 86
Milwaukee brace, 514, 518

Mineral deficiency, 537
Mineral supplements, 537
Mitochondrial respiratory chain
        defect, 276
MMR vaccine. *See* Measles,
        mumps, and rubella vaccine
Mobility, 559
Monoplegia, 64
MOPP drug regimen, 222
Moral development
    adolescent (postconventional
        stage), 698
    infant, 681
    preschooler (preconventional
        stage), 689
    school-aged child (conventional
        stage), 693
    toddler (preconventional stage),
        684
Moraxella catarrhalis, 443
Morbidity, 417
Moro (startle) reflex, 677*t*
Morphine, 563*t*, 585, 736*t*
Mortality, 417
Motor development
    fine; *See* Fine motor development
    gross; *See* Gross motor
        development
Mouth ulcers, 352*t*-353*t*
MRI. *See* Magnetic resonance
        imaging
Mucolytics, 113
Mucopolysaccharidoses, 277
Multiorgan transplantation, 539
Murmur, 584
Muscle biopsy, 387
Muscular dystrophy, 385-390
Musculoskeletal assessment, 671-672
Mycoplasma pneumoniae, 460, 462*b*
Myelomeningocele, 552-553, 555-
        556
Myringotomy
    bilateral, 447
    for otitis media, 446
    postoperative care, 449

Mysoline (primidone), 524
Mythical-literal stage, 693

N

Naproxen (Naprosyn), 310, 738*t*
Narcotics, 196, 563*t*
Nasal non-Hodgkin's lymphoma, 423
Nasopharyngeal culture, 365
National Center for Education in Maternal and Child Health, 419*b*
National Child Abuse Reporting Hotline, 75*b*
National Clearinghouse on Child Abuse and Neglect Information, 75*b*, 420*b*
National Crime Victims Research and Treatment Center, 75*b*
National Data Archive on Child Abuse and Neglect, 75*b*
National SAFEKIDS Campaign, 420*b*
National Sudden Infant Death Syndrome Foundation, 574*b*
Native Alaskans, 70
Natural rubber allergy, 559-560
Nausea and vomiting, 351*t*
Near-drowning, 144-149
Near-miss sudden infant death syndrome, 20
NEC. *See* Necrotizing enterocolitis
Necrosis, tissue, 355*t*
Necrotizing enterocolitis, 391-399
Nedocromil, cromolyn sodium and, 33
Needle aspiration biopsy, direct, 439
Neglect, 68-76, 72*b*
Neisseria meningitidis, 362
Nembutal (pentobarbital), 654
Nemours Foundation, 451
Neomucosa, 539
Neonatal hemochromatosis, 276

Nephritis, 182
Nephrotic syndrome, 400-409
   primary, 401*b*
   secondary, 401*b*
Nerve conduction velocity studies, 279
Neuroblastoma, 410-415
Neurologic assessment, 668-669
Neurologic function, decreased, 475
Neuron-specific enolase, 412
Neuropathic pain, 732*t*
Neuropathy, uremic, 482
Neuropsychologic tests, 40
Newborn feeding, 87
Newborn screening
   guidelines for, 273-274
   for sickle cell anemia, 544*b*-545*b*
Newborns
   calorie requirements, 87
   hemochromatosis in, 276
   Hirschsprung's disease in, 212-213
   meningitis in, 363
   nonpharmacologic pain management techniques for, 740*t*
   pain assessment in, 733
NHL. *See* Non-Hodgkin's lymphoma
Nicotinamide adenine dinucleotidase (NADase), 509
Nicotine, 563*t*
Nipples, sore, 769
Nipride (sodium nitroprusside), 96
Nitrogen mustard (mechlorethamine), 222
Nodular sclerosis, 219
Non-Hodgkin's lymphoma, 422-428
Nonsteroidal anti-inflammatory drugs, 310, 737*t*-738*t*
Norwalk virus, 167, 168*t*
Nursing action, general, 637-638

Nursing assessment(s), 667-672.
*See also specific conditions,
procedures*
  cardiovascular, 667-668
  endocrine, 672
  gastrointestinal, 670
  general, 637
  hematologic, 672
  musculoskeletal, 671-672
  neurologic, 668-669
  renal, 670-671
  respiratory, 668
Nursing interventions. *See also
specific conditions,
procedures*
  general, 637-638
Nutritional support
  for acute renal failure, 477-478
  for acute rheumatic fever, 511
  for burns, 57
  for chronic lung disease of
     infancy, 80
  for cleft lip and cleft palate,
     88-90
  for congestive heart failure, 103
  for cystic fibrosis, 115
  for nephrotic syndrome, 407
  for osteomyelitis, 439
  for short bowel syndrome,
     537-538
  Special Supplemental Nutrition
     Program for Women,
     Infants, and Children
     (WIC), 765

O

Obstruction, intestinal, 28
Octreotide acetate (Sandostatin),
  536
Older children
  developmental dysplasia of the
     hip in, 124
  hydrocephalus in, 239
  meningitis in, 364
Oncovin (vincristine), 222, 425

Opioids, 563*t*, 736*t*-737*t*
OPV. *See* Oral poliovirus vaccine
Oral injuries, 71*b*
Oral non-Hodgkin's lymphoma,
  423
Oral poliovirus vaccine, 702
  immunization
     recommendations, 701*b*
  recommended ages for, 701*b*
Oral rehydration solutions, 173
Oral stage, 679-680
Orbital cellulitis, 61*b*
Organ transplantation, 603-607
  heart-lung, 113-114
  liver and small bowel, 539
  lung, 113-114
  multiorgan, 539
  postoperative care, 606
  postoperative evaluation, 605
  preoperative care, 605
  preoperative evaluation, 604
  small bowel, 539
Organic acidemias, 272*b*, 275, 276,
  277
Orthoplast jacket, 518
Ortolani's maneuver, 125*b*
Osmolality, serum, 719
Osmolality, urine, 402, 719
Osmolarity, urine, 365
Osteogenic sarcoma, 429-436
Osteomyelitis, 437-442
Ostomy care, 297
Otitis media, 443-451
  acute, 443-444, 445, 448-449,
     449
  with effusion, 444, 445, 449
Oucher Scale, 733, 734*f*
Ova and parasites, fecal, 719
Oxycodone, 737*t*
Oxygen
  arterial partial pressure of
     (Pao_2), 493
  partial pressure of (Po_2), 714
Oxygen saturation, normal, 640*b*
Oxygen therapy, 106, 585

P

Pacific Islanders, 70, 766
Packed red blood cells, 12, 142, 190
Paco₂ (arterial partial pressure of
        carbon dioxide), 493
Pain, 730-742
    acute, 732*t*, 736*t*-738*t*
    chronic persistent, 732*t*
    modulation of, 731, 731*f*
    nature of, 732*t*
    neuropathic, 732*t*
    nursing interventions related to
            child undergoing
            chemotherapy and
            radiotherapy, 353*t*-354*t*
    psychogenic, 732*t*
    recurrent, 732*t*
    transduction of, 730, 731*f*
    transmission of, 730, 731*f*
Pain assessment, 731-735
    Oucher Scale, 733, 734*f*
Pain management, 735-740
    for arthralgia, 510
    for burns, 57
    for hepatitis, 206
    for JRA, 313
    for nephrotic syndrome, 408
    nonpharmacologic, 740, 740*t*-741*t*
    for osteomyelitis, 440
    pharmacologic, 735-740
    for scoliosis, 517
    for sickle cell anemia, 549
Paired Associates Learning Task, 40
Palate, cleft, 85-92
Palatoplasty, 86
Palivizumab (Synagis), 80, 498
Palmar (grasp) reflex, 677*t*
Pancreatic enzyme supplements,
        113
Pao₂ (arterial partial pressure of
        oxygen), 493
Parachute reflex, 677*t*
Paranasal non-Hodgkin's
        lymphoma, 423

Parenteral nutrition, 537
Parenting issues, 755
Partial thromboplastin time
    activated, 719
    normal values, 719
    in Reye's syndrome, 503
Participation, 686
PASS. *See* Plan for Achieving
        Self-Support
Patent ductus arteriosus, 452-459
Patient-controlled analgesia, 739
Pauciarticular juvenile rheumatoid
        arthritis, 308, 311*t*
Pavlik harness, 126
PCA. *See* Patient-controlled analgesia
Pco₂ (partial pressure of carbon
        dioxide), 714
PCP (phencyclidine
        hydrochloride), 564*t*
PCR. *See* Polymerase chain
        reaction
PCV7, 700*b*
PDA. *See* Patent ductus arteriosus
Pedialyte, 173
D-Penicillamine, 332
Penicillamine (Cuprimine), 312
Penicillin, 403
Pentobarbital (Nembutal), 654
Pericardiocentesis, 509
Perineal anoplasty, 265-266
Periorbital cellulitis, 61*b*
Peristalsis, 216
Peritoneal dialysis, 656-660
    in acute renal failure, 473
    indications for, 190-191, 656-657
Peritonitis, 28
pH
    gastric, 535
    normal, 662, 714-715
pH probe monitoring, 661-662
Phallic stage, 688
Pharmacologic pain management,
        735-740
Pharyngeal non-Hodgkin's
        lymphoma, 423

Phencyclidine hydrochloride (PCP), 564*t*
Phenobarbital, 524, 536, 563*t*
Phenylketonuria, 270, 273
Phenytoin (Dilantin), 524
Phlebitis, 355*t*
Phosphatidylglycerol levels, 492
Phosphorus, serum, 719
Phototherapy, 246
Physical abuse, 68
Physical changes
    in adolescence, 695
    during puberty, 693, 694*t*
Physical development, delayed, 355*t*
Placing reflex, 677*t*
Plan for Achieving Self-Support (PASS), 767
Plantar reflex, 677*t*
Plaquenil (hydroxychloroquine), 312
Plasma renin activity study, 250
Plasminogen, plasma, 719
Platelet antibody tests, 260
Platelet count
    in hemolytic-uremic syndrome, 188
    in idiopathic thrombocytopenic purpura, 259
    in Kawasaki disease, 319
    in leukemia, 343
    in nephrotic syndrome, 403
    normal values, 719
    in tetralogy of Fallot, 585
Platelets
    for aplastic anemia, 12
    for disseminated intravascular coagulation, 142
    for hemolytic-uremic syndrome, 190
Pleural fluid culture, 463
Pneumococcal infection, 703
Pneumocystis carinii pneumonia, 233
Pneumogram sleep studies, 663

Pneumonia, 460-465
    bacterial, 461*b*
    mycoplasmal, 462*b*
    viral, 461*b*
Po₂ (partial pressure of oxygen), 714
Poison management, 468
Poisoning, 466-468
    acute, 467
    lead, 325-333
Poison-proofing, 468
Polio immunization recommendations, 701*b*
Poliomyelitis vaccines, 702
Polyarticular juvenile rheumatoid arthritis, 307-308, 311*t*
Polymerase chain reaction, 119, 231
Polysomnography, 663
Pompe's disease, 276
Positioning after amputation, 433
Positron emission tomography, 523
Postconventional stage, 698
Postoperative or postprocedural care
    for amputation, 433-435
    for appendectomy, 28-29
    for cardiac catheterization, 641
    for cleft lip and cleft palate, 90-91
    for coarctectomy, 97-98
    for foreign body aspiration, 159
    general nursing interventions, 638
    for hernia repair, 210-211
    for Hirschsprung's disease, 214, 215-216
    for hydrocephalus, 241-242
    for hypertrophic pyloric stenosis, 256-257
    for imperforate anus, 267-268
    for inflammatory bowel disease, 296-297
    for intravenous pyelogram, 652
    for necrotizing enterocolitis, 398

Postoperative or postprocedural care *(Continued)*
for organ transplantation, 605, 606
for otitis media, 449
for patent ductus arteriosus, 458-459
for scoliosis, 516-517, 518
for spina bifida, 558
for tetralogy of Fallot, 589-591
for ventricular septal defects, 625-626
for Wilms' tumor, 631-632
Potassium (K⁺), serum, 717
Potassium-sparing diuretics, 585
Preconventional stage, 684, 689
Prednisolone, 403
Prednisone
for Hodgkin's disease, 222
for leukemia, 343-344
for nephrotic syndrome, 403
for non-Hodgkin's lymphoma, 425
side effects, 343-344
Preoperational stage, 686
Preoperative or preprocedural care
for amputation, 432-433
for appendectomy, 27-28
for cardiac catheterization, 640-641
for cleft lip and cleft palate repair, 88-90
for coarctectomy, 96-97
emotional support, 432
for foreign body aspiration, 158
general interventions, 637
for hernia repair, 210
for Hirschsprung's disease, 214-215
for hydrocephalus, 241
for hypertrophic pyloric stenosis, 255-256
for imperforate anus, 266-267
for inflammatory bowel disease, 295

Preoperative or preprocedural care *(Continued)*
for intravenous pyelogram, 651-652
for necrotizing enterocolitis, 397-398
for organ transplantation, 604, 605
for patent ductus arteriosus, 457
psychosocial interventions, 750-752
routine testing, 555
for scoliosis, 516
for spina bifida, 557
for tetralogy of Fallot, 589
for ventricular septal defects, 625
for Wilms' tumor, 631
Preschoolers (3 to 6 years)
cognitive development, 686
faith development, 689
fine motor development, 685
gross motor development, 684-685
growth and development, 684-689
Head Start, 765-766
language development, 686-687
mental retardation in, 377-378
moral development, 689
nonpharmacologic pain management techniques for, 741*t*
pain assessment in, 733
phallic stage, 688
physical characteristics, 684
preoperational stage, 686
psychosexual development, 688
psychosocial development, 688-689
sensory development, 685
socialization behavior, 689
stature-for-age and weight-for-age percentiles, 746*f*, 749*f*
urinary tract infections in, 617

Prevent Child Abuse America, 420*b*

Primidone (Mysoline), 524

Probiotics, 536

Procarbazine (Matulane), 222

Propionate metabolism, disorders of, 272*b*

Propranolol (Inderal), 96, 585

Prosthetic devices, 433-434

Protection and advocacy activities, 381*b*

Protein, serum
  in hemolytic-uremic syndrome, 188
  in inflammatory bowel disease, 291
  in meningitis, 365
  normal values, 719

Protein, urine, 719

Protein replacement, 403

Proteinuria, 402

Prothrombin time, 503, 719

Prozac (fluoxetine), 373

Pseudomonas aeruginosa, 110

Psychogenic pain, 732*t*

Psychosexual development
  adolescent (genital stage), 696-697
  infant (oral stage), 679-680
  preschooler (phallic stage), 688
  school-aged child (latency stage), 691-692
  toddler (anal stage), 683

Psychosocial development
  adolescent (identity *versus* role confusion), 697-698
  infant (trust *versus* mistrust), 680
  preschooler (initiative *versus* guilt), 688-689
  school-aged child (industry *versus* inferiority), 692-693
  toddler (autonomy *versus* shame and doubt), 683-684

Psychosocial dysfunction, 482

Psychosocial interventions, 750-753

Puberty, changes during, 693, 694*t*

Pulmonary function testing, 112, 260

Pulmonary infection, 405

Pulmonary toilet, intensive, 458

Pulse oximetry, 157, 359

Pulses, 667

Pupillary reaction, 669

Purine metabolism, disorders of, 273*b*

Purinethol (mercaptopurine), 346

Pyloric stenosis, hypertrophic, 253-258

Pyloromyotomy, 254-255

Pyridoxine, 279

Pyruvate carboxylase complex, disorders of, 272*b*

Pyruvate dehydrogenase complex, disorders of, 272*b*

Pyruvate dehydrogenase deficiency, 277-278

Pyruvate kinase deficiency, 272*b*, 276

Q

Quadriparesis, 64

R

Radiation somnolence, 350

Radiography
  abdominal; *See* Abdominal radiography
  anteroposterior lateral, 430
  chest; *See* Chest radiography
  in osteomyelitis, 438
  skull studies, 120
  xeroradiography, 157

Radiology, 120, 394

Radionuclide studies, 221, 251

Radiotherapy
  external-beam radiation, 222
  for Hodgkin's disease, 222
  for neuroblastoma, 414

Radiotherapy *(Continued)*
  nursing interventions, 223-224,
    351*t*-355*t*
  side effects of, 224
  total nodal radiation, 222
Range-of-motion limitations,
  322-323
Ranitidine (Zantac), 536
Rapid Automatized Naming Test,
  337
Rapid-sequence intravenous
  pyelography, 250
RDS. *See* Respiratory distress
  syndrome
Reading disorder, 335*b*
Reading tests, standardized, 337
Recombinant immunoblot assay 2,
  204
Recombivax HB (hepatitis B
  vaccine), 205
Rectal pull-through procedure, 213
Red blood cell distribution width,
  302
Red blood cells, 719-720
Reflexes, infant, 677*t*-678*t*
Reflexive stage, 698
Remicade (infliximab), 312
Renal agenesis, 264*t*
Renal assessment, 670-671
Renal biopsy, 183, 188, 260
Renal failure
  acute, 469-479, 470*b*
  chronic, 480-489
Renal function, deteriorating, 187*b*
Renal function tests, 220
Renal scan, 188, 343
Reserpine, 96
RespiGam, 498
Respiratory assessment, 668
Respiratory distress syndrome,
  490-496
Respiratory status, 98
Respiratory syncytial virus, 43, 80,
  497-499
Reticulocyte count, 302, 720

Retrograde pyelography, 618
Reye's syndrome, 500-506
  staging, 502*t*
Rheumatic fever, acute, 507-512
  revised Jones criteria for, 508*b*
Rheumatoid arthritis, juvenile,
  306-316
Rheumatoid factor assay, 119, 309
Ribavirin, 498
Ricelyte, 173
Righting reflex, 677*t*
Ringer's solution, lactated, 173
Ritalin (methylphenidate), 40, 373
Rofecoxib (Vioxx), 310
Role confusion, 697-698
Rooting reflex, 678*t*
Rotavirus, 168*t*, 172
RSV. *See* Respiratory syncytial virus
Russell's sign, 49

S

Sabin vaccine, 702
Sacrum, agenesis of, 264*t*
Safety, anticipatory guidance for,
  526
Safety activities, 380*b*
Salmonella infection, 167,
  168*t*-169*t*, 173, 174
Salter-Harris classification, 160,
  161*b*
Sandostatin (octreotide acetate),
  536
Sarcoma, osteogenic, 429-436
SBS. *See* Short bowel syndrome
Scald burns, 56
Scalp lacerations, 610
SCHIP. *See* State Children's Health
  Insurance Program
School problems, 314
School referral, 754-755
School-aged children (7 to 12 years)
  cognitive development, 690-691
  concrete operational stage,
    690-691
  conventional stage, 693

School-aged children *(Continued)*
faith development, 693
fine motor development, 690
gross motor development, 690
growth and development, 689-693
language development, 691
mental retardation in, 378-382
moral development, 693
mythical-literal stage, 693
nonpharmacologic pain management techniques for, 741*t*
pain assessment in, 733-735
physical characteristics, 689-690
psychosexual development, 691-692
psychosocial development, 692-693
stature-for-age and weight-for-age percentiles, 746*f,* 749*f*
urinary tract infections in, 617
Sclerosis, nodular, 219
Scoliosis, 513-519
Screening(s)
blood coagulation tests, 194
Early and Periodic Screening, Diagnosis, and Treatment Program (EPSDTP), 763-764, 766
for inborn errors of metabolism, 273-274
lead poisoning screening guidelines, 327-328, 330*t*-331*t*
for maple syrup urine disease, 273
newborn, 273-274, 544*b*-545*b*
recommended ages for, 701*b*
for sickle cell anemia, 544*b*-545*b*
Secobarbital, 563*t*
Secondary brain injury, 611-612
Sedatives, nonbarbiturate, 563*t*
Seizure disorders, 520-527
evaluation strategies, 376*t*

Seizures
absence, 521*b*
atonic, 522*b*
complex partial, 521*b*
generalized (convulsive or nonconvulsive), 521*b*-522*b*
idiopathic, 520
international classification of, 521*b*-522*b*
myoclonic, 521*b*
nursing interventions, 525
partial (focal, local), 521*b*
simple partial, 521*b*
tonic-clonic (grand mal), 521*b*-522*b*
types of, 521*b*-522*b*
Selective serotonin reuptake inhibitors, 7
Self-care responsibilities, 197
Self-injurious behavior, 373
Self-perception of disability, 553
Sensorimotor stage, 676-679
Sensory development
infant, 675-676
preschooler, 685
Sepsis, 394
Septal defects, ventricular, 621-627
Septicemia, 528
Septra (trimethoprim sulfamethoxazole), 233
Sequestration crisis, 545
Serologic tests, 119
Seroreverters, 231
Serum glutamic-oxaloacetic transaminase levels
in hepatitis, 203
in Kawasaki disease, 319
normal values, 720
in Wilms' tumor, 629
Serum glutamic-pyruvic transaminase levels
in hepatitis, 203
in Kawasaki disease, 319
normal values, 720
in Wilms' tumor, 629

Sexual abuse, 68, 72*b*
Sexual development, delayed, 355*t*
SGOT levels. *See* Serum
      glutamic-oxaloacetic
      transaminase levels
SGPT levels. *See* Serum
      glutamic-pyruvic
      transaminase levels
Shaken baby syndrome, 72*b*
Shame and doubt, 683-684
Shigella, 167, 169*t*, 173
Shigella dysenteriae, 186
Shock, 27, 57
Short bowel syndrome, 532-542
    acquired, 533*b*
    congenital, 533*b*
    etiology, 533*b*
Shunt insertion
    complications, 240
    for hydrocephalus, 239-240
    postoperative care, 241-242
    preoperative care, 241
Sickle cell anemia, 543-551
    early detection of, 544*b*-545*b*
    newborn screening programs,
      544*b*-545*b*
Sickle cell crisis, 544, 548
Sickle cell disease
    heterozygous (Hb AS), 543
    homozygous (Hb SS), 543
Sickle cell trait, 543, 544
SIDS. *See* Sudden infant death
    syndrome
Sigmoidoscopy, 291
Skeletal bone scans, 430
Skeletal deformities, 264*t*
Skeletal survey, 343
Skin, 668
Skin biopsy, 260
Skin injuries, 71*b*
Skull fractures, 610
Skull radiography, 120
Sleep studies, pneumogram, 663
Slit-lamp examinations, 260, 311*t*
Small bowel transplantation, 539

Smith-Lemli-Opitz syndrome, 275,
    276, 278
Social activities, 381*b*
Social disadvantage, 376*t*
Social Security Administration
    (SSA), 767, 768
Socialization behavior
    infant, 680-681
    preschooler, 689
Sodium (Na+), serum, 716
Sodium bicarbonate, 585
Sodium nitroprusside (Nipride),
    96
Sodium restriction, 403
Solid tumors, 594*b*
Solvents, volatile, 564*t*
Spastic cerebral palsy, 64
Special education services, 757
Special health care needs, Title V
    Program for, 764-765
Special Supplemental Nutrition
    Program for Women,
    Infants, and Children
    (WIC), 765
Spica cast care, 127
Spina bifida, 552-561
    with imperforate anus, 264*t*
Spina bifida cystica, 552
Spina bifida occulta, 552
Spleen scans, 343
Sputum culture, 463
Squatting position, 583
SSA. *See* Social Security
    Administration
SSI. *See* Supplemental Security
    Income
Staging procedure, 223
Standardized math tests, 337
Standardized reading tests, 337
Standardized written expression
    tests, 337
Stanford Diagnostic Reading Test,
    337
Stanford-Binet IV, 372
Staphylococcus aureus, 60, 110, 444

Startle reflex, 677*t*
State Children's Health Insurance Program (SCHIP), 762-763
Stature-for-age and weight-for-age percentiles
  for boys, 749*f*
  for girls, 746*f*
Status epilepticus, 522*b*, 525-526
Steroids, 405
Stimulants, 41, 563*t*
Stomatitis, 352*t*-353*t*
Stool culture, 172, 291
Stool hematest, 291
Stool softeners and laxatives, 556
Stool tests in short bowel syndrome, 535
STP (dimethoxy-4-methylamphetamine), 564*t*
"Strawberry" tongue, 318
Streptococci
  group A, 60, 444, 507
  group B, 362, 460
Streptococcus pneumoniae, 529
  in cellulitis, 60
  in meningitis, 362
  in otitis media, 443
  in pneumonia, 460
Streptozyme, 509
Subarachnoid hemorrhage, 611
Subluxation of hip, 123
Substance abuse, 567
Substance dependence, 562
Substance-related disorders, 562-569
Succimer, 332
Sucking reflex, 678*t*
Sudden infant death syndrome, 570-575
  modifiable risk factors for, 574*b*
  near-miss, 20
  resources, 574*b*
  risk factors for, 571*b*
Sudden Infant Death Syndrome Clearing House, 574*b*

Suicide, 576-581
Sulfasalazine (Azulfidine), 312
Supplemental Security Income (SSI), 767-768
Supportive care, 752-753
Suprapubic aspiration, 618
Surgical management. *See also* Postoperative or postprocedural care; Preoperative or preprocedural care
  appendectomy, 26-27
  cleft lip and cleft palate repair, 86
  coarctectomy, 94-96
  definitive repair of tetralogy of Fallot, 586
  hernia repair, 209
  of Hirschsprung's disease, 213
  of hydrocephalus, 239-240
  of hypertrophic pyloric stenosis, 254-255
  of inflammatory bowel disease, 292-293
  of myelomeningocele, 555-556
  of necrotizing enterocolitis, 395, 396
  of neuroblastoma, 413-414
  of patent ductus arteriosus, 455-456
  psychosocial preparation for, 750-752
  rectal pull-through procedure, 213
  of scoliosis, 515
  of short bowel syndrome, 538-539
  shunt insertion for hydrocephalus, 239-240
  of spina bifida, 555-556
  of tetralogy of Fallot, 585-586, 590-591
  ventricular septal defect repair, 623-624
Surgical staging laparotomy, 221

Sweat test, 112, 720
Swimming reflex, 678*t*
Synagis (palivizumab), 80, 498
Syncretism, 686
Synovial fluid analysis, 309

T

Tay-Sachs disease, 273
TBI. *See* Traumatic brain injury
Teaching and educational activities, 379*b*
Tegretol (carbamazepine), 373, 524
Test of Awareness of Language Segments, 337
Test of Written Spelling—Second Edition, 337
Tet spells, 583
Tetanus toxoid, adult, 701*b*
Tetralogy of Fallot, 582-592
Thermal injuries. *See also* Burns
deliberate or unexplained, 71*b*
Thermoregulation, 441
Thiopental sodium, 563*t*
Thioridazine (Mellaril), 373
Thought, formation of, 686
Thought characteristics, 686, 695
3TC (lamivudine), 233
Throat culture, 509
Thrombocytopenia, 354*t*, 394
Thrush, 771-772
Thyroid-stimulating hormone, serum, 720
Tissue biopsy, 260, 430
Title V Program for Children with Special Health Care Needs, 764-765
Toddlers (1 to 3 years)
anal stage, 683
developmental dysplasia of the hip in, 124
early intervention services for, 759
faith development, 684
fine motor development, 682-683

Toddlers *(Continued)*
gross motor development, 682
growth and development, 681-684
head circumference-for-age and weight-for-length percentiles, 745*f*, 748*f*
intuitive-projective stage, 684
length-for-age and weight-for-age percentiles, 744*f*, 747*f*
mental retardation in, 377-378
moral development, 684
nonpharmacologic pain management techniques for, 740*t*-741*t*
pain assessment in, 733
physical characteristics, 681
preconventional stage, 684
psychosexual development, 683
psychosocial development, 683-684
serious bacterial infection in, 528
stature-for-age and weight-for-age percentiles, 746*f*, 749*f*
TOF. *See* Tetralogy of Fallot
Tolerance, 562
Tolmetin (Tolectin), 310
Tonic-clonic (grand mal) seizures, 521*b*-522*b*
Total airway obstruction, 158
Total nodal irradiation, 222
Toxic-metabolic disorders, 376*t*
Toxoids, 699, 702-703
Toxoplasmosis, other infections, rubella, CMV infection, and herpes (TORCH) screen, 119, 720
Tracheostomy care, 153
Tranquilizers, 563*t*
Transaminase, serum, 503
Transcranial Doppler ultrasound, 547

Transduction, 686
Transferrin, serum, 720
Transferrin saturation, 302
Transfusion reaction, 549
Transition planning, 761-762
Transplantation
    bone marrow, 593-602
    heart, 603
    heart-lung, 113-114
    liver and small bowel, 539
    lung, 113-114
    multiorgan, 539
    organ, 603-607
    small bowel, 539
Transsulfuration of amino acids,
        disorders of, 272*b*
Trauma, nonaccidental, 416-421
    resources for, 419*b*-420*b*
Traumatic brain injury, 608-615
Traumatic hair loss, 71*b*
Trendelenburg's test, 125*b*
Triamcinolone hexacetonide, 312
Triglycerides, serum, 250, 403,
        720
Trimethoprim sulfamethoxazole
        (Septra, Bactrim), 233, 536
Trust *versus* mistrust, 680
Tuberculin skin test, 463
    recommended ages for, 701*b*
Tumor necrosis factor inhibitors,
        312
Tumors
    solid, 594*b*
    Wilms', 628-633
Tympanostomy tubes, 447, 449

U

Ulcerative colitis
    clinical manifestations,
        289-290
    complications, 290
    incidence, 289
    medical management, 291
    pathophysiology, 288-289
Ulcers, mouth, 352*t*-353*t*

Ultrasonography
    abdominal, 412
    in acute renal failure, 472
    in short bowel syndrome, 535
    in Wilms' tumor, 629
United Nations Background Note
        on Children's Rights, 420*b*
United Ostomy Association, Inc.,
        298
Universal Nonverbal Intelligence
        Test (UNIT), 373
Upper gastrointestinal tract
        radiographic series, 291
Upper respiratory tract infection
        symptoms, 497
Urea cycle defects, 275, 276, 277
Uremia
    hemolytic-uremic syndrome,
        186-191
    signs and symptoms of, 475, 485
Uremic neuropathy, 482
Uric acid, serum, 720
Urinalysis
    in Hodgkin's disease, 220
    in hypertension, 250
    in JRA, 309
    normal values, 720
    in short bowel syndrome, 535
    in Wilms' tumor, 629
Urinary tract infections, 616-620
Urine culture, 250, 365, 618
Urine dipstick test, 402, 535
Urine specific gravity, 402
Urine tests. *See also specific tests*
    in acute renal failure, 472
    in chronic renal failure, 483-484
    in glomerulonephritis, 183
    in nephrotic syndrome, 402
Ursodiol (Actigall), 536
U.S. Department of Agriculture,
        765
U.S. Department of Health and
        Human Services
    Children's Bureau, 420*b*
    Head Start Bureau, 766

"U.S. Newborn Screening System Guidelines II: Follow-Up of Children, Diagnosis, Management, and Evaluation: Statement of the Council of Regional Networks for Genetic Services (CORN)", 273-274
UTIs. *See* Urinary tract infections
Uveitis, 308-309

V

Vaccines, 700, 702-703
Valproic acid (Depakene), 524
Vanillylmandelic acid, 411
Varicella vaccine, 703
    immunization recommendations, 701*b*
    recommended ages for, 701*b*
Vascular volume depletion, 481
Vasoocclusive crisis, 544-545
Venograms, excretory, 250
Ventricular septal defect repair, 623-624
    postoperative care, 625-626
    preoperative care, 625
Ventricular septal defects, 621-627
Ventricular-peritoneal shunt, 240
Verbalization of feelings, 58
Vinblastine, 222
Vincristine (Oncovin)
    for Hodgkin's disease, 222
    for ITP, 260
    for leukemia, 344
    for non-Hodgkin's lymphoma, 424-425
    side effects, 344
Vineland Adaptive Behavior Scales, 373
Vioxx (rofecoxib), 310
Viral cultures, 119
Viral pneumonia, 461*b*
Visual-perceptual skills, 337
Vital signs, 668, 670
Vitamin B₁₂, 279

Vitamin deficiency, 537
Vitamin K supplements, 113
Vitamin supplements, 113
Vitamin therapy, 279
Voiding cystourethrogram, 618
Volatile solvents, 564*t*
Voltaren (diclofenac sodium), 310
Vomiting. *See* Nausea and vomiting
VP (ventricular-peritoneal) shunt, 240
VP-16 (etoposide), 413

W

WAIS-III. *See* Wechsler Adult Intelligence Scale III
Walking reflex, 678*t*
Warfarin (Coumadin), 320
Wechsler Adult Intelligence Scale III (WAIS-III), 372
Wechsler Intelligence Scale of Children—Third Edition (WISC-III), 336, 372
Wechsler Preschool and Primary Scale of Intelligence (WPPSI-R), 372
Weight
    growth curves, 744*f*-749*f*
    West nomogram, 728*f*-729*f*
Weight-for-age percentiles
    for boys, 747*f*, 749*f*
    for girls, 744*f*, 746*f*
Weight-for-length percentiles
    for boys, 748*f*
    for girls, 745*f*
West nomogram, 728*f*-729*f*
Western blot test, 230
White blood cell counts
    in acute rheumatic fever, 509
    in idiopathic thrombocytopenic purpura, 260
    in inflammatory bowel disease, 291
    in meningitis, 364
    normal values, 721

White blood cell differential, 721

Whites, 766

Whole blood, fresh, 142

WIC. *See* Special Supplemental Nutrition Program for Women, Infants, and Children

Wilms' tumor, 628-633

WISC-III. *See* Wechsler Intelligence Scale of Children—Third Edition

Woodcock-Johnson Psycho-Educational Battery—Revised Tests of Cognitive Ability, 336

Wound healing, 58
postoperative, 28-29

WPPSI-R. *See* Wechsler Preschool and Primary Scale of Intelligence

Written expression, disorder of, 335*b*

Written expression tests, standardized, 337

X

Xeroradiography, 157

Y

Yersinia, 167

Yersinia enterocolitica, enteropathogenic, 171*t*

Z

Zalcitabine (DDC), 233

Zantac (ranitidine), 536

Zarontine (ethosuximide), 524

ZDV (zidovudine), 233

Zellweger syndrome, 275, 276

Zidovudine (AZT, ZDV), 226-227, 233

Zyloprim (allopurinol), 347